## GASTROINTESTINAL SYSTEM

**Check for:**
• vomiting and abdominal distention, possibly indicating bowel obstruction, peptic ulcer, or internal bleeding
• tachycardia, hypotension, diaphoresis, or pallor, possibly indicating occult bleeding and impending hypovolemia
• pain, guarding, or rigidity, possibly indicating peritoneal irritation.

## MUSCULOSKELETAL SYSTEM

**Check for:**
• deformity, local swelling, decreased range of motion, immobility, or bruises, possibly indicating fracture or dislocation
• poor capillary refill, absent or diminished pulses, pallor, or cool skin, possibly indicating vascular compromise
• paralysis, numbness, or decreased sensation, possibly indicating nerve injury.

## EYES, EARS, NOSE, AND THROAT

**Check for:**
• limited extraocular movements, decreased sensation, facial asymmetry, and hearing or vision loss, possibly indicating neuromuscular damage
• local swelling, redness, drainage, fever, tenderness, and lesions, possibly indicating infection
• nasal or neck swelling and stridor, dyspnea, or tachypnea, indicating respiratory compromise.

open the airway immediately.
• *Look* for chest expansion, *listen* for air flow, and *feel* for expired air. Provide assisted ventilation immediately if your patient's not breathing.
• Check his pulse (the carotid pulse in an adult or child; the brachial pulse in an infant). If you can't feel a pulse, start cardiac compressions immediately.

Once you've stabilized your patient's ABCs and he's out of immediate danger, move on to the secondary phase of your emergency assessment. Focus your efforts on determining your patient's chief complaints, intervening as necessary to prevent his emergency problems from worsening. *Always* be prepared to immediately interrupt your assessment, and to intervene as necessary, if complications develop that threaten your patient's ABCs.

## GENITOURINARY SYSTEM

**Check for:**
• ecchymoses in the flank area, possibly indicating retroperitoneal bleeding
• a suprapubic mass or perineal mass, possibly indicating urine extravasation
• severe colicky flank pain, possibly indicating renal calculi.

## SHOCK

**Check for:**
• altered mental status, possibly indicating decreased cerebral tissue perfusion (early sign)
• tachycardia, possibly indicating decreased cardiac output (early sign)
• tachypnea, possibly indicating poor tissue perfusion (early sign) or acidosis (late sign)
• pale, cool, and clammy skin, possibly indicating compensatory sympathetic response (early sign); or warm, flushed, dry skin, possibly indicating early septic shock.

## BURNS

**Check for:**
• stridor, coughing, hoarseness, black or sooty sputum, and singed nasal hairs, possibly indicating inhalation injury
• decreased blood pressure and increased pulse rate, possibly indicating impending shock
• diminished peripheral pulses, possibly indicating impaired circulation from edema or thrombosis
• fractures, hemorrhage, or other injuries from falls or tetanic contractions.

# NURSE'S REFERENCE LIBRARY®

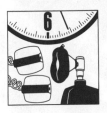

# Emergencies

*Nursing85* Books™
Springhouse Corporation
Springhouse, Pennsylvania

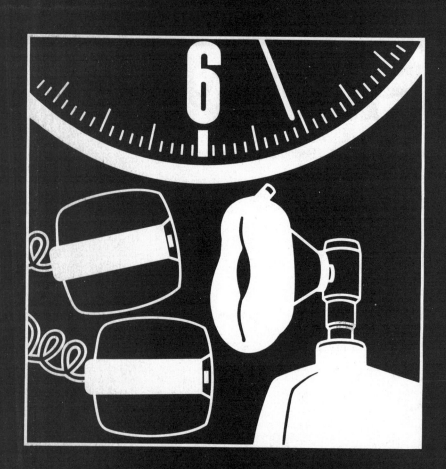

# NURSE'S REFERENCE LIBRARY®

# Emergencies

*Nursing85* Books™
Springhouse Corporation
Springhouse, Pennsylvania

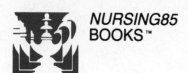

*NURSING85*
BOOKS™

## Springhouse Corporation Book Division

**CHAIRMAN**
Eugene W. Jackson

**PRESIDENT**
Daniel L. Cheney

**VICE-PRESIDENT AND DIRECTOR**
Timothy B. King

**VICE-PRESIDENT, BOOK OPERATIONS**
Thomas A. Temple

**VICE-PRESIDENT, PRODUCTION AND PURCHASING**
Bacil Guiley

**PROGRAM DIRECTOR, REFERENCE BOOKS**
Stanley E. Loeb

© 1985 by Springhouse Corporation, 1111 Bethlehem Pike, Springhouse, Pa. 19477

NRL8-011284

Library of Congress Cataloging in Publication Data
Main entry under title:

Emergencies.

    (Nurse's reference library)
    "Nursing84 books."
    Includes bibliographies and index.
    1. Emergency nursing—Handbooks, manuals, etc.
I. Springhouse Corporation.    2. Series.    [DNLM:
1. Emergencies—nurse's instruction.    WY 150
E515]
RT120.E4E42    1984    616'.025    84-14122
ISBN 0-916730-85-9

# NURSE'S REFERENCE LIBRARY®

# Staff for this volume

**EDITORIAL DIRECTOR**
Diana Odell Potter

**CLINICAL DIRECTOR**
Minnie Bowen Rose, RN, BSN, MEd

**ART DIRECTOR**
Sonja Douglas

**Editorial Manager:** Jill S. Lasker
**Clinical Editor:** Carole Arlene Pyle, RN, BSN, MA, CCRN
**Clinical Editorial Consultants:** Donna L. Hilton, RN, CCRN, CEN; Paulette Schank, RN, CCRN, CEN
**Contributing Clinical Editors:** Margaret L. Belcher, RN, BSN; Nan Cameron, RN, BSN; Marlene McNemar Ciranowicz, RN, MSN; Mary Chapman Gyetvan, RN, BSEd; Sandra Ludwig-Nettina, RN, BSN; Linda J. Spicer, RN, BSN; Nina Poorman Welsh, RN
**Senior Editor:** Andrea F. Barrett
**Associate Editors:** Kevin J. Law, Elizabeth L. Mauro
**Contributing Editors:** Sandra E. Cherrey, Nancy J. Priff, Rebecca S. Van Dine, Roger Wall
**Editorial Assistant:** Roberta E. Weller
**Acquisitions:** Bernadette M. Glenn, Thomas J. Leibrandt
**Drug Information Manager:** Larry Neil Gever, RPh, PharmD
**Copy Supervisor:** David R. Moreau
**Copy Editors:** Dale A. Brueggemann, Diane M. Labus
**Contributing Copy Editors:** Laura Dabundo, Reni Fetterolf, Max A. Fogel, Tim Gaul, Linda A. Johnson, Jane Paluda, Doris Weinstock, William J. Wright
**Production Coordinator:** Kathleen P. Luczak
**Senior Designer:** Jacalyn Bove Facciolo
**Designer:** Christopher Laird
**Contributing Designers:** Maryanne Buschini, Lynn Foulk
**Illustrators:** Michael Adams, Dimitrios Bastas, Jean Gardner, Tom Herbert, Robert Jackson, Robert Phillips, George Retseck, Dennis Schofield
**Art Production Manager:** Robert Perry
**Art Assistants:** Diane Fox, Don Knauss, Bob Miele, Robert Renn, Sandy Sanders, Louise Stamper, Bob Wieder
**Typography Manager:** David C. Kosten
**Typography Assistants:** Cynthia Gray, Ethel Halle, Debra Lee Judy, Diane Paluba, Nancy Wirs
**Senior Production Manager:** Deborah C. Meiris
**Production Manager:** Wilbur D. Davidson
**Production Assistant:** Tim A. Landis
**Assistants:** Mary Ann Bowes, Maree E. DeRosa, Caroline M. Swider
**Indexer:** Tony Greenberg, M.D.
**Researchers:** Vonda Heller, Elaine Shelly

Special thanks to Holly Ann Burdick; Elizabeth J. Cobbs; Regina Daley Ford, RN, BSN, MA; Alice Loxley, RN, BA, MSN; Judith A. Schilling McCann, RN, BSN; Loy Wiley Associates, Inc.: Loy Wiley; Julie M. Beck, SRN; Pat Madden; Karen Nappi; Theresa Reynolds; Leslie Smith; Cynthia B. Springer, RN; Norma Wiesman; who assisted in the preparation of this volume.

# Contents

## 1 Approaches to Emergency Care

## 2 Legal Concerns in Emergencies

# 3 Emergency Assessment and Intervention

# 4 Respiratory Emergencies

# 5 Cardiovascular Emergencies

# 6 Neurologic Emergencies

# 7 Gastrointestinal Emergencies

# 8 Musculoskeletal Emergencies

# 9 Eye, Ear, Nose, and Throat Emergencies

# 10 Endocrine and Metabolic Emergencies

# 11 Hematologic Emergencies

# 12 Obstetric and Gynecologic Emergencies

# Emergency! Atlas of Major Injuries

# 13 Genitourinary Emergencies

# 17 Poisoning and Substance Abuse Emergencies

# Appendices and Index

*NURSING85*
BOOKS™

# NURSE'S REFERENCE LIBRARY®

This volume is part of a series conceived by the publishers of *Nursing85*® magazine and written by hundreds of nursing and medical specialists. This series, the NURSE'S REFERENCE LIBRARY, is the most comprehensive reference set ever created exclusively for the nursing profession. Each volume brings together the most up-to-date clinical information and related nursing practice. Each volume informs, explains, alerts, guides, educates. Taken together, the NURSE'S REFERENCE LIBRARY provides today's nurse with the knowledge and the skills that she needs to be effective in her daily practice and to advance in her career.

## *Other volumes in the series:*

Diseases          Drugs          Procedures          Practices
Diagnostics     Assessment     Definitions

## *Other publications:*

**NEW NURSING SKILLBOOK™ SERIES**
Giving Emergency Care Competently
Monitoring Fluid and Electrolytes Precisely
Assessing Vital Functions Accurately
Coping with Neurologic Problems Proficiently
Reading EKGs Correctly

Combatting Cardiovascular Diseases
    Skillfully
Nursing Critically Ill Patients Confidently
Dealing with Death and Dying
Managing Diabetics Properly

**NURSING PHOTOBOOK™ SERIES**
Providing Respiratory Care
Managing I.V. Therapy
Dealing with Emergencies
Giving Medications
Assessing Your Patients
Using Monitors
Providing Early Mobility
Giving Cardiac Care
Performing GI Procedures
Implementing Urologic Procedures

Controlling Infection
Ensuring Intensive Care
Coping with Neurologic Disorders
Caring for Surgical Patients
Working with Orthopedic Patients
Nursing Pediatric Patients
Helping Geriatric Patients
Attending Ob/Gyn Patients
Aiding Ambulatory Patients
Carrying Out Special Procedures

**NURSING NOW™ SERIES**
Shock                     Cardiac Crises                Neurologic Emergencies
Hypertension         Respiratory Emergencies
Drug Interactions   Pain

**NURSE'S CLINICAL LIBRARY™**
Cardiovascular Disorders
Respiratory Disorders
Endocrine Disorders

Neurologic Disorders
Renal and Urologic Disorders
Gastrointestinal Disorders

*Nursing85* **DRUG HANDBOOK™**

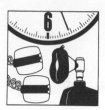

# Advisory Board

*At the time of publication, the advisors, contributors, and clinical and legal consultants held the following positions:*

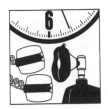

# Clinical and Legal Consultants

**Lindsay Staubus Alger, MD,** Assistant Professor, Department of Obstetrics and Gynecology, School of Medicine, University of Maryland, Baltimore

**Garrett E. Bergman, MD, FAAP,** Associate Professor, Department of Pediatrics, The Medical College of Pennsylvania, Philadelphia

**Heather Boyd-Monk, SRN, RN, BS,** Educational Coordinator, Wills Eye Hospital, Philadelphia

**Linda Buschiazzo, RN, CEN,** Nurse Manager, Emergency Department, Albert Einstein Medical Center—Northern Division, Philadelphia

**Susan Diane Chenowith, RN, BS, JD,** Trial Attorney, Bernstein, Bernstein & Harrison, P.C., Philadelphia

**James L. Combs, MD, FACEP,** Emergency Physician, St. Elizabeth Medical Center, Covington, Ky.

**Carmelle Pellerin Cournoyer, RN, MA, JD,** Attorney, Health Law Educator, and Consultant, Manchester, N.H.

**Brian B. Doyle, MD,** Clinical Professor of Psychiatry and Community and Family Medicine, School of Medicine, Georgetown University, Washington, D.C.

**Thaddeus P. Dryja, MD,** Assistant Professor of Ophthalmology, Harvard Medical School, Boston

**Anna Gawlinski, RN, MSN, CCRN,** Cardiovascular Clinical Nurse Specialist, UCLA Medical Center, Los Angeles

**Joan Holter Gildea, RNC, MA,** Clinical Assistant Director of Nursing, Department of Pediatrics, New York University Medical Center, New York

**John D. Gorry, MD, FACEP,** Chairman, Department of Emergency Medicine, Crozer-Chester Medical Center, Chester, Pa.

**Joyce P. Griffin, RN, MSN, CCRN,** Instructor, School of Nursing, University of Pennsylvania, Philadelphia

**Otis Mark Hastings, MD,** Attending Emergency Department Physician/CME Coordinator, Good Samaritan Hospital, Suffern, N.Y.

**Tobie Hittle, RN, BSN, CCRN,** Head Nurse, Intensive Care Unit, The Genesee Hospital, Rochester, N.Y.

**Nancy M. Holloway, RN, MSN, CCRN, CEN,** Director and Critical Care Emergency Nursing Consultant, Nancy Holloway & Associates, Oakland, Calif.

**Irving Huber, MD,** Medical Director, Walk-in Medical Center; Clinical Assistant Professor, Department of Medicine, Division of Emergency Medicine, Hahnemann University, Philadelphia

**Jacquelyn A. Huebsch, RN, MS,** Cardiovascular Nurse Clinician, St. Paul Ramsey Medical Center

**William M. Keane, MD, FACS,** Assistant Professor of Otorhinolaryngology, School of Medicine, University of Pennsylvania; Surgeon, Pennsylvania Hospital, Philadelphia

**Jane Sinnott Klucsik, RN, MS, CCRN,** Critical Care Clinical Nurse Specialist, Montgomery General Hospital, Olney, Md.

**Barbara Knezevich, RN, MS, CEN, TNS,** Nurse Manager, Emergency Department/Outpatient Department, St. Anne's Hospital, Chicago

**Mary R. LaBove, RN, MSN,** Medical Surgical Nurse Clinical Specialist, Diagnostic Cardiology Associates, Collingswood, N.J.

**Maureen McNamara Laraia, RN, MSN,** Clinical Consultant, Private Practice, Exton, Pa.

**Susan Little, RN,** Adult Ambulatory Urology Nurse, Department of Urology, New England Medical Center Hospital, Boston

**Alice A. K. Loxley, RN, BA, MSN,** Clinical Specialist, Independent Practice, Coatesville, Pa.

**Ann Butler Maher, RN, MS,** Instructor of Nursing, County College of Morris, Randolph, N.J.

**Hedy Freyone Mechanic, RN, BSN, MEd,** Associate Professor, School of Nursing, College of Human Services, San Diego State University, California; formerly Major, ANC and Clinical Nurse Researcher at USAISR, Fort Sam Houston, San Antonio, Tex.

**Linda Mowad, RN, MA,** Clinical Nurse Specialist, East Orange (N.J.) General Hospital

**Steve Nitenson, RN, BSN, CCRN, MICN,** Education Coordinator, Stanford University Hospital and Medical Center, Daly City, Calif.

**Valerie Novotny-Dinsdale, RN, BSN, CEN,** Emergency Nursing Staff Developer, Emergency Department, Northwest Hospital, Seattle

**Maureen O'Reilly-Bertneskie, RN, BSN, CEN,** Staff Nurse/Preceptor, Emergency Department, Good Samaritan Hospital, Suffern, N.Y.

**Janet Gren Parker, RN, MS,** Assistant Director of Ambulatory Nursing/Assistant Professor of Medical-Surgical Nursing, Vanderbilt University Hospital, Nashville, Tenn.

**Patricia Ann Payne, RN, MPH,** High Risk Maternity Coordinator, Maryland Institute for Emergency Medical Services Systems/Department of Obstetrics-Gynecology, University of Maryland, Baltimore

**Bette Alexandria Perkins, RN, BSN, CCRN,** Staff Nurse, U.S. Army, Institute of Surgical Research (Burn Unit), Fort Sam Houston, San Antonio, Tex.

**Peter T. Pons, MD,** Attending Physician, Emergency Department, Denver General Hospital and St. Joseph Hospital, Denver

**Grannum R. Sant, MD, FRCS,** Assistant Professor of Urology, School of Medicine, Tufts University, Boston

**Kay Freeman Sauers, RN, BSN, MS,** Clinical Nurse Specialist in Orthopedics, University of Maryland Medical Systems/Hospital, Baltimore

**Eric Zachary Silfen, MD,** Staff Emergency Physician, National Hospital, Arlington, Va.; Clinical Attending, Departments of Emergency and Internal Medicine, Georgetown University Hospital, Washington, D.C.

**Paulette J. Strauch, RN,** Community Outreach Program Coordinator, Good Health Mobile, Metropolitan Hospital Corporate for Metropolitan Hospital, Philadelphia

**Timothy L. Turnbull, MD,** Assistant Professor of Clinical Emergency Medicine, University of Illinois Medical School at Chicago/Mercy Hospital and Medical Center, Chicago

**Joseph B. Warren, RN, BSN,** Nurse Clinician, Head Injury Clinical Center, Division of Neurosurgery, Medical College of Virginia, Richmond

**Kathleen M. Wruk, RN, BSN,** Head Nurse, Rocky Mountain Poison Center, Denver General Hospital

**Joseph A. Zeccardi, MD,** Director, Emergency Department, Thomas Jefferson University Hospital, Philadelphia

# Contributors

**Carol R. Beaugard, RN, MA, CS,** Private Practice; Adjunct Professor/Instructor, Herbert Lehman College, Bronx, New York

**Pamela W. Bourg, RN, MS, CEN,** Assistant Director of Nursing, Emergency Medical Services and Outpatient Department, Denver General Hospital

**Georgia Lee Caven, RN, BS, CCP, CCRN, CEN,** Clinical Nurse, Emergency Medical Services, Denver General Hospital

**Carmelle Pellerin Cournoyer, RN, MA, JD,** Attorney, Health Law Educator, and Consultant, Manchester, N.H.

**Dudley Culver, RN, BSN,** Clinical Nurse, Emergency Medical Services, Denver General Hospital

**Janie B. Daddario, RN, MSN,** Instructor, Vanderbilt University School of Nursing, Nashville, Tenn.

**Carol Solomon Dalglish, RN, MSN,** Clinical Nurse Specialist in Obstetric-Gynecologic Infertility, Vanderbilt University Hospital, Nashville, Tenn.

**Alice M. Donahue, RN, MSN,** Supervisor, Emergency Department, Sacred Heart Hospital, Norristown, Pa.

**Judy Donlen, RN, MSN,** Assistant Director for Nursing Education, Children's Hospital of Philadelphia

**Deborah A. Doyle, RN, MSN, JD,** Risk Manager, Chester County Hospital, West Chester, Pa.

**Linda M. Duffy, CURN, CANP, MS,** Clinical Specialist/Nurse Practitioner for Urology, Minneapolis Veterans Administration Medical Center

**Judith T. Evangelisti, RN,** Staff Nurse, Glenbrook Hospital, Glenview, Ill.

**Janice M. Fitzgerald, RN, MSN,** Clinical Unit Instructor, St. Agnes Medical Center, Philadelphia

**Terry Matthew Foster, RN, CEN, CCRN,** Staff Nurse, Emergency Department, Our Lady of Mercy Hospital, Cincinnati; Codirector, Midwest Nursing Seminars, Cincinnati; Staff Nurse, Emergency Department, St. Elizabeth Medical Center, Covington, Ky.

**Nancy M. Holloway, RN, MSN, CCRN, CEN,** Director and Critical Care/Emergency Nursing Consultant, Nancy Holloway & Associates, Oakland, Calif.

**Barbara Lamp, RN, CEN,** Clinical Nurse, Emergency Medical Services, Denver General Hospital

**Terri Hendler Lipman, RN, MSN,** Clinical Nurse Specialist in Diabetes/Endocrinology, St. Christopher's Hospital for Children, Philadelphia

**Melanie L. Lobdell, RN,** Flight Nurse, Survival Flight, University of Michigan Hospitals, Ann Arbor

**Alice A. K. Loxley, RN, MSN,** Clinical Specialist, Independent Practice, Coatesville, Pa.

**Sandi Martin, RN, BSN, CCRN,** Critical Care Instructor, Wyandotte (Mich.) General Hospital

**Christine M. May, RN, MSN,** Education Coordinator, Ambulatory Services, Kettering (Ohio) Medical Center

**Alice P. MacLarnon, RN, CEN,** Clinical Nurse, Emergency Medical Services, Denver General Hospital

**Margaret Miller, RN, BSN, MSEd,** Chairperson, Department of Continuing Education, School of Nursing, Creighton University, Omaha

**Jean Marie Montonye, RN,** Clinical Nurse, Emergency Medical Services, Denver General Hospital

**Linda Mowad, RN, MA,** Clinical Nurse Specialist, East Orange (N.J.) General Hospital

**Maureen O'Reilly-Bertneskie, RN, BSN, CEN,** Staff Nurse/Preceptor, Emergency Department, Good Samaritan Hospital, Suffern, N.Y.

**Patricia M. Orr, RN, MBA,** Head Nurse, Burn Treatment Center, St. Agnes Medical Center, Philadelphia

**Marie T. O'Toole, RN, MSN,** Assistant Professor, Department of Baccalaureate Nursing, Thomas Jefferson University, Philadelphia

**Janice Overdorff, BSN,** Administrative Nurse III, University of Illinois Hospital, Chicago

**Patricia L. Radzewicz, RN, BSN,** Head Nurse, University of Illinois Eye and Ear Infirmary, Chicago

**Sharon Reilly, RN, CEN,** Clinical Nurse, Emergency Medical Services, Denver General Hospital

**Jacqueline Rhoads, RN, MSN, CEN, CCRN,** Assistant Professor in Critical Care, School of Nursing, University of Texas Health Science Center, San Antonio

**Dorothy Schulte, RN, BS, CEN,** Clinical Nurse, Emergency Medical Services, Denver General Hospital

**Juliana H. Smith, RN, CEN,** Assistant Head Nurse, Emergency Medical Services, Denver General Hospital

**Gloria Y. Sonnesso, RN, MSN, CCRN,** Consultant in Critical and Pulmonary Care, Skilled Nursing, Inc., Springhouse, Pa.

**Margaret M. Stevens, RN, BSN, CNP, ACNN,** Neurosurgery Nurse Practitioner, Maryland Institute of Emergency Medical Services Systems, University of Maryland, Baltimore

**Frances J. Storlie, ANP, PhD,** Director, Personal Health Services, Southwest Washington Health Department, Vancouver

**Constance J. Thorpe, RN, CCRN, CANP,** President, C.J. Thorpe & Associates, Arlington Heights, Ill.

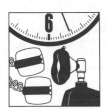

# Foreword

"Emergency!" The very word conjures up drama and excitement. What comes to *your* mind when you imagine an emergency scene? Do you clearly picture a skilled emergency team smoothly performing complex lifesaving procedures? Or do you picture a less well-focused scene, suggesting that the persons responding to the emergency are unsure of their roles or actions? Perhaps most important, which scene do you see yourself in?

Of course, as a nurse, you know that only the first scene will do. But you probably also know that anxiety and uncertainty—inevitable in emergency situations—can cause even the most skilled nurses and doctors to make errors. What can you do to keep the pressure-cooker atmosphere of an emergency from overwhelming your judgment? This book, EMERGENCIES, can help.

In EMERGENCIES, you'll find the answers to your questions about emergency assessment and intervention. Questions like these:
- Does this patient have an emergency problem?
- If he has multiple emergency problems, which ones take priority over others? Where should I start?
- What emergency interventions should I perform?
- Do I need a doctor's order, or may I legally act on my own to provide the emergency care this patient needs?

EMERGENCIES will give you the confidence you need to skillfully manage emergencies on the unit *and* in the ED—for patients with virtually all types of major emergency problems.

Chapters 1 through 3 of EMERGENCIES cover the fundamentals of emergency care. In Chapter 1, you'll find in-depth coverage of how emergencies are handled outside the hospital, in the ED, and on the unit, along with full discussions of the principles of triage and the roles of emergency team members. And here, for the first time anywhere, you'll find a definitive discussion of your role as a staff nurse in managing emergencies.

Chapter 2 reviews the legal principles that apply in emergencies. Legal "gray areas" abound when you have to act fast—and the guidelines here will help you avoid costly mistakes. Particularly interesting is a discussion of your responsibilities when the police ask you to gather evidence from a patient in their custody.

Chapter 3 shows you how to perform a step-by-step

emergency assessment, detailing the differences between primary and secondary assessment and showing you just where to focus your attention during those first few critical minutes. This chapter also includes special sections on multiple-trauma patients, pediatric patients, geriatric patients, and pregnant patients.

Following Chapter 3, you'll find a special section, "Life Support: Performing Basic and Advanced Techniques." You'll turn to this illustrated section often to refresh your life-support skills.

Chapters 4 through 13 provide detailed information on emergencies affecting specific body systems. Each chapter opens with a sample patient presentation. Then, detailed entries describe:

• what you need to know about the emergency care your patient may have received, from rescue personnel, *before* he reached the hospital.

• what you should do *first* to stabilize your patient's vital life functions (airway, breathing, and circulation—the so-called ABCs). For each body system, you'll learn about specific problems that can threaten your patient's ABCs during emergency care.

• what you should do *next* to assess for the patient's chief emergency problems and to intervene initially—*even before the doctor's made a diagnosis.*

• what you should consider when caring for pediatric and geriatric patients with emergencies.

• how you should care for patients with emergency conditions *after a diagnosis has been made.* Each such entry starts with a summary of initial emergency care and then takes you through your nursing priorities and your continuing assessment and intervention steps.

As you can see, EMERGENCIES helps you to understand the entire *process* of your patient's care. You may not follow your patient through the whole course of his emergency—you won't move with him from the ED to the ICU to the unit, and you may not be trained to perform all the procedures described. But, with this book's unique timeline format, you'll understand what happened to the patient *before* he arrived at the hospital, what to do *while* you're seeing him, and what might happen *after* you've seen him.

Chapters 14 through 17 show you how to manage emergencies affecting multiple body systems: shock, burns, environmental emergencies, and poisoning and substance abuse. In these chapters, too, you'll find the helpful timeline format—leading you from initial acute assessment through definitive management.

Throughout the chapters, numerous illustrations, charts, and supplementary text pieces enlarge your understanding and clarify difficult points. Emergency assessment checklists, emergency patient-care procedures, drug information, legal pointers, and explanations of pathophysiology are just some of the important information presented this way.

But that's not all you'll find in EMERGENCIES. The special four-color section following Chapter 12—"Emergency! Atlas of Major Injuries"—graphically depicts how injuries occur from different causes (mechanisms of injury) and presents numerous illustrations of injuries requiring emergency intervention. In the Appendix, following Chapter 17, you'll discover:

• a comprehensive chart covering pediatric emergencies
• a chart describing the uses of colloid and crystalloid solutions
• a quick-reference guide to coping with psychiatric emergencies.

You'll find this information useful in many emergency situations.

EMERGENCIES is a clearly written, comprehensive reference book that you'll turn to day after day. Its easy-to-use format makes a wealth of emergency information quickly accessible. And, because it was written by currently practicing clinical specialists, you can be sure that the information contained in its pages is correct and clinically relevant.

This book can help you achieve the satisfaction of knowing that, in the next emergency you face, you'll function calmly and expertly.

Nancy M. Holloway, RN, MSN, CCRN, CEN

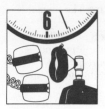

# Overview

Few of us work in an ED everyday; fewer still have the in-depth training required to qualify as a Certified Emergency Nurse (CEN). But you *become* an "emergency nurse" anytime your patient has an emergency and you're the primary person caring for him. Can you meet this challenge with confidence in your skills?

Make no mistake—the demands on you may be enormous. You may have to function as part of an emergency team, interacting with a physician, a respiratory therapist, an X-ray technician, and others who will scrutinize your decisions and even question them. Or you may simply be alone, on a medical-surgical unit or in a small hospital ED, when a patient urgently needs your help. Wherever you are, alone or not, you'll have much to do and little time to do it.

Fortunately, these situations—and emergencies in general—don't happen often in medical-surgical nursing practice. But, when any emergency occurs, you don't want to simply *react* to the frightening urgency of the situation—this response puts you a crucial step behind events as they unfold. Instead, you want to *act* decisively and correctly—to be a step ahead, prepared to meet each of the patient's emergency needs the moment it's identified. This book, EMERGENCIES, can be your "silent partner" in those first critical minutes. In EMERGENCIES, you'll discover techniques for performing rapid emergency assessments and on-the-spot interventions. The minutes you save may save a patient's life.

I've "been there." The first time was about a year into my nursing career when a patient went into anaphylactic shock on my unit. If he'd been in the ED, he'd have had the full support of an emergency team and all the appropriate equipment. But on the unit, at that moment, he had only *me.* I'd gone into nursing because I considered myself a calm, capable person who could learn to manage any nursing situation. Well, I learned more about myself that day! Somehow, I did manage to assess the patient's situation, to set the necessary priorities, to call the doctor, and to intervene until he arrived. But I've never forgotten the life-or-death urgency of that moment.

A situation like that one is enough to make any nurse feel insecure. Of course, you're comfortable within the

limits of medical-surgical nursing practice. But if you're
not an emergency specialist, then fast-paced drama
and the chance to participate in innovative procedures
may be more frightening than exciting. Even worse
may be the self-inquisition once an emergency's over:
Did I do enough? Should I have done something differently? Here again, EMERGENCIES can be your silent
partner, validating your decisions and your care.

In my opinion, to be prepared to act confidently in
any emergency, you need to construct a set of self-
expectations based on your skills and knowledge and on
the expectations of at least four other groups of people. I
call these groups the "four Ps": peers, physicians, patients, and patients' families.

Your peers and the physicians you work with have the
right to expect that you:
• have accurate, up-to-date information
• can make the correct decisions in an emergency situation
• have the professional expertise to follow through on
those decisions
• have the interpersonal skills to communicate effectively
with team members in a tension-filled environment.
They expect, in short, a quality performance.

Patients and their families also expect a quality performance—and more. If you hide your insecurities behind
a wall of clinical expertise, you'll be letting them down.
They expect you, quite rightly, to *care*—to be their
"angel of mercy" in a terrifying situation. Patients expect
the swift touch, the comforting word that lets them
know you're not another impersonal cog in the hospital
machinery. Families relegated to corridors and waiting
rooms expect you to know what's going on—what the
sudden burst of activity means, what the unfamiliar
equipment is doing to help the patient. At the most critical times, you're their strongest link to him.

Meeting all these expectations is a formidable task.
The best way to achieve it is by learning—and learning,
and learning more. And that's where EMERGENCIES fits
your needs perfectly. It will help you become thoroughly
familiar with emergency assessment and intervention
procedures. When a patient has an emergency, you'll have
the satisfaction of knowing what to do and doing it correctly—no small reward in itself. And, when your patient
takes a turn for the better, you'll experience the added
reward of having played a vital role in his survival.

So, in managing emergencies, as in many areas of life,
nothing can substitute for knowledge and experience.
Experience, of course, comes only gradually. But knowledge lies always at our fingertips; *we* make the choice
to acquire and to use it. EMERGENCIES is at your fingertips
now. Choose to use it.

Frances J. Storlie, RN, PhD, ANP

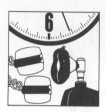

# How to Use This Book

Can a book help you in an emergency, when seconds count and a patient's life may depend on the decisions you make? EMERGENCIES can, because it has a unique *timeline format.* This means that chapters 4 through 17 follow patients' emergency care directly from transport to the hospital through ED care and unit care. So EMERGENCIES will prepare you to intervene at any point when a real emergency occurs.

For example, if you're interested in what care a patient with a body-system emergency may have received before arriving in the ED, consult the "Prehospital Care: What's Been Done" entry in the "Initial Care" section of the chapter covering that body system. If ED care is your concern—or if you don't know the patient's diagnosis, just that he has an emergency involving that particular body system—turn to the "What to Do First" and "What to Do Next" entries. Here you'll find initial and secondary priorities for emergency care clearly spelled out. What if you do know the patient's diagnosis? Then you can turn directly to the "Care after Diagnosis" section of the relevant body-system chapter and locate the entry that covers that diagnosis. The entry will recap prehospital and ED care briefly, then tell you just what emergency-care procedures a patient with that diagnosis will undergo—and what your nursing concerns and actions must be.

The chapters covering shock, burns, environmental emergencies, and poisoning and substance abuse are similarly organized. The difference is that in these conditions the diagnosis will probably be made, and definitive care will probably begin, more quickly than is possible in body-system emergencies. So in these four chapters, the section "Definitive Care" covers specific types of emergencies.

Look for special learning aids in each chapter,

too. These are designed to clarify your understanding so you can sharpen your emergency care skills. For example, "Emergency Assessment Checklist" helps you organize your approach to your patient and keep your care on track. "Case in Point" illustrates legal principles you'll want to keep in mind during emergencies. "Procedures" takes you step-by-step through emergency patient-care procedures. "Pathophysiology" clearly describes the underlying causes and pathophysiologic processes of emergencies. "Drugs" highlights important considerations to keep in mind when administering certain drugs to patients with emergencies. You'll also find numerous additional illustrations and graphs in each chapter. And each chapter ends with a list of selected references; use these as a guide to further reading.

EMERGENCIES also has special features, besides its chapter content, that make the book uniquely valuable. For example, following Chapter 3 you'll find a multipage section, "Life Support: Performing Basic and Advanced Techniques." Here, in precisely illustrated detail, is all the information you need to keep your life-support skills fresh. And following Chapter 12, a special four-color section, "Emergency! Atlas of Major Injuries," illustrates mechanisms of injury as well as many of the serious injuries that require emergency intervention. EMERGENCIES also contains a well-selected appendix with charts that will improve your management of pediatric emergencies and your understanding of how colloids and crystalloids are used. You'll also find a concise set of guidelines for dealing with psychiatric emergencies.

To protect your patients, your institution, and yourself, use the information in EMERGENCIES in strict accordance with your personal employment situation. Be sure to follow your institution's policies on managing emergencies, as well as your state nurse practice act and all other laws, rules, regulations, or policies that may apply to your nursing care in an emergency.

You can use EMERGENCIES as an on-the-job resource *and* as a learning or teaching tool. Whenever and wherever you use it, you'll be ensuring that your patients receive first-quality emergency care.

# 1

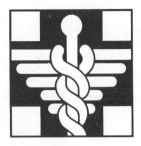

# Approaches to Emergency Care

## Introduction

*Emergency.* It can happen anytime, to anyone, anywhere. If you're the first person to respond—at the scene, in the ED, or on the medical-surgical unit—you face the ultimate challenge of your nursing skills. Why? Because you may not know what happened or exactly what's wrong with your patient, you may have only minutes to intervene, and a slip in judgment may be disastrous.

You probably can recall times on the unit when you thought you had everything under control—breakfast over, baths and medications given, beds made—and suddenly one of your patients had a seizure or became very short of breath and cyanotic. What did you do? Were you satisfied with the way you responded and with the outcome? Or do you wish you'd done something—maybe several things—differently?

EMERGENCIES is designed to increase your self-confidence and effectiveness in an emergency. How? By increasing your preparedness to assess and intervene appropriately. This chapter first introduces you to today's sophisticated network of emergency services (including prehospital and ED care). Then, it describes how the ED and the medical-surgical unit are organized to care for patients with serious emergency problems. Finally, this chapter explains how you, as a nurse on the unit, fit into the plan for emergency care in your hospital.

### Emergency: Some definitions

*Emergency* means different things to different people. Traditionally, health-care professionals have defined a *true emergency* as "any trauma or sudden illness that requires immediate intervention to prevent imminent severe damage or death."

At first glance, from your perspective as a nurse, this definition may seem complete. But what about your patient? What if he believes he needs emergency care, but you don't assess the situation the same way? Must he prove to you that he has an emergency? Strange as this may seem, sometimes a patient *does* have trouble convincing a nurse or doctor that he's really sick. But in general, health-care personnel are becoming more sensitive to the patient's viewpoint.

The American Hospital Association's definition of *emergency* incorporates this modern viewpoint: "any condition that—in the opinion of the patient, his family, or whoever assumes the responsibility of bringing the patient to the hospital—requires immediate medical intervention. This condition continues until a determination has been made that the patient's life or well-being is not threatened."

# EMERGENCY: THE MEDICAL-SURGICAL UNIT'S ROLE

If you think ED care's remote from care on your unit, think again. Chances are you can recall a number of patients you've cared for on your unit who were first admitted via your hospital's ED. The fact is, no matter where else such a patient may be cared for during his time in the hospital, he'll end up on the medical-surgical unit before discharge. This chart gives you an overview of the various routes patients who need emergency care may follow in the hospital.

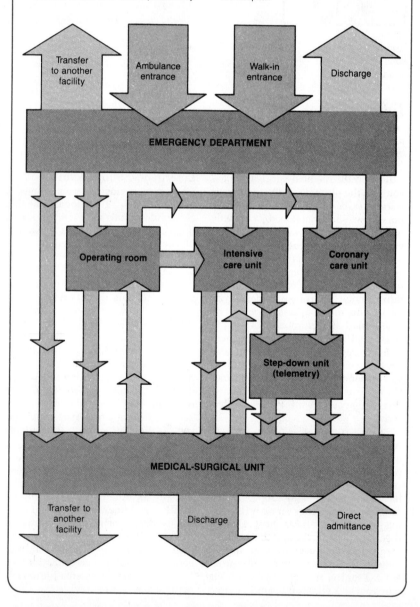

Obviously, these two definitions are both correct. How can they be brought together? Your skilled approach to managing an emergency is the key. When you simultaneously assess the patient's emergency problem *and* his perspective on it, then intervene appropriately, you're providing definitive emergency care.

### The Emergency Medical Services systems

Not so long ago—as late as the 1960s—communities had few or no organized ways to transport emergency patients, much less to care for them en route. Ambulances weren't commonly staffed with medical or nursing personnel, and local EDs were sometimes poorly equipped and understaffed. (See *Emergency Transport to the Hospital: Then and Now,* pages 6 and 7.) Police, fire fighters, and first-aiders provided the only prehospital care available. Sometimes hearses brought patients to the ED!

Today, this situation's been replaced with coordinated community systems for aiding and transporting emergency patients. The 1966 National Highway Safety Act, which authorized the U.S. Department of Transportation to establish Emergency Medical Services (EMS) guidelines, began this trend. Under the new law, funds were made available to community agencies for the purchase of ambulances, the installation of rescue personnel communication networks, and the development of emergency medical technician (EMT) training programs. Then, in 1970, the National Registry of Emergency Medical Technicians was formed to unify the educational and examination requirements and the certification criteria for EMTs. The next step was passage of the Emergency Medical Services Systems Act in 1973. This act divided the nation into 304 administrative regions and provided additional EMS funds for qualifying communities. Its purpose? To stimulate regional EMS systems to upgrade and standardize their emergency services.

Today, virtually all U.S. communities are tied into the EMS network. This means that each community has a plan for providing comprehensive emergency rescue and medical care, from first response through completion of specific emergency procedures. Stages in this plan include:

● *first rescue response,* involving trained rescue personnel (including police and fire fighters) who may use specialized *rescue* equipment
● *first medical response,* involving trained personnel who give *care* at the scene and during transport
● *continued care in the hospital* by emergency doctors and nurses and (if the patient's admitted) by staff in other hospital units.

## REVIEWING PREHOSPITAL EMERGENCY CARE

# How Field Teams May Be Structured

Today, trained rescue vehicle personnel provide most on-site and in-transit emergency care—although police and fire fighters remain part of the prehospital emergency-care networks. (See *How Did Your Patient Come to the E.D.?*, page 5.) The emergency vehicles they use include standard ambulances, mobile intensive care units (MICUs), and, sometimes, helicopters.

The care that rescue vehicle personnel give ranges from basic to advanced life support, depending on the community's size, overall plan for prehospital emergency care, and amount of EMS funding. These elements are related to each other, of course. For example, to provide prehospital advanced life support on a routine basis, a community usually needs a population base of 50,000 or more. (Many areas provide services combining basic and advanced life support.)

In most EMS systems, field teams—consisting of dispatchers, EMTs, nurses and doctors, fire and police departments, and citizens—are organized to respond to communities' prehospital emergency-care needs. The field teams may work for the hospitals, which administer the overall prehospital-care programs and serve as communication centers for their rescue vehicles.

Communication is a vital component of prehospital emergency care. A large community may have a main communication center, coordinating all calls requesting prehospital emergency care, as well as hospital-to-rescue-unit or hospital-to-hospital communication. In such a community, the *dispatcher* (usually an EMT) answers all the calls that come into the local EMS system. (Many communities now use the "911" telephone code for people to summon medical as well as police help.) His responsibilities include gathering pertinent information from the caller, assessing the information, and communicating with the rescue vehicle that goes to the scene.

EMTs are mainly categorized as EMT (EMT-1) and EMT-Paramedic (EMT-P). The *EMT-1* is trained to recognize life-threatening conditions and qualified to give first aid and basic life support, including closed-chest cardiac massage. He may also help in emergency childbirth. His training ranges from 80 to 150 hours and includes on-the-job training and hospital work, usually in the ED.

The EMT-1 may work together with an *EMT-P*, who's qualified to give advanced life-support care, to manage certain cardiac dysrhythmias, to defibrillate, to intubate, and to start an I.V. In an MICU, the EMT-P communicates with the hospital base, relating his assessment findings and receiving orders from the doctor or nurse. EMT-P training is more advanced than EMT-1

training—up to 2,000 hours.

In states where the *mobile intensive care nurse* (MICN) is part of the prehospital-care team, she rides with EMTs in the MICU, provides advanced life-support care, and trains and supervises paramedics.

In some EMS regions, *specially trained and certified nurses* communicate by radio with EMT-Ps in the field. These nurses give instructions for care of patients being transported to the hospital in the MICU. (Usually this sophisticated and expensive rescue vehicle can be fielded only when the hospital is a major center for emergency care in a heavily populated region.)

Standards for *police and fire fighter* emergency medical training vary widely. Because they're often the first to arrive on the emergency scene, most police officers and fire fighters must have at least some training in first aid. Some fire departments employ EMT-Ps as part of their own rescue teams.

In some EMS systems, *doctors, nurses,* and even *respiratory therapists* may care for patients en route to the hospital. (See *Comparing Types of Field Teams,* pages 8 and 9.)

If you ever work in a hospital ED, you'll have three major responsibilities to the EMTs who bring in patients:

• *to continue the care they began.* For example, they may have been performing CPR on the patient for 20 minutes or more. They expect—and deserve—to have that care continued until the doctor orders different care.

• *to be receptive to information they provide about the patient.* The EMTs' assessment and intervention helped stabilize the patient's condition—perhaps even kept him alive—until he could reach the ED. Make the best use of this by recording all the information they can provide about the patient. Of course, this information will also be needed for his continuing care.

• *to continue their training* and *to ensure the continued quality of their care* by tactfully correcting flaws in their techniques or procedures.

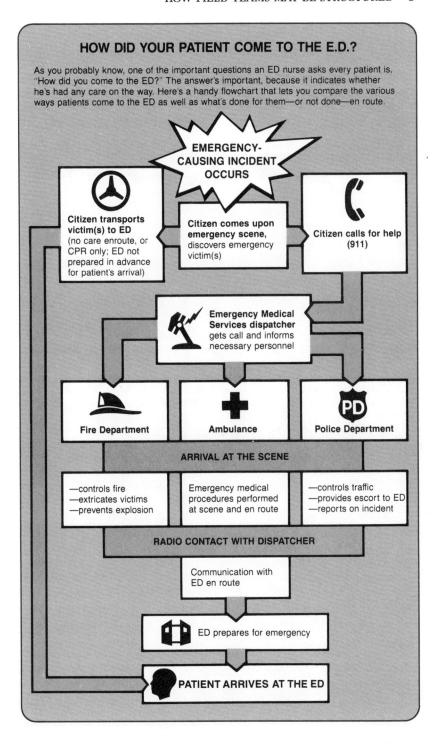

## HOW DID YOUR PATIENT COME TO THE E.D.?

As you probably know, one of the important questions an ED nurse asks every patient is, "How did you come to the ED?" The answer's important, because it indicates whether he's had any care on the way. Here's a handy flowchart that lets you compare the various ways patients come to the ED as well as what's done for them—or not done—en route.

**EMERGENCY-CAUSING INCIDENT OCCURS**

**Citizen transports victim(s) to ED** (no care enroute, or CPR only; ED not prepared in advance for patient's arrival)

**Citizen comes upon emergency scene,** discovers emergency victim(s)

**Citizen calls for help (911)**

**Emergency Medical Services dispatcher** gets call and informs necessary personnel

**Fire Department**

**Ambulance**

**Police Department**

ARRIVAL AT THE SCENE

—controls fire
—extricates victims
—prevents explosion

Emergency medical procedures performed at scene and en route

—controls traffic
—provides escort to ED
—reports on incident

RADIO CONTACT WITH DISPATCHER

Communication with ED en route

ED prepares for emergency

**PATIENT ARRIVES AT THE ED**

# EMERGENCY TRANSPORT TO THE HOSPITAL: THEN AND NOW

 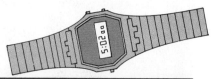

| THEN (20 years ago) | | NOW |
|---|---|---|
| Edgar Mellon, age 50, previously in good health, awakens with crushing substernal chest pain and shortness of breath. | 2:00 a.m. | Joe Edge, age 50, previously in good health, awakens with crushing substernal chest pain and shortness of breath. |
| His wife is frightened and not sure whom to call for help. She grabs the telephone book and begins to search. | 2:01 a.m. | Joe's wife, frightened, quickly dials 911, the city's well-publicized emergency telephone number. |
| Still searching. | 2:02 a.m. | An Emergency Medical Services dispatcher questions her to obtain pertinent information. He assures her that help will be on the way in a matter of seconds. |
| She's found seven ambulance companies listed in the yellow pages; she calls the one at the top of the list. | 2:03 a.m. | The dispatcher notifies the fire department and mobile intensive care unit (MICU) nearest the emergency. |
| The ambulance company answers and tells her they don't offer 24-hour service. | 2:05 a.m. | The fire rescue unit, at the same time as the MICU, "rolls code 3" (with red lights and siren), on their way to the Edges' home. |
| She calls the next ambulance company on the list. They tell her all the ambulances are out right now, but one will respond as soon as possible. | 2:05 a.m. | On the way. |
| Still waiting. | 2:06 a.m. | Trained fire fighter emergency medical technicians (EMTs) arrive in their rescue unit. They administer oxygen to Joe, assess his condition, and get his vital signs. |
| The ambulance hasn't arrived. Edgar's wife is even more frightened now. She returns to the bedroom to check on him and finds he's sweating profusely and having considerable difficulty breathing. | 2:10 a.m. | The MICU arrives. Two EMT-Paramedics (EMT-Ps) quickly take over Joe's care and evaluate his condition. He's ashen, profusely diaphoretic, and in moderately severe respiratory distress, with rales in both lungs. The cardiac monitor reveals frequent multifocal premature ventricular contractions (PVCs). |

| THEN (20 years ago) | | NOW |
|---|---|---|
| Still waiting. | 2:10 a.m. | The EMT-Ps establish radio and telemetry contact with their base hospital. A doctor, specially trained in emergency medicine, takes the information and issues instructions: an I.V. (dextrose 5% in water), morphine, oxygen, and lidocaine. |
| Still waiting. | 2:12 a.m. | The EMT-Ps start the I.V. and administer the medications. |
| The ambulance arrives at the Mellons' house. The crew begins to place Edgar on a stretcher. | 2:16 a.m. | While Joe's being prepared for transport, one of the EMT-Ps notifies base that the PVCs have stopped and the patient appears stable. After receiving cardiac monitor telemetry, the doctor requests a "code 2" transport (no red lights or siren) to the nearest ED. |
| The ambulance crew has loaded Edgar into the ambulance; now they begin to speed to the nearest hospital with the red lights flashing and the siren on. On the way, Edgar loses consciousness, stops breathing, and has no pulse. One of the attendants tries cardiopulmonary resuscitation. | 2:16 a.m. | The doctor at the base hospital calls the ED at the receiving hospital and provides a complete patient report on Joe to the triage nurse there. |
| Still in transit. | 2:21 a.m. | In transit, one of the EMT-Ps reports to the receiving hospital, by radio, that Joe's pain and shortness of breath have decreased, and his color has improved. |
| The ambulance arrives at the ED. The doctor must be called at home and asked to come in. The duty nurse is reluctant to initiate definitive medical care. | 2:25 a.m. | The MICU arrives at the receiving hospital's ED. Joe's quickly cared for by specially trained emergency doctors and nurse specialists. |
| The doctor arrives and tries heroic resuscitative efforts that prove futile. | 2:33 a.m. | Joe's transferred to the coronary care unit (CCU). |
| Edgar's pronounced dead. | 3:00 a.m. | Joe's resting comfortably in the CCU. |

Adapted with permission from Aspen Systems Corporation, from Barbara Secord-Pletz, "Prehospital Emergency Care and Transportation" in *Emergency Medicine*, edited by T. Kravis and C. Warner: Rockville, Maryland, 1983.

# UNDERSTANDING THE EMERGENCY DEPARTMENT

You may never work in your hospital's ED. But if you do, you'll need to know how the ED's organized and what your role is in providing emergency care. If you work on a medical-surgical unit, maybe the ED seems pretty remote. It isn't, though—because some of your patients will have been admitted through the ED. You'll be able to give them better care now if you understand the care they've already had. (See *Emergency: The Medical-Surgical Unit's Role*, page 2.)

## COMPARING TYPES OF FIELD TEAMS

As you may know, an ED's response to a patient's need for emergency care depends, in part, on the prehospital care (if any) he's received. The ED team may receive a patient who's had no care, some care, or sophisticated care similar to what the ED itself would provide. If you work in your hospital's ED, be sure you're familiar with how your area's field teams work. This will prepare you to care for patients when they arrive and help you evaluate the care they received. Here's a chart that compares the three basic types of emergency-care field teams and indicates the extent of the care each can provide.

| | FIRST-AID SQUAD (NONINVASIVE CARE) | FIRST-AID SQUAD (INVASIVE CARE) |
|---|---|---|
| **Personnel** | Advanced first-aider, first responder, or both (may also carry an emergency medical technician [EMT]) | Usually two EMTs; may be EMT and EMT-Paramedic (EMT-P) |
| **Certifying group** | American Red Cross or state (first-aider); National Registry of Emergency Medical Technicians or state | National Registry of Emergency Medical Technicians or state |
| **Equipment** | Ambulance with: <br>• radio transmitter (voice only) <br>• litter <br>• portable suction unit <br>• portable oxygen equipment <br>• bandages and dressings <br>• splints and backboards | Ambulance with all equipment on first-aider ambulance, plus: <br>• tools for extricating trapped accident victims |
| **Treatment** | • Responds, gives care at scene, transports <br>• Administers first aid and CPR <br>• Splints fractures <br>• Assists with childbirth <br>• Stabilizes patient's spine <br>• Gives oxygen <br>• Provides basic care for victims of poisoning | • Responds, gives care at scene, transports <br>• Administers first aid and CPR <br>• Uses oral airway <br>• Performs suction <br>• Assists with extricating accident victims (using tools) <br>• Uses medical antishock trousers (MAST suit) <br>• Splints fractures <br>• Assists with childbirth <br>• Stabilizes patient's spine <br>• Gives oxygen <br>• Provides basic care for victims of poisoning |

# ED Facilities

State regulatory agencies categorize EDs, within EMS regions, according to facilities, services, and staff. This helps to ensure that high-quality medical and nursing emergency care are available

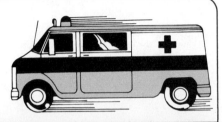

**MOBILE INTENSIVE CARE UNIT (INVASIVE CARE)**

Usually two EMT-Ps; may also carry a doctor, nurse, and/or respiratory therapist

National Registry of Emergency Medical Technicians or state

Ambulance with all equipment on first-aider ambulance, plus:
• tools for extricating trapped accident victims
• radio transmitter for both voice and cardiac telemetry
• advanced airway equipment
• I.V. equipment
• cardiac telemetry unit
• portable defibrillator
• drug box

• May respond and give care at scene only or respond, give care, and transport
• Does all treatment procedures that first aid squads do (invasive and noninvasive)
• Uses esophageal obturator airway and endotracheal tube
• Initiates I.V.s
• Uses cardiac monitor
• Transmits EKG data to ED doctor or nurse
• Administers medication per doctor's orders or standard orders, based on voice and monitor radio contact with hospital-based personnel

to entire regional populations. It also serves to avoid needless duplication of emergency equipment and services.

The design of an ED is based on:
• the community's specific emergency-care needs
• the size and facilities of nearby EDs
• whether a trauma center's nearby
• the size of the patient population.

Typically, a hospital ED exercises no control over the patient population it serves. Anyone can walk in (or be brought in) for help for any ailment. So an ED must be staffed and equipped to manage or refer all kinds of emergencies, 24 hours a day. A rural hospital's ED may provide mainly primary care, with referral to the patient's private doctor. In contrast, a large city hospital's ED may provide a full spectrum of emergency care.

Whatever their capacity to provide care, all EDs have the same broad objectives:
• diagnosis, treatment, and stabilization of all life-threatening and all urgent emergency conditions
• symptomatic care of nonurgent conditions and/or referral to patients' private doctors.

The ED's design must allow for easy, organized movement of patients from the entrance (and the ambulance entrance), through triage, to the waiting room and treatment rooms. EDs typically have separate treatment rooms for various kinds of emergencies. Some EDs also have specialized treatment areas for such services as dialysis, burn treatment, and trauma care. How many rooms an ED has, and the types of care given in them, depend on the size of the patient population it serves. (See *Viewing a Typical E.D. Floor Plan*, page 14.) If the patient population is very large (for example, in a big inner-city hospital), the ED may be correspondingly large, with additional specific treatment areas: a psychiatric quiet room, for example, or an X-ray department.

Within some EMS regions, regional trauma centers have been established to care for patients with serious multiple injuries. These trauma centers are usually separate from hospital EDs and are staffed 24 hours a day solely to care for trauma victims. In some EMS regions, however, certain hospitals have trauma rooms (or areas) as part of their emergency-care facilities.

An ED's efficient organization includes having specialized equipment and crash carts available in specific areas for immediate use. (See *Crash Cart Crash Course,* page 13.)

# ED Staff

Increasingly, ED staffs are made up of doctors, nurses, and other personnel specifically educated and trained to give emergency care. The role of *nurses* in the ED has expanded accordingly. Through education and certification, the Emergency Department Nurses Association (EDNA) and other special-interest groups are actively promoting the practice of emergency nursing as a specialty. Not all ED nurses are EDNA-certified, of course—but they're all specially trained. This is necessary because an ED nurse must have highly developed and specialized skills that only on-the-job training can provide.

Many large EDs have one nurse per shift assigned to do triage on incoming patients. This helps to determine which patients need immediate care for severe illnesses or injuries—and which patients can wait. (See *What Is Triage?*) The *triage nurse* may give preliminary care (such as wound care) before a patient goes to a treatment area. She may also answer the EMS hotline, handling requests for rescue vehicle services from her hospital.

The *emergency doctor* has the ultimate responsibility for patient care in the ED. Not all hospitals are able to staff their EDs with doctors trained in emergency medicine, however. In fact, many hospitals are unable to provide

## WHAT IS TRIAGE?

The word *triage* comes from the French word for "sort out." Triage *is* a sorting process, developed originally to classify victims of war and disasters according to the urgency of their medical needs and their likelihood of survival if treated. In the ED, nurses increasingly are performing triage to decide which patients should be treated before others and where treatment should take place. On the medical-surgical unit, *you* sort your patients, too. In fact, all nurses use the principles of triage when planning care for more than one patient. You use your nursing knowledge and skills to decide which patient to care for first and what you need to do first. And throughout your shift, you know who's at risk for sudden development of an emergency problem.

**Purpose**
The purpose of triage is to make the best possible use of the available medical and nursing personnel and facilities. In the ED, triage ensures that the patients who need immediate care receive it. On the medical-surgical unit, triage ensures that you're making proper patient assignments and closely observing unstable patients.

**Triage categories**
To determine priorities of care, patients are divided into three categories: *emergent, urgent,* and *nonurgent.* Here are definitions and examples of patients in each category, both in the ED and on the medical-surgical unit. (Note the similarities *and* the differences between the lists for each category.)

24-hour coverage by a doctor in the ED. In hospitals with residency training programs, residents may work in the ED under supervision of the attending staff. In hospitals with no full-time coverage by doctors in the ED, area doctors may take turns being "on call" to manage emergencies in the ED.

Obviously, administrators of an ED that lacks 24-hour coverage by a doctor are depending heavily on nurses to provide ED services. This means that the ED nurse, like the unit nurse, spends most of her time with patients and may provide most of their care.

| CATEGORY | ED PATIENTS WITH: | MEDICAL-SURGICAL PATIENTS WITH: |
|---|---|---|
| **EMERGENT** | | |
| The patient has a life-threatening emergency and will probably die without immediate attention. In the ED, this patient is seen *first*. On the unit, you stop whatever you're doing and care for this patient *now*. | • cardiac arrest<br>• airway and breathing problems<br>• chest pain with acute dyspnea and/or cyanosis<br>• active seizures<br>• obvious or suspected severe bleeding<br>• severe head injury and/or a comatose state<br>• open chest or abdominal wound<br>• severe shock<br>• excessively high temperature (over 105° F., or 40.6° C.) | • cardiac arrest<br>• airway and breathing problems<br>• chest pain with acute dyspnea and/or cyanosis<br>• active seizures<br>• obvious or suspected severe bleeding<br>• a change in level of consciousness<br>• injury from a fall<br>• sudden alteration in vital signs<br>• excessively high temperature (over 105° F., or 40.6° C.) |
| **URGENT** | | |
| The patient has a condition requiring medical attention within a few hours; if he doesn't receive treatment, he may die or suffer irreversible injury. In the ED, this patient has second priority. On the unit, you call the doctor for this patient, then probably stay with him. | • cerebrovascular accident or transient ischemic attack<br>• persistent nausea and vomiting and/or diarrhea<br>• any type of pain the patient describes as severe<br>• fever above 102° F. (38.9° C.)<br>• circulatory deficit in a limb<br>• severe or sudden headache | • sudden numbness or paralysis<br>• persistent nausea and vomiting and/or diarrhea<br>• any type of pain the patient describes as severe<br>• sudden fever above 102°F. (38.9° C.)<br>• circulatory deficit in a limb<br>• severe or sudden headache |
| **NONURGENT** | | |
| The patient has a condition that probably doesn't require the resources of an ED. Referral may be made to a private doctor or clinic. On the unit, you won't need to observe this patient constantly. | • sprains, strains<br>• mild headache<br>• minor lacerations | • no acute problem—hospitalized for diagnostic tests<br>• no acute problem—waiting for discharge or waiting for transfer to an extended-care facility |

## PROVIDING EMERGENCY CARE ON THE UNIT

# Responding in an Emergency: Are You Prepared?

Did you know that, as a nurse on the medical-surgical unit, you have an important dual role in providing emergency care? That's right. You have assessment and intervention skills that let you *manage* many emergencies, and you're in a unique position to *prevent* some emergencies from ever happening.

Consider the ED nurse's perspective on a seriously ill or injured patient. This patient's *already* seriously ill or injured: the ED nurse rarely, if ever, sees a patient at the onset of his emergency. She cares for him only briefly, perhaps concentrating so hard on his emergency problem that she never learns anything else about him. She doesn't have a role in his follow-up care; in fact, she may never learn what ultimately happens to him.

Your situation is different. On the medical-surgical unit, you spend more time with patients. than anyone else does. Of course, this means you're likely to be right there, or nearby, if an emergency occurs. But it also means that you have constant opportunities to observe your patient. So you're able to note a change in his status that, even though slight, may signal an impending emergency. By alerting the patient's doctor to the problem, or by intervening yourself, you may prevent the emergency from occurring—or at least reduce its damaging effects.

Successful intervention in an emergency typically depends on your knowledge of basic life-support methods—and on your skill in applying them. When one of your patients has an emergency (an obvious example is cardiac arrest), your job is to summon help while doing what you can to keep him alive until the help arrives. Clearly, routine assessment and intervention techniques are inadequate for this—you need to do a rapid-fire assessment with simultaneous intervention as necessary. EMERGENCIES will teach you how to do this, using the skills and training you already have.

But this isn't the whole story: you must also prepare yourself, in advance, to respond appropriately. Here are four basic steps you can take to make sure you're prepared for emergencies:

### Know your facility

Always make sure you're thoroughly familiar with the emergency procedures and equipment in your ED or on your unit. Where are the various pieces of equipment kept? Does your unit have its own crash cart, or does the code team bring it to the scene? If your unit has a crash cart, where is it kept? (See *Crash Cart Crash Course.*) Are oxygen and suction available from wall outlets in your unit, or do you have to bring equipment in?

Be sure you know how all the equipment works, too—and your unit's protocols for using it. Remember, stress—the kind of stress that every emergency situation brings—can make the simplest tasks confusingly complex. If you're unprepared, if you're not absolutely sure where everything you need is, you'll be *looking* for something when you should be *doing* something. You could find yourself trying to figure out *how* a piece of equipment (such as a defibrillator) works, when you should be *making* it work.

Here's a list of specific items you should be able to locate and use (or assist with) in an emergency, with no wasted effort:
- Ambu bag
- artificial airways
- intubation equipment
- I.V. equipment
- central venous pressure kits
- tracheostomy trays
- emergency drugs.

Many hospital units keep certain emergency drugs—for example, epinephrine—in a locked drug box. If you aren't completely familiar with the contents of your unit's drug box, open it (ask permission first, if necessary) and familiarize yourself with what's inside. (Protocol usually dictates that the box must be returned to the pharmacy whenever it's been opened.)

### Know the proper scope of your emergency care

Basic nursing procedures in an emergency include:
- deciding when to call the doctor
- calling a code
- performing emergency assessment and intervention procedures
- assisting with other emergency procedures
- coordinating your care with what the other emergency team members are doing.

Of course, you're aware that an important part of being prepared is know-

## CRASH CART CRASH COURSE

Here's a typical crash cart, one that might be used in an ED or on a medical-surgical unit. The crash cart's stocked with equipment, drugs, tray sets, and other supplies needed to manage common emergencies.

As you're probably aware, crash cart contents vary from hospital to hospital and from unit to unit. Be sure you're familiar with your unit's crash cart. Check it at least once every shift, and after each emergency, to restock supplies and to test the defibrillator/monitor unit. Also check the drugs' expiration dates, and stock the cart with fresh drugs if necessary.

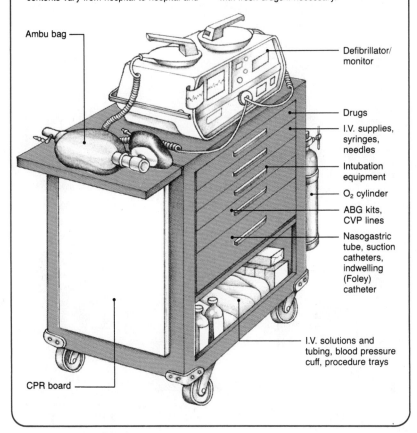

Ambu bag

Defibrillator/ monitor

Drugs

I.V. supplies, syringes, needles

Intubation equipment

$O_2$ cylinder

ABG kits, CVP lines

Nasogastric tube, suction catheters, indwelling (Foley) catheter

I.V. solutions and tubing, blood pressure cuff, procedure trays

CPR board

ing what's expected of you in emergency situations. Emergency protocols vary greatly from hospital to hospital, so be sure you know exactly what your hospital and state nurse practice act allow you to do in an emergency. Be sure, too, that you're thoroughly familiar with your responsibilities on the unit— to patients and to other staff members—in an emergency.

If you're the staff member who discovers a patient with an emergency, *stay with him*. Call for help while you begin primary care—such as CPR. The first nurse who arrives to help should assist you while others bring needed equipment, call specialists (if needed), document how the emergency is managed, and keep tabs on the other patients. When the doctor arrives, he'll take over primary care. Then your role will be to assist.

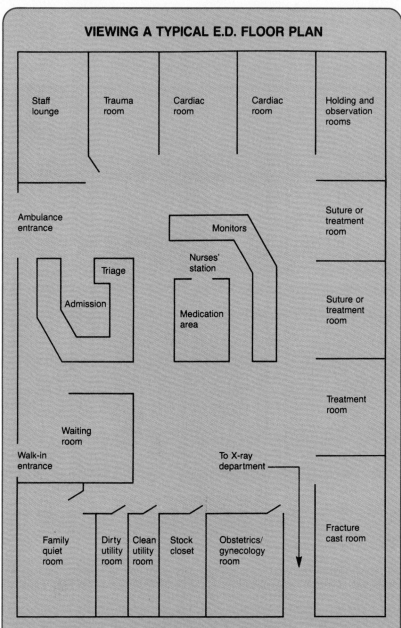

## VIEWING A TYPICAL E.D. FLOOR PLAN

Staff lounge

Trauma room

Cardiac room

Cardiac room

Holding and observation rooms

Ambulance entrance

Monitors

Nurses' station

Triage

Admission

Medication area

Suture or treatment room

Suture or treatment room

Treatment room

Waiting room

Walk-in entrance

To X-ray department

Family quiet room

Dirty utility room

Clean utility room

Stock closet

Obstetrics/ gynecology room

Fracture cast room

This floor plan shows the layout of a typical ED in a medium-size hospital. (Of course, an ED may be smaller or much larger than this.) Note how the ambulance and walk-in entrances and the triage, waiting, and treatment areas flow into each other for maximum efficiency in caring for patients with emergencies. In each treatment area, equipment and supplies are also arranged for most efficient use.

## Know your patients

Your assessment of every new patient on your unit should include determining whether he's at risk for a specific emergency. For example:

• A patient on anticoagulant therapy is at risk for excessive bleeding.

• A patient recovering from a myocardial infarction may suddenly develop chest pain, dysrhythmias, or congestive heart failure.

• A patient with thrombophlebitis is at risk for pulmonary emboli.

If you or the doctor considers one of your patients on the unit is at risk for an emergency, make sure you have the appropriate resuscitative equipment nearby. Then you'll be able to act quickly if an emergency does occur.

## Stay prepared

Once you're confident of your role in an emergency on your unit, be sure you *stay* prepared. How? By regularly reviewing your hospital's and your unit's policies, procedures, and assignments, as well as where the emergency equipment is located and how to use it. When your response in an emergency becomes a well-organized reflex action, you'll know you're always ready to manage emergencies confidently.

## A FINAL WORD

Most hospitalized patients—whether they're admitted through the ED or not—will eventually receive nursing care on a medical-surgical unit. And any of them can go from stable to emergency status in the blink of an eye. To manage such emergencies, be sure your emergency assessment and intervention skills are sharp. Be sure, too, that you're thoroughly familiar with your unit's plan for responding in an emergency. Finally, be sure you always consider which of your patients is at risk for an emergency. If it happens, you'll be prepared. If it doesn't happen, you'll still be prepared. Either way, you—and your patients—benefit.

## Selected References

*Accreditation Manual for Hospitals: 1982 Ed.* Chicago: Joint Commission on Accreditation of Hospitals, 1981.

Bowers, John F., and Purcell, Elizabeth, eds. *Emergency Medical Services: Measures to Improve Care.* New York: J. Macy Foundation, 1980.

Boyd, David R., and Edlich, Richard F. *Systems Approach to Emergency Medical Care.* East Norwalk, Conn.: Appleton-Century-Crofts, 1983.

Budassi, Susan A., and Barber, Janet. *Emergency Nursing: Principles and Practice.* St. Louis: C.V. Mosby Co., 1980.

Eckert, Charles, ed. *Emergency-Room Care,* 4th ed. Boston: Little, Brown & Co., 1981.

Harvey, J.C. "The Emergency Medical Ser-

vice Systems Act of 1973," *New England Journal of Medicine* 292(10):529-30, March 6, 1975.

Hughes, M.M. "Nursing Theories and Emergency Nursing," *Journal of Emergency Nursing* 9(2):95-7, March/April 1983.

Lanros, Nedill E. *Assessment and Intervention in Emergency Nursing,* 2nd ed. Bowie, Md.: Robert J. Brady Co., 1982.

Montgomery, B.J. "Emergency Medical Services: A New Phase of Development," *Journal of the American Medical Association* 243(10):1017-21, 1980.

U.S. Department of Health, Education, and Welfare. "EMS Systems: Program Guidelines" (HSA-76-2028). U.S. Government Printing Office, 1976.

# 2

# Legal Concerns in Emergencies

## Introduction

When you respond to a patient's need for care in an emergency, his urgent clinical needs will naturally take precedence over your concerns about legal risks. You've no time to ponder legalities: With your nursing judgment and skill on the line, your response must be immediate and decisive.

But—you can't afford to ignore the threat of liability inherent in every emergency-care situation.

The solution to this dilemma? Take the time *now* to learn about the laws, court-case decisions, legal principles, and institutional rules and regulations that can influence your care in an emergency. For example, here are some questions you should know the answers to:

• Is the potential for negligence increased in emergency situations?
• Do hospitals have a duty to provide emergency care?
• What is the extent of your responsibility, as a nurse, for providing emergency care in the hospital? What about outside the hospital—beyond the scope of your employment?
• Does the patient's right to give informed consent change in an emergency situation?
• How do the various reporting laws affect your care in an emergency?
• What's your responsibility for fulfilling police requests? For example, if a police officer asks you to search a suspected criminal's belongings for evidence, or to obtain a blood or urine sample from a patient in police custody, do you have to comply?

This chapter provides answers to these questions. It also tells you how to respond in an emergency with actions that minimize your legal liability but don't jeopardize the quality of your care.

Emergencies aren't everyday occurrences on the unit, so you don't have regular opportunities to practice your emergency assessment skills. This leaves you vulnerable to emergency pitfalls—actions or inactions commonly cited in lawsuits alleging nursing negligence:

• failure to recognize an emergency
• failure to respond appropriately to an emergency
• failure to communicate adequately
• failure to administer medications properly
• failure to detect and correct preventable equipment failure.

When you've finished reading this chapter, you'll be better prepared to recognize these pitfalls and to avoid them. Then, when the next emergency occurs—whether you're at the scene, on the unit, or in the ED—you'll have increased confidence in your ability to meet the challenge.

## PROVIDING EMERGENCY CARE IN THE HOSPITAL

# A Hospital's Duty to Provide Emergency Care

Until about 25 years ago, no legally supported right to receive emergency care existed. Today, however, as a result of federal legislation, state laws, and influential court-case decisions, a special right for persons to receive emergency care in hospital EDs prevails.

### Federal legislation

The Hill-Burton Act of 1946 provided federal funding to communities for constructing or modernizing healthcare facilities. To obtain funding, the sponsoring health-care institutions had to promise they'd give some "uncompensated care" and also provide some unspecified "community services." The 1970 amendments to the Hill-Burton Act included funding of emergency services. This meant that, within a particular state, each hospital's ED could now be considered for funding, as part of development of the federally mandated state plan for providing emergency care for its citizens. With federal funding available, more and more states began requiring hospitals to provide emergency services.

The "uncompensated care" called for in the Hill-Burton Act was generally limited to care given in hospital EDs until 1979, when further amendments to the act gave hospitals the option to decide which departments would provide such service.

### State laws and regulations

In some states, laws (or hospital-licensing regulations) now require that all hospitals provide necessary emergency care to anyone who requests it in the ED—whether he can pay for it or not. In fact, in certain states, if a doctor in a publicly funded hospital has diagnosed a patient in the ED as seriously ill or injured, the hospital must provide the emergency services the patient needs, even if he can't pay for them. If the hospital withholds the services, it may be prosecuted.

### Common law influence

The courts have also recognized a right to emergency services; this right generally prevails even in states that don't have laws requiring emergency care. The most influential court-case decision is *Wilmington General Hospital v. Manlove* (1961). The lawsuit charged a hospital with the wrongful death of an infant who was refused treatment in the hospital's ED and subsequently died at home. The child's parents were the plaintiffs in the case. Here's what happened:

When the parents arrived in the ED with the infant, who was seriously ill with diarrhea and a high fever, the nurse in charge didn't examine him. Instead, her first response was an attempt to contact the infant's doctor. Why? Because hospital policy required ED personnel to obtain a patient's doctor's permission before treating the patient in the ED. The nurse was unable to contact the infant's doctor, so—still without examining the infant—she recommended that the parents take their child home and return to the hospital's pediatric clinic the next morning. The parents did return home. Although they were able to contact the child's doctor and make an appointment with him for that evening, their efforts were in vain—the child died that afternoon.

The ensuing lawsuit reached the Delaware Supreme Court, which ruled: "Should a person in need of emergency care request such treatment from a private hospital in reliance upon its accepted custom of providing it, the hospital cannot turn that person away

## DOES YOUR E.D. PATIENT RELINQUISH ANY OF HIS RIGHTS?

The answer to this question is a resounding *no*. Never forget that even in the sometimes chaotic environment of the ED, you must observe all your patient's rights—or you may face a charge of negligence. Most hospitals design their own patient's bills of rights. The American Hospital Association's bill of rights is shown below.

### A PATIENT'S BILL OF RIGHTS

**1** The patient has the right to considerate and respectful care.

**2** The patient has the right to obtain from his physician complete, current information concerning his diagnosis, treatment, and prognosis in terms the patient can be reasonably expected to understand. When it is not medically advisable to give such information to the patient, the information should be made available to an appropriate person in his behalf. He has the right to know, by name, the physician responsible for coordinating his care.

**3** The patient has the right to receive from his physician information necessary to give informed consent prior to the start of any procedure and/or treatment. Except in emergencies, such information for informed consent should include but not necessarily be limited to the specific procedure and/or treatment, the medically significant risks involved, and the probable duration of incapacitation. Where medically significant alternatives for care or treatment exist, or when the patient requests information concerning medical alternatives, the patient has the right to such information. The patient also has the right to know the name of the person responsible for the procedures and/or treatment.

**4** The patient has the right to refuse treatment to the extent permitted by law and to be informed of the medical consequences of his action.

**5** The patient has the right to every consideration of his privacy concerning his own medical care program. Case discussion, consultation, examination, and treatment are confidential and should be conducted discreetly. Those not directly involved in his care must have the permission of the patient to be present.

**6** The patient has the right to expect that all communications and records pertaining to his care should be treated as confidential.

**7** The patient has the right to expect that within its capacity a hospital must make reasonable response to the request of a patient for services. The hospital must provide evaluation, service, and/or referral as indicated by the urgency of the case. When medically permissible, a patient may be transferred to another facility only after he has received complete information and explanation concerning the needs for and alternatives to such a transfer. The institution to which the patient is to be transferred must first have accepted the patient for transfer.

**8** The patient has the right to obtain information as to any relationship of his hospital to other health-care and educational institutions insofar as his care is concerned. The patient has the right to obtain information as to the existence of any professional relationships among individuals, by name, who are treating him.

The patient has the right to be advised if the hospital proposes to engage in or perform human experimentation affecting his care or treatment. The patient has the right to refuse to participate in such research projects.

**10** The patient has the right to expect reasonable continuity of care. He has the right to know in advance what appointment times and physicians are available and where. The patient has the right to expect that the hospital will provide a mechanism whereby he is informed by his physician or a delegate of the physician of the patient's continuing health-care requirements following discharge.

**11** The patient has the right to examine and receive an explanation of his bill, regardless of source of payment.

**12** The patient has the right to know what hospital rules and regulations apply to his conduct as a patient.

without acting reasonably under the circumstances." This decision, which has become known as the "reliance principle," established the people's right to rely on their community hospitals for emergency treatment. If a hospital refuses such treatment, its liability will be based on the court's presumption that the patient's condition will worsen unnecessarily during the time he spends trying to find another hospital.

The court limited such liability, however, to situations when persons with frank or unmistakable emergencies (who would routinely rely on the hospital to provide care) are denied medical attention. Who decides whether a patient's emergency is "frank or unmistakable"? An ED triage nurse or doctor.

The reliance theory was also involved in *Stanturf v. Sipes* (1969). In this lawsuit, the Missouri Supreme Court reversed a judgment in favor of a hospital administrator who'd refused to admit a patient to the ED because he couldn't pay the $25 admission charge. The patient had requested treatment for frostbite of both feet. The hospital was the only one in the immediate area. The court ruled that the public had reason to rely on the hospital for necessary emergency care, and that the plaintiff's condition worsened during his futile efforts to obtain treatment elsewhere.

In *Guerrero v. Copper Queen Hospital* (1975), the court stated that if a law requiring emergency facilities exists, presumably it also imposes a duty on those facilities to aid persons seeking emergency care and treatment. The Arizona court ruled that the privately owned hospital, operated solely for one company's employees, nevertheless was obligated to provide emergency care in an unmistakable emergency—even to illegal aliens.

Some emergency-care laws define "emergency," but courts will probably continue to decide, on a case-by-case basis, whether an emergency existed.

This means that hospital EDs must have written protocols that doctors and triage nurses can use to identify and treat patients seeking necessary emergency care.

# What's a Nurse's Legal Duty in an Emergency?

In a lawsuit charging a nurse with negligence, the plaintiff-patient attempts to prove that the defendant-nurse had a duty to the plaintiff, that she breached that duty, and that the breach of duty caused injury to the plaintiff. These elements—duty, breach of duty, injury, and causation—are usually incorporated into state malpractice or medical injury laws.

A legal duty exists when a nurse is working within the scope of her employment—including when she's responding to an emergency in the ED or on a hospital unit. The employer-employee relationship creates the duty. If a nurse responds to an emergency outside her place of employment, the general rule is that no duty exists.

## Standards of care
In a lawsuit, before a charge of breach of duty can be proved or disproved, the scope of a nurse's duty—the standard of care that the duty imposes on her—must be determined. The court will apply the "reasonable nurse" standard, which says that the scope of any nurse's duty in a particular situation includes what the reasonably prudent nurse with similar skills and training would do in the same or similar circumstances. Because no two nurse-patient situations are exactly alike, the courts evaluate each case individually. How? By matching its unique circumstances with expert-witness testimony and other pertinent information to derive the appropriate standard of care for judging the defendant-nurse's actions.

## LEGAL TERMS USED IN THIS CHAPTER

**battery** • The unauthorized touching of a person by another person, such as when a health-care professional treats a patient beyond what the patient consented to.

**borrowed servant doctrine** • A legal doctrine that courts may apply in cases when an employer "lends" his employee's services to another employer who, under this doctrine, becomes liable for the employee's wrongful conduct.

**common law** • Law derived from previous court decisions, not from statutes. Also called case law.

**corporate negligence** • Failure by a hospital to provide reasonable care to its patients, by failing to follow its own policies and procedures, or to adequately supervise its staff.

**damages** • An amount of money a court orders a defendant to pay the plaintiff, in deciding the case in favor of the plaintiff.

**defendant** • The party that is named in a plaintiff's complaint and against whom the plaintiff's allegations are made. The defendant must respond to the allegations.

**dual servant doctrine** • A legal doctrine, derived from the borrowed servant doctrine, that allows a court to hold both the hospital and doctor liable for a nurse's negligent act.

**duty** • A legal obligation owed by one party to another. Duty may be established by statute or other legal process, as by contract or oath supported by statute, or it may be voluntarily undertaken. Every person has a duty of care to all other people to avoid causing harm or injury by negligence.

**informed consent** • Permission obtained from a patient to perform a specific test or procedure after the patient has been fully informed about the test or procedure.

**liability** • Legal responsibility for failure to act, so causing harm to another person, or

for actions that fail to meet standards of care, so causing another person harm.

**malpractice** • A professional person's wrongful conduct, improper discharge of professional duties, or failure to meet standards of care—any such actions that result in harm to another person.

**negligence** • Failure to act as an ordinary prudent person; conduct contrary to that of a reasonable person under similar circumstances.

**plaintiff** • A person who files a civil lawsuit initiating a legal action. In criminal actions, the prosecution is the plaintiff, acting in behalf of the people of the jurisdiction.

**proximate cause** • A legal concept of cause and effect, which says an act produces a sequence of natural and continuous events, resulting in an injury that wouldn't have otherwise occurred.

**reasonably prudent nurse** • The standard a court uses to judge whether any other nurse would have acted similarly under similar circumstances.

**reliance theory** • The theory that a community relies on a hospital to give emergency care. Therefore, a hospital cannot deny emergency medical attention to people who request it.

**reporting laws** • Laws that require health-care professionals (and others) to report certain deaths and types of illness and injury to governmental agencies.

**respondeat superior** • "Let the master answer." A legal doctrine that makes an employer liable for the consequences of his employee's wrongful conduct while the employee is acting within the scope of his employment.

**triage nurse** • A nurse assigned to the ED to sort patients according to their need for care. The kind of illness or injury, the severity of the problem, and the facilities available govern the process she uses to decide.

(See *Working in the E.D.: Protecting Yourself Against Lawsuits,* page 22.)

If a nurse assists a doctor with a medically related task, and a lawsuit charging negligence results, the court will evaluate her actions according to the standard of care, for that task, that a doctor would be expected to meet.

## WORKING IN THE E.D.:
## PROTECTING YOURSELF AGAINST LAWSUITS

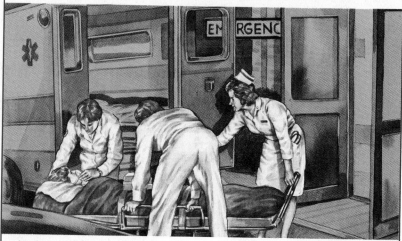

As you know, when you work in your hospital's ED, your expanded responsibilities may make you extra vulnerable to malpractice lawsuits. To protect yourself, take the following precautions:

• Request a clear, written definition of your role in the ED. Your hospital should have an overall policy and an individual, written job description for you that specifies the limits of your nursing role.

• Be sure you know who's responsible, in your ED, for making administrative decisions. Always consult this person when you're caught in a conflict involving a patient and police, his family, or the doctor. Remember, this person speaks for the hospital; if you act without her approval, you'll involve the hospital in the consequences of your actions.

• Document everything you do, so there's no question later about your actions. Your notes, of course, should reflect the nursing process: document your assessment of the ED patient, your care plan, your actual care, and your evaluation of the plan's effectiveness.

• Make sure of your own competence. If your role expands, your skills have to grow, too. If this requires advanced courses and supervised clinical experience, make sure you get both.

• Insure yourself. Damages awarded to patients can be very high, and high legal fees may mean you can't afford even to win a lawsuit. If you don't have your own professional liability insurance and your hospital doesn't help defend you against a lawsuit, you could face a startling bill even after all claims against you are proven groundless and dropped.

Few guidelines exist for deciding which nursing actions are legally appropriate in an emergency situation. Most state nurse practice acts don't list specific procedures, let alone *emergency* procedures, that a nurse may or may not perform. Some state boards of nursing, however, do take clear positions on which nursing acts they do—or don't—consider to be within the scope of nursing practice. (For example, in Pennsylvania, releasing a tension pneumothorax isn't considered within the scope of nursing practice.) To protect yourself, be sure you're familiar with your state's nurse practice act and with the regulations promulgated under its authority.

Nurses who work in specialty areas are expected to meet the standard of the reasonably prudent nurse with similar skills and training in the specialty area. The recent trend toward certification of ED nurses has the effect of upgrading the presently required skills and training; this may eventually result in the expectation of a higher standard of care from ED nurses.

In a lawsuit, the plaintiff's attorney will attempt to prove that the defendant-nurse's actions were below the standard of care that her duty to the patient required. How will he do this? By introducing expert-witness testimony and relevant published standards (such as those of the American Nurses' Association, the Emergency Department Nurses Association, and the particular state's nurse practice act). He may also introduce the relevant policies and procedures of the defendant-nurse's hospital because they represent the standard of care the hospital would expect her to meet.

A negligent action that *doesn't* cause provable injury—for example, if a nurse administers the wrong drug but the patient isn't harmed—can't be used as the basis of a lawsuit charging negligence. This means that the plaintiff must be prepared to prove that the nurse's negligence injured him. Damages the patient can claim include financial loss, bodily injury, and (in some states) psychological or emotional injury.

The degree of proof required for a plaintiff to show that the legal cause of his loss or injury is the defendant's breach of duty (negligence) varies from state to state. In some states, proof that the defendant's action increased the risk that the claimed injury would occur may be sufficient to establish liability. Here's an example:

Suppose a nurse is proved to have negligently given the wrong drug to a patient who shortly afterward suffered respiratory arrest, with ensuing complications. Although the drug itself may not pharmacologically have caused the plaintiff's injury, it may have increased the likelihood that the arrest would occur. Or, by impairing the patient's capacity to resist the onset of arrest, the drug may have reduced the likelihood that he'd survive it.

If a plaintiff-patient's injury can't be directly related in this way to a defendant-nurse's negligent act, the nurse can't be found liable.

## Who gets sued?

How does a plaintiff-patient decide whom to sue? Technically, every individual is personally responsible for his negligent acts, so he can be made to pay damages to a plaintiff who wins a lawsuit against him. In lawsuits charging medical or nursing negligence, however, the issue of who's liable is more complicated. Before naming a defendant (or defendants), the plaintiff-patient and his attorney must first examine the employment relationship of the nurses, doctors, and hospital involved in his case. For example, courts have sometimes ruled that a hospital owes a duty of reasonable care to its patients and can be held "personally" liable, as a corporation, for its negligence. This method of assigning liability is called the *corporate negligence doctrine*. Courts most commonly invoke it in lawsuits when a hospital's failure to follow its own policies and procedures and failure to adequately supervise its staff are proved.

A hospital can also be held vicariously liable for the negligent acts of its employees under the *respondeat superior doctrine*. This means that although, like anyone else, a nurse is personally liable for her own negligent actions, the hospital can be named as a defendant in a lawsuit against her. The hospital can be made to pay the damages, too, if the nurse is found liable for injury to a plaintiff-patient. Respondeat superior can only be invoked, however, if the court proceedings establish that the nurse was an employee of the hospital and was acting within the proper scope of her employment at the time the negligent act occurred.

Most doctors are independent contractors who can be held solely liable for their negligent acts. Some, however—particularly ED doctors—are hospital employees to whom the respondeat superior doctrine can also apply. But increasingly, the *dual servant doctrine*—derived from the *borrowed servant doctrine*—applies when a team of professionals responds to an emergency situation, in the ED or on a unit. Under the dual servant doctrine, a court can hold both the doctor and the hospital liable for a nurse's negligent act.

# Preparing for Emergencies

In an emergency, you must *quickly* and *simultaneously* perform an accurate assessment, make correct nursing judgments (in situations when you may not get a second chance), and implement proper actions. The urgency of the emergency situation obviously increases the chances that you'll make a mistake. How can you avoid emergency pitfalls? By anticipating the challenges and problems emergencies present and preparing yourself to handle them properly when they occur.

### Emergency pitfall #1: Failure to recognize an emergency and respond appropriately

ED nurses with triage responsibilities are particularly vulnerable to charges of negligence. To assist its nurses and avoid legal problems, the ED should establish and maintain written protocols that specify the types of complaints the ED will routinely handle and the types that the triage nurse should usually refer elsewhere. Then, using these protocols as guidelines, the triage nurse must exercise her professional nursing judgment to decide which patients should be admitted to the ED and which should be referred, according to the protocols.

If you're in the position of making such a decision, you must consider whether the referral for treatment could

aggravate the patient's condition or threaten his life or well-being. If you do decide to transfer the patient, keep in mind that your hospital, as the transferring institution, is responsible for the transfer's successful completion. Take the following steps to ensure that the transfer goes smoothly:

● *Determine how long the patient's evaluation and treatment will be delayed because of the transfer.* Could the delay worsen his condition? If a good chance exists that the delay would be harmful, you probably should admit the patient. Otherwise, you may be liable for a charge of abandonment. For the protection of its staff, your ED's policy on transferring patients should provide specific guidelines. Areas the policy should cover include *acceptable reasons for transfer* (whether the patient *or* the hospital requests it); necessity for an *initial examination* of the patient, as a basis for the decision to transfer him or not; *rules, regulations, and laws* regarding transfer that staff should take into account; and details of any *interhospital agreements* that may apply in the transfer decision.

● Before transferring the patient, *contact the referral institution to be sure it will accept the patient.* Be prepared to provide a *transfer summary* detailing the patient's emergency status, the reason for his transfer, and any additional pertinent information.

● *Make sure the patient is protected during the transfer* and that he receives continuity of care, which meets the proper standard, until he reaches the referral institution.

This is a very common area of liability, as the following court cases illustrate:

● A pediatric outpatient director overruled a medical resident's decision to admit a patient with a head injury to the ED—and failed to provide the written sheet, containing instructions and signs and symptoms to watch for, that was customarily provided in such situations (*Niles v. City of San Rafael*, 1974).

## POSSIBLE DEFENSES AGAINST MALPRACTICE CHARGES

Suppose a patient who was injured while in your care decides to sue you. If your attorney can establish one of the following defenses, the court will either dismiss the charges against you or reduce the amount of any damages.

| DEFENSES | RATIONALE |
|---|---|
| **Lack of proof** | Does the plaintiff have legally sufficient proof that your actions caused his injuries? If he doesn't, the court will dismiss the case against you. |
| **Contributory negligence** | Did the plaintiff, through carelessness, contribute to his injury? If he did, some states permit the court to charge the plaintiff with failing to meet the standards of a reasonably prudent patient, barring him from recovering *any* damages. |
| **Comparative negligence** | A few states permit the court to apportion liability— barring the plaintiff from recovering *some*, but not all, of the damages he claims. |
| **Assumption of risk** | Did the plaintiff understand the risk involved in the treatment, procedure, or action that allegedly caused his injury? Did he give proper informed consent and so voluntarily expose himself to that risk? If he did, the court may rule that the plaintiff assumed the risk, knowingly disregarding the danger, and so relieved you of liability. |

• An ED nurse transferred a bleeding patient without getting any information from him, without advising the ED doctor of the extent of the bleeding, and without taking any action to stop it (*New Biloxi Hospital v. Frazier*, 1962).

A nurse's actions in responding to an emergency are also subject to charges of unprofessional conduct and resulting censure by her state board of nursing. For example, a nurse who examined a pregnant patient in her hospital's parking lot referred her to a hospital 20 miles away (*Murphy v. Rowland et al.*, 1980). The patient died en route of a ruptured uterus. The unprofessional conduct charge was upheld even though the nurse had offered to obtain a police escort and testimony showed that the hospital was limited in its capacity to perform the necessary surgery.

When have hospitals *not* been held liable for alleged mismanagement of patients in the ED? Here are some examples:

• Members of a hospital's medical staff refused to admit a pregnant patient when, in their judgment, no critical emergency was apparent (*Hill v. Ohio County*, 1971). Their decision was in accord with their institution's admission policies.

• ED nurses referred a patient to another hospital that had facilities—lacking in the first hospital—to test for the drug the patient had allegedly taken (*Nance v. Archer Smith Hospital*, 1976). While in the first hospital's ED, the patient showed no behavior that would have led the nurses to foresee, as the subsequent lawsuit charged, that the patient would run away en route to the referral hospital and later stab the plaintiff's husband.

## Emergency pitfall #2: Failure to communicate adequately

An emergency, in the ED or on a hospital unit, typically involves the fast-paced actions of several health professionals working both individually and as a team, each according to his knowledge and training. These circumstances complicate the assembling of an *accurate and timely record* of the patient's treatment. But these circumstances also *are* the record—and if the record's not complete, or not fully accurate, it can give a distorted picture of what was done for the patient.

The ED record is both similar to and different from the nurse's notes you keep for patients on the unit. This is because state laws, Medicare and Medicaid regulations, and accrediting agencies require comprehensive documentation. For example, the Joint Committee on Accreditation of Hospitals (JCAH) standards require that the ED record contain:

• patient identification (if not obtainable, the reason must be recorded)

• the time and means of the patient's arrival

• pertinent history of the patient's illness or injury and detailed physical findings, including vital signs

• any emergency care the patient received prior to his arrival in the ED

• the treatment the doctor ordered

• clinical observations, including the results of treatment

• reports of procedures, tests, and their results

• diagnostic impressions

• conclusions following the patient's evaluation and treatment—including final disposition, the patient's condition on discharge or transfer, and any instructions given to the patient or his family for follow-up care

• a detailed description of the circumstances, if a patient leaves the ED against medical advice.

The ED record's *medical significance* is, of course, familiar to you: it documents the patient's diagnosis, describes his signs and symptoms, indicates the treatment and nursing care he received, and serves as a basis for his continued care. The *legal significance* of the ED record may be less familiar to you—but it's no less important. Courts view the ED record (if it was made during the regular course of ED business and at or near the time the patient received treatment, and if the source and method of information are reliable) as evidence that identifies the professional persons involved, documents their medical and nursing decisions, and reflects the standard of care they provided. The record also documents the obtaining of informed consent from the patient, together with his reactions and comments. So you can see that a clear, contemporaneous, accurate ED record is invaluable in supporting a hospital's defense against a charge of negligence. And remember, 3 to 5 years may pass before an allegedly negligent incident is examined in court. The ED record may prove invaluable for jogging witnesses' memories and reconstructing what happened.

*Absence of crucial notes* in a plaintiff-patient's ED record can be very damaging to a hospital's defense during a lawsuit. In *Collins v. Westlake Community Hospital* (1974), the court ruled that a jury could conclude that the absence of specific notes indicated that the corresponding observations did not take place. A court is particularly likely to make this ruling if the treatment or observation in question is one that other professionals would usually record. Recording any ED discharge instructions and follow-up clinic appointments is essential, too—and provides a defense against a patient's charge of negligence.

The following court cases show how the failure of health professionals to document their emergency care adequately can expose them to liability. (Note that some of these cases involve emergency situations that occurred in hospital units other than the ED.)

• A hospital was held liable when a nurse failed to check a patient's vital signs every 30 minutes as ordered *and* failed to notify the doctor when the patient's condition became life-threatening (*Cline v. Lund*, 1973).

• A nurse refused to call a doctor even when signs of imminent delivery of an infant were apparent (*Hiatt v. Groce*, 1974).

• A nurse waited for 6 hours before notifying the doctor that a patient had signs and symptoms of heart failure (*Duling v. Bluefield Sanitarium, Inc.*, 1965).

• An obstetric nurse, believing that the doctor wouldn't respond if she called him, waited 3 hours—until the patient had gone into shock—to notify him that a postpartum patient was bleeding heavily from an incision made to assist in the delivery (*Goff v. Doctors General Hospital of San Jose*, 1958).

• Nurses failed to notify the department chairman when an attending doctor didn't respond adequately to a patient's worsening condition (*Utter v. United Hospital Center, Inc.*, 1977). Reporting such events to the chairman was re-quired by hospital policy and stipulated in the hospital's nursing manual.

• A nurse's ambiguous charting misled the doctor and may have caused him to make an incorrect diagnosis (*Baldwin v. Knight*, 1978). The chart stated, "The patient has a puncture-type wound obtained when mowing the grass from a broken bottle." Assuming that the glass had caused the laceration, the doctor didn't suspect an imbedded foreign object and didn't order tests and X-rays that might have uncovered it.

• A nurse neglected to tell a doctor treating two infant boys, brought to the ED with high fevers and head and chest rashes, that she had earlier removed ticks from one of them. In the ensuing lawsuit (*Ramsey v. Physicians Memorial Hospital, Inc.*, 1977), the court held that her omission contributed to the doctor's misdiagnosis of measles instead of the correct diagnosis, Rocky Mountain spotted fever. One of the boys died.

Clear and concise communication in the ED isn't limited to what goes into the medical record, however. Nurses, doctors, patient, family—all should clearly understand the nature of the emergency and the actions taken to assess and treat it.

*Telephone communications,* as you know, are particularly hazardous where liability for nurses is concerned. Diagnosis and treatment via telephone is a high-risk process under any circumstances, but particularly in an emergency. Hospital policy must clearly indicate actions you should take when you feel a doctor's response to your telephoned assessment findings is inadequate to ensure your patient's safety and welfare. As always, clear communication of your assessment findings—and accurate recording of the doctor's response and orders—are vital, as is full documentation of the telephone conversation and your subsequent nursing actions. Then, if a misunderstood telephone communication results in a charge of negligence, this documentation will help the court decide whether the applicable standard of care was breached—and by whom. In this situation, you're protecting your hospital's interests as well as your own.

The following court-case decisions show the importance of documentation when doctors and nurses disagree in court about the content of emergency-related telephone conversations.

• A hospital and doctor were held liable for the death of a patient struck by a car (*Thomas v. Corso,* 1972). A nurse telephoned the doctor, who was on call, and described the patient's condition. The doctor, a surgeon, ordered the patient admitted and scheduled X-rays for the following morning. Because the hospital was full, however, the patient was placed on a stretcher near the nurse's station. He died 3 hours later. The nurse and doctor contradicted each other concerning the content of the telephone conversation about

## UNDERSTANDING TORT CLAIMS

When a patient decides to sue a nurse or other health-care professional who cared for him, he must select the charge that applies—and that he hopes to prove. The law recognizes six possible charges—also called *tort claims.* The law also classifies each of those six torts as either an intentional tort—a direct invasion of someone's legal right—or an unintentional tort—a civil wrong from the defendant's negligence. This chart shows you both intentional and unintentional torts and examples of improper nursing actions that could lead a patient to use each claim in a lawsuit.

| TORT CLAIMS | EXAMPLES OF IMPROPER NURSING ACTIONS |
|---|---|
| **UNINTENTIONAL TORT** | |
| **Negligence** | • Leaving foreign objects inside a patient following surgery<br>• Failing to observe a patient as the doctor ordered<br>• Failing to ensure that a patient's informed consent has been obtained<br>• Failing to report a change in a patient's vital signs<br>• Failing to report a staff member's negligence that you witnessed |
| **INTENTIONAL TORTS** | |
| **Assault** | • Threatening a patient |
| **Battery** | • Forcing a patient to ambulate without his consent<br>• Forcing a patient to submit to treatment he's specifically refused |
| **False imprisonment** | • Confining a patient in a psychiatric unit without a doctor's order<br>• Refusing to let a patient return home |
| **Invasion of privacy** | • Releasing private information about a patient to newspaper reporters<br>• Allowing unauthorized persons to read a patient's medical records<br>• Allowing unauthorized persons to observe a procedure<br>• Taking pictures of the patient without his consent |
| **Slander** | • Making false accusations about a patient in front of newspaper reporters |

the patient, and this contributed to the court's assignment of liability. The doctor was found liable for failing to personally examine the patient. The hospital was also found liable. Why? Because the nurses who were attending the patient failed to notify the doctor that the patient's condition was deteriorating.

• A nurse denied ED admission to a woman in active labor; her child was born while she was en route to another hospital (*Childs v. Greenville Hospital Authority*, 1972). During the ensuing lawsuit, the nurse testified that the ED doctor had indicated the patient should see her own doctor. The doctor's version was that he'd told the nurse to have the patient call her doctor to learn what he wanted done.

• An ED nurse examined a patient and found nothing apparently wrong with him except that he'd been drinking (*Citizens Hospital Association v. Schoulin*, 1972). She communicated this information by telephone to the on-call doctor, who ordered the patient medicated and released. In fact, the man had a broken back. The hospital was held liable in the resulting lawsuit. Why? Because the court found that the ED nurse failed to discover the patient's true condition within a reasonable period of time after he arrived in the ED, and failed to communicate his condition to the doctor properly.

The doctor, who was not found liable for the patient's injuries, testified that he'd ordered the patient admitted for tests and X-ray; he denied that the nurse told him the patient was complaining of a back injury and having difficulty walking.

## Emergency pitfall #3: Medication errors

In an emergency, the risk of making a medication error is compounded by the hectic environment and the need for speed as well as accuracy in drug administration. Errors can stem from a multitude of wrong choices: wrong drug, wrong dose, wrong concentra-

tion, wrong site, wrong patient. All these types of errors have spawned litigation. For example:

• A nurse was held liable for an infant's death because she administered 3 cc of digitalis by injection instead of 3 cc of the pediatric elixir the doctor's order indicated (*Norton v. Argonaut Insurance Co.*, 1962).

• A nurse instilled hydrochloric acid into a patient's nose—instead of the nose drops the doctor ordered (*Neel v. San Antonio Community Hospital*, 1959).

To avoid making a medication error in an emergency, make sure you're familiar with the types of drugs commonly used in typical emergency situations—and that you completely understand every medication order before you administer any drug. If the order's unclear or you know—or have reason to believe—that the patient will suffer harm if the drug is administered as ordered, seek clarification. If you aren't satisfied with the answer you get, you can refuse to administer the drug. Just be sure to immediately advise the patient's doctor and your nursing supervisor of your decision.

## Emergency pitfall #4: Preventable equipment failure

Today's EDs and other hospital units use equipment that's highly complex and sophisticated—and correspondingly susceptible to malfunction. Often a nurse is the first person to become aware that a piece of equipment is malfunctioning. Or she may have the responsibility of checking a piece of equipment (for example, a defibrillator) to be sure it's functioning properly. Of course, no nurse can be expected to have the expertise of an engineer or an electrician. But a baseline standard of care might stipulate that:

• she can reasonably be expected to note defects and problems that any reasonable nurse would note.

• she also can be expected to follow procedures that ensure maintenance, repair, and replacement of equipment when necessary.

Of course, a hospital can't guarantee that all its equipment will function correctly during proper use, but courts have held that an obligation exists for that equipment to be "reasonably adequate, inspected, and maintained." If equipment has a hidden defect, the manufacturer will generally be held liable; however, if the defect is visible or could be detected by reasonable inspection, or if the user knows the equipment isn't functioning properly, then the hospital may be held liable.

• A clinic was held liable when a patient was burned because a technician continued to use an electrotherapy machine he knew wasn't working properly (*Orthopedic Clinic v. Hanson,* 1966).

• A doctor was held liable for using contaminated sutures because he had reason to know they were contaminated (*Shephard v. McGinnis,* 1964).

• A hospital was held liable for a patient's death due to lack of proper oxygen equipment (*Bellaire General Hospital v. Campbell,* 1974). The patient's transfer to a private room took place without the aid of portable oxygen equipment, so no backup was immediately available when the oxygen equipment intended for the patient was discovered to be incompatible with the room's wall plug.

# RESPONDING TO EMERGENCIES AT THE SCENE

## Your Responsibility to Help

In *Malloy v. Fong* (1951), the court upheld the generally prevalent axiom that no one is legally obliged to assist a stranger, "even though he could do so by a word and without the slightest danger to himself." But, the court ruled, once he has undertaken to give assistance, he has a lawful duty to care for that person. This ruling extends to nurses who encounter emergency situations away from the places where they work. A nurse has no legal duty to give care to a person in an emergency, but if she voluntarily assumes this duty, then she must provide care that is "reasonable under the circumstances." She can be held liable if she provides substandard care. "Reasonable care" includes not abandoning the patient once she's volunteered her assistance; she must remain with him until qualified persons assume responsibility for his care.

### Good Samaritan laws

Every state (except Wisconsin) plus the District of Columbia, the Virgin Islands, and some of the Canadian provinces have enacted Good Samaritan laws. (See *Comparing Good Samaritan Laws,* pages 32 to 37.) These laws don't compel persons to stop and assist in emergencies. Instead, these laws provide limited immunity from liability to such "Good Samaritans," so they'll be encouraged to provide aid.

Good Samaritan laws vary widely, and many don't specify protection for nurses. So be sure you know who's protected—and under what emergency circumstances—under your state's law.

Most Good Samaritan laws specify a standard of care to be met in order to qualify for immunity from liability. Some laws, however, simply require that the person act in "good faith" or with "due care," or give aid without "gross negligence" or "willful or wanton misconduct." In most states, the scope of protection that Good Samaritan laws provide consists of immunity from liability for ordinary negligence in rendering assistance.

Only the state of Vermont mandates emergency assistance. Vermont's "Duty to Aid the Endangered" act, passed in 1968, requires a person to assist others exposed to grave physical harm if he can do so without danger to himself. Persons violating the Vermont law can be fined up to $100.

To date, no lawsuit against a nurse or doctor who offered non-employment-related emergency assistance has been successful. In part, this is because Good Samaritan laws nullify the duty of reasonable care that otherwise exists under common law. But this situation may also reflect the courts' understanding of the purpose of Good Samaritan laws: to encourage citizens to stop and help others, in good faith and without fear of litigation that might ensue.

### Do Good Samaritan laws ever protect hospital nurses?

Because more than 25 states' Good Samaritan laws require that aid be given without compensation, and others stipulate that aid must be given outside a person's employment situation, no organized ED service comes under Good Samaritan laws' protection. A few courts have granted Good Samaritan protection to individual doctors, but this is very rare because immediate care is ED doctors' expected work in their place of employment. In *Colby v. Schwartz* (1978), the court affirmed this opinion, suggesting that granting Good Samaritan immunity to hospital staff doctors would lower the standard of care to the point where injured plaintiffs would no longer have the option to sue for alleged negligence.

## OBTAINING EMERGENCY CONSENT

## Considerations in Obtaining Consent

As a nurse, you know that treating a patient who hasn't given proper in-

---

### THERAPEUTIC PRIVILEGE: WHEN WITHHOLDING INFORMATION IS ALLOWED

The doctrine of informed consent assumes that an informed patient can act in his own best interests. But what if information about his condition seems likely to act against his interests—if just giving the patient the information would jeopardize his health?

In these situations, the courts recognize a doctor's *therapeutic privilege*. This legal concept permits the doctor to temporarily withhold information he believes would jeopardize the patient's health. This concept of therapeutic privilege may be extended to allow the doctor to provide care to the patient before obtaining his informed consent. But after the risk has passed, the doctor must inform the patient.

---

formed consent is technically a battery—an unlawful touching. If you treat such a patient, you could be liable. For the required written consent to be legally valid, it must meet certain specific criteria:

• It must be signed voluntarily.

• It must show that the procedure performed was the one the patient consented to.

• It must show that the person giving the consent understood the nature of the procedure, the risks involved, the probable consequences, and the available alternatives.

The patient's age and mental and physical well-being determine whether he may give consent himself or whether someone else should give consent for him.

In an emergency, the patient may be unconscious and unable to consent to treatment. Or he may be so badly injured or seriously ill that his competence to give informed consent is questionable. In these circumstances, with these patients, *the requirement to obtain informed consent doesn't change*—but how it's obtained, and from whom, may.

# COMPARING GOOD SAMARITAN LAWS

| | ALABAMA | ALASKA | ARIZONA | ARKANSAS | CALIFORNIA | COLORADO | CONNECTICUT | DELAWARE | DIST. COLUMBIA | |
|---|---|---|---|---|---|---|---|---|---|---|
| Date of act or last amendment | 1981 | 1976 | 1978 | 1979 | 1963 | 1975 | 1978 | 1974 | 1977 | |
| Covers "any person" | | ● | ● | ● | | ● | | ● | ● | |
| Covers in-state nurses only | | | | | ● | | | ● | | |
| Includes out-ot-state nurses in coverage | ● | | ● | | | ● | ● | ● | ● | |
| Requires acts in good faith | ● | | ● | ● | ● | ● | | ● | ● | |
| Covers only gratuitous services | ● | ● | ● | ● | | ● | ● | ● | ● | |
| Covers aid at scene of emergency, accident, disaster | ● | ● | ● | ● | ● | ● | ● | ● | ● | |
| Covers only roadside accidents | | | | | | | | | | |
| Covers emergencies outside place of employment, course of employment | | | | | ● | | ● | | | |
| Covers emergencies outside of hospital, doctor's office, or other places having medical equipment | | | | | | | | | ● | |
| Protects against failure to provide or arrange for further medical treatment | ● | ● | ● | | | | | ● | | |
| Covers transportation from the scene of the emergency to a destination for further medical treatment | | | | | | | | | | |
| Specifically mentions that acts of gross negligence or willful or wanton misconduct are not covered | | ● | ● | ● | ● | | ● | ● | ● | |

Use this chart to familiarize yourself with your area's Good Samaritan laws. Your state or province may also have motor vehicle statutes or nurse practice acts with overlapping Good Samaritan content. Check with your board of nursing to see how "any person" is defined and to see if new statutes or amendments have been passed since 1984.

| | FLORIDA | GEORGIA | HAWAII | IDAHO | ILLINOIS | INDIANA | IOWA | KANSAS | KENTUCKY | LOUISIANA | MAINE | MARYLAND |
|---|---|---|---|---|---|---|---|---|---|---|---|---|
| | 1978 | 1962 | 1979 | 1980 | 1980 | 1973 | 1969 | 1977 | 1980 | 1964 | 1977 | 1977 |
| | ● | ● | ● | ● | | ● | ● | ● | | ● | ● | |
| | | | | | | | | | ● | | | |
| | | | | ● | | | ● | | | ● | | ● |
| | ● | ● | ● | ● | ● | ● | ● | | | ● | | |
| | ● | ● | ● | | ● | ● | ● | ● | ● | ● | ● | ● |
| | ● | ● | ● | ● | ● | ● | ● | ● | ● | ● | ● | ● |
| | | | | | | | | | | | | |
| | | | | | | | | | | | | |
| | ● | | | | | | | | | | | |
| | ● | ● | | | | ● | | | | ● | | |
| | | | | ● | | | | | | | | ● |
| | | | ● | ● | ● | ● | ● | ● | ● | ● | ● | ● |

(continued)

**COMPARING GOOD SAMARITAN LAWS** *(continued)*

| | MASSACHUSETTS | MICHIGAN | MINNESOTA | MISSISSIPPI | MISSOURI | MONTANA | NEBRASKA | NEVADA | NEW HAMPSHIRE |
|---|---|---|---|---|---|---|---|---|---|
| Date of act or last amendment | 1969 | 1978 | 1978 | 1979 | 1979 | 1970 | 1971 | 1975 | 1977 |
| Covers "any person" | | | ● | | ● | ● | ● | ● | ● |
| Covers in-state nurses only | | | | | | | | | ● |
| Includes out-of-state nurses in coverage | ● | ● | | ● | ● | | | ● | ● |
| Requires acts in good faith | ● | | ● | ● | ● | ● | | ● | ● |
| Covers only gratuitous services | ● | | | | | ● | ● | ● | |
| Covers aid at scene of emergency, accident, disaster | ● | ● | ● | ● | ● | ● | ● | ● | ● |
| Covers only roadside accidents | | | | | | | | | |
| Covers emergencies outside place of employment, course of employment | | | | | | | | | ● |
| Covers emergencies outside of hospital, doctor's office, or other places having medical equipment | | | ● | | | | | | |
| Protects against failure to provide or arrange for further medical treatment | ● | | | | | | ● | ● | ● |
| Covers transportation from the scene of the emergency to a destination for further medical treatment | | | ● | ● | | | | | |
| Specifically mentions that acts of gross negligence or willful or wanton misconduct are not covered | | ● | | ● | ● | ● | ● | ● | |

| | NEW JERSEY | NEW MEXICO | NEW YORK | NORTH CAROLINA | NORTH DAKOTA | OHIO | OKLAHOMA | OREGON | PENNSYLVANIA | RHODE ISLAND | SOUTH CAROLINA | SOUTH DAKOTA |
|---|---|---|---|---|---|---|---|---|---|---|---|---|
| | 1968 | 1972 | 1975 | 1975 | 1977 | 1981 | 1979 | 1981 | 1978 | 1969 | 1964 | 1976 |
| | ● | ● | | ● | ● | ● | ● | | | | ● | |
| | | | | | ● | | | | | | | |
| | ● | | ● | | | | ● | ● | ● | ● | | ● |
| | ● | ● | | | ● | | ● | | ● | | ● | ● |
| | | ● | ● | | | ● | ● | ● | | ● | ● | |
| | ● | ● | ● | ● | ● | ● | ● | ● | ● | ● | ● | ● |
| | | | | ● | | | | | | | | |
| | | | | | | | | | | | | |
| | | | ● | | | ● | | | ● | ● | | |
| | | | | | | | | | | | ● | |
| | | | | | | | | | | | | |
| | | | | | | | | | | | | |
| | | ● | ● | ● | | ● | ● | ● | ● | ● | ● | |

*(continued)*

## COMPARING GOOD SAMARITAN LAWS *(continued)*

| | TENNESSEE | TEXAS | UTAH | VERMONT | VIRGINIA | WASHINGTON | WEST VIRGINIA | WISCONSIN | WYOMING |
|---|---|---|---|---|---|---|---|---|---|
| Date of act or last amendment | 1976 | 1977 | 1979 | 1968 | 1980 | 1975 | 1967 | | 1977 |
| Covers "any person" | ● | ● | | ● | ● | ● | ● | | ● |
| Covers in-state nurses only | | | ● | | | | | | |
| Includes out-ot-state nurses in coverage | | | | | | | | | |
| Requires acts in good faith | ● | | | ● | | ● | ● | | ● |
| Covers only gratuitous services | ● | ● | | ● | ● | ● | ● | NO GOOD SAMARITAN ACT | ● |
| Covers aid at scene of emergency, accident, disaster | ● | ● | ● | ● | ● | ● | ● | | ● |
| Covers only roadside accidents | | | | | | | | | |
| Covers emergencies outside place of employment, course of employment | | ● | | | | | | | |
| Covers emergencies outside of hospital, doctor's office, or other places having medical equipment | | | | | | | | | |
| Protects against failure to provide or arrange for further medical treatment | ● | | | | | | | | |
| Covers transportation from the scene of the emergency to a destination for further medical treatment | | | | | ● | ● | | | |
| Specifically mentions that acts of gross negligence or willful or wanton misconduct are not covered | ● | ● | | ● | | ● | | | ● |

* Doctors only

| | ALBERTA | BRIT. COLUMBIA | MANITOBA | NEW BRUNSWICK | NEWFOUNDLAND | NOVA SCOTIA | ONTARIO | PRINCE EDWARD IS. | QUEBEC | N.W. TERRITORIES | SASKATCHEWAN | YUKON TERR. |
|---|---|---|---|---|---|---|---|---|---|---|---|---|
| | 1970 | 1979 | | | 1971 | 1969 | | | | | 1978 | 1976 |
| | ● | ● | | | ● | ★ | | | | | ● | ● |
| | ● | | | | | | | | | | | |
| | | | | | | | | | | | | |
| | | | | | | | | | | | | |
| | | ● | | | ● | ● | | | | | | |
| | ● | ● | | | ● | ● | | | | | ● | ● |
| | | | NO GOOD SAMARITAN ACT | NO GOOD SAMARITAN ACT | | | NO GOOD SAMARITAN ACT | NO GOOD SAMARITAN ACT | NO GOOD SAMARITAN ACT | NO GOOD SAMARITAN ACT | | |
| | | ● | | | | | | | | | | |
| | ● | | | | ● | ● | | | | | ● | |
| | | | | | | | | | | | | |
| | | | | | | | | | | | | |
| | ● | ● | | | | ● | | | | | ● | ● |

Adapted from *NursingLife*, March/April 1982.

# Implied Consent

If a patient needs emergency medical treatment but can't give his consent immediately, his doctor may delay treatment until the patient can consent, if the delay doesn't increase the patient's risk of harm. But when a "true emergency" exists and the patient isn't able to give his consent to treatment—for example, because he's unconscious—his consent is said to be "implied" so he can be given the care he needs. Implied consent is based on the belief that, if the patient understood the situation and was competent to give consent, he would do so.

A "true emergency" is one where the threat to the patient is immediate and treatment must be undertaken at once to save his life or to prevent permanent bodily injury. In this situation, delaying treatment could constitute negligence.

A patient's extreme pain can be a justification for treatment via implied consent, but you should be aware that court opinions on this have varied. In *Sullivan v. Montgomery* (1935), the court endorsed pain as a justifiable premise for treatment without informed consent. But in *Cunningham v. Yankton Clinic* (1978), the court found pain an insufficient emergency to allow treatment via implied consent.

A doctor who decides to treat a patient with an emergency condition without obtaining his informed consent, especially if the patient requires surgery, usually will consult with another doctor for corroboration of his decision. In lieu of a formal consultation, the doctor may obtain a concurring progress note from a second doctor prior to performing the surgery.

If you're ever involved in a situation involving a patient's implied consent, check your hospital's policy closely. It may require notifying an administrator prior to treating the patient—particularly if he's a minor.

## Burden of proof: Who has it?

Remember, if you're ever named as a defendant in a lawsuit centering on a patient's implied consent, *you'll* have the "burden of proof." This means that, to avoid being held liable for the plaintiff-patient's injuries, you'll be required to establish, by a "preponderance of the evidence," that a true emergency existed.

## Importance of documentation

As always, the best evidence is timely and accurate documentation of the event. For example, if you make several unsuccessful telephone calls in an effort to contact family members to obtain consent to operate on a patient, document them. Then, if the patient's family later files a lawsuit charging that the operation was a battery, your documentation will become part of the hospital's defense. Document *all* efforts to obtain consent, including:

- who called whom
- what telephone numbers were tried
- what time the calls were made
- what response (if any) was received
- how many attempts to make contact were made
- any alternate means used (such as sending police to the patient's home, leaving a note there, or contacting neighbors).

Finally, keep in mind the fact that implied consent is a *legal doctrine* applicable only when a patient needs specific emergency treatment for a specific period of time. Once the patient's out of danger, the doctor must obtain his formal written consent for any further treatment procedures.

# How Valid Is Oral Consent?

When a patient's able to give proper informed consent, but taking time to write it may increase his danger from injuries or illness, he may give oral consent to treatment. Oral consent is as legally valid as written consent. However, with oral consent, the hospital must be prepared to prove the patient consented. (With written consent, of course, the signed consent form constitutes proof.) Your documentation of the event, detailing the doctor's explanation of the treatment he'll provide and the patient's oral consent to that treatment, constitutes proof that the patient gave his informed consent. Be sure your documentation is witnessed.

You may also find yourself in a situation where a patient, although conscious and coherent, can't sign an informed consent because of an injury. Oral consent is valid here, too. Or, if the patient can't sign his name but can write an X, have him do this in the presence of a countersigning witness.

# What About Blanket Consent Forms?

Consent obtained for an emergency procedure, just as for any other form of treatment, should specify the procedure the patient will undergo. A general or "blanket" consent form, such as a patient customarily signs on admission to most EDs and hospitals, clearly isn't valid for this purpose. As you probably know, these consents mainly serve to show that the patient willingly presented himself for examination and treatment. (This protects the hospital from a charge of battery related to examining the patient.) The reason blanket consent can't be substituted for informed consent is that, when the patient signs a blanket consent form, his treatment hasn't been determined yet— so he can't be "informed" about it, much less consent to it. He can only give informed consent once he's been told what treatment is planned, the reasons for it, the risks involved, the prob-

able consequences, and the available alternatives.

Of course, the patient doesn't need to sign a form for each procedure he undergoes in the ED or on a unit. But, although written consent may not always be required, consent itself is. The patient should be "informed" before he allows the nurse to draw blood or start an I.V., and before he allows an X-ray to be taken. He has the right to be told, before any procedure is carried out, its nature, its purpose, and why it's necessary for him.

Remember that, once the patient gives his informed consent (whether written or oral), the treatment he receives must conform exactly to the treatment he consented to. For example, consent to type and cross-match blood doesn't mean consent to transfusion; surgery by Dr. X doesn't permit Dr. Y to operate. Nor does a patient under anesthesia relinquish any of his rights to the exact treatment he consented to— except when an unforeseen emergency determines that the patient's given his implied consent to a change in treatment plan.

# Special Consent Issues

To give a valid informed consent, a person must be of legal age, competent, and able. These criteria exclude (among others) minors and intoxicated, comatose, or mentally incompetent persons.

### Minors
Unless a person has reached the state's established age of majority, he usually can't legally consent to medical treatment. Instead, his parents or guardian must do so, and their consent must be properly informed. If you must call a child's parents in an emergency to obtain their consent, have another hospital employee listen to the conversation on another extension. (Tell the parents

# CAN YOUR PATIENT (OR HIS FAMILY) ALWAYS REFUSE LIFESAVING TREATMENT?

As you know, a court will usually respect a patient's right to refuse treatment if he's capable of making a reasoned decision. Or, if the patient's a child, typically his parents may decide on his care. But courts will intervene in some instances when a patient or parent refuses to allow lifesaving treatment. Here are some court cases illustrating how courts have handled such situations:

• In *Collins v. Davis* (1964), the court overruled a wife's refusal of surgery for her unconscious husband, even though such a refusal is frequently ruled valid.

• A court may view a patient's responsibility for a child as reason to overrule the patient's refusal of lifesaving treatment. In *Application of the President and Directors of Georgetown College, Inc.* (1964), the court ordered a blood transfusion for a Jehovah's Witness, mother of an infant, who refused to consent to the transfusion.

• If a patient's pregnant and refuses lifesaving treatment so that her child's life is also endangered, a court may reverse the patient's decision. In *Jefferson v. Griffin Spalding County Hospital Authority* (1981), a pregnant woman with a complete placenta previa, who had refused to consent to a cesarean section, was denied the right to refuse the surgery. The court awarded custody of her unborn child to a state agency, which then had full authority to consent to the surgery.

• The courts will not normally permit a child's parent or legal guardian to refuse consent for treatment that will save the child's life. *In re Sampson* (1972) was such a case.

Besides its concern for preservation of a patient's life or protection of his dependents, a state may ask a court to intervene to prevent a patient's irrational self-destruction, to preserve the ethical integrity of health-care providers, or to protect public health. You should be aware, however, that each such case must be decided individually. Courts don't always rule that the state's interest overrides the patient's rights under common law and the U.S. Constitution.

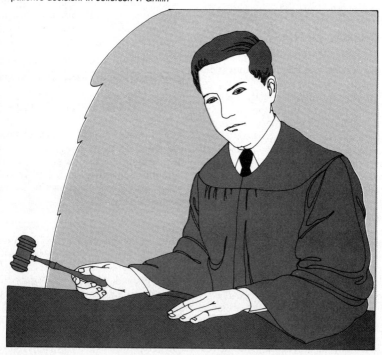

you're doing this.) This person is your witness to the consent given. If possible, verify the identity of the person you're speaking to and his relationship to the child. Explain the circumstances and planned treatment thoroughly. Have the parent repeat this information back to you. Document the entire conversation, and have your telephone witness sign it, too. Then, as soon as possible, be sure to have the child's parents sign a written consent form confirming their earlier oral consent.

In a true emergency, for a minor as well as for an adult, lack of informed consent isn't a reason to delay treatment. If the parents refuse to consent to lifesaving measures for their child—for example, on religious grounds—treatment should proceed, and the hospital should seek a court order simultaneously.

In some circumstances, a minor may give informed consent. Most states recognize the *emancipated minor,* usually a minor who has a home separate from his parents and is responsible for his own financial support. (A married minor is a good example.) In most states, an emancipated minor must be at least 16. In some states (for example, Pennsylvania), minors who are pregnant, parents, or high school graduates are considered legally emancipated.

The courts are also beginning to recognize the concept of a *mature minor,* one who's emotionally mature and sufficiently intelligent to understand adult issues. If such a minor and his parents disagree on whether the minor may give his informed consent for emergency treatment, a court may honor the minor's wishes. If possible, the doctor should obtain the mature minor's *and* his parents' consent and be sure all are properly informed.

### Incompetent adults

When an adult's mentally unable to execute a valid informed consent and a true emergency exists, a close relative or other authorized individual should be contacted for consent, if possible. If

time doesn't permit this, however, then the doctor may proceed with the patient's implied consent, as he would if the patient were simply unconscious.

## Is Informed Consent Revocable?

Once a patient consents to treatment, he can change his mind, and his doctor and others caring for him must honor his wishes. If a patient says he wants to withdraw his consent, notify his doctor immediately, and document the incident. Be sure that the patient understands the risks involved in discontinuing or postponing the treatment, and that he's given an opportunity to reconsider his decision.

This approach also applies when a patient who's voluntarily admitted himself to the hospital decides to leave against medical advice. He has the legal right to do so. If possible, have him sign a form stating not only that he's leaving against medical advice but also that the risks involved have been explained to him. If he refuses to sign the form, don't try to force him, but be sure to document his refusal in his record.

## REPORTING LAWS AND EMERGENCY CARE

## Why Are Reporting Laws Necessary?

Reporting laws reflect our society's determination that certain problems must be exposed for the protection of the public. These problems include suspicious deaths, certain types of infectious diseases, incidents of child abuse, and criminal acts or their results—such as a gunshot or stab wound. Depending on her hospital's size and location, an ED nurse may see a high percentage of patients with these problems. So she (or the ED doctor) may frequently have to report to the agencies specified in the various reporting laws of her state.

Reporting laws vary from state to state concerning:
• what must be reported
• who should receive the report
• what degree of protection from liability the law offers to the person making the report.

Many of the reporting laws don't contain wording that promises immunity from lawsuits for unauthorized disclosure. However, a nurse making a report in good faith and without malice, and according to the procedures set forth in the applicable reporting law, will be able, in court, to claim a qualified privilege to disclose the information. This means she probably won't be found liable.

If you work in an ED, be sure you're familiar with the federal, state, and local laws and regulations that may apply when you must make a report. Be sure, too, that your ED's policies and its procedure manual are current, complete, and unambiguous about ED personnel's reporting responsibilities.

# When to Make a Report

## Gunshot wound laws

*Gunshot wound laws* require healthcare personnel to report injury (including self-inflicted injuries) caused by lethal weapons. Other incidents that are reportable under gunshot wound laws may include drug overdoses, poisonings, suspected criminal abortions, and animal bites. (Some gunshot wound laws classify automobiles as lethal weapons, making injuries due to automobile accidents reportable.)

Your ED's procedures for making reports under this law should also reflect an awareness of federally mandated reporting laws. For example, a patient's death due to a blood transfusion must be reported to the Food and Drug Administration.

## Child and elderly abuse laws

All states and the District of Columbia have laws to protect children from *child abuse*, and most such laws provide immunity from liability for persons required to report the suspected abuse. State-law definitions of child abuse vary, but all the definitions include physical abuse inflicted by other than accidental means. Some laws also cite psychological and emotional abuse, moral neglect, or immoral associations. These laws require health-care professionals to report *all* cases of suspected or substantiated child abuse.

Courts have been very strict in interpreting child abuse laws, which usually impose a fine or a short jail term—or both—as criminal penalties for a person's failure to report. In *Landeros v. Flood* (1976), a doctor was found liable for discharging an abused child, age 11 months, to the abusing parents without making a report, which would have given the state an opportunity to intervene. The court in this case also ruled that under common law, civil charges could be brought against a person failing to report, even if the reporting law didn't address the issue of civil liability. This means that a person fined according to reporting-law penalties may then be sued by the child's guardian in a civil action. To avoid this and other problems associated with reporting incidents of child abuse, be sure you understand and fulfill all of the reporting requirements in your state. You may want to make an immediate telephone call to the appropriate agency, followed by a written report.

Some states have also enacted *elderly neglect and abuse* reporting laws.

These laws reflect society's increasing awareness that a number of elderly persons are now living alone or in circumstances where they suffer abuse. In some states, licensing regulations specifically require the reporting of incidents of patient abuse in nursing homes.

### Requirement to report certain diseases

In all states, public health laws and regulations require that *certain diseases,* such as sexually transmitted diseases, be reported to appropriate health agencies. The doctor who diagnoses the disease is usually responsible for reporting it, but a nurse may be involved in processing the report. Remember, state *and* local laws may apply in this situation.

### Which deaths are reportable?

All states have laws requiring the legal investigation and reporting of deaths from other than "normal" causes—so-called suspicious deaths. Usually, the doctor in attendance is required to report the death to a medical examiner or coroner. The laws vary from state to state, but in general, the following deaths are reportable:

• all deaths when the patient's "dead on arrival"
• all suicides
• all deaths resulting from violent acts
• all deaths from poisoning
• all deaths occurring in the course of pregnancy
• all deaths occurring within 24 hours of admission to a hospital, when a diagnosis has not been made
• all deaths occurring without prior medical care
• all deaths resulting from accidents.

The report to the medical examiner must state the time, place, manner, circumstances, and cause of the person's death. This information may be transmitted initially by telephone and then put into the written report.

If you're ever involved when a patient's death must be reported, be sure

## CONSENT TO PHOTOGRAPH AN ABUSED CHILD

You're on duty in your hospital's ED when a social worker brings in a girl, age 6, who's a possible victim of child abuse. The social worker asks you to photograph the girl's injuries to document them.

Can you legally take photographs of the patient?

No, but you can arrange for it. In most states, either an agency caseworker or the local police can photograph child abuse injuries without parental consent. In states that don't specifically grant the right to photograph, the examining doctor has the responsibility to authorize photographs, because the duty to report implies a responsibility to preserve any evidence. If the parents are present and object to photographs, the doctor should contact law enforcement officials to secure a court order.

All 50 states now have laws requiring that doctors and social workers (among other professionals) report suspected child abuse in children under age 16 or 18, depending on the state. These laws also offer professional care givers some immunity from liability, as long as they act in good faith.

Some states have designated reporting agencies. These agencies have 24-hour-a-day coverage and will send a caseworker to investigate night or day. Find out the appropriate agency you should contact when you suspect child abuse, and post the number near the ED telephone.

Child abuse reporting laws are far from standardized, so ED personnel should request a specific procedure from the hospital administration. Obviously, the administration should design a procedure that meets all state reporting laws.

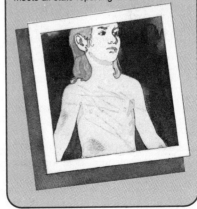

you don't move the body, or permit it to be moved, without the medical examiner's permission—except as authorized by law. (Some states authorize the moving of bodies under certain conditions, such as a need to preserve the body or to protect the health and safety of others.) State laws also determine whether tubes, catheters, and other paraphernalia can be removed prior to the medical examiner's postmortem examination.

In all states, the rule is that the person entitled to possession of the body for burial has a legally protected interest. If anyone interferes with that interest, he can be held liable for damages for the emotional and mental suffering that result. A suspicious death is the medical examiner's responsibility; this means that his authority, by law, supersedes that of the ED doctor, the attending doctor, the patient's spouse, or any other family member. Signing the death certificate and performing autopsy procedures are also the sole responsibility of the medical examiner. If you work in your hospital's ED, be sure that its policies and procedures incorporate state-law requirements that apply when a patient's death becomes the medical examiner's responsibility. Be sure, too, that you know what action to take if a patient dies in the ED.

# OBTAINING EVIDENCE: LEGAL IMPLICATIONS

## When Police Ask for Your Help

The Fourth Amendment to the United States Constitution guarantees the right of persons to be free from unreasonable search and seizure. *This right applies* *everywhere, including the ED.* So what should you do if a police officer asks you to search a patient who may have committed a crime, or to search his belongings for contraband or evidence? What if he asks you to draw blood or obtain urine to test the patient for use of an illegal drug or for excessive levels of alcohol in his blood?

Before you do *anything,* remind yourself that hospitals and health-care professionals have no legal duty to perform tests on patients, or to search patients for contraband or evidence, at police request. If you perform such a test or search, your action may violate the patient's legal rights and expose you to liability for invasion of privacy, assault and battery, or both. Furthermore, the evidence thus uncovered may be inadmissible in court.

## Protecting your patient's rights during a search

What makes searching a patient's belongings for evidence "reasonable"? You may legally proceed with a police-requested search, without the patient's consent, only if he's under arrest *and/ or* a valid search warrant is in effect. In all other circumstances, *don't make the search.* Refer the police request to your supervisor.

What if you're going through a seriously injured and unconscious patient's belongings, looking for items of identification, when you unexpectedly find a gun in his pocket? What should you do? You know that the patient was injured attempting to flee the scene of a robbery he allegedly committed. Can you remove the gun without violating your patient's constitutional protection against unreasonable search and seizure? Generally speaking, the answer is yes. Why? Because the purpose of your search was *not* to look for evidence. You may legally remove the gun and turn it over to your supervisor, who should maintain custody of it. (If it's turned over to the police, the officer who takes it should provide a receipt.)

## When can you test a patient for evidence?

Two problems arise when police ask ED personnel to perform a test on a patient without his consent:

• The hospital and ED staff are concerned about becoming involved in a civil suit for battery.

• The police are concerned about whether the information obtained will be admissible as evidence in criminal proceedings against the patient.

A good example is when the police request that ED personnel take a blood or urine sample from a person arrested on suspicion of drunken driving. If the patient consents *and* a doctor gives an order for the test, you may take the sample. If the patient refuses his consent for the sample to be taken, *don't take it*. Instead, refer the police request to your supervisor. *This isn't a front-line decision.* If you do take the samples against the patient's will, you'll expose yourself and your hospital to liability. And the evidence the police obtain will probably be inadmissible in court.

In a similar situation, if a police officer suspects that a person has swallowed illegal drugs encased in a capsule or balloon, he may request that ED personnel perform procedures or administer medication that will facilitate retrieval. Almost invariably, when this has been done and the evidence retrieved has been presented later as evidence in court proceedings, the court has ruled that forcing emetics or laxatives on a person without his consent is a violation of his constitutional rights and an invasion of his privacy. (One such case was *Rochin v. California*, 1952.)

Some states (Louisiana, for example) have laws that protect hospitals and hospital personnel from liability for damages when a sample's been taken from a nonconsenting patient at a police officer's request. If your state has such a law, it should be reflected in your hospital's policy covering such situations. However, keep in mind that these laws only apply when the sam-

---

### HANDLING EVIDENCE PROPERLY

When police ask you to obtain evidence or to take charge of it in the ED, follow these general guidelines for identifying and preserving it:

• Identify and label *each piece* of evidence.

• Give the patient a receipt for *all* personal property taken from him. Be sure the hospital keeps a copy of this receipt.

• Preserve the evidence in its original state as much as possible—by taking steps to protect it while handling it as little as possible.

• Maintain the necessary "chain of custody" over the evidence, while it's in your custody, by obtaining the signature of each person who handles it. When *you* relinquish custody of the evidence, be sure to obtain a receipt for it.

• Protect a rape victim's legal rights by ensuring that all specimens are carefully labeled and that transfer of the evidence from the nurse or doctor to the police is carefully documented.

---

pling procedure is done correctly. They don't protect you from the consequences of negligent actions.

If a person does consent to a test performed to obtain evidence against him, be sure the consent is in writing and the person has been fully informed of the risks involved in the test. If the test may harm the person in any way, it probably shouldn't be done. Some courts, such as in *State v. Overstreet* (1971), have required a finding of minimal risk of permanent injury before they would even permit surgical removal of a bullet, which would become evidence.

## A FINAL WORD

Your patient's medical emergency problem is his alone—but his legal problems may easily become yours if they arise from the care you give him.

In an emergency, as you know, speedy actions and quick decisions can save your patient's life or prevent serious complications. But they also can increase your risk of liability.

To protect your interests as well as your patient's in an emergency, don't wait until the emergency to think about them. Instead, be sure you continually keep abreast of changes in the laws and regulations that define your professional responsibilities. Then, in the possible turmoil of meeting a patient's emergency needs, you'll feel confident that you're acting within the legal scope of nursing practice in your state and within the proper scope of your employment.

You can further increase your confidence about decision-making in an emergency by actively working to clarify your ED's (or unit's) written policies and procedures. These should be unambiguously set forth for all personnel to follow in an emergency. Then you and your colleagues won't have the burden of making administrative decisions when you should be concentrating on your patient's urgent need for medical and nursing care.

---

## Court Cases Cited in This Chapter

**Application of the President and Directors of Georgetown College, Inc.,** 331 F. 2d 1000 (D.C. Cir. 1964); cert. denied, 377 U.S. 978 (1964).

**Baldwin v. Knight,** 569 S.W. 2d 450 (1978).

**Bellaire General Hospital v. Campbell,** 510 S.W. 94 (Tex. Civ. App. 1974).

**Childs v. Greenville Hospital Authority,** 479 S.W. 2d 399 (Texas 1972).

**Citizens Hospital Association v. Schoulin,** 48 Ala. 101, 262 So. 2d 303 (1972).

**Cline v. Lund,** 31 Cal. App. 3d 755; 107 Cal. Rptr. 629 (1973).

**Colby v. Schwartz,** 78 Cal. App. 3d 885, 144 Cal. Rptr. 624 (1978).

**Collins v. Davis,** 44 Misc. 2d 622; 254 N.Y.S. 2d 666 (1964).

**Collins v. Westlake Community Hospital,** 312 N.E. 2d 1964 (Ill. 1974).

**Cunningham v. Yankton Clinic,** 262 N.W. 2d 500 (S.D. 1978).

**Duling v. Bluefield Sanitarium, Inc.,** 149 W.Va. 467; 142 N.E. 2d 754 (1965).

**Goff v. Doctors General Hospital of San Jose,** 166 Cal. App. 2d 314; 333 P. 2d 29 (1958).

**Guerrero v. Copper Queen Hospital,** 537 P. 2d 1329 (Ariz. 1975)

**Hiatt v. Groce,** 215 Kan. 14, 523 P. 2d 320 (1974).

**Hill v. Ohio County,** 468 S.W. 2d 306 (Ky. 1971).

**Jefferson v. Griffin Spalding County Hospital Authority,** 247 Ga. 86; 247 S.E. 2d 457 (1981).

**Landeros v. Flood,** 17 Cal. 3d 399, 551 P. 2d 389 (1976).

**Malloy v. Fong,** 37 Cal. 2d 356; 220 P. 2d 48; 223 P. 2d 241 (1951).

**Murphy v. Rowland et al.,** 609 S.W. 2d 292 (1980).

**Nance v. Archer Smith Hospital,** 329 So. 2d 377 (Fla. Dist. Ct. App. 1976).

**Neel v. San Antonio Community Hospital,** 1 Cal. Rptr. 313 (1959).

**New Biloxi Hospital v. Frazier,** 245 Miss. 185, 146 So. 2d 882 (1962).

**Niles v. City of San Rafael,** 42 Cal. App. 3rd 230 (1974).

**Norton v. Argonaut Insurance Co.,** 144 So. 2d 249 (Ct. App. La. 1962).

**Orthopedic Clinic v. Hanson,** 415 P. 2d 991 (Olka. 1966).

**Ramsey v. Physicians Memorial Hospital, Inc.,** 36 Md. App. 42; 373 A. 2d 76 (1977).

**Rochin v. California,** 342 U.S. 165 (1952).

In re Sampson, 29 N.Y. 2d 900; 328 N.Y.S. 2d 686 (1972).

Shephard v. McGinnis, 251 Iowa 35, 131 N.W. 2d 475 (1964).

Stanturf v. Sipes, 447 S.W. 2d 558 (Mo. 1969).

State v. Overstreet, 551 S.W. 2d 621 (Mo. 1971).

Sullivan v. Montgomery, 155 Misc. 448, 279 N.Y.S. 575 (1935).

Thomas v. Corso, 288 A. 2d 379 (Md. 1972).

Utter v. United Hospital Center, Inc., 236 S.E. 2d 213 (W.Va. Sup. Ct. App., 1977).

Wilmington General Hospital v. Manlove, 54 Del. 15, 174 A. 2d 135 (1961).

## Selected References

Bertolet, Mary M., and Goldsmith, Lee S., eds. *Hospital Liability: Law and Tactics*, 4th ed. New York: Practising Law Institute, 1980.

Cazalas, Mary W. *Nursing and the Law*, 4th ed. Rockville, Md.: Aspen Systems Corp., 1983.

Creighton, Helen. *Law Every Nurse Should Know*, 4th ed. Philadelphia: W.B. Saunders Co., 1981.

Fiesta, Janine. *The Law and Liability: A Guide for Nurses.* New York: John Wiley & Sons, 1983.

Hemelt, Mary D., and Mackert, Mary E. *Dynamics of Law in Nursing and Health Care*, 3rd ed. Reston, Va.: Reston Publishing Co., 1982.

Mancini, Marguerite R., and Gale, Alice T. *Emergency Care and the Law.* Rockville, Md.: Aspen Systems Corp., 1981.

Miller, Robert D. *Problems in Hospital Law*, 4th ed. Rockville, Md.: Aspen Systems Corp., 1983.

*Practices.* Nurse's Reference Library. Springhouse, Pa.: Springhouse Corp., 1983.

Rosoff, Arnold J. *Informed Consent: A Guide for Health Care Providers.* Rockville, Md.: Aspen Systems Corp., 1981.

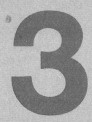

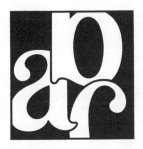

# Emergency Assessment and Intervention

## Introduction

If you're like most nurses, you consider responding correctly in a serious emergency the ultimate test of your nursing skills.

You need an extra-organized approach to managing emergencies. Why? Because you may have so little time to intervene successfully and so much chaos and confusion around you.

A patient with an emergency has acute problems that demand immediate intervention. You don't have the luxury of performing a separate routine assessment, evaluating your data at leisure, pondering a care plan, implementing it over time, and evaluating the result from a perspective of days or weeks. (Of course, this is an exaggerated view of the steps of the nursing process—but it's how these steps appear in contrast to their application in an emergency.) Instead, you need to know how to do a rapid emergency assessment, which dominates your entire approach to the patient. Your emergency assessment findings tell you when to *stop* assessing so you can intervene for urgent problems, and your assessment continues until you've identified *all* the patient's emergency problems and intervened as necessary.

Even knowing all this isn't enough. You must also be able to fill different nursing roles during emergencies. For example, on the unit, you may start CPR

for a patient in cardiac arrest, then switch to documenting the incident when the code team arrives. Or, at the scene of an accident, you may intervene to stabilize a patient's fractured leg by improvising a splint from a piece of board you find along the roadside. Wherever you are, whatever facilities you have available when an emergency happens, you must be prepared to think quickly, to assess your patient's problems rapidly, to prioritize them accurately, and to intervene skillfully.

Here are the steps to follow in performing an emergency assessment; this chapter covers them in detail. Keep in mind that, while you're performing *each* of these steps, you're simultaneously assessing, planning, implementing, and evaluating:

*Step 1:* Perform a *primary assessment* of his airway, breathing, and circulation (the ABCs), intervening to stabilize each function as necessary. Check his mental status and general appearance, too.

*Step 2:* Perform a *secondary assessment*, combining subjective and objective evaluation and focusing on the patient's chief complaint. Here, too, you intervene as necessary, for each complaint, to prevent the patient's emergency problems from worsening. The patient's airway, breathing, and circulation may also become compromised at this later step in your assessment, so be prepared to intervene for these problems, as well.

*Step 3:* Begin definitive care and obtain laboratory tests, remembering that test results may alter your interventions.

While you're performing these steps, you'll also be forming a first impression, determining the urgency of your patient's condition, deciding on priorities for his care, and controlling his emotional environment, if necessary.

As you read this chapter and expand your understanding of how to assess and intervene during emergencies, keep in mind that, as a staff nurse, you're in a position to *prevent* many emergencies. Make sure you're aware of which of your patients on the unit are at risk for emergency complications of illness, injury—or even treatment. Then you can take precautions to help ensure that some emergencies, at least, never happen.

## SETTING THE STAGE

Set the stage for your emergency assessment by reviewing these basic concepts:
• forming a first impression
• determining urgency.

These important concepts affect all the steps of your emergency care. Why? Because if you don't heed, or fully evaluate, your first impressions, you may overlook important information. If you don't accurately determine the urgency of your patient's condition, his care may not meet all his emergency needs. And these concepts help you set priorities for your patient's care.

Of course, forming a first impression and determining urgency aren't really steps, the way that performing a primary or secondary assessment is a step. Don't think of them as things to do

first—instead, think of them as things you do continually, *throughout* your emergency assessment and intervention.

## Forming a First Impression

A first impression—it may not seem very important compared to the rush and seriousness of an emergency assessment. But don't underestimate its value. Embodied in your first impression is a wealth of information, based on your knowledge and experience, that will help you make your way confidently through your primary and secondary emergency assessments.

Remember, your first impression may coincide with the first actions of your primary assessment, so be prepared to intervene *immediately* if your first impression is that your patient has a life-threatening problem.

Obtaining a first impression is simply *looking* and *listening*. In an emergency, even though your instinctive reaction is to *do*—to start right in with those vital assessment and intervention steps—you still need to take a few moments to observe the whole patient.

If your patient on the unit has suddenly developed an emergency, consider how he was before and what's changed now. Has one of his vital signs changed suddenly? Has his level of consciousness decreased? Did he have a preexisting infection, or does he have a urinary catheter, a central venous pressure (CVP) line, or other invasive device that may have caused sepsis? On the unit, you usually have the advantage of knowing the patient, his diagnosis, and his progress.

If you're in the ED, you usually don't know your patients, and the information you can obtain before you begin your assessment may be incomplete and even inaccurate. You have to depend

## WHEN YOUR PATIENT CAN'T COMMUNICATE

The best way to get information about your patient with an emergency, of course, is for *him* to tell you about his history and what happened to him. But suppose your patient can't talk—for example, what if he's unconscious? Here are some suggested ways to get the emergency assessment information you need:

• Question anyone who may be able to provide information—for example, family members or friends, witnesses, or rescue personnel.

• Is he wearing a Medic Alert bracelet (or necklace)? Be sure to check for this and—if he's wearing one—to note what it says about the patient's medical status.

• Has he been transferred from a nursing home, outpatient clinic, or referral agency? Call them for information.

• Does he have any prescription medica-

tions with him? If he does, call the pharmacy listed on the bottle. Most pharmacies keep patient profile cards containing significant medical information, including other medications their customers may be taking.

• What is the medication? It may indicate a preexisting condition. For example, if he's taking procainamide hydrochloride (Pronestyl), you know he's probably had prior episodes of cardiac dysrhythmias.

• Who is his doctor? Is the name on a medication bottle? If it is, call the doctor for more information. Is the doctor a cardiologist, a neurosurgeon, a psychiatrist? The answer will help you define your patient's problem or illness.

• Has he been in your hospital before? You may be able to locate the old chart or ED record.

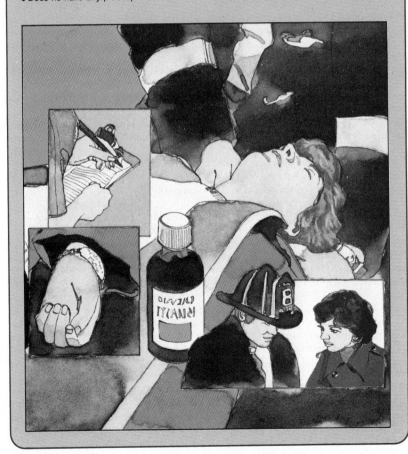

heavily on your first impression for clues to his emergency problems. Look at him closely—does he look sick? You can notice airway or breathing problems immediately; circulation problems aren't so obvious, but you may see bleeding or signs of severe trauma or of shock. His facial expression, skin color and moisture, and ease of breathing are also important clues. Trust your nursing instincts. Remember, you're not diagnosing your patient; you're trying to determine which of his problems need your immediate attention.

Here's an important point: If you have a gut feeling that your patient's seriously ill or injured, *he probably is.* Acting on this assumption, even if you overestimate the seriousness of his condition, is certainly better than finding out your instincts were correct after the patient's condition deteriorates.

Is your patient anxious? Or, if he's a child, are his parents anxious? (See *Dealing with Anxiety,* pages 60 and 61.) Trust *his* instincts, too. Your patient knows his body. If he says he's frightened and he's never felt like this before—or your pediatric patient's mother says she's scared because she knows her child is really sick—these fears may well be justified. Don't make the patient *prove* he's sick, hurt, or dying. (See *"I Think I'm Gonna Die."*)

*Listen* to what your patient initially says—he may give clues that alert you to a serious problem. For example, if your patient on the unit says that he thinks his surgical wound has opened, he may well be right, despite the fact that the surface of the wound is still closed. Throughout these first few moments of caring for your patient (in fact, throughout your emergency assessment and intervention), show your concern by maintaining eye contact, touching him supportively, and letting him know you're willing to listen.

If your patient's unconscious, you must base first impressions on what you can observe and what you can find out from other sources. (See *When Your Patient Can't Communicate,* page 51.)

# Determining Urgency

Determining the urgency of your patient's condition is a process that continues throughout your emergency assessment. Of course, you don't actually stop and say to yourself, "Now I'm going to determine urgency," because determining urgency is a thought process, not an assessment step. But it's no less important. The fact is, the urgency of your patient's condition will determine the depth of your assessment *and* when you'll have to stop your assessment to intervene. So you need to keep urgency constantly in mind.

## Primary assessment clues
Your *first impression* and *primary assessment* provide initial clues to the urgency of your patient's emergency problems. (See the "Primary Assessment: What to Do First" entry in this chapter.) Obviously, significantly altered vital signs and life-threatening conditions, such as cardiac arrest, multiple trauma with shock, or airway obstruction, tell you your patient needs immediate intervention. In other patients, however, urgency may be much more subtle.

## Secondary assessment clues
During your secondary assessment, listen first for *subjective* clues to urgency. (See the "Secondary Assessment: What to Do Next" entry in this chapter.) Your patient may report things you wouldn't be able to notice initially. Suppose, for instance, that you've examined a middle-aged man, in no obvious distress, who came into the ED because he'd had sharp chest pain an hour before (but none on arrival). Your first impression was that he didn't look sick and that his airway, breathing, and circulation weren't compromised. But now, as you're interviewing him, he reports that he had an episode of chest pain early that morning and another—

more severe—episode in midafternoon; and he tells you that the pain he had an hour before coming into the ED was the most severe of all. As a nurse, you know that this sequence of increasing chest pain is classic for preinfarction angina and that your patient's at immediate risk for a massive myocardial infarction. Recognizing that this patient's condition is much more urgent than it originally seemed, you adjust your interventions accordingly.

Of course, subjective clues may also *downgrade* urgency. For example, suppose you have a patient with vaginal bleeding who initially appears very anxious and fearful. Because you never want to underestimate the severity of any patient's condition, you initially assess her condition as urgent, based on her complaint of bleeding. But as you work through your subjective assessment, you find that—frightened by the bleeding—she's greatly exaggerated the amount of blood she's lost. (She's saturated just one perineal pad in the past 4 hours.) Now her condition seems less urgent. You know you can safely continue your assessment and obtain more information before you intervene. And you know that controlling her anxiety is now a priority (see *Dealing with Anxiety*, pages 60 and 61).

Try to use the subjective information you obtain during your secondary assessment to uncover links between *cause* and *effect*. What happened first? For example, if the patient had an accident, was it because he fainted or felt ill? Or suppose your elderly patient falls in her hospital room and injures her wrist. You note the obvious deformity immediately—but as you care for her wrist you ask her how she fell. When she says, "I don't know—I was walking to the bathroom and I blacked out," her response tells you her condition's more urgent than just an injured wrist. She may have had a transient ischemic attack or a cardiac dysrhythmia that caused her to faint.

Use the *objective* clues you obtain during your secondary assessment of the patient to finalize or reclassify your determination of urgency. Of course, your patient's vital signs will be a factor: if his pulse, blood pressure, or temperature has changed significantly, you know his condition may be more urgent than you initially thought. Consider laboratory tests in your determination of urgency, as well. Your patient may have vomited a small amount of blood at home, for example, but has no signs or symptoms in the ED. He appears to be stable and has no complaints. Yet, when you test his hematocrit and hemoglobin levels, you note they're decreased, indicating that the patient may be bleeding from another site or bleeding more than you originally thought. Immediately, you have to upgrade your determination of urgency and to rethink your assessment and intervention priorities for this patient.

## Other clues to urgency

Your patient may have preexisting health problems that affect your determination of urgency. Check for Medic Alert jewelry, for medications or prescriptions in his pockets, for an EKG

### "I THINK I'M GONNA DIE"

You've probably heard this and similar statements many times, from patients with many different disorders. But how often do you take such a patient seriously?

Rather than being a cry for extra attention, a statement like this may be a valuable clue to your patient's condition—a clue that only he can provide. For example, a keen sense of impending doom often accompanies the persistent chest pain that precedes a myocardial infarction.

So *listen* to your patient, and take any statement he makes about his condition as a signal to assess him extra carefully. Don't let his premonitions become reality.

strip in his wallet, and for any other indications of preexisting disease. (Find out all you can about these before you include the information in your emergency assessment.) Be alert, in particular, for a history of:
• an organ transplant
• recent open-heart surgery
• cancer
• systemic lupus erythematosus
• pregnancy
• paraplegia or quadriplegia
• diabetes
• renal dialysis
• heart or lung conditions.
You'll usually manage patients with these preexisting health problems as urgent, no matter what their specific emergency complaints may be.

Remember: *Whenever you're in doubt, assume your patient's condition is urgent.*

# PERFORMING ASSESSMENT AND INTERVENTION

In an emergency, before you do anything else, you need to assess the adequacy of your patient's *a*irway, *b*reathing, and *c*irculation—the ABCs of emergency care (see *ABCs: Your First Priority*, page 58). This sounds obvious—but all too often you may be tempted to overlook this *primary assessment* because of the patient's other urgent problems. *Don't!* No matter what else is wrong, your patient will die if his airway, breathing, or circulation is severely compromised. Think of primary assessment as a separate step you always do *first* in an emergency—even for patients with seemingly minor complaints or with major problems in other body systems. If you find a problem and intervene to correct it, you will have saved your patient's life. Or, if you find that your patient's airway, breathing, and circulation

aren't compromised, you can move on and complete your primary assessment with a quick survey of your patient's general appearance and mental status. Here, too, you may need to intervene, especially if your patient has obvious signs of trauma or a severely altered level of consciousness.

Next, perform a *secondary assessment.* This is when you gather essential subjective and objective data, similar to the data you gather in a nonemergency assessment. The difference lies in the *amount* of information you gather, the *way* you gather it, and the fact that you may need to intervene for urgent problems at any time.

In a nonemergency situation, you obtain subjective information about your patient by taking a complete nursing history that includes these components:
• biographical data (including source)
• chief complaint
• history of present illness
• past history
• family history
• psychosocial history
• activities of daily living
• review of systems.
Then, you obtain objective information by performing a complete physical examination, using the head-to-toe or the major-body-systems method.

You can't follow these detailed procedures when you're performing a secondary assessment for a patient with an emergency—you simply don't have the time. Instead, you must focus your assessment efforts on identifying the patient's *chief complaints,* then organizing the rest of your secondary assessment around them. Ask open-ended questions to determine what those chief complaints are and to clarify them. As you identify each complaint, perform appropriate physical assessment procedures related to it and ask additional history questions related to the complaint (reviewing portions of the patient's past history, history of present illness, and so forth). As always, *be prepared to stop your assessment at any point to intervene as necessary for life-threatening chief complaints,* such as chest pain. Throughout your secondary assessment, assess the status of your patient's airway, breathing, and circulation frequently, intervening as necessary.

So, during your emergency assessment, you don't go into the same depth as you do during a nonemergency assessment. You may omit certain steps and combine others, depending on the urgency of your patient's condition and the nature of his chief complaints. Remember that, although the steps of an emergency assessment are discussed separately in this chapter, you perform them just about simultaneously when you're caring for a patient with an emergency.

# Primary Assessment: What to Do First

During your primary emergency assessment, you may identify life-threatening problems involving your patient's airway, breathing, or circulation. *These problems require your immediate intervention.* Stop your assessment, and immediately begin using the techniques of basic life support (BLS) and/or advanced cardiac life support (ACLS).

BLS includes establishing that the patient's unresponsive and has cardiac or respiratory arrest, then using CPR to restore:
- a patent airway
- breathing
- adequate circulation.

In the hospital setting, you'll also use ACLS techniques, which employ:
- airway adjuncts
- ventilatory adjuncts
- circulatory adjuncts
- monitors
- drugs
- defibrillation or cardioversion equipment.

(You'll find the BLS/ACLS sequence and techniques discussed in detail in the special "Life Support" section of this chapter.)

Here are the steps to follow during your primary emergency assessment, whether you're working on the unit, in an ED, or in a critical-care area.

## Airway
Begin your primary assessment by checking the patency of your patient's airway. Look and listen for such signs and symptoms as gurgling, stridor, wheezing, noisy breathing, circumoral or nail-bed cyanosis, obvious neck trauma, deviated trachea, and decreased level of consciousness. If your patient's *unconscious,* place your ear close to his nose and mouth—you should *hear* his breathing and *feel* his breath on your cheek.

If your patient's airway is patent, you can move on to assess his breathing—the second step in your primary assessment. But if it isn't, you need to take *immediate* steps to open it.

If your conscious patient clutches his throat and starts to cough, you know that he's choking. Ask him if he can speak. If he can speak or cough, leave him alone while he attempts to expel the obstruction, and encourage him to cough (or to continue coughing). However, if he can't speak or cough, or if he begins to make crowing noises, assume his airway's obstructed and intervene immediately. (See *Aiding a Choking Victim,* pages 94 to 97.)

If your patient isn't choking, but you still don't hear or feel air movement, position him on his back and use the *head-tilt/chin-lift* method or the *head-tilt/neck-lift* method to try to open his airway. Use the *jaw-thrust without head-tilt* method if you have *any* reason to suspect cervical spine injury; use the *"sniff" position* if your patient is an infant. (See *Opening the Airway,* page 98.) Then, use a finger sweep to clear any foreign body from the oral cavity, and suction him if necessary. Check again for air flow from his nose and

# USING AN EMERGENCY DEPARTMENT FLOW SHEET

Emergency care flow sheets *aren't* just for ED nurses. Of course, if you're floated to the ED, you'll want to be familiar with your hospital's flow sheet and how to use it. But you may find yourself dealing with flow sheets every day, even if you never leave your unit.

Why? Because more and more hospitals are using these forms to ensure that critical information is documented quickly and efficiently, in *one* easily located place, so it's readily available to other members of the health-care team. When you receive a patient from the ED, a form like the one shown here may accompany him. If it's filled out correctly, it can provide

## EMERGENCY DEPARTMENT FLOW SHEET

Patient name _____

Time in _____ Brought by _____ From _____

Accompanied by family: No _____ Yes ___ Who? _____

Chief complaint: _____

Allergies _____ Current meds _____

_____

**PREHOSPITAL CARE:**

Vital signs: BP _____ P _____ R _____

CPR ☐ Airway ☐ _____MAST ☐

Time of arrival on scene _____

Rhythm observed _____ I.V. fluids _____

Loss of consciousness: Yes ☐ No ☐ Backboard/splints ☐

C-Collar ☐ Restraints ☐ O$_2$ ☐ Amt. _____

Bloods drawn ☐ Meds _____

**INITIAL ASSESSMENT:**

Mental status: Alert ☐ Awake, but confused ☐ Lethargic ☐ Unresponsive ☐
Behavior: Cooperative ☐ Uncooperative ☐ Combative ☐ Other _____
Skin: Dry ☐ Diaphoretic ☐ Pink ☐ Pale ☐ Cyanotic ☐
Head: Wounds ☐ Pupils: Size R ___ L ___React R ___ L ___
Chest: Wounds ☐ Paradoxical movements ☐
Breath sounds: Present R ☐ L ☐ Diminished R ☐ L ☐ Adventitious R ☐ L ☐
Abd: wounds ☐ Distended ☐ Bowel sounds ☐ Rigidity
Extremities: Wounds/deformities ☐
Movement present: Upper R ☐ L ☐ Lower R ☐ L ☐

| Vital signs | | | | | | Glasgow Coma Scale | | | | Pupils | | | | I N T A K E | O U T P U T | |
|---|---|---|---|---|---|---|---|---|---|---|---|---|---|---|---|---|
| | | | | | | Eyes open | Verbal | Motor | T O T A L | Size | | React | | | | |
| Time | B/P | T | P | R | CVP | | | | | R | L | R | L | | | |
| | | | | | | | | | | | | | | | | |
| | | | | | | | | | | | | | | | | |
| | | | | | | | | | | | | | | | | |
| | | | | | | | | | | | | | | | | |
| | | | | | | | | | | | | | | | | |

Physician's signature _____ Totals _____ _____

you with a wealth of well-organized baseline data concerning your patient.

You only need minutes to fill out a flow sheet; you don't need much longer to interpret one. And that's the big advantage. Flow sheets vary from hospital to hospital, but they're usually designed so that information can be recorded by checks, plus and minus signs, or a few quick numbers or words. The key details captured here may be vital to the care you provide later. Make yourself familiar with the ED flow sheets where you work, so you know how to fill one out and, if you receive one, how to interpret the information it contains.

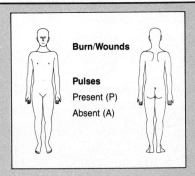

**Burn/Wounds**

**Pulses**

Present (P)

Absent (A)

### ACLS DRUGS AND PROCEDURES
Times

| | | | | | | | |
|---|---|---|---|---|---|---|---|
| NaHCO$_3$ | | | | | | | |
| Epinephrine | | | | | | | |
| Atropine | | | | | | | |
| Ca | | | | | | | |
| Lidocaine | | | | | | | |
| Defib. | | | | | | | |

### CRITICAL LAB VALUES

| Time | WBC/HCT | GLUC | K | Na | pH | PCO$_2$ | FIO$_2$/PO$_2$ | Other | Other |
|------|---------|------|---|----|----|---------|-----------------|-------|-------|
| | | | | | | | | | |
| | | | | | | | | | |
| | | | | | | | | | |

**Procedures (give time):**

Foley ___ EKG ___ NG ___

Guaiac ___ Airway ___ Other ___

Lab: ABG ___ SMA-6 ___

CBC ___ U/A ___ BS___

BUN ___ Creatinine ___

C&S ___ Tox. ___ Amylase ___

T&C ___ Other ___

**RHYTHM STRIP**
(Attach EKG)

| Monitor patterns | Medications |
|---|---|
| | |
| | |
| | |
| | |
| | |

### OBSERVATIONS AND ASSESSMENTS

Primary nurse _____

## ABCS: YOUR FIRST PRIORITY

**A**

**Airway**
First, check the victim's airway for patency. If it's occluded, remove any obstruction and open it immediately. Remember, in addition to a foreign object, his tongue or secretions (or swelling) also may occlude his airway; don't overlook any possibility.

**B**

**Breathing**
Check his breathing by *looking* for chest expansion, *listening* for air flow, and *feeling* for expired air. If he's not breathing, provide assisted ventilation immediately.

**C**

**Circulation**
Check the *carotid* pulse in an adult or child; check the *brachial* pulse in an infant. If you don't feel a pulse, start cardiac compressions immediately.

mouth. Using the appropriate head position may be enough to open his airway and to restore his breathing—especially if his tongue caused the obstruction.

If he still isn't breathing, close your patient's nostrils with your thumb and index finger and deliver four quick mouth-to-mouth ventilations. (See *Giving Mouth-to-Mouth Resuscitation,* page 102.) Watch for chest movement as you deliver these—if his chest doesn't rise and then fall after the fourth ventilation, you know air isn't flowing through his lungs, his airway's not open, and you'll have to try airway adjuncts. You may insert an oropharyngeal airway if he's unconscious, or a nasopharyngeal airway if he's semiconscious. Or (in a patient over age 15) you may use an esophageal obturator airway (EOA) or an esophageal gastric tube airway (EGTA), a modification of an EOA that has a port for passage of a nasogastric (NG) tube (see *Inserting an Artificial Airway,* page 99). These airways are most commonly used outside the hospital, by rescue personnel. Inside the hospital, endotracheal in-

tubation is preferred, so you're more likely to *remove* an EOA or an EGTA from a patient in the ED than to insert one. If you do remove an EOA or an EGTA, remember this: *Don't* take it out until the doctor's successfully performed endotracheal intubation. Have suction equipment ready, because the patient will probably vomit, and he may aspirate his vomitus. (Maintain the patient in the correct head position no matter which airway you use.)

The doctor may decide to insert an endotracheal tube rather than another type of airway adjunct, especially if:
• the patient is apneic and unconscious or has areflexia.
• you can't ventilate the patient successfully by mouth or with an Ambu bag.
• the patient needs tracheal suctioning.
• the doctor wants to avoid the gastric distention that may occur with other airways and with Ambu bag ventilation.
• the doctor anticipates a need for prolonged mechanical ventilation.

Endotracheal intubation has the advantages of providing airway control, protecting the patient from aspiration, allowing visualization and easy suctioning of the trachea, and providing access for hand-held or mechanical ventilation. Assist the doctor with intubation as necessary (see *Assisting with Endotracheal Intubation*, pages 120 and 121). After the tube's inserted, quickly auscultate your patient's chest to confirm correct tube placement—if he has absent breath sounds on the left side, you know the tube's been incorrectly placed in the right main-stem bronchus.

If your patient has problems that may make airway insertion or endotracheal intubation impossible (such as facial injuries, cervical spine injuries, or an obstruction that can't be bypassed), you and the doctor will have to open his airway quickly using some other procedure. If you're on the unit, have someone call a code *immediately*. If you're in the ED, expect to assist with percutaneous transtracheal catheter ventilation or cricothyrotomy. This will provide a temporary airway until your patient can be tracheally intubated or until he can be taken to the operating room for a tracheotomy. (See *Performing Cricothyrotomy and Percutaneous Transtracheal Catheter Ventilation*, pages 100 and 101.) During percutaneous ventilation, the doctor will insert a large-bore cannula into the patient's trachea and attach it to high-flow oxygen, which is delivered rhythmically. The doctor will perform cricothyrotomy by making a quick incision into the cricothyroid membrane and inserting an endotracheal or tracheostomy tube for Ambu bag oxygenation.

### Breathing
Once you've established that your patient has an open airway (or you've intervened as necessary to open it), check his breathing. If he's breathing, quickly assess the rate, depth, and quality of his respirations, noting if they're unusually fast or slow, shallow or deep, or irregular. Observe him for chest-wall expansion, abnormal chest-wall motion, and accessory muscle use.

Provide supplemental oxygen by nasal cannula or mask if he's breathing but short of breath, or if he has:
• chest pain
• signs and symptoms of poor cardiac output (decreased pulse and blood pressure)
• signs and symptoms of hypoxemia (such as confusion, anxiety, or restlessness)
• profuse bleeding
• nausea.

Remember, never give oxygen by mask at a flow rate less than 5 liters/minute. If you do, the patient will rebreathe carbon dioxide, decreasing the effectiveness of oxygen therapy.

If he's breathing adequately, move on to assess his *circulation*—the third step in your primary assessment.

If he *isn't* breathing, ventilate him immediately. Close his nostrils and deliver four quick breaths (see *Giving Mouth-to-Mouth Resuscitation*, page 102). Or, if you're using an Ambu bag, deliver four quick ventilations (see *Using an Ambu Bag*, page 103). If this doesn't restore his breathing, continue delivering ventilations at the rate of 12 breaths/minute, and expect the doctor to intubate him. Continue to ventilate him with an Ambu bag before and after intubation—you can't safely interrupt ventilations for more than 15 to 20 seconds at the most. If the doctor can't successfully intubate him within this time, he'll stop the procedure and ask you to deliver ventilations for a few minutes; then he'll try again.

### Circulation
Assess your patient's circulatory status by first checking his pulses, starting with the carotid. If they're strong and regular, check his blood pressure. If it's stable, quickly check his *mental status* and *general appearance*—the last steps in your primary assessment. Intervene *immediately*, however, if you note any of these problems:
• *no pulse*, indicating cardiac arrest
• *irregular or abnormal pulse*, possi-

## DEALING WITH ANXIETY

In an emergency situation, your patient and his family members experience varying degrees of anxiety. You should always try to alleviate it.
This isn't strictly an issue of providing emotional support. Your first responsibility to a

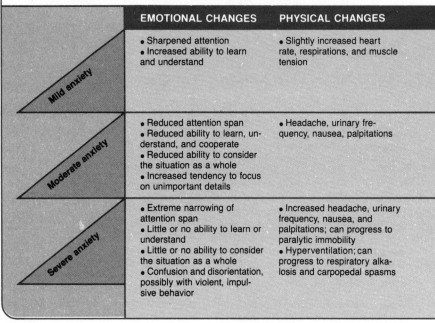

| | EMOTIONAL CHANGES | PHYSICAL CHANGES |
|---|---|---|
| **Mild anxiety** | • Sharpened attention<br>• Increased ability to learn and understand | • Slightly increased heart rate, respirations, and muscle tension |
| **Moderate anxiety** | • Reduced attention span<br>• Reduced ability to learn, understand, and cooperate<br>• Reduced ability to consider the situation as a whole<br>• Increased tendency to focus on unimportant details | • Headache, urinary frequency, nausea, palpitations |
| **Severe anxiety** | • Extreme narrowing of attention span<br>• Little or no ability to learn or understand<br>• Little or no ability to consider the situation as a whole<br>• Confusion and disorientation, possibly with violent, impulsive behavior | • Increased headache, urinary frequency, nausea, and palpitations; can progress to paralytic immobility<br>• Hyperventilation; can progress to respiratory alkalosis and carpopedal spasms |

bly indicating dysrhythmias
• *weak, rapid, thready pulse* and *decreased blood pressure,* possibly indicating shock.

If your patient has *no pulse,* he's in cardiac arrest; begin CPR *immediately,* and have someone call a code. Open his airway and ventilate him by mouth or with an Ambu bag, as described previously. If he's on mechanical ventilation, expect that it will be discontinued and that you'll start ventilating him with an Ambu bag. (Mechanical ventilators aren't effective during chest compressions.)

Be sure he's placed on a cardiac arrest board or some other firm surface. To perform chest compressions, position your hands correctly (depending on whether the patient's an adult, a small child, or an infant). Deliver chest compressions at the appropriate rate

(see *Continuing CPR with Chest Compression and Ventilation,* pages 104 to 106). Mechanical chest compressors are available, but you probably won't use one unless you must give CPR for a long time and all available rescuers tire. If you're giving CPR alone, ventilate the patient with 2 breaths after every 15 compressions. If another person's assisting you, have her deliver 1 breath after every 5 compressions. After you've performed CPR for 1 minute, check your patient's pulse for 5 seconds. If you don't feel a pulse, continue CPR.

If you're in a critical-care area, expect to assist with ACLS procedures, such as giving emergency drugs or assisting with cardioversion or defibrillation (see *Performing Defibrillation and Emergency Synchronized Cardioversion,* pages 107 to 109). If you're on

patient with an emergency is rapid assessment and intervention, but you'll be less than fully effective if the emotional side of the situation isn't under control. Remember, you assess and intervene here, too. This chart shows you how to recognize the three basic levels of anxiety and how to intervene appropriately.

## NURSING CONSIDERATIONS

- Observe the patient or family member closely.
- Offer reassurance and emotional support.
- Explain all procedures, to prevent escalation of anxiety.
- Watch for any increase in anxiety.

- Provide a quiet environment.
- Maintain eye contact when speaking.
- Express your concern and support.
- Encourage crying and other expressions of feelings.
- Provide simple explanations, when asked (more detailed explanations will increase his anxiety).
- Inform the doctor of the patient's or family member's degree of anxiety.

Same as for moderate anxiety, *plus:*
- Intervene immediately to prevent the patient or family member from harming himself or others.
- Set limits in a firm, calm, and clear manner, to maintain control and to reduce the patient's or family member's anxiety.
- Request an order for antianxiety medication.

the medical-surgical unit, continue CPR until the code team responds. Expect them to take over CPR without interruption, to connect the patient to a cardiac monitor, and to begin ACLS procedures (see *Knowing Your Role in a Code,* pages 62 and 63). *Don't stop CPR for any reason* until someone else takes over.

Code-team members will give oxygen and cardiac drugs, perform endotracheal intubation, deliver chest compressions, and defibrillate or cardiovert the patient as necessary (see *Emergency Cardiac Drugs,* pages 110 to 113, and *Performing Defibrillation and Emergency Synchronized Cardioversion,* pages 107 to 109). Help them by continuing basic CPR or by documenting procedures and the medications given. Monitor the patient's femoral pulse, if asked, to determine

the effectiveness of CPR and when his pulse is restored. Make sure you get a 12-lead EKG when his cardiac rhythm returns, and check his blood pressure.

If your patient has an *irregular or abnormal pulse,* he may be experiencing cardiac dysrhythmias. Expect to start cardiac monitoring, insert an I.V. for medication administration, and take a 12-lead EKG (see *Electrocardiograms: Measuring the Heart's Electrical Current,* pages 172 and 173). Expect the doctor to ask you to administer antiarrhythmic drugs specific to your patient's dysrhythmia. Draw blood for necessary laboratory tests, and watch the monitor carefully to detect any changes.

If your patient has *weak, rapid, thready pulses and decreased blood pressure,* he's probably in shock. Look for these signs and symptoms:

## KNOWING YOUR ROLE IN A CODE

Imagine this scene: the unit's quiet at 2:15 a.m., so Marge Dwyer, RN, decides to go get a cup of coffee. As she starts down the corridor, she hears a thud in one of the rooms ahead. Fearing the worst, Marge rushes to the room and finds Earl Storey, a cardiac patient, age 55, collapsed on the floor. She calls his name and shakes his shoulders, but gets no response. Knowing she has to have assistance immediately, Marge calls to another nurse, "Chris, I need your help *right away!*"

Then Marge turns back to Earl and opens his airway using the head-tilt/chin-lift technique. She can't hear or feel any breathing or see any chest movement, so she pinches his nostrils closed, makes a tight seal around his mouth, and—without allowing him to exhale—gives him four quick breaths. As she pauses briefly to palpate for his carotid pulse, Chris bursts into the room. "What is it? What can I do?" she asks. "He's got no pulse—call a code!" Marge orders.

Suppose you were Marge. Would you know how to proceed, with Chris' help, with efforts to resuscitate Earl? Would you know what to do once the code team arrived? If you're not sure, review this list of roles that health-team members may assume during a code situation. Keep in mind, however, that these descriptions are somewhat idealized. In "real life," you or other team members may be expected to fill more than one role. (For example, when Basic Rescuer Number One is relieved from ventilating the patient, she may become the Recorder Nurse or the Medication Nurse.) Or your hospital may modify this version of a code team. (For example, a respiratory therapist may provide ventilatory support for patients.) Be sure you know your unit's procedures and your role(s) when you hear, "It's a code!"

**Recorder Nurse**
• Observes and documents resuscitation efforts, using special code forms if required

**Medication Nurse**
• Prepares all I.V. medications as ordered
• May administer I.V. medications as ordered

**Equipment Nurse**
• Sets up emergency equipment
• Assists with emergency procedures

**Director**
(usually a doctor)
• Directs all major life-saving interventions
• Oversees resuscitation efforts

**Basic Rescuer Number One**
(usually the person who finds the patient)
• Calls for help
• Starts one-man CPR

**Basic Rescuer Number Two**
• Calls for advanced life-support personnel
• Performs two-man CPR with Basic Rescuer Number One

**Anesthetist/Anesthesiologist**
• Intubates patient
• Ventilates patient

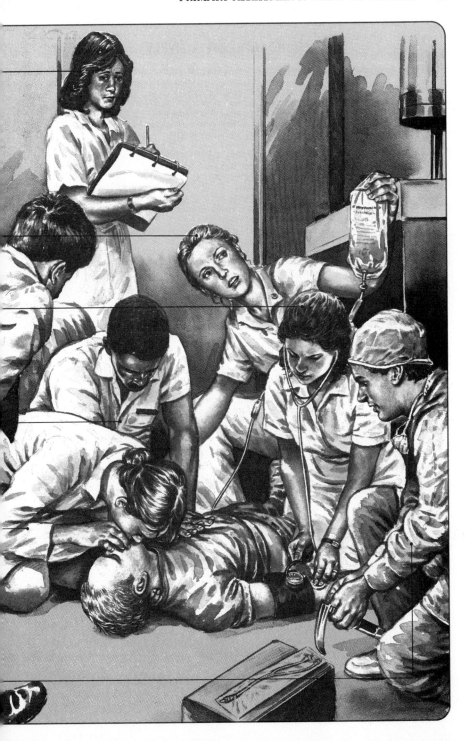

## COMMUNICATING EFFECTIVELY

In an emergency, one of your most important functions is communicating—you're the vital link between the patient, his family, the doctor, and other health-care workers. But communication is a two-way street, with potential barriers for everyone involved. Because you're the patient's advocate, you'll need to recognize and help overcome these barriers to make sure he receives the best possible emergency care.

When communicating with your patient, concentrate on removing *your* barriers by:
- sharpening your emergency assessment skills.
- reducing your own anxiety level.

Help your patient overcome *his* communication barriers by:
- providing information that's clear to him.
- answering his questions.
- helping him deal with his pain and fear.
- maintaining a calm and caring attitude.
- finding a translator, if needed.

To communicate effectively with your patient's family, remove your barriers by reminding yourself how important his family is to his recovery. They may be able to give you crucial information about the patient, and they can provide him with vital emotional support.

Of course, *his family* may have communication problems that you can relieve by:
- providing them with easy-to-understand information.
- answering their questions.
- letting them vent their guilt and anxiety to a sympathetic, nonjudgmental person—you.

When dealing with *doctors and other health-care workers*, you can foster good communication by:
- documenting your care thoroughly.
- relaying pertinent information regarding your patient's condition.
- double-checking doctor's orders that are unclear.
- seeking clear and accurate information from other members of the health-care team.

- restlessness
- dizziness or syncope
- thirst
- pallor
- diaphoresis.

You may apply medical antishock trousers (a MAST suit) if your patient's severely hypovolemic; this will increase blood flow to his vital organs. And you'll always insert at least one large-bore (14G to 16G) I.V. catheter for fluid and drug administration—more than one if you anticipate a need for rapid fluid administration to support the patient's circulation. Start cardiac monitoring (see *Positioning Electrodes for Hardwire Monitoring*, page 175). Assist the doctor as necessary if he inserts a CVP line, an arterial line, or a Swan-Ganz catheter. Draw blood as ordered for necessary laboratory tests (see Chapter 14 for a complete discussion of how to care for a patient in shock).

### General appearance and mental status

You will have observed your patient's general appearance and mental status while you assessed his airway, breathing, and circulation. Obviously, if one or more of these vital functions was compromised, his general appearance was poor and his mental status was altered. But even if the patient's vital functions were stable, take a few seconds to assess him for obvious wounds and deformities, abnormal breath or body odors, altered skin color, diaphoresis, tremors, and facial expressions indicating distress or anxiety. Determine the patient's level of con-

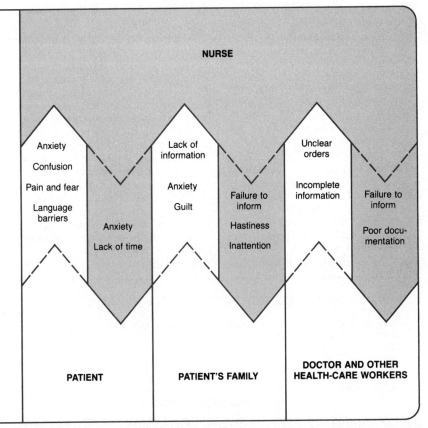

**NURSE**

Anxiety
Confusion
Pain and fear
Language barriers

Anxiety
Lack of time

Lack of information
Anxiety
Guilt

Failure to inform
Hastiness
Inattention

Unclear orders
Incomplete information

Failure to inform
Poor documentation

**PATIENT**

**PATIENT'S FAMILY**

**DOCTOR AND OTHER HEALTH-CARE WORKERS**

sciousness in response to verbal communication, touch, or painful stimuli, and use the Glasgow Coma Scale, if necessary, to determine his degree of unresponsiveness (see *Assessing Your Patient's Level of Consciousness Using the Glasgow Coma Scale,* page 229). You'll assess these factors more completely during your secondary assessment.

# Secondary Assessment: What to Do Next

When you've stabilized your patient's airway, breathing, and circulation, you're ready to use your emergency as-

sessment skills to identify your patient's most serious problems. Your assessment will include:
• *subjective factors* (the information the patient provides about himself, including answers to history questions)
• *objective factors* (the information you uncover with inspection, palpation, percussion, and auscultation in the course of your physical examination).

When you perform an actual emergency assessment, you'll combine these factors to save time, using your patient's chief complaints to focus your physical examination. Here, they're discussed separately only to make each step clearly understandable.

### Subjective assessment

When you collect subjective data, you put the focus on the *patient's* perception of his problem. Even if you have time for only a few critical questions, the answers may provide significant clues to his condition. And asking these questions helps you provide a kind of emotional support, through communicating with him during his crisis, even while you're proceeding with your emergency assessment.

Remember, you won't have time in an emergency to include all the components of a regular history. Instead, focus on the most important information. Make sure you have appropriate *biographical data.* Usually, this information will already be on your patient's chart. But check what's there to make sure you have the patient's full name, address, telephone number, and age. If the information's incomplete, try to obtain the remainder from the patient or his family.

Document the *source of your information,* whether it's the patient, his family, or a friend. If you have reason to suspect that your source is unreliable (for example, if your elderly patient's confused), document this, too, and attempt to confirm the information later.

Place your main focus on your patient's *chief complaint and history of present illness or injury.* Normally two separate steps, these are closely linked in an emergency and can be covered at the same time. Don't skimp here—determining your patient's chief complaint and history of present illness or injury is the heart of your subjective assessment. Ask open-ended questions designed to elicit as much information

## GUIDELINES FOR TETANUS PROPHYLAXIS

Proper wound care *always* includes appropriate tetanus prophylaxis. To determine the correct immunization for your patient, you must know:
• his wound classification (tetanus-prone or non-tetanus-prone)
• his history of tetanus immunization.
First, use the chart below to classify your patient's wound. Then, after determining his history of tetanus immunization, use the immunization schedule on the right to identify the prophylaxis he'll need now.

### WOUND CLASSIFICATION

| CLINICAL FEATURES OF WOUND | TETANUS-PRONE WOUNDS | NON-TETANUS-PRONE WOUNDS |
|---|---|---|
| Age | Greater than 6 hours | Less than 6 hours |
| Configuration | Stellate wound, avulsion, abrasion | Linear wound |
| Depth | Greater than 1 cm (⅜″) | Less than 1 cm (⅜″) |
| Mechanism of injury | Missile, crush, burn, frostbite | Sharp surface (for example, a knife or a piece of glass) |
| Signs of infection | Present | Absent |
| Devitalized tissue | Present | Absent |
| Contaminants (for example, dirt, feces, soil, saliva) | Present | Absent |
| Denervated and/or ischemic tissue | Present | Absent |

as possible. Remember to ask about the *location, duration, chronology,* and *intensity* of the chief complaint and whether the patient's noticed any *influencing factors* or *associated symptoms* (see *How Bad Is It?* page 68). Do this no matter what the chief complaint is—these factors are as significant for nausea, for example, as they are for dyspnea. Of course, if your patient on the unit develops an emergency, his chart will list his initial chief complaints and his diagnosis. But remember—his emergency may be unrelated to his initial problem, so you still want to focus on his *current* chief complaints.

Keep in mind that you may have to stop your assessment and to intervene if your patient's chief complaint (or anything else) suddenly threatens his airway, breathing, or circulation.

When you've assessed your patient's chief complaint and history of present illness or injury, take a few minutes to quickly review his *past medical history.* You need cover only these important points:

• illnesses he's being treated for
• major surgery he's had—for what condition(s), and when
• medications he's taking (including over-the-counter medications)
• allergies, including a description of the reaction(s) he's had
• his last tetanus immunization, if he has an open wound (see *Guidelines for Tetanus Prophylaxis*).

If your patient's female, ask her when she had her last menstrual period. Tell

## TETANUS PROPHYLAXIS

| HISTORY OF TETANUS IMMUNIZATION (number of doses) | TETANUS-PRONE WOUNDS | | NON-TETANUS-PRONE WOUNDS | |
|---|---|---|---|---|
| | Td* | TIG** | Td | TIG |
| Uncertain | Yes | Yes | Yes | No |
| 0 to 1 | Yes | Yes | Yes | No |
| 2 | Yes | No (*yes* if 24 hours since wound was inflicted) | Yes | No |
| 3 or more | No (*yes* if more than 5 years since last dose) | No | No (*yes* if more than 10 years since last dose) | No |

*Td = Tetanus and diphtheria toxoids adsorbed (for adult use), 0.5 ml
**TIG = Tetanus immune globulin (human), 250 units

When Td and TIG are given concurrently, separate syringes and separate sites should be used.

NOTE: For children under age 7, diphtheria and tetanus toxoids, and pertussis vaccine adsorbed (D.P.T.), is preferred to tetanus toxoid alone. If pertussis vaccine is contraindicated, administer tetanus and diphtheria toxoids adsorbed (D.T.).

Adapted from American College of Surgeons, Committee on Trauma, *Prophylaxis against Tetanus in Wound Management,* April 1984

## HOW BAD IS IT?

As a nurse, you know that quantifying pain is very difficult, because what's excruciating for one patient may be merely uncomfortable for another. Of course, this happens because everyone's pain threshold is different.

Here's a tip for obtaining an accurate baseline assessment of your patient's pain: Try asking him to rate his pain on a scale of 1 to 10, 1 representing no pain and 10 representing the worst pain he's ever felt. This technique gives your patient a way of measuring and expressing his pain. It also involves him actively in the assessment, which may have the added benefit of helping to reduce his anxiety. And it provides baseline data that you can use when you assess his pain again.

the doctor *immediately* if a possibility exists that she's pregnant, so he can decide whether or not to order X-rays.

Ask the patient's family or friends these questions if the patient's unconscious or unable to speak. The answers will influence his care and may provide clues to his diagnosis.

If you can obtain information for these important history components, you'll establish a baseline and help determine the urgency and causes of your patient's problem. Later, when your patient is stabilized, you'll be able to fill in the other components of a normal health history—childhood diseases, immunization history, prior injuries, previous hospitalizations, family history, psychosocial history, and a review of systems. These things are important, too—but in an emergency you must set priorities. And part of setting priorities is knowing *what* to ask and *when* to ask it.

### Objective assessment

Collect objective assessment data concerning your patient's emergency by performing a rapid head-to-toe physical assessment, concentrating most on the areas relating to his chief complaint. (See *Head-to-Toe Emergency Assessment Checklist*, pages 72 and 73.) You'll usually do this in preference to a body-systems examination, because head-to-toe is quicker. However, either method is fine, as long as you're consistent and you perform the examination the same way each time. (See *Body-System Emergency Assessment Checklist*, pages 70 and 71.)

If possible, undress your patient completely. You won't have time for a detailed assessment—instead, you'll rapidly but systematically assess each area of the patient's body, paying particular attention to those areas related to the patient's chief complaint or history of present illness or injury.

When you examine your patient, don't skip areas or jump to conclusions about what you should or shouldn't assess. Instead, use your experienced nursing judgment to adjust the extent of your examination appropriately for each area. For example, if your patient's chief complaint is abdominal pain with vomiting lasting for 3 days, you *won't* test his vision or palpate his face and neck, but you *will* perform a thorough abdominal examination. Similarly, if your patient's chief complaint is severe headache with blurred vision, you *won't* perform a rectal examination, but you *will* perform a pupil check and a visual acuity test.

Remember—you're not diagnosing the patient. Your goal is to widen your base of information about your patient's chief complaint, not to narrow it toward a diagnosis. You want to gather as much pertinent information as possible, because your findings provide an important baseline. And the doctor may rely on them heavily when he's making a diagnosis—especially if you're on the unit when one of your patients develops an emergency problem, and you must convey your findings by phone. The key to performing an emergency physical examination is flexibility: while still being thorough, you need to attune yourself to your pa-

## ASSESSING EXTRAOCULAR MUSCLE FUNCTION

Test your patient's extraocular muscle function if he's suffered facial or eye trauma or has a suspected neurologic deficit. If any of the six extraocular muscles or three pairs of cranial nerves (III, IV, and VI) that control eyeball movements is impaired (because of edema, orbital fracture, or impingement), he'll have improper eye alignment, impaired eye movement, and diplopia. Here's how to check for impaired extraocular muscle function.

First, check your patient's corneal light reflex by shining a penlight directly between his eyes, holding it 12″ to 15″ (30.5 to 38.1 cm) away. You'll see a small dot of light at the same spot on each cornea, equidistant from his nose. If the dots are asymmetrical, suspect muscle impairment.

Next, check specific muscle and nerve function. Ask your patient to follow your finger (or a pencil) with his eyes as you trace the six cardinal fields of gaze in front of his face (see the illustration). Stop at each field and observe your patient's eyes. If both eyes don't deviate fully into each field of gaze, suspect muscle entrapment or paralysis, with possible nerve damage.

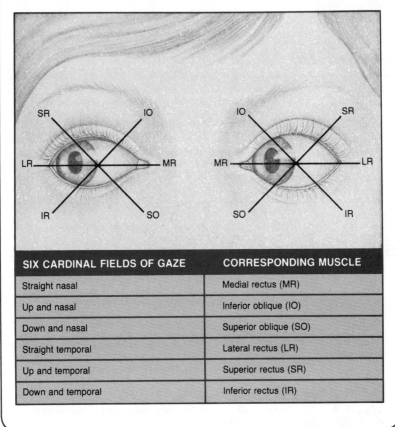

| SIX CARDINAL FIELDS OF GAZE | CORRESPONDING MUSCLE |
|---|---|
| Straight nasal | Medial rectus (MR) |
| Up and nasal | Inferior oblique (IO) |
| Down and nasal | Superior oblique (SO) |
| Straight temporal | Lateral rectus (LR) |
| Up and temporal | Superior rectus (SR) |
| Down and temporal | Inferior rectus (IR) |

tient's problems.

As you know, your findings during an emergency head-to-toe physical examination may relate to possible disturbances in a number of body systems. For example, a respiratory problem, a cardiovascular problem, an endocrine problem, or shock may cause alterations in skin color, temperature, and turgor.

The overview of secondary objective assessment that follows concentrates on what you should assess. Remember that you won't necessarily perform *all* these assessment procedures for *every* emergency patient.

Start your head-to-toe examination by taking your patient's *vital signs*. You

# BODY-SYSTEM EMERGENCY ASSESSMENT CHECKLIST

| BODY SYSTEM | WHAT TO ASSESS |
|---|---|
| **(Vital signs)**  | • Auscultate or palpate the patient's blood pressure.<br>• Note the rate, depth, pattern, and symmetry of his respirations.<br>• Palpate his radial pulse and note its rate, rhythm, and strength.<br>• Take his temperature. |
| **Neurologic** 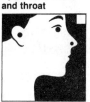 | • Determine the patient's level of consciousness.<br>• Inspect his pupils for size, symmetry, and reaction to light.<br>• Observe him for abnormal posture (decorticate or decerebrate).<br>• Inspect and palpate his scalp for trauma or deformities.<br>• Assess the sensory and motor responses of each affected body part.<br>• Observe him for facial asymmetry, and listen for slurred speech.<br>• Assess deep tendon reflexes. |
| **Eyes, ears, nose, and throat** 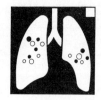 | • Inspect the patient's eyes for burns.<br>• Inspect and palpate his face and his eyes, ears, nose, and throat for trauma or deformities.<br>• Assess his speech for dysphonia or aphonia.<br>• Inspect his ears and nose for bleeding, drainage, and foreign objects.<br>• Inspect his oral mucosa for color, hydration, inflammation, and bleeding.<br>• Inspect and palpate his thyroid gland for tenderness and enlargement.<br>• Inspect his oropharynx for signs of burns due to ingestion of caustic agents.<br>• Assess his gross visual acuity and eye movements. |
| **Respiratory** | • Observe the patient for use of accessory muscles, for paradoxical chest movements, and for respiratory distress.<br>• Inspect his chest for contour, symmetry, and deformities or trauma.<br>• Auscultate his lungs for adventitious sounds and increased or decreased breath sounds.<br>• Palpate his chest for tenderness, pain, and crepitation. |

checked these during your primary assessment—but check them again frequently throughout your secondary assessment, because they're a significant indication of your patient's improvement, stability, or deterioration. Palpate his peripheral and central pulses for rate, rhythm, and quality. Auscultate his blood pressure and take his temperature. Count the rate of his

| BODY SYSTEM | WHAT TO ASSESS |
|---|---|
| **Cardiovascular**  | • Palpate the patient's peripheral pulses—especially of each affected body part—for rate, rhythm, quality, and symmetry.<br>• Inspect him for jugular vein distention.<br>• Inspect and palpate his extremities for edema, mottling and cyanosis, and temperature change.<br>• Auscultate his heart sounds for timing, intensity, pitch, and quality, and note the presence of murmurs, rubs, or extra sounds.<br>• Auscultate blood pressure in both arms. |
| **Gastrointestinal**  | • Inspect the patient's abdomen for obvious signs of trauma.<br>• Inspect any vomitus or stool for amount, color, presence of blood, and consistency.<br>• Inspect his abdomen for distention.<br>• Auscultate his abdomen for bowel sounds.<br>• Palpate his abdomen for pain, tenderness, or rigidity.<br>• Percuss his abdomen for possible ascites. |
| **Genitourinary** 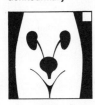 | • Inspect the patient's external genitalia for bleeding, ecchymoses, edema, or hematoma.<br>• Palpate his abdomen for suprapubic pain.<br>• Palpate his external genitalia for pain or tenderness.<br>• Palpate for costovertebral angle (CVA) tenderness. |
| **Musculoskeletal** 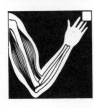 | • Inspect the patient's body for trauma and deformities.<br>• Gently palpate his cervical spine for tenderness and deformities.<br>• Palpate his vertebral spine and percuss his costovertebral areas for tenderness.<br>• Inspect his skin for color, ecchymoses, pigmentation, and discoloration.<br>• Palpate his pulses distal to any injury.<br>• Palpate the area of suspected injury for tenderness, pain, and edema.<br>• Assess his motor and sensory responses.<br>• Observe the range of motion of his injured extremity.<br>• Inspect his skin for needle marks.<br>• Assess for nuchal rigidity. |

# HEAD-TO-TOE EMERGENCY ASSESSMENT CHECKLIST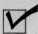

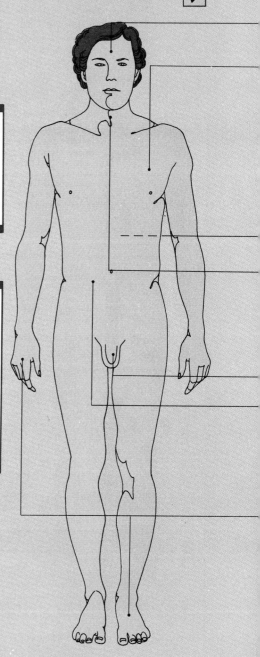

## VITAL SIGNS
• Auscultate or palpate the patient's blood pressure.
• Note the rate, depth, pattern, and symmetry of his respirations.
• Palpate his radial pulse and note its rate and rhythm (regular/irregular).
• Take his temperature.

## GENERAL SURVEY
• Observe the patient's level of consciousness, behavior, and mental status.
• Inspect his body for obvious deformities due to trauma.
• Observe him for severe, moderate, or mild distress and anxiety.
• Inspect his skin for color, moisture, turgor, temperature, and ecchymoses.
• Note the presence of any distinctive odors on his breath, such as alcohol or acetone.
• Note his degree of mobility.

## CHEST

- Inspect the patient's chest for contour, symmetry, and deformities or trauma.
- Palpate his chest for tenderness, pain, and crepitation.
- Auscultate his lungs for increased or decreased breath sounds or the presence of adventitious sounds.
- Auscultate his heart sounds for timing, intensity, pitch, and quality, and note the presence of murmurs, rubs, or extra sounds.

## NECK

- Gently palpate the patient's cervical spine for tenderness and deformities.
- Inspect him for jugular vein distention.
- Inspect and palpate his thyroid gland for tenderness and enlargement.

## ABDOMEN

- Inspect the patient's abdomen for deformities, trauma, bleeding, abnormal drainage, or abnormal pulsations.
- Ascultate for bowel sounds.
- Palpate the four quadrants for pain, tenderness, and rigidity.
- Percuss his abdomen for ascites.

## HEAD

- Inspect the patient's eyes for injuries or burns.
- Inspect his oropharynx for burns.
- Observe him for nasal flaring.
- Inspect and palpate his scalp and face for trauma and deformities.
- Inspect his pupils for size, symmetry, and reaction to light.
- Inspect his ears and nose for bleeding, drainage, and foreign objects.
- Inspect his oral mucosa for color, hydration, inflammation, and bleeding.

## BACK

- Inspect the patient's back for deformities or trauma.
- Palpate for tenderness in his vertebral spine and percuss his costovertebral areas.
- Palpate his flanks for tenderness.

## EXTERNAL GENITALIA

- Inspect the patient's genitalia for bleeding, ecchymoses, edema, or hematoma.
- Palpate the genitalia for pain and tenderness.

## EXTREMITIES

- Inspect and palpate the patient's extremities for trauma, deformities, and edema.
- Inspect his arms for needle tracks.
- Palpate the distal pulses of an injured extremity.
- Assess the motor and sensory responses of an injured extremity.
- Palpate his extremities for pain and tenderness.

respirations, and evaluate their depth and rhythm.

Note your patient's *general appearance and mental status*. You quickly checked these in your primary assessment, but do this in more depth now. Note if he's well-nourished, cachectic, or obese, and whether he appears generally healthy. Pay attention to his personal hygiene and dress—they may reflect his general well-being. Inspect his skin for color, moisture, turgor, and temperature. Check for alterations in his level of consciousness, and note any signs of decreased mentation, inappropriate behavior, distress, or anxiety. Observe his posture, body position, and mobility, and note any impairments.

Inspect and palpate his *head* for wounds, bruises, or other signs of trauma. Look for facial symmetry, and palpate the scalp carefully—he may have wounds that his hair is covering. Inspect his eyes, and perform a pupil check for size, symmetry, and reaction to light (see *Understanding Pupillary Changes*, page 230, and *Documenting Pupil Size*, page 231). See if he can move his eyes in all directions and if he can raise both eyebrows (see *Assessing Extraocular Muscle Function*, page 69). If he's complained of an eye problem, check his vision (one eye at a time), using a Snellen test, or have him read something handy like the label on the I.V. bottle. If he's unconscious, note if his eyes are open or closed. Inspect his ears and nose for bleeding, cerebrospinal fluid (CSF) leakage, or foreign objects. Check his oral mucosa for color, hydration, bleeding, and inflammation, and note any unusual mouth odors such as a fecal, alcoholic, or fruity smell. Expect the doctor to perform an ophthalmoscopic or otoscopic examination if indicated. He may also order skull X-rays or a computerized tomography (CT) scan, if necessary.

Inspect your patient's *neck* and note if he has jugular vein distention. Palpate his cervical spine gently, and note any tenderness and deformities that may indicate a spinal injury that you didn't detect during your primary assessment. Call the doctor *immediately* if you note any of these. Why? Because you'll need to manage this patient with special care until the doctor can rule out spinal injury after an X-ray (using portable equipment). Palpate the patient's lymph nodes and thyroid gland, noting if they're enlarged.

Inspect your patient's *chest* for wounds, bruises, contusions, and discolorations. Palpate his rib cage and compress it lightly from side to side—note any swelling, tenderness, or crepitation that may indicate fractured ribs. Also palpate his clavicles, sternum, and shoulders for indications of fractures. If his chief complaints lead you to suspect a respiratory problem, auscultate his lung sounds; if you note any abnormalities, expect that the doctor will order a chest X-ray and arterial blood gases (see Chapter 4, RESPIRATORY EMERGENCIES). If the patient's chief complaints lead you to suspect a cardiac problem, auscultate his heart sounds (see Chapter 5, CARDIOVASCULAR EMERGENCIES). Expect to do an EKG and, possibly, to draw blood for cardiac enzyme levels.

Palpate your patient's *back* along the vertebrae and over the flanks, and palpate or percuss the costovertebral angles. Note any tenderness or signs of injury. Expect the doctor to order X-rays if you detect any problem.

Remember that your patient's *abdomen* may be very sensitive if he has a GI complaint, so inspect and auscultate it thoroughly before you palpate or percuss it. Look for signs of trauma, such as wounds or discoloration around the umbilicus or along the flanks, sacrum, or perineum, because these may indicate internal bleeding. Note any distention, bulging flanks, or abnormal pulsations over the aorta. If appropriate, auscultate the bowel sounds in all four quadrants and note if the sounds are increased, decreased, or absent. Palpate the patient's abdomen for tenderness and rigidity, and note any guarding. (If the patient complains of abdominal pain, begin your palpation *away* from the painful quadrant, and palpate it last.) If you noted distention or bulging flanks, percuss for a fluid-motion wave. Obtain a urine sample for analysis and culture, and note if the patient has difficulty urinating. If necessary, assist the doctor with a rectal examination, and obtain a stool specimen.

Inspect your patient's *genitals* for obvious lesions or abnormalities, bleeding, or discharge. If you find a discharge, prepare a Thayer-Martin plate for the doctor so he can test for gonorrhea, and expect to draw blood for a Venereal Disease Research Laboratory (VDRL) or rapid plasma reagin (RPR) test for syphilis. The doctor may decide to obtain a specimen of the discharge for culture. If your female patient requires a pelvic examination, be prepared to assist the doctor.

Check your patient's *extremities* for obvious wounds, deformities, or edema, and assess his muscle tone. Look for needle marks, possibly indicating drug abuse. Palpate his extremities for tenderness and swelling, and compare his pulses and skin temperature in all four extremities. Pay particular attention to skin color and pulses in an injured extremity, and test sensation, strength of movement, and range of motion where applicable. If the patient has an injured extremity, expect the doctor to order X-rays and, possibly, an arteriogram or venogram.

When you've completed your head-to-toe assessment, document your findings and take a few minutes to think about how the information you've obtained relates to the patient's chief complaints. Have you uncovered new information unrelated to his complaints? If you have, question him further about these findings. Remember to repeat your examination periodically to detect any changes and to compare your findings with your baseline data. Arrange for any appropriate diagnostic tests, as the doctor orders.

# ASSESSING SPECIAL PATIENTS

Multiple trauma patients, pediatric patients, geriatric patients, and pregnant patients present special problems that require refinements of your emergency assessment and intervention skills. The basics remain the same: a rapid primary assessment—to secure your patient's airway, breathing, and circulation—followed by a more detailed secondary assessment. But you need to be aware of certain important factors for each of these groups of patients and to consider these factors during your emergency assessment.

# Multiple Trauma Patients

If your patient's suffered trauma to multiple body systems, expect to combine a speedy assessment (even faster than your normal emergency assessment) with aggressive intervention and a high index of suspicion. Remember that your patient's under severe physical (as well as emotional) stress—with multiple trauma, the seriousness of his condition is more than just the sum of his external and internal injuries. For example, morbidity and mortality risks are high in a patient with multiple trauma, because he can easily go into shock. The resulting secondary hypoxemia and hemorrhage—added to the primary injury—take their toll on vital organs: your patient risks both organ failure and sepsis.

No matter where in the hospital you're working, you can expect to care for a patient with multiple trauma. You may be:
• in the ED (even if he has to be trans-

# USING ACCIDENT INFORMATION TO PREDICT INJURIES

When you're assessing an accident victim, every second counts. You simply don't have time to do a complete head-to-toe assessment and to obtain a detailed health history. So how can you make the most of every second? As quickly as you can, find out what type of accident caused the damage. Then, knowing that each major type of accident has a distinctive mechanism of injury, you can predict the types of injuries your patient's likely to have and focus your assessment accordingly.

This chart shows you the mechanisms of injury and related possible injuries for major types of accidents and for assaults.

| TYPE | MECHANISM OF INJURY | POSSIBLE INJURIES |
|---|---|---|
| **MOTOR VEHICLE COLLISIONS (OCCUPANT INJURIES)** | | |
| • Head-on | • Body travels down and under, striking knees on dashboard, then chest on steering wheel *or* • Body travels up and over, snapping head forward (hitting windshield) and striking lower chest or upper abdomen on steering wheel | • Knee dislocation, femur fracture, posterior fracture or dislocation of hip, cardiac contusion, aortic tears and dissection • Head trauma, hyperflexion or hyperextension, cervical spine injuries, rib fractures, intraabdominal injuries |
| • Rear-end | • Body travels forward as head remains in place, then snaps back across backrest or headrest • If frontal impact's also involved, body travels forward and hits dashboard and steering wheel | • Whiplash injuries of third to fourth cervical vertebrae • Injuries from frontal impact (such as cardiac contusion, rib fractures, intraabdominal injuries, intrathoracic injuries) |
| • Lateral impact | • Body slams into door, injuring chest, pelvis, and neck | • Chest injuries with or without humerus fracture, pelvic or femur fractures, contralateral neck injuries (tears or sprain of neck ligaments) |
| • Rotational force | • Body reacts to collision as vehicle hits stationary object and rotates around it | • Combination of head-on and lateral impact collision injuries |
| • Rollover | • Body stays in place (if restrained) or bounces around as vehicle rolls over | • Various collision injuries, similar to rotational-force injuries |
| • Seat belt | • Body compresses against lap belt worn too high (above anterior superior iliac spine) • Body compresses against shoulder belt | • Abdominal organ injuries, thoracic or lumbar spine injuries • Shoulder and neck injuries |

| TYPE | MECHANISM OF INJURY | POSSIBLE INJURIES |
|---|---|---|
| **MOTOR VEHICLE ACCIDENTS (PEDESTRIAN INJURIES)** | | |
| • **Head-on** (Waddell's triad) | • Body impacts with bumper and hood | • Femur and chest injuries |
| | • Force propels victim toward third point of impact (when body comes to rest) | • At third point of impact, contralateral skull injuries |
| • **Lateral impact** | • Lower and upper leg impact with bumper and hood | • Tibia, fibula, and femur fractures<br>• Ligament damage in opposite knee because of excess stress |
| **MOTORCYCLE COLLISIONS** | | |
| • **Head-on** | • Body (head and chest) strikes handlebars | • Head, chest, and abdominal injuries, bilateral femur fractures |
| • **Angular** | • Motorcycle falls on body | • Crush injuries to lower limbs, open fractures |
| • **Ejection** | • Body is thrown from motorcycle into an object | • Head and spine injuries, deceleration injuries |
| **ASSAULTS** | | |
| • **Beating** | • Body—especially head, neck, abdomen—is struck by blunt object or fist | • Soft tissue injuries, major organ injuries in specific area of blunt trauma |
| • **Stab wound** | • Body—usually chest or abdomen—is stabbed with sharp weapon | • Major blood loss, sucking chest wound, organ penetration, heart or major vessel penetration (location and direction of attack, length and type of weapon, and height and strength of attacker determine severity) |
| • **Missile injuries** | • Projectile from a pistol, rifle, shotgun, or explosion enters and exits body, or enters and lodges in body<br>*and* | • Range from minor puncture to life-threatening wound of chest, abdomen, or head |
| | • Projectile follows path of least resistance<br>*and* | • Lacerated tissue in bullet's path, possible injury to remote organs |
| | • Projectile forms cavity as it releases energy into tissues in its path<br>*and* | • Initial wound, subsequent tissue injury (not necessarily in direct path of bullet), secondary infection |
| | • Energy travels through affected tissues and injures other tissues<br>*and* | • Internal tissue and bone damage |
| | • Close contact may cause muzzle blast injury | • Internal tissue and bone damage |

*(continued)*

| USING ACCIDENT INFORMATION TO PREDICT INJURIES *(continued)* | | |
|---|---|---|
| **TYPE** | **MECHANISM OF INJURY** | **POSSIBLE INJURIES** |
| **JUMPS AND FALLS** | | |
| • **Compression force** (Don Juan syndrome) | • Person falls from a height and lands on his heels <br> • Forward momentum causes acute flexion of lumbar spine, then continued forward momentum causes person to land on outstretched hands | • Bilateral fractures of calcaneus <br> • Compression fractures of vertebrae <br> • Colles' fracture of wrists |
| • **Indirect force** | • Person falls backward and lands on back and head | • Spine and head injuries, tibia and fibula fractures |
| • **Twisting force** | • Person falls (usually during sports activity) and twists legs | • Tibia and fibula fractures |

ferred to a trauma center)
• in the intensive-care unit or the coronary-care unit
• on the medical-surgical unit (possibly for long-term care).
Don't let the complexity of his injuries overwhelm you. Your key to preventing this is understanding the *mechanisms of trauma* so that you consider all possible associated injuries during your assessment. (See *Using Accident Information to Predict Injuries,* pages 76 to 78, and *Emergency! Atlas of Major Injuries,* pages 548 to 565.)

Give this patient as much emotional support as you can. *You're* the constant factor in his otherwise chaotic and frightening new environment. Let him rely on you to protect his interests and to act as a buffer between him and the many other health-care workers and procedures involved in his care.

### Mechanisms of trauma

Even as you stabilize your patient's airway, breathing, and circulation and gather vital assessment data, consider the way your patient was injured. Obtain a brief history from your patient, his family, friends, rescue personnel, bystanders—anyone who may know something of how the trauma occurred.

Why is this important? Because knowing how the trauma occurred provides you with information about the severity of the patient's injuries, alerts you to possible hidden injuries, helps prevent iatrogenic injury, and increases your ability to provide definitive care.

As you know, injury occurs whenever the force applied to a tissue exceeds the tissue's ability to absorb or deflect it. For a patient with multiple trauma, consider the *type* of force that caused his injuries (blunt or penetrating), its *magnitude,* and whether it was applied *directly* or *indirectly.*

If your patient has a *penetrating injury,* you can commonly expect less secondary trauma than if he has a blunt injury, because a penetrating injury usually involves less energy. Stab wounds, in particular, are relatively low-energy wounds, which may involve only one or two body systems.

When you examine your patient, look at the entrance wound and imagine the organs that lie in the path of the penetrating object. Remember to consider *all* possibilities. For example, an abdominal penetrating wound can also involve the thoracic cavity if the diaphragm was penetrated, or a penetrating thoracic wound may involve the abdominal cavity. You don't know where the patient's diaphragm was at the time of injury—up during expiration or down during inspiration. So the doctor may perform peritoneal lavage for any wound below the nipple line, and he may insert a chest tube for any injury high in the abdomen. Similarly, a small puncture wound to the patient's abdomen may also have caused multiple punctures of his intestines and colon. These can rapidly lead to peritonitis and death.

When you've learned to keep a clear picture of your patient's internal structures in mind, you'll be less likely to underestimate the severity of his injuries.

If a bullet caused your patient's penetrating injury, you need to consider more than just the path the bullet followed. This is because, unlike stab wounds, gunshot wounds are associated with high energy that creates pressure waves within the patient's body. These pressure waves may create a cavity many times the actual size of the bullet. Additionally, combustion burns from gunpowder may cause serious internal tissue and bone destruction. To estimate damage accurately, you need to consider the caliber of the weapon used and the range at which it was fired—a large-caliber gun, such as a .45, will cause much more damage than a small-caliber gun, such as a .22, especially when fired at close range. So don't let a small, neat entrance wound mislead you—your patient may have massive internal injuries. And always look for an *exit* wound—its position and size may help you determine the bullet's path and force.

A device capable of injecting a substance under the skin at high pressure—such as a paint gun—may cause severe muscle and soft tissue damage. Yet, you may see only a small puncture wound. In fact, your patient's history of the event and complaint of pain may be your only other clues.

If your patient has a *blunt injury*, you may have difficulty determining which organs are injured and whether he has secondary injuries. This is because blunt trauma involves indirect as well as direct forces, so it may cause injuries at some distance from the site where the major force was applied. In assessing your patient, picture the organs that lie underneath the injured site. Solid organs, such as the liver and kidneys, may be crushed or compressed against an unyielding structure, such as the vertebral column. Hollow, air-filled organs, such as the intestines and the lungs, may burst when compressed or subjected to blast forces, because the gas inside transmits force equally in all directions.

Consider the areas of stress in your patient's body where relatively mobile body parts join relatively fixed body parts. The blunt force transmits motion to your patient's body. The result? His mobile body parts tend to keep moving and can rupture at the point where they're fixed. A blow to your patient's head, for example, may bruise his brain, which is relatively mobile, against his fixed skull, or it may create a subdural hematoma due to rupture of the fixed dural veins. Or, as the mobile brain moves, it may rip fixed cranial nerves. Similarly, blunt or twisting forces applied to his upper chest may rupture his mobile lower trachea where it joins his fixed upper trachea or may rupture his mobile descending aorta where it joins his fixed ascending aorta and aortic arch.

Also consider the areas of weakness and susceptibility in your patient's body. Look for skeletal injuries not just at the point of impact but at nearby, less stable joints and along the axis of the bone; consider organ injuries *under* broken bones, too, especially under the pelvis, skull, and rib cage. (Remember that nerves and blood vessels may be injured, as well.)

You can use your knowledge of how your patient's multiple trauma occurred to help predict the types of injuries he may have. Motor vehicle accidents, for example, tend to cause

## WHEN THE WORST HAPPENS

Grief—as a nurse, you see it all the time. A patient who's dying or who's lost a body part or function will naturally grieve; a dead or dying patient's family may grieve just as intensely. You can help a grieving person make the climb from despair toward acceptance by recognizing the five stages of grieving and intervening appropriately. (Of course, not all people progress through the grief process in the same sequence—the stages may overlap, or a person may revert to an earlier stage.)

In most emergency situations, you'll see only the first two stages—denial and anger. Encourage your patient or his family members to express their feelings, and assure them that these feelings are normal and acceptable. By doing so, you'll help them work through their grief and eventually come to terms with their loss.

**THE FIVE STAGES OF GRIEVING**

**STAGE 1**

**Denial**
*Characterized by:*
• overwhelming shock
• disbelief
• rejection of reality ("No, not me!")
*Assist by:*
• being receptive to his need to talk
• listening sympathetically
• sharing your feelings if you think it could help him
• making it possible for him to continue communicating.

**STAGE 2**

**Anger**
*Characterized by:*
• impatience
• uncooperativeness
• bitterness
• jealousy
• helplessness
• increasing awareness ("Why me?")
*Assist by:*
• letting him express his feelings
• remembering that you're not expected to answer unanswerable questions like "Why me?"
• not taking his anger personally. (He's not angry with you, but with his own painful situation.)

certain combinations of injuries to occupants, depending on how fast the vehicle was traveling, its point of impact, and whether individual occupants were wearing seat belts. If a vehicle struck your patient, he'll probably have a different set of injuries, such as Waddell's triad—a combination of femur and chest injuries, from the impact of the bumper and hood, and a third injury from the fall after the impact. A patient who's fallen from a height and landed on his feet may suffer a combination of heel fractures, vertebrae compression fractures (as he flexes forward), and wrist fractures (as he attempts to catch himself on his outstretched hands). (See *Using Accident Information to Predict Injuries,* pages 76 to 78, and *Emergency! Atlas of Major Injuries,* pages 548 to 565.)

Be sure you're alert to the forces involved and their patterns of possible injury when you assess your multiple trauma patient. Then you'll be confident that you haven't missed anything.

**Primary assessment pointers**
When you assess a patient with multiple trauma, you'll be part of a team working on him simultaneously. This approach is designed to ensure that he quickly receives the multiple treatments he may need for survival. As you carry out your role in stabilizing your patient's airway, breathing, and circulation, follow the steps discussed in the "Primary Assessment: What to Do

## STAGE 3

**Bargaining**
*Characterized by:*
• depression
• exhaustion
• final attempt to avoid reality ("If you will..., I will....")
*Assist by:*
• helping him to complete any unfinished business
• making time to be with him and caring enough to listen.

## STAGE 4

**Depression**
*Characterized by:*
• quietness
• withdrawal
• melancholy ("What's the use?")
*Assist by:*
• supporting his grief
• not interrupting his grieving process
• sharing any sad feelings you may have.

## STAGE 5

**Acceptance**
*Characterized by:*
• contemplativeness
• serenity
• ability to discuss his condition ("I can handle it.")
*Assist by:*
• not deserting him
• respecting his acceptance of his loss.

First" entry in this chapter. Also consider the following important points.

Your patient may have maxillofacial fractures or direct laryngeal or tracheal trauma that disrupts his airway or occludes it with blood, bone, loose teeth, or dentures.

*Don't* use the head-tilt/chin-lift or head-tilt/neck-lift maneuvers to open his airway—you *must* suspect cervical spine injury until X-ray rules it out. Make sure your patient's secured to a backboard, and remember to immobilize his chest *first*. (If you immobilize his head first, you create a giant lever if his body moves before you stabilize it, possibly causing further serious injury.) Immobilize his head and neck by taping his forehead to the backboard or by applying a hard collar and sandbags. (See *Handle with Care*, page 82.)

If his airway's not open, insert a nasopharyngeal or oropharyngeal airway until the doctor can perform endotracheal or nasotracheal intubation or emergency cricothyrotomy. If the doctor chooses intubation, he may ask you to apply traction to the patient's cervical spine while he inserts the tube, preventing hyperflexion and hyperextension. Suction any foreign material from the airway. Insert an NG tube, if ordered, to suction the patient's stomach contents, to prevent aspiration, and to test for blood.

Your patient's breathing may be disrupted by anything that affects his airway, by central respiratory depression resulting from a central nervous system (CNS) injury, or by trauma that disrupts his chest wall or lungs. Cover an open ("sucking") chest wound immediately to prevent pneumothorax, and check for blunt chest trauma that may have produced a flail chest, pulmonary or myocardial contusion, hemothorax, or pneumothorax. (See these entries in Chapters 4 and 5.) If your patient has central respiratory depression, expect the doctor to intubate him; provide immediate ventilations by Ambu bag or mechanical ventilation. If the patient's chest wall is disrupted or the doctor suspects hemothorax or pneumothorax, expect to assist with insertion of a chest tube to drain fluid and air and to allow normal lung expansion. Provide supplementary oxygen by nasal cannula or mask or through the endotracheal tube. And be sure you check the patient's arterial blood gases (ABGs) frequently.

Expect to maintain your patient's circulation by using direct pressure to halt any external hemorrhage and by replacing lost fluids and blood. But check your patient's carotid pulse first—he may be in cardiac arrest from:
• direct cardiac injury
• respiratory failure and resulting hypoxia
• cardiac tamponade
• tension pneumothorax
• hypovolemic shock.

*Start CPR immediately if you don't feel a pulse* (see the "Life Support" section of this chapter). Remember, however, that CPR won't be effective until you've restored fluid volume in a patient who's suffered massive hemorrhage. Why? Because he has no blood to pump. To restore his fluid volume, insert large-bore I.V. lines immediately—at least two and, for some patients, as many as four, one in each extremity. The doctor may perform a venous cutdown if he can't find an adequate peripheral vein and can't insert a central venous line. Infuse fluids as ordered, and assist the doctor as necessary with insertion of a CVP line to monitor the patient's fluid balance. Insert an indwelling (Foley) catheter to measure his urine output. (If you see blood at the meatus, expect the doctor to call a urologist to evaluate the patient before catheterization.) Draw blood for necessary laboratory tests and for typing and cross matching; transfuse blood as ordered. Take an EKG, and start the patient on a cardiac monitor.

Your patient with multiple trauma is at risk for hypovolemic shock even if his cardiac status is initially stable. Monitor his pulse and blood pressure frequently. If you suspect severe internal bleeding, apply a MAST suit, as ordered, to increase his blood flow to his vital organs.

Quickly check your patient's *mental status.* Look for an altered level of consciousness, which may indicate neurologic damage, inadequate perfusion, or inadequate oxygenation. Perform a quick pupil check and assess his extraocular movements (see *Assessing Extraocular Muscle Function,* page 69). Note decorticate (abnormal flexion) or decerebrate (abnormal extension) posturing, indicating CNS damage. Examine his ears, nose, and mouth for CSF drainage.

## HANDLE WITH CARE

*Always* assume cervical spine injury in any patient who's been in a serious traffic or diving accident or who's fallen from a significant height. Remember, improper handling *can* damage his spinal cord. To prevent this, be sure to immobilize his chest first, then his head and neck, and maintain immobilization until X-rays rule out spinal injury. Use a cervical backboard, a cervical collar, or sandbags, or tape his forehead and chest to the stretcher.

If you must open his airway, *don't* use the head-tilt/chin-lift or head-tilt/neck-lift methods—you don't want to hyperextend his neck. Instead, use the jaw-thrust without head-tilt method.

## Secondary assessment pointers

Your secondary assessment of a patient with multiple trauma will focus more on *objective* findings and less on *subjective* findings than with other emergency patients. This is because you're not determining a chief complaint. Instead, you're quickly assessing all his major injuries.

Use the five questions of the AMPLE mnemonic to provide you with essential *subjective* history information. You need to know about the patient's:

• *Allergies.* He'll be receiving many medications, and you want to avoid an allergic reaction or anaphylaxis.

• *Medications.* Certain medications (especially anticoagulants) will affect his care; others provide clues to specific health problems.

• *Previous diseases.* If he has diseases such as diabetes, renal disease, coronary artery disease, or asthma, he may need special drug therapy or monitoring.

• *Last meal eaten.* If he's eaten recently, he may vomit and aspirate his stomach contents, especially if he's given an anesthetic for surgery.

• *Events leading to trauma.* A history of the injury-causing event may help you predict some of the patient's injuries.

Perform a quick head-to-toe assessment, using your understanding of the mechanisms of trauma to help you focus your rapid examination. (See *Head-to-Toe Emergency Assessment Checklist*, pages 72 and 73, and *Using Accident Information to Predict Injuries*, pages 76 to 78.) Remember, be particularly alert to the possibility of associated and secondary injuries in patients with multiple trauma.

# Pediatric Patients

Both your primary and secondary emergency assessments will be different if your patient is a child. Why? Because his developing body predisposes him to special problems that threaten his airway, breathing, and circulation. Also, his anxiety and (if he's very young) inability to communicate make secondary assessment more difficult. You'll use the same basic skills you reviewed in the "Primary Assessment: What to Do First" and "Secondary Assessment: What to Do Next" entries in this chapter, with the following important differences.

## Primary assessment pointers

Airway obstruction and breathing difficulties, especially in infants and young children, are most often the result of viral infection. But remember, children commonly aspirate food, such as candy or peanuts, or small objects, such as toys or buttons. A young child's tongue, proportionately larger than an adult's, is more likely to block his airway if he's unconscious or has a seizure. And swelling or mucus—for example, in a child with croup or epiglottitis—may easily occlude his narrow airway. Be alert for signs of respiratory distress in any child with an emergency. These signs include:

• tachypnea (probably the first sign)
• intracostal, subcostal, or suprasternal retractions
• expiratory grunts
• nasal flaring
• wheezing
• cyanosis
• paradoxical breathing.

If the child's airway is occluded, use the head-tilt/neck-lift technique or use the 'sniff' position to try to open it (see *Opening the Airway*, page 98). If these methods don't work, insert an appropriate-size artificial airway. The doctor may decide to intubate the child or, if the obstruction can't be bypassed, to perform an emergency cricothyrotomy. (See *Performing Cricothyrotomy and Percutaneous Transtracheal Catheter Ventilation*, pages 100 and 101.)

As you probably know, infants are obligate nose-breathers. So if an in-

# ASSESSING A PEDIATRIC PATIENT'S BLOOD PRESSURE, PULSE, AND RESPIRATORY RATE

When examining a newborn (NB), an infant, a child, or an adolescent, use these charts as a guide to normal parameters.

**KEY:** Upper limit _ _ _ _ _ _ _ _ _ _ _    Mean _____    Lower limit ● ● ● ● ● ● ● ●

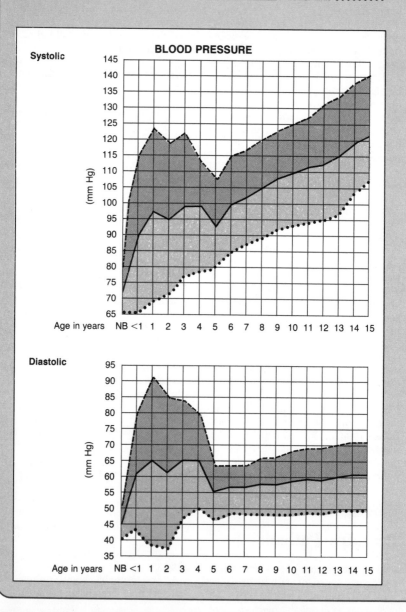

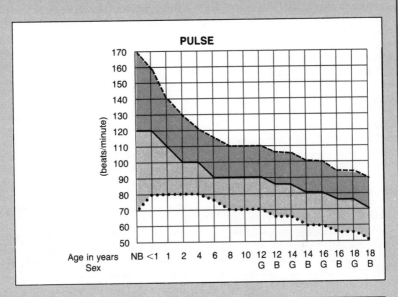

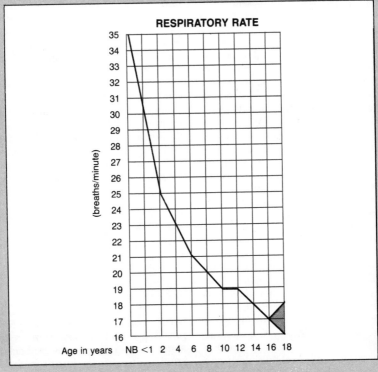

fant's cold is congesting or obstructing his nostrils, he'll have to breathe through his mouth, and this can create breathing difficulties. Assess his respiratory rate, remembering that, in infants and young children, breathing is primarily diaphragmatic and thoracic excursion is minimal. You may find it easier to obtain a respiratory rate if you observe *abdominal* rather than *thoracic* excursion. Assess the rate for more than the usual 30 to 60 seconds to obtain an accurate count, because infants may have periodic breathing with variable rates, changing every 15 to 30 seconds. Also, a child's respiratory rate is more responsive than an adult's to illness, emotion, and exercise—it may double if he's stressed.

When you assess your pediatric patient's circulation, remember that you can feel a carotid pulse in an older child, but you may *not* be able to feel it in an infant. Auscultate his apical pulse, or palpate his brachial pulse, because these are easier to assess. Note any increase, decrease, or irregularity, remembering that heart rate in infants and children is labile and more sensitive to stressful events. Keep in mind that many children normally have sinus arrhythmia, in which heart rate increases with inspiration and decreases with expiration. If your patient's able to cooperate, ask him to hold his breath for a few seconds—his heart rate will become regular if he has sinus arrhythmia but will continue to be irregular if he has a true dysrhythmia.

When you interpret your patient's blood pressure readings, remember that systolic blood pressure increases gradually during childhood. (See *Assessing a Pediatric Patient's Blood Pressure, Pulse, and Respiratory Rate*, pages 84 and 85.) First, try to auscultate his blood pressure. If your patient's younger than age 1, auscultation may be difficult. Use a Doppler device, if available, which gives you a more accurate and reliable reading. If a Doppler device isn't available, determine his systolic pressure by *palpating* the

radial artery and recording the point at which you first feel a pulse. Typically, your reading will be about 10 mm Hg lower than if you'd auscultated the child's systolic blood pressure.

If your patient's an infant, and none of the above methods for taking his blood pressure worked, use the flush technique, which allows you to obtain a value somewhere between his systolic and diastolic pressures. To do this, place a blood-pressure cuff on the infant's arm or leg, and then wrap it snugly in an elastic bandage. Inflate the cuff to a pressure above a normal systolic pressure and remove the bandage. Reduce the cuff pressure slowly until color returns, flushing the extremity. Note the pressure reading.

If your patient has an external wound or suspected internal bleeding, be careful that you don't underestimate the degree of his blood loss—even minor blood loss may be significant. The child's compensatory mechanisms (particularly increased vasoconstriction) may mask signs of blood loss by maintaining pulse rate and blood pressure within a normal range until his blood loss is extreme. You may not be aware of this until the child enters severe and refractory shock.

More often than an adult, an infant or young child may experience dehydration and shock from excessive diarrhea or vomiting, polyuria, fever, or burns—his greater surface area–to–weight ratio makes his obligatory water losses greater. And he'll lose water more rapidly because a larger proportion of his total body water is maintained as extracellular fluid. If your patient's an infant, check his anterior fontanelle—if it's depressed, you know he's dehydrated. (If it's tense and bulging, notify the doctor *immediately*—this may be a sign of increased intracranial pressure and serious CNS illness.) Assess his hydration by gently pinching a fold of loose skin on his abdomen: if it doesn't bounce back to normal after you lift it, he's probably dehydrated.

Give your patient oral or I.V. fluids, as ordered, at the first signs of dehydration. Remember, however, that an infant or young child is also more susceptible to iatrogenic *over*hydration than an adult, so monitor his fluid balance carefully.

**Secondary assessment pointers**
Take your patient's temperature as soon as you've stabilized his airway, breathing, and circulation. When you take your patient's temperature, remember that this vital sign is more labile in infants and young children than in older children and adults. (For example, a child's normal rectal temperature may rise as high as 101° F. [38.3° C.] in the late afternoon.) An infant with a severe infection may have a normal or even a subnormal temperature, and a young child may have a very high temperature from even a minor infection. So the degree of his fever does not always correlate with the severity of his illness.

Pay attention to the child's mental status—a sick infant may be extremely irritable or listless, whereas a toddler may sulk or scream. An older child who's sick may be tearful, withdrawn, or irritable. Watch how the child uses his eyes—if he looks around and curiously observes his environment, his illness probably isn't too severe. Ask your patient's parents how the child's behavior differs from normal—unusual behavior tells you something's wrong.

Remember that your approach to the patient and his family may determine your success in obtaining useful information. If possible, given the emergency situation, take a few moments to get acquainted with both the child and his family. Be attentive to the needs of both—they'll be anxious and unsure of what's happening. If your patient's a young child, you'll have to rely on the parents to provide most of the subjective information. But don't exclude the child. Keep him in the room while you obtain essential information, and let

him describe how he feels if he's willing and able to do so.

When you examine your patient, you may need to alter your usual head-to-toe emergency assessment approach. Consider the maneuvers you need to perform, and try to proceed from the least threatening to the most threatening. This will keep his level of distress as manageable as possible for as long as possible. For example, try to examine his eyes, ears, and mouth *later* in your examination, and take his blood pressure last of all (if possible); these procedures can be frightening. Examine the child's respiratory and cardiovascular function *first,* when he's quiet. Auscultate his bowel sounds next (if appropriate). Keep your patient warm throughout the examination and, if it's helpful, have the child's parents hold him or stay nearby and within sight while you examine him.

# Geriatric Patients

When you assess an elderly patient in an emergency, you'll use the same techniques you would for any other adult. However, you need to take into account the physiologic and biological changes that are a normal part of the aging process. Decreased respiratory and cardiovascular function may make your patient more susceptible to airway, breathing, and circulation difficulties; decreased function in other body systems may compound the effects of an emergency condition. And your elderly patient may have one or more chronic diseases that complicate his management and care.

**Primary assessment pointers**
When you assess your patient's airway, remember that he may have a diminished gag reflex and be more likely than a younger adult to aspirate stomach contents if his level of consciousness decreases. Expect the doctor to ask you

## SLOWDOWN AT SUNDOWN

In an elderly patient, *sundown syndrome*—diminished mental capacity late in the day—can seriously hinder your emergency assessment. Why? On the one hand, a patient who's confused or disoriented may give inaccurate or misleading answers to your assessment questions. On the other hand, you may mistake his slowed responses for signs indicating illness or injury.

You need to use your best communication skills in this situation. Speak to your elderly patient slowly and clearly, then give him time for organizing his thoughts and for responding to your questions. Reassure him with a calm attitude, a comforting touch, and regular eye contact. If you can, double-check the accuracy of his information by asking a family member or friend.

to insert an NG tube in an effort to reduce this risk. Your patient's diminished ciliary activity and decreased ability to cough mean he's also more likely to have a small-airway disorder or pulmonary infection that makes breathing difficult; the doctor may need to intubate an elderly patient and to provide ventilatory assistance more commonly than for a younger adult.

Other factors that affect your geriatric patient's breathing include:
• decreased maximum breathing capacity
• decreased inspiratory reserve volume
• decreased vital capacity
• decreased forced expiratory volume
• increased residual volume.

The result? Lowered tolerance for oxygen debt.

If your patient isn't breathing, start CPR as described in the "Life Support" section, and have someone call a code. Remember: Don't be timid when you give chest compressions—although you may fear breaking his ribs because of his osteoporosis and decreased muscle mass, you must give compressions strong enough to perfuse his vital organs.

If he is breathing, check his respirations for rate, depth, and pattern—and, of course, report any abnormalities to the doctor.

If he has respiratory distress, expect to provide supplemental oxygen, even though he may have chronic obstructive pulmonary disease. Your patient's decreased ventilatory capacity and decreased erythrocyte mass mean he's at high risk for hypoxemia, and you *must* oxygenate him to prevent tissue damage.

Your patient's advanced age affects his circulation, too. He probably has:
• decreased cardiac output (decreased by as much as 35% in many patients older than age 70)
• decreased arterial wall elasticity
• arterial and venous insufficiency.
So he's more likely than a younger adult to have chronic heart disease, hypertension, and atherosclerosis—all posing additional risks for him in an emergency. Expect him to have a slower heart rate because of his increased vagal tone; if he has a sclerosed aorta, you may also note elevated systolic blood pressure with normal diastolic pressure.

When you take your elderly patient's pulse and blood pressure, try to evaluate your results against what's normal for your patient. Take his blood pressure in both arms. Remember that his peripheral pulses may *normally* be decreased if he has chronic venous and arterial insufficiency—so weak or absent peripheral pulses don't necessarily indicate shock or circulatory impairment in this patient.

### Secondary assessment pointers

Data collection for your *secondary assessment* may be difficult if your elderly patient has decreased mental function. This is because:
• He may have syncope or be confused as the result of cerebral hypoperfusion.
• Neuron degeneration may be causing decreased sensory function and men-

tation. (See *Slowdown at Sundown.*)

Remember to sit close to your patient, to face him, and to speak to him slowly. (He may have both vision and hearing loss—and his emergency problem may be affecting his ability to communicate.) Help him focus on the most important history information. He'll probably have an extensive past medical history—and difficulty relating it chronologically. Help him by asking questions that keep him on track. For example, you might ask him if he had a particular illness, injury, or operation before or after his last birthday or another chronological landmark, such as a holiday or a major news event.

If possible, obtain a detailed medication history that includes over-the-counter medications (he may be taking a number of different drugs). See if he has a list of his medications and dosages or has brought his bottles into the hospital. Make sure you ask how and when he takes his medications. When he *last* took medication is particularly important if he's diabetic and taking insulin or has heart disease and is taking cardiac drugs. Remember, his chief complaint may be related to:
• failure to take his medications as prescribed.
• overdoses of medications, such as digitalis or antiarrhythmics.

Your elderly patient's pain tolerance may be increased, or his pain sensations may be different from a younger adult's if he has sensory loss. Make sure you don't underestimate the urgency of his emergency condition because he isn't reporting severe pain.

When you examine your patient, remember that he may have decreased function in all his body systems. Expect him to have decreased intestinal motility, decreased renal function, decreased sensation and reflexes, reduced muscle mass, and weakened joints and bones. If he's suffered trauma, be particularly alert to the possibility that even a small amount of force may have caused a hip or pelvic fracture or other trauma-related injuries.

# Pregnant Patients

If your patient's pregnant, the emergency may threaten both her and her child's life and well-being. For example, if your patient becomes hypoxemic or develops shock, her child is at risk, as well. And any injury may trigger a spontaneous abortion.

Certain normal body changes during pregnancy may complicate management of her emergency condition. Her breathing may be hindered if she's near term, with her uterus displacing the diaphragm upward. She'll have an increased respiratory rate—although her vital capacity won't change—because increased hormone levels allow ligament relaxation and an increase in her anteroposterior dimension. Make sure to provide supplemental oxygen at the first signs of respiratory distress, to make sure both your patient and the fetus are adequately oxygenated.

She'll also have decreased stomach emptying time, and she may be subject to reflux of stomach contents—so expect to insert an NG tube if her level of consciousness is decreased and you're afraid she may vomit and aspirate.

When you assess your pregnant patient's circulation, remember that her systolic and diastolic blood pressures will fall in midpregnancy and return to normal in her third trimester. Find out what her normal pressure is—a rise of 30 mm Hg systolic or 15 mm Hg diastolic above her normal pressure is abnormal, and you should report this to the doctor *immediately*. Her pulse rate will be elevated by about 10 beats/minute above her normal rate; her heart will be enlarged and displaced upward and to the left. If she's suffered trauma, remember that she may not develop signs and symptoms of shock as quickly as a nonpregnant woman, because her blood volume during pregnancy is normally increased by as much as 1,500 ml. Her body will eventually respond to decreased blood volume with vasoconstriction to the uterus, assuring perfusion of her vital organs. However, this means that the *fetus* is at high risk for hypoxia. Your patient may also have dependent edema without underlying cardiovascular problems, because she has increased venous pressure in her legs and feet from compression of her pelvic veins.

During your *secondary assessment,* consider the position of the fetus if your patient's experienced trauma to the abdomen. Early in pregnancy, the fetus lies within the bony pelvis, which protects it. Later, however, the uterus rises above the pelvis, making the fetus more vulnerable to trauma. Paradoxically, the enlarged uterus protects the mother's abdominal organs to some degree if she suffers blunt or penetrating trauma. And her major blood vessels are *posterior* to the uterus, so they're less likely to be injured by a penetrating object.

If your patient's unconscious and you can't determine the gestational age of her fetus, estimate it by evaluating fundal height. Measure from the mother's symphysis pubis to the top of the uterine fundus: between week 18 and week 32 of pregnancy, fundal height in centimeters is equivalent to gestational age in weeks. Of course, you'll note any vaginal bleeding and report it to the doctor *immediately.* (See Chapter 12 for a complete discussion of obstetric emergencies.)

## A FINAL WORD

When you're working on the unit, you may not get a chance to use your emergency assessment skills every day. Nevertheless, you can't afford to be unprepared when one of your patients does have an emergency. And from time to time, you may be floated to the ED or a critical-care unit, where emergency assessment skills are a must. What you need, to feel sure of your ability to manage an emergency, is *practice*. It may not make you perfect—but it will make you ready. And as a nurse on the medical-surgical unit, you have more opportunities to practice emergency assessment skills than you're probably aware of. For example, a fast and accurate emergency assessment depends heavily on a thorough understanding of what's *normal*. This means that the more you practice and refine your everyday assessment skills, the more familiar you'll become with the range of normal assessment findings in many types of patients. The experience you gain will give you a more critical eye. Then, in an emergency, when you're obtaining a first impression and determining urgency, problems that might have gone undetected will leap out at you.

You can practice emergency nursing *process* on the medical-surgical unit, too. As you know, every patient who's admitted to the hospital via the ED is cared for on the unit before being discharged. When you're caring for such a patient, study his chart to learn what happened to cause his emergency, what treatment he has received (and is receiving), and what progress he's made. Then ask yourself: What if this patient's condition suddenly became critical? What would I assess him for? How would I probably intervene—for what types of problems? For example, suppose your patient on the unit has a thromboembolism; you should watch him closely for signs and symptoms of a developing pulmonary embolism. Similarly, learn to watch for signs and symptoms of diabetic ketoacidosis in a diabetic patient who develops an infection. When you've already given thought to your patient's risk of developing an emergency condition and prepared yourself to recognize clues to its development, you'll be well prepared to manage it—if it ever happens.

Don't forget to practice BLS/ACLS procedures, as well. Of course, no practice procedure has the same value as performing BLS procedures on the unit or, in a critical-care area, assisting with ACLS procedures as part of a code team. But you *can* keep yourself up to date by taking courses, by becoming certified in these life-saving techniques, and by observing and participating in as many codes as possible.

Learn to think about emergency care as part and parcel of your comprehensive nursing skills. Then, you'll always respond confidently when an emergency occurs.

## Selected References

Barber, Janet M., and Budassi, Susan A. *Mosby's Manual of Emergency Care: Practices and Procedures.* St. Louis: C.V. Mosby Co., 1979.

Budassi, Susan A., and Barber, Janet M. *Emergency Nursing: Principles and Practice.* St. Louis: C.V. Mosby Co., 1980.

Holloway, Nancy M., ed. *Core Curriculum.* Chicago: Emergency Department Nurses Association, 1980.

Kravis, Thomas C., and Warner, Carmen G. *Emergency Medicine: A Comprehensive Review.* Rockville, Md.: Aspen Systems Corp., 1982.

McIntyre, Kevin M., and Lewis, A. James, eds. *Textbook of Advanced Cardiac Life Support.* Dallas: American Heart Association, 1983.

McSwain, N. "To Manage Multiple Injury... Consider Mechanisms... in a Traffic Accident," *Emergency Medicine* 14(20):206-18, November 30, 1982.

McSwain, N. "To Manage Multiple Injury... Establish Priorities," *Emergency Medicine* 14(20):223-32, Nov. 30, 1982.

Molyneux-Luick, M. "The ABCs of Multiple Trauma," *Nursing77* 7:30-36, October 1977.

Rund, Douglas A., and Rausch, Tondra S. *Triage.* St. Louis: C.V. Mosby Co., 1981.

"Standards and Guidelines for Cardiopulmonary Resuscitation (CPR) and Emergency Cardiac Care (ECC)," *The Journal of the American Medical Association* 244(5):453-508, August 1, 1980.

Turner, S.R. "Golden Rules for Accurate Triage," *Journal of Emergency Nursing* 7:153-55, July/August 1981.

Warner, Carmen G. *Emergency Care: Assessment and Intervention,* 3rd ed. St. Louis: C.V. Mosby Co., 1982.

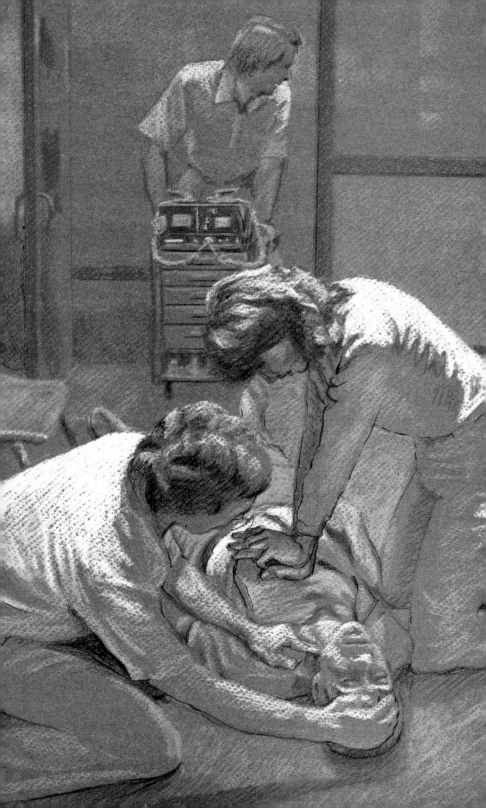

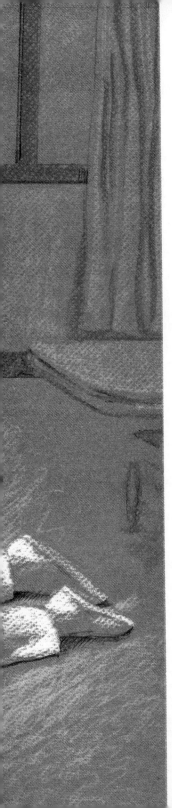

# Life Support: Performing Basic and Advanced Techniques

"Help—someone's choking!"

"He's not breathing—quick, call a code!"

Life-threatening emergencies—to a nurse, they're the ultimate challenge. You must bring all your nursing skills into action swiftly and expertly to save your patient's life.

Do you know what to do if faced with such a situation? This special section on emergency life support will teach you the procedures you need to know—or refresh your memory if you're already familiar with them. In this section, you'll learn how to:

- aid a choking victim (pages 94 to 97)
- open an obstructed airway (page 98)
- insert an artificial airway (page 99)
- assist with cricothyrotomy and percutaneous transtracheal catheter ventilation (pages 100 and 101)
- give mouth-to-mouth resuscitation (page 102)
- use an Ambu bag (page 103)
- give chest compressions (pages 104 to 106)
- perform defibrillation and cardioversion (pages 107 to 109).

The American Heart Association designates two types of emergency life-support procedures: basic life support (BLS) and advanced cardiac life support (ACLS). BLS is emergency first aid focused on recognizing respiratory or cardiac arrest and providing CPR to maintain life until the victim recovers or until ACLS is available. You can perform BLS procedures quickly, in almost any situation, without assistance or equipment. The critical factor is *time*—the quicker you start BLS, the better your patient's chances of survival.

ACLS consists of BLS plus procedures requiring special equipment (such as a defibrillator or an artificial airway) or medications. ACLS is done in hospitals, in other health-care settings, or in mobile intensive care units and requires more than one person.

As you know, life support *always* follows the "ABC" sequence: open the victim's *airway* and restore his *breathing* and *circulation,* as necessary. You'll find the procedures in this section presented in the same sequence, for easy reference.

Make sure you're familiar with BLS and ACLS procedures. One way to ensure BLS mastery is to become certified in CPR through a course sponsored by the American Heart Association or the American Red Cross. For some of your patients, it could mean the difference between life and death.

# Aiding a Choking Victim

**1.** If the victim can speak or cough, let him try to expel the obstruction on his own. If he can't speak or cough, however, he has little or no air exchange—he needs your help *immediately.*

**2.** If the victim's *conscious,* quickly move to his side and slightly behind him. Place one hand on his sternum, the other on his back, and lean him forward so his head's lower than his chest. (If the victim's a child age 1 to 8, kneel and lay him across your thighs—with his head lower than his trunk—and support his head and chest with one hand.) With the heel of your hand, deliver four rapid, sharp, forceful blows over his spine between his shoulder blades.

**3.** If the back blows don't dislodge the foreign body, prepare to deliver abdominal thrusts to the adult victim (chest thrusts to a child).

To deliver abdominal thrusts, move behind the victim and wrap your arms around his waist, making a tight fist with one hand and grasping it firmly with your other hand. Now place your clasped fist, thumb in, against his abdomen between his navel and rib cage. *Don't* tighten your arms around his rib cage.

*Back blows for a conscious victim*

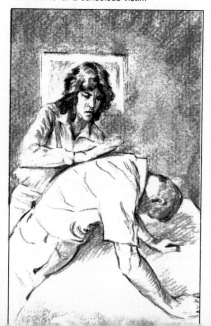

Quickly and forcefully thrust your fists up and into his abdomen, at an angle toward your own chin. Deliver four thrusts, if necessary.

If the victim's a child, you'll have to deliver chest thrusts. To do this, roll the child gently onto his back on the floor, and kneel beside him. Place the heel of one hand on his chest, at approximately the midpoint of his sternum. Deliver four chest thrusts. (Chest thrusts are preferred for infants and children because this technique's less likely to injure internal organs.)

**4.** If the victim's obese or pregnant, deliver chest thrusts instead of abdominal thrusts. To do this, stand behind the victim and wrap your arms around his or her chest. Clasp your fists as you would for abdominal thrusts, and place them in the middle of the sternum, thumbs in. Make sure your fists are above the xiphoid process and lower rib cage—improper fist placement could result in internal injuries when you thrust.

Quickly and forcefully thrust your fists into the chest, straight back toward you. *Don't* tighten your arms around the chest. Deliver a total of four thrusts, if necessary.

**5.** Reassess the victim's air exchange. If it's not adequate, repeat the series of back blows and abdominal or chest thrusts until he either expels the foreign body or becomes unconscious. (Do this for a child, as well, using back blows and chest thrusts.)

**6.** If an adult or child victim *loses consciousness,* his throat muscles may relax, partially opening his airway. If this happens, roll him onto his back and attempt to ventilate him.

**7.** If you can't ventilate the victim, prepare to deliver more back blows. Kneel at the victim's side, roll him toward you, and support him against your thighs. With the heel of your hand, deliver four sharp back blows over his spine between his shoulder blades.

**8.** Roll him onto his back and check his air exchange. If it's not adequate, you'll have to deliver abdominal thrusts (for an adult) or chest thrusts (for a child or an obese or pregnant adult).

**9.** To deliver abdominal thrusts when the victim's unconscious, kneel at his side

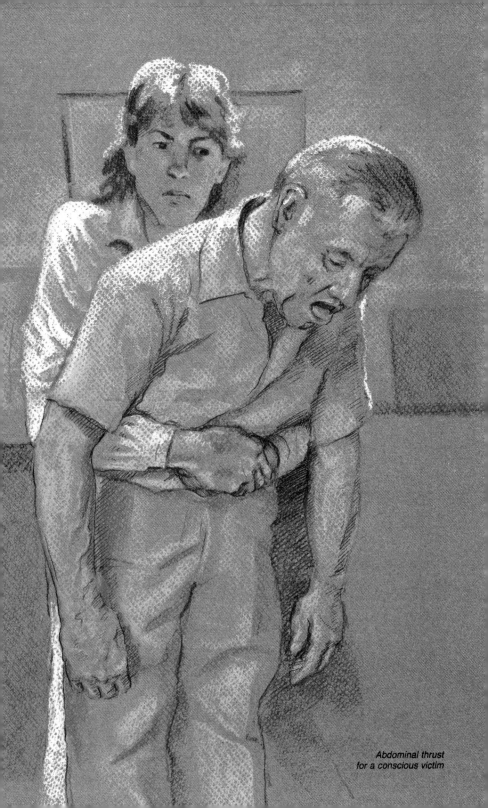

Abdominal thrust
for a conscious victim

(or straddle him) at hip level. Place the heel of one hand on his abdomen, halfway between navel and rib cage. Cover it with your other hand, and interlock your fingers. Lean forward so your shoulders and hands are in line, and deliver four sharp thrusts in and up.

**10.** If you must deliver chest thrusts when the victim's unconscious, kneel beside him at his chest level. Position your hands as you would for cardiac compression, and deliver four sharp downward thrusts.

**11.** Reassess his air exchange. If it's inadequate, prepare to do a finger sweep to find and remove any foreign object. (Caution: *Never* do a blind finger sweep on an infant or child—you could force a foreign object

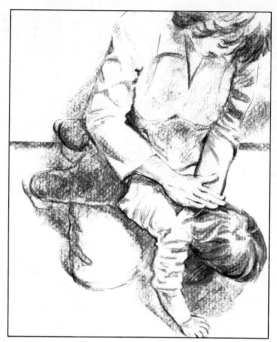

*Back blows for a child*

deeper into his throat, completely obstructing the airway.)

**12.** Position the victim on his back and open his mouth using the tongue-jaw-lift technique. Grasp his lower jaw and his tongue between your thumb and fingers and lift. This technique pulls his tongue away from the back of his throat and may partially relieve the obstruction.

If you can't open his mouth with the tongue-jaw lift, try the crossed-finger technique. Cross your thumb and index finger; place your thumb on his upper teeth and your finger on his lower teeth. Then open his mouth by pushing up with your thumb and down with your finger.

Once his mouth's opened, insert the index

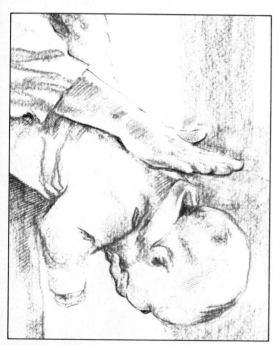

*Back blows for a choking infant*

finger of your other hand down along the inside of his cheek to the base of his tongue. If you feel the obstruction, use a hooking motion to dislodge it and lift it out. *Be extremely careful to avoid pushing it deeper.*

**13.** Reposition his head and try to ventilate him. If you can't, repeat the series of back blows, abdominal or chest thrusts, and finger sweeps until he has adequate air exchange or until advanced life support is available.

**14.** To aid a choking *infant* (under age 1), first turn him onto his abdomen and lay him along one of your arms, keeping his head lower than his trunk. Support his head in your hand.

With the heel of your other hand, deliver four back blows between his shoulder blades. Deliver each blow less forcefully than you would for a child or adult.

Check his air exchange. If it's inadequate, gently turn him over, keeping his head and neck supported in your hand.

Lay him on his back across your thigh, with his head lower than his trunk. Place your index and middle fingers of one hand on his chest, between his nipples. Deliver four chest thrusts, being careful not to use too much force.

Check his air exchange again. Has it improved? If not, repeat the series of back blows and chest thrusts. If your efforts are unsuccessful and the infant becomes unconscious, you'll have to open his airway and ventilate him (see *Opening the Airway,* page 98, and *Giving Mouth-to-Mouth Resuscitation,* page 102).

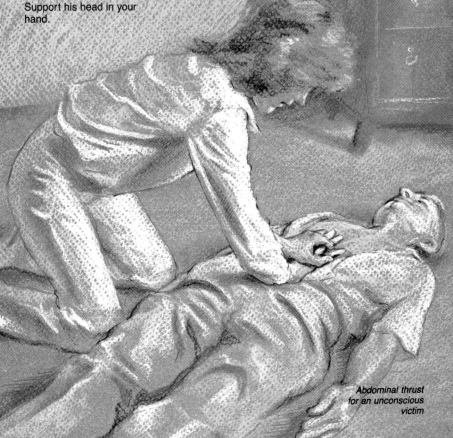

*Abdominal thrust for an unconscious victim*

# Opening the Airway

If your unconscious patient's tongue falls back and occludes his airway, place him on his back and use one of the following methods to open his airway. (Use only the third method if you suspect neck or spine injury.)

To use the *head-tilt/chin-lift* method, hyperextend your patient's neck by placing one hand on his forehead and tilting his head back slightly. Gently lift his chin up with the fingertips of your other hand, being careful not to close his mouth completely.

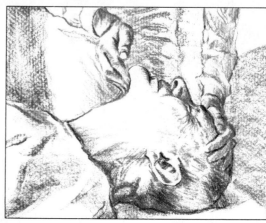
*Head-tilt/chin-lift method*

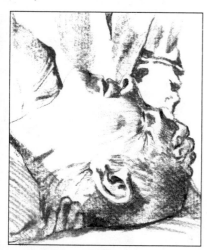
*Head-tilt/neck-lift method*

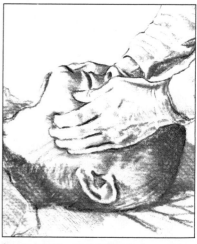
*Jaw-thrust without head-tilt method*

To use the *head-tilt/neck-lift* method, place one hand on the patient's forehead and your other hand under his neck close to the back of his head. Push his forehead back while gently lifting up and supporting his neck.

To use the *jaw-thrust without head-tilt* method (when you suspect a neck or spine injury), place yourself behind the victim's head. Grasp his lower jaw by placing your thumbs on his mandibles near the corners of his mouth, pointing your thumbs toward his feet. Your fingertips should be at the angles of his jaw. Lift his lower jaw upward with your index fingers while pushing your thumbs down. This action causes the patient's jaw to jut forward without hyperextending his neck.

After opening the victim's airway, check to see if his breathing's restored.

*Reminder:* Don't hyperextend an infant's neck as much as you would an adult's. Overextension may block the infant's airway or damage his spinal cord.

# Inserting an Artificial Airway

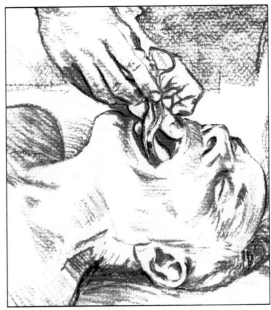

*Insertion of an oropharyngeal airway*

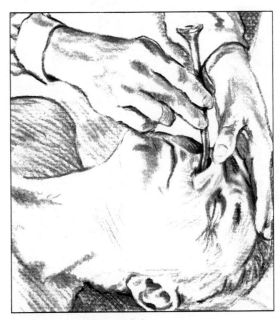

*Insertion of a nasopharyngeal airway*

When the doctor isn't available or when he doesn't choose to perform endotracheal intubation, use these techniques to keep an unconscious victim's tongue from falling back and occluding his airway. (Note: If paramedics have inserted an esophageal obturator airway, *don't* remove it to insert one of these other airways—wait until the doctor arrives.)

*To insert an oropharyngeal airway,* you may use the crossed-finger or the tongue-blade technique. For the crossed-finger technique, place your thumb on the victim's upper teeth and your index finger on his lower teeth, and gently push his mouth open. Then, slide the tip of the curved rubber or plastic airway back over the patient's tongue upside down. (Attempting to insert the airway in its "normal" position is likely to push the tongue back, further obstructing the airway.) Or, point the tip toward his cheek, push gently, and then rotate the airway until it's pointing down.

For the tongue blade technique, open the victim's mouth and depress his tongue with a tongue blade. Guide the artificial airway in the normal position over the back of his tongue until it's in place.

*To insert a nasopharyngeal airway,* push up the tip of his nose and gently slide the lubricated soft-rubber or plastic tube into his nostril. Secure the airway.

# Performing Cricothyrotomy and Percutaneous Transtracheal Catheter Ventilation

If all your efforts to relieve your patient's airway obstruction fail, and he still has inadequate air exchange, you may have to perform cricothyrotomy or percutaneous transtracheal catheter ventilation to gain rapid entry into the patient's airway until the doctor can establish a definitive airway. (Of course, you'd do this only if you were specially trained and if no doctor was available.) Cricothyrotomy is the more effective method of providing short-term ventilation, but the procedure may interrupt cardiac compression. Transtracheal catheter ventilation takes only about 30 seconds to perform and can be done without hindering CPR.

To begin either procedure, place the patient on his back and hyperextend his head and neck. Locate the cricothyroid membrane by palpating his neck, starting at the top. (The first prominence you'll feel is the thyroid cartilage; the second, the cricoid cartilage. The space between the two is the cricothyroid membrane.) Prepare the incision site with a broad-spectrum antimicrobial, such as povidone-iodine. Then proceed as follows, depending on the procedure you're performing:

**Cricothyrotomy**
**1.** Make a horizontal incision, less than

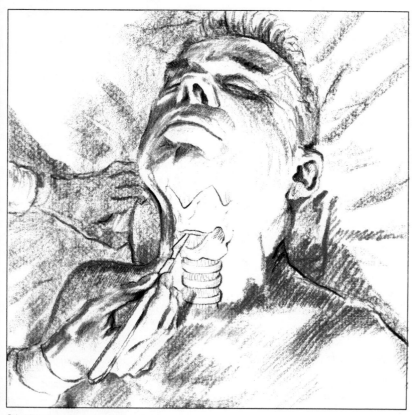

*Cricothyrotomy performed with scapel*

½″ (1.3 cm) long, with the scalpel, cutting through the patient's skin and the membrane. Then insert the scalpel handle and rotate it 90° to spread the cartilage.

**2.** Insert a small tube (#6 tracheostomy tube or similar-sized device) into the opening, and secure it.

**3.** Attach the tube to an Ambu bag or other ventilation device to provide positive-pressure ventilation with high oxygen concentration.

**Percutaneous Transtracheal Catheter Ventilation**

**1.** Attach a 14G (or larger) plastic I.V. catheter with a needle to a 10-ml syringe.

**2.** Carefully insert the needle and catheter through the patient's skin and membrane, aiming downward and caudally at a 45° angle to the trachea.

**3.** Maintain negative pressure on the syringe as you advance the needle and catheter. You'll know the needle has entered the patient's trachea when air enters the syringe.

**4.** When the needle's in his trachea, advance the catheter over the needle and carefully remove both needle and syringe.

**5.** Here's how to provide *jet insufflation* (a temporary technique of providing intermittent ventilation to a patient with a percutaneous transtracheal catheter). Attach I.V. extension tubing to the hub of the catheter and attach a hand-operated release valve and then a pressure-regulating adjustment valve to the other end of the I.V. tubing. Connect the entire assembly to an oxygen source.

**6.** Press the release valve to introduce an oxygen jet into the patient's trachea to inflate his lung. When his lungs are visibly inflated, release the valve to allow passive exhalation. Adjust the pressure-regulating valve to the minimum pressure needed for adequate lung inflation.

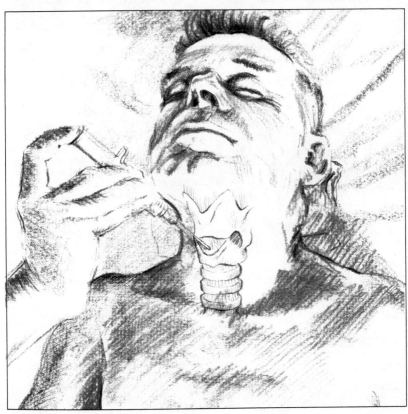

*Insertion of transtracheal catheter*

# Giving Mouth-to-Mouth Resuscitation

If you've opened the victim's airway, but he's still not breathing, begin artificial respiration immediately.

**1.** If the victim's an *adult* or *child*, keep his neck hyperextended. (If you suspect cervical spine injury, use the jaw-thrust without head-tilt method instead of hyperextension.)

**2.** With your hand on the victim's forehead, pinch his nostrils closed. Maintain pressure on his forehead. (If you're using the jaw-thrust without head-tilt method, seal his nostrils by pressing your cheek against them.)

**3.** Take a deep breath, then make a tight seal by placing your mouth around his mouth.

**4.** Quickly breathe into his mouth four times, completely refilling your lungs after each breath. Don't allow his lungs to deflate fully between breaths. This maintains positive pressure in his lungs.

**5.** Watch for his chest to rise and then fall with each breath, confirming that air is entering and leaving his lungs. If you don't see chest movement, recheck

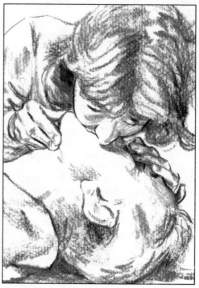

*Mouth-to-mouth resuscitation for an adult or child*

his head position and make sure your mouth seal is tight. Try to ventilate him again. If you're still unsuccessful, assume his airway is obstructed and begin using back blows and the abdominal or chest-thrust procedure.

**6.** If you do see chest movement, check his carotid pulse.

**7.** If you feel a pulse, but he's still not breathing, give him one breath every 5 seconds. Until he begins to breathe again, check for a carotid pulse after every 12 ventilations.

**8.** If you can't feel a pulse, initiate cardiac compressions with ventilations immediately.

For an *infant,* modify the adult resuscitation procedure slightly, as follows:

**1.** Tilt his head back *only slightly,* to prevent tracheal collapse.

**2.** Place your mouth over his mouth *and* nose.

**3.** Inflate his lungs with small puffs of air—just enough to make his chest rise. (Use about as much air as it takes to fill your cheeks.)

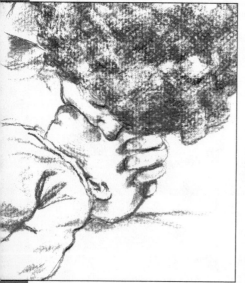

*Mouth-to-mouth-and-nose resuscitation for an infant*

# Using an Ambu Bag

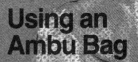

With a bag-valve-mask device, such as an Ambu bag, you can ventilate a patient with oxygen or room air.

To ventilate with oxygen (the preferred method when a source is available), attach the bag to the mask and connect the resuscitator to the oxygen tank or wall unit if either is available. (For room air, just attach the bag to the mask.) Position yourself near the vic-tim's head and hyperextend his neck (unless hyperextension's contraindicated). Place the mask over his face. Use firm pressure to seal the mask tightly, keeping his neck hyperextended. Use your free hand to compress the bag.

The resuscitator bag delivers about 1 liter of air per full compression to an adult victim. If you're ventilating an infant or small child, you'll need to use a smaller bag.

Each time you compress the bag, watch for the victim's chest to rise and fall. If it doesn't, the mask may not be sealed properly or the victim's airway may not be open. If necessary, reposition his head and check for airway obstruction.

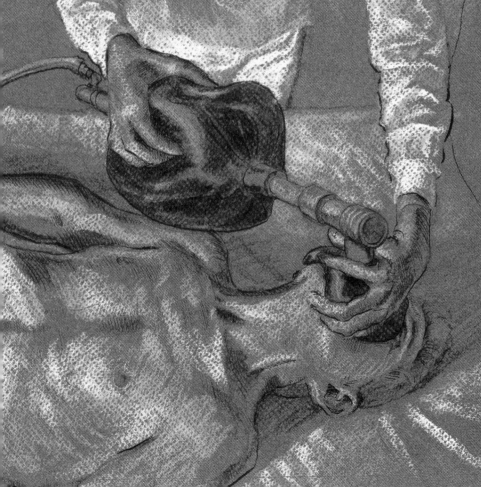

# Continuing CPR with Chest Compression and Ventilation

**For one-rescuer CPR:**
**1.** *With an adult victim,* locate his xiphoid process. Then measure up 1½" to 2" (3.8 to 5.1 cm), or about two finger widths, and place the heel of your hand at this point, on the long axis of the sternum, for chest compressions. Be careful to place your hands correctly, or you may lacerate his liver or fracture his ribs when you deliver compressions.
**2.** Place one hand on top of the other and interlock your fingers to keep them off the victim's ribs. Keeping your elbows straight, lean forward so that your hands and shoulders are in direct alignment to make full use of your body weight when delivering downward compressions.
**3.** With the heels of your hands, apply steady, smooth pressure to depress the victim's sternum 1½" to 2" (3.8 to 5.1 cm).

*(continued)*

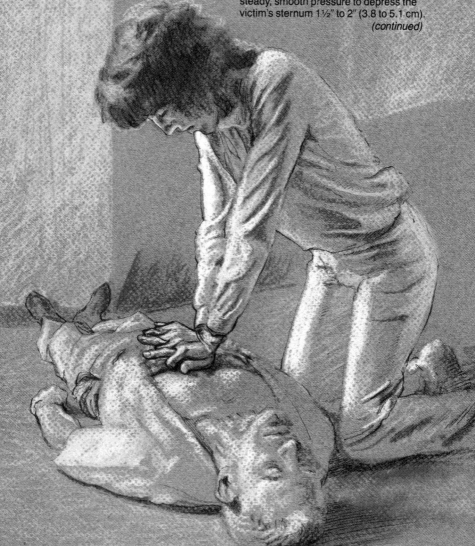

*Chest compressions for an adult*

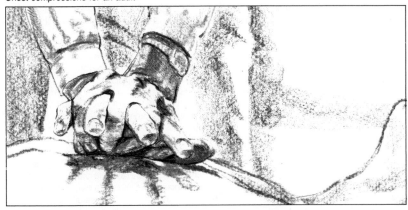

*Chest compressions for an infant*

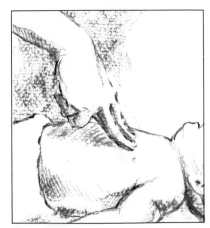

*Chest compressions for a child*

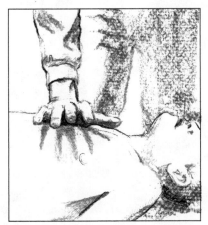

This forces blood from the heart's chambers. Then relax the pressure completely to allow the victim's heart to fill with blood. Don't let your hands leave his chest when you release the pressure, or you may lose the correct hand position.

**4.** Time your compressions at a rate of 80 per minute. To keep these compressions smooth and rhythmic, count aloud, "One and, two and, three and...." After every 15 chest compressions, give the victim two quick lung inflations without allowing him to exhale fully between breaths. (Actually, you'll be delivering 60 compressions per minute because of the time lost while ventilating your patient.)

**5.** After performing CPR for 1 minute, check his carotid pulse for 5 seconds. If it's absent, give him two more ventilations, to ensure adequate oxygenation, and resume CPR.

*If your patient's a child,* locate the pressure point using the same technique you would use for an adult. Then, using the heel of *one* hand, depress his sternum about 1" to 1½" (2.5 to 3.8 cm). Give 80 compressions per minute, counting "One and, two and, three and...." Give a breath after every fifth compression.

*With an infant,* check his brachial pulse (located on the inside of his upper arm at the midpoint)—his carotid pulse is hard to detect. For chest compressions, place the tips of your index and middle fingers of one hand in the middle of his chest, between his nipples. Deliver 100 compressions per minute, depressing the sternum ½" to 1" (1.3 to 2.5 cm). Give a breath after every fifth compression. Usually, one rescuer alone can handle this.

**For two-rescuer CPR:**
**1.** Position yourself and the other rescuer on opposite sides of the victim, facing each other.
**2.** As your partner opens the victim's airway and tries to locate his carotid pulse, continue giving compressions.
**3.** If she feels a pulse, she'll confirm that your compressions are adequate but will tell you to stop compressions for 5 seconds so she can check to see if the victim's heart is beating on its own.
**4.** If she can't feel a pulse, she'll deliver one breath, then tell you to continue chest compressions. Deliver approximately 60 compressions per minute while your partner delivers a full breath on the upstroke of every fifth compression. You should count out loud, "one-one thousand, two-one thousand, three-one thousand..." to maintain the right rhythm for two-man CPR. Your partner should check the victim's carotid pulse every few minutes.
**5.** If you get tired of giving chest compressions, you can switch positions with your partner. When you want to switch, say "*Change*-one thousand, two-one thousand, three-one thousand...." On the fifth compression, your partner gives one lung inflation and moves into place for chest compressions. You move up to the victim's head and check his pulse and breathing for 5 seconds. If you don't feel a pulse, inform your partner and continue CPR.

*Two-rescuer CPR*

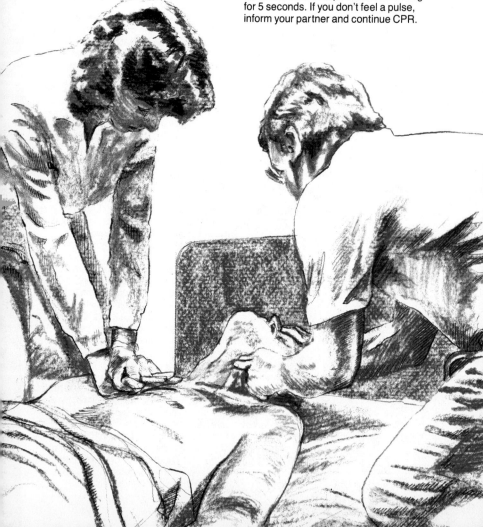

# Performing Defibrillation and Emergency Synchronized Cardioversion

Severe cardiac dysrhythmias demand immediate attention. Ventricular fibrillation, the most disorganized dysrhythmia, can stop cardiac output, causing death. If you observe that your patient's heart is in ventricular fibrillation as shown on the cardiac monitor, and the dysrhythmia doesn't revert with a precordial thump, he'll need an immediate defibrillation countershock. You'll use emergency synchronized cardioversion (employing a defibrillator) to correct less serious ventricular or supraventricular dysrhythmias.

In an emergency, you may have to do these procedures, depending on your hospital's protocol and your own specific training. Remember that defibrillators vary in their setup and operation—be sure to familiarize yourself with your hospital's equipment *before* an emergency situation arises and you have to use it.

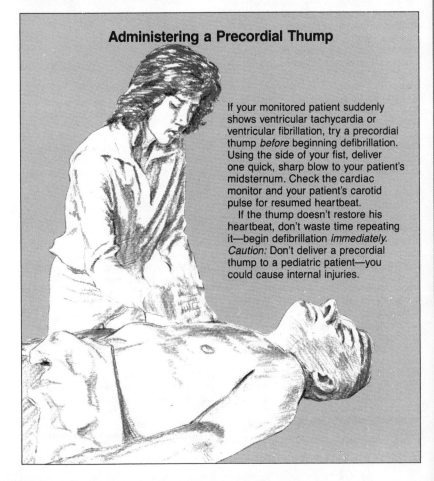

## Administering a Precordial Thump

If your monitored patient suddenly shows ventricular tachycardia or ventricular fibrillation, try a precordial thump *before* beginning defibrillation. Using the side of your fist, deliver one quick, sharp blow to your patient's midsternum. Check the cardiac monitor and your patient's carotid pulse for resumed heartbeat.

If the thump doesn't restore his heartbeat, don't waste time repeating it—begin defibrillation *immediately*. *Caution:* Don't deliver a precordial thump to a pediatric patient—you could cause internal injuries.

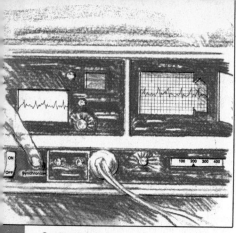

*Cardioversion*

## Here's how to defibrillate a patient with ventricular fibrillation:

**1.** You may use standard or anteroposterior (A/P) paddles. Apply special defibrillator pads if available. Otherwise, apply conductive jelly around the rim of each paddle's surface, then rub the paddles together to coat them evenly. *Never* use alcohol pads as an electrical conductor—they might ignite when the current is applied.

**2.** If you apply jelly, use just enough to coat the paddles—excess jelly may produce arcing, which can cause burns.

**3.** Turn on the defibrillator, making sure the machine is not in the synchronous mode.

**4.** Charge the paddles, selecting the correct electrical charge (200 to 300 joules, or watt-seconds, for an adult; 2 to 3.5 joules per kilogram of body weight for an infant or child).

**5.** When the paddles are fully charged, position them on your patient. To position standard paddles on a man, a child, or an infant, place one paddle to the right of his upper sternum, just below his clavicle; place the other paddle immediately to the left of his left nipple. If your patient's a woman, don't place the paddles on her breasts; position them at the mid- or anterior-axillary level.

To position A/P paddles, place the flat paddle under your patient, behind his heart and just below his left scapula. Place the other paddle directly over his heart, over the left precordium.

**6.** Recheck the rhythm on the monitor to be sure the patient's still in ventricular fibrillation.

**7.** Make sure the oxygen's turned off (if it's in use), and that the floor where

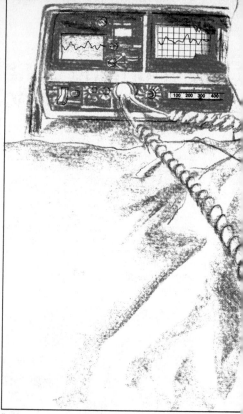

*Defibrillation*

you're standing is *dry.* Check that no one's touching the patient or his bed and make sure you're standing clear, as well.

**8.** When you're ready to discharge the paddles, loudly announce "stand clear" and give other members of the code team time to step away.

**9.** Apply firm arm pressure on each paddle to ensure good contact, and discharge the paddles by pressing both discharge buttons simultaneously (the discharging control may be on only one handle). Be sure to keep the paddles firmly in position during discharge. But don't lean on them—they could slip.

**10.** After the first discharge, check the patient's cardiac monitor. If *fibrillation has stopped,* check the patient's carotid pulse; if you can't detect an effective pulse, resume CPR. If *ventricular fibrillation persists,* defibrillate him again at the same setting as soon as possible. Continue CPR while waiting for the paddles to recharge.

**11.** If the second defibrillation doesn't stop the ventricular fibrillation, continue CPR with supplemental oxygen (to ensure

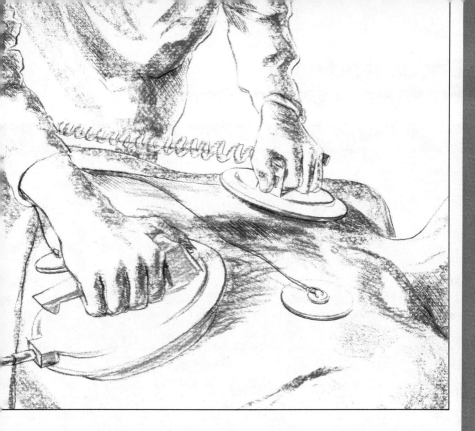

maximum oxygenation of myocardial tissue). You may also administer sodium bicarbonate I.V., as ordered (to correct metabolic acidosis), and epinephrine I.V., as ordered (to convert fine ventricular fibrillation to a higher amplitude that's more amenable to defibrillation).

**12.** Wait a few moments for the drugs to take effect; then prepare to defibrillate the patient for the third time. Apply more jelly to the paddles and reposition them. Increase the energy level (up to 360 joules for an adult). *Make sure the oxygen is shut off before you discharge the paddles.*

**13.** If the patient doesn't have an organized cardiac rhythm after three defibrillation attempts, the doctor will probably order additional drugs, such as bretylium.

**14.** If the paddles have been recharged but not used again, clear the charge by turning off the machine and turning the discharge control to zero or by pressing the "bleed" button if there is one. Don't discharge paddles into each other or into the air.

**15.** Using soap and water, clean the lubricant off the patient's skin and the paddles.

The equipment and procedure for *emergency cardioversion* is the same as that used for defibrillation, with these important differences:

● If your patient is conscious, give him I.V. diazepam, as ordered, to make him drowsy.

● Make sure the monitor's QRS complex is upright. The lead should have a maximum R-wave height.

● *Activate the synchronizer circuit.*

● For the initial countershock, deliver 200 joules of energy (for an adult), unless a lower dose is ordered.

● Press and *hold* the paddles' discharge buttons until you deliver the countershock. Remember that the countershock will synchronize with the R wave and *may not* occur exactly when you push the discharge button. Use defibrillation-level energy for additional attempts if your first try isn't successful.

● If ventricular fibrillation occurs, immediately turn off the synchronizer circuit and begin defibrillation as described.

# Understanding Emergency Cardiac Drugs

| | INDICATIONS | MECHANISM OF ACTION/EFFECTS | DOSE/ROUTE |
|---|---|---|---|
| atropine sulfate | • Used for treating excessive vagus-induced bradycardia, first degree atrioventricular (AV) block, and Mobitz I AV block | Cholinergic blocker (parasympatholytic) <br>• Inhibits action of acetylcholine <br>• Increases heart rate <br>• Decreases salivation and respiratory secretions <br>• Decreases smooth muscle spasm | • I.V. push: administer 0.5 to 1 mg over 1 to 2 minutes. Can be repeated every 5 minutes; total dose should not exceed 2 mg. |
| bretylium tosylate (Bretylol, Bretylate**) | • Used for treating ventricular dysrhythmias that are unresponsive to lidocaine | Antiarrhythmic <br>• Prolongs the refractory period <br>• Has positive inotropic effect | • I.V. push: rapidly administer 5 mg/kg; can be repeated every 15 to 30 minutes until 30 mg/kg has been given. <br>• Infusion: 500 mg diluted to at least 50 ml with dextrose 5% in water ($D_5W$) or normal saline solution; infuse at 1 to 2 mg/minute. |
| calcium chloride | • Used for treating asystole and electromechanical dissociation of the heart <br>• Used for treating hyperkalemia | Electrolyte <br>• Replaces and maintains serum calcium levels <br>• Has positive inotropic effect | • I.V. push: administer 5 to 10 ml at 1 ml/minute; can be repeated every 10 minutes. <br>• Infusion: can add to $D_5W$ or normal saline solution; flow rate should not exceed 1.5 mEq/minute. |
| digoxin (Lanoxin*, Masoxin) | • Used for treating atrial fibrillation and flutter, paroxysmal atrial tachycardia, and congestive heart failure (CHF) | Cardiotonic glycoside <br>• Increases force of myocardial contraction by promoting myocardial calcium concentration <br>• Slows conduction through AV node <br>• Prolongs AV node refractory period | • I.V. push: administer 0.5 to 1 mg divided over 24 hours, then 0.125 to 0.5 mg daily. |
| dobutamine hydrochloride (Dobutrex) | • Used in short-term treatment to increase cardiac output in cardiogenic shock and heart failure | Adrenergic (sympathomimetic) <br>• Directly stimulates the heart's beta-adrenergic receptors, increasing cardiac contractility and output | • Infusion: reconstitute with $D_5W$ or normal saline solution, then prepare standard dilution; administer 2.5 to 10 mcg/kg/minute. |
| dopamine hydrochloride (Intropin*) | • Used for treating cardiogenic shock and other hemodynamic problems, hypotension, and decreased cardiac output | Adrenergic (sympathomimetic) <br>• Stimulates adrenergic receptors (dopaminergic, alpha, and beta) <br>• Increases cardiac contractility and output <br>• Increases renal perfusion | • Infusion: standard dilution; may use with $D_5W$, dextrose 5% in normal saline solution, or dextrose 5% in ½ normal saline solution; administer 2 to 5 mcg/kg/minute, up to 50 mcg/kg/minute. |

*Available in U.S. and Canada. **Available in Canada only. All other products (no symbol) available in U.S. only.

During a code, seconds are crucial and the margin for error is narrow. You can increase your effectiveness during a code by making sure you're familiar with the drugs used to treat life-threatening cardiac conditions. You need to know each drug's mechanism of action, usual dose, and route of administration. The chart below provides this information, along with important precautions and nursing considerations to keep in mind when you administer emergency cardiac drugs.

| PRECAUTIONS | NURSING CONSIDERATIONS |
|---|---|
| • Lower doses (less than 0.5 mg) may *cause* bradycardia rather than *correct* it.<br>• Higher doses (more than 2 mg) may cause full vagal blockage.<br>• Contraindicated for glaucoma patients (isoproterenol should be used instead).<br>• May increase ischemic area in patients with acute myocardial infarction (MI); use only if bradycardia is severe and symptomatic.<br>• Use cautiously in patients with benign prostate hypertrophy. | • Monitor cardiac rhythm for heart rate greater than 110 beats/minute and for premature ventricular contractions (PVCs).<br>• Monitor for urine retention.<br>• Maintain hydration and oral moisture. |
| • Generally not used to treat PVCs unless other drugs fail.<br>• May increase digitalis toxicity.<br>• May potentiate hypotension. | • Keep your patient supine to minimize orthostatic changes.<br>• Be prepared for vomiting after rapid administration of undiluted drug.<br>• Monitor blood pressure, pulse, and cardiac rhythm. |
| • Contraindicated in patients with hypercalcemia.<br>• Infiltration may produce severe tissue damage.<br>• Use cautiously in patients receiving digoxin; may cause dysrhythmias.<br>• Do not give to patients with high serum phosphate levels; may produce fatal calcium phosphate deposits in vital organs.<br>• Do not mix with any other medications—it will precipitate. | • Monitor for normal serum calcium levels (8.5 to 10.5 mg/100 ml, or 4.5 to 5.8 mEq/liter).<br>• Remind the doctor if your patient is receiving digoxin.<br>• Monitor for bradycardia and for decreased QT interval. |
| • Toxic levels may cause life-threatening dysrhythmias, hypotension, or severe CHF.<br>• Do not administer calcium salts to a digitalized patient.<br>• Use with caution in elderly patients and patients with MI, incomplete AV block, renal insufficiency, or hypothyroidism.<br>• Do not administer to patients with ventricular tachycardia (unless caused by CHF or ventricular fibrillation). | • Monitor EKG, blood pressure, electrolytes, blood urea nitrogen, and serum creatinine.<br>• Monitor the serum digoxin level.<br>• Obtain a 12-lead EKG to document significant changes in cardiac rate or rhythm.<br>• Withhold 1 to 2 days before performing cardioversion. |
| • Do not use with beta-blockers, such as propranolol.<br>• Incompatible with alkaline solutions.<br>• Patients with atrial fibrillation should receive digoxin first, to prevent rapid ventricular response.<br>• Infiltration may produce severe tissue damage. | • Monitor blood pressure, central venous pressure (CVP), pulmonary artery wedge pressure (PAWP), cardiac rhythm, and urine output.<br>• Always use an infusion pump. |
| • Do not use to treat uncorrected tachydysrhythmias or ventricular fibrillation.<br>• May precipitate dysrhythmias.<br>• Infiltration may produce severe tissue damage.<br>• Solution deteriorates after 24 hours.<br>• Do not mix other drugs in bottle.<br>• Do not give alkaline drugs through the same I.V. line as dopamine. | • Titrate to maintain desired systolic blood pressure and urine output.<br>• Always use an infusion pump.<br>• Monitor cardiac rhythm, urine output, blood pressure, CVP, and PAWP.<br>• Use a large vein to minimize risk of severe tissue damage from extravasation. |

*(continued)*

# Understanding Emergency Cardiac Drugs (continued)

| | INDICATIONS | MECHANISM OF ACTION/EFFECTS | DOSE/ROUTE |
|---|---|---|---|
| **epinephrine hydrochloride (Adrenalin Chloride)** | • Used for treating asystole and ventricular fibrillation | Adrenergic (sympathomimetic) • Stimulates both alpha and beta receptor cells • Increases cardiac output and systolic blood pressure, relaxes bronchial spasms, and mobilizes liver glycogen stores | • I.V. push: administer 5 to 10 ml of 1:10,000 solution (0.5 to 1 mg) over 1 minute. • Intracardiac: administer 1 to 10 ml of 1:10,000 solution (0.1 to 1 mg). • Intratracheal: instill 1 to 2 mg per 10 ml sterile water (1 ml of 1:10,000, or 1 ml of 1:5,000) directly into endotracheal tube. • Infusion: can mix 2 to 4 mg in 500 ml $D_5W$; administer at 1 to 4 mcg/minute. |
| **isoproterenol hydrochloride (Isoprenaline**, Isuprel*)** | • Used for treating complete heart block, asystole, and cardiogenic shock | Adrenergic (sympathomimetic) • Affects beta receptors only, not alpha receptors | • Infusion: use standard dilution; administer at 0.5 to 20 mcg/minute and titrate as needed. |
| **lidocaine hydrochloride (Lignocaine**, Xylocaine*)** | • Used for treating PVCs and ventricular tachycardia | Antiarrhythmic • Increases electrical stimulation threshold, controlling ventricular dysrhythmias • Does not affect contractility | • I.V. push: administer 50 to 100 mg; can be repeated every 5 minutes; total dose should not exceed 200 mg. • Infusion: standard dilution; administer at 1 to 4 mg/minute. • Intratracheal: infuse 50 to 100 mg per 10 ml sterile water. |
| **procainamide hydrochloride (Pronestyl*)** | • Used for treating PVCs and ventricular fibrillation when lidocaine is not effective | Antiarrhythmic • Depresses the myocardium's response to electrical stimulation and slows conduction through the AV node | • I.V. push: administer 100 mg at 20 mg/minute; can be repeated every 5 minutes; total dose should not exceed 1 g. • Infusion: infuse 2 to 6 mg/minute. |
| **propranolol hydrochloride (Inderal*)** | • Used for treating supraventricular, ventricular, and atrial dysrhythmias and excessive tachydysrhythmias | Beta-blocker • Blocks effects of catecholamines • Slows heart rate • Relaxes myocardial muscle tension | • I.V. push: administer 1 to 3 mg at a rate not greater than 1 mg/minute; may be repeated in 2 minutes. |
| **sodium bicarbonate** | • Used for treating cardiac arrest | Alkalizer • Facilitates defibrillation by reversing metabolic acidosis | • I.V. push: rapidly administer 44.6 mEq in 50 ml $D_5W$ (1 mEq/kg); repeat doses according to blood gas values. |
| **verapamil (Isoptin*, Calan)** | • Used for treating supraventricular tachydysrhythmias | Calcium channel blocker • Selectively inhibits movement of calcium ions during depolarization • Delays impulse transmission through the AV node • Depresses rhythmicity of the SA node • Restores normal sinus rhythm and temporarily controls the rate of atrial fibrillation or flutter | • I.V. push: administer 5 to 10 mg (0.075 to 0.15 mg/kg) over a minimum of 2 minutes; for older patients, administer over 3 minutes; can be repeated in 30 minutes. |

*Available in U.S. and Canada. **Available in Canada only. All other products (no symbol) available in U.S. only.

| PRECAUTIONS | NURSING CONSIDERATIONS |
|---|---|
| • Increases intraocular pressure.<br>• May exacerbate CHF, dysrhythmias, angina pectoris, hyperthyroidism, and emphysema.<br>• May cause headache, tremors, or palpitations. | • Monitor blood pressure every 2 to 5 minutes until it's stable.<br>• Monitor cardiac rhythm.<br>• Watch for signs of overdose: cold and diaphoretic skin, cyanosis of nail beds, tachypnea, and changes in mental status. If any occur, discontinue the drug immediately. |
| • Use cautiously in patients with heart failure.<br>• Do not administer with epinephrine.<br>• Use cautiously when administering together with propranolol.<br>• Do not administer for preexisting dysrhythmias induced by digitalis toxicity. | • Monitor intraarterial pressure, if possible.<br>• Using an infusion pump, titrate as ordered.<br>• Check blood pressure every 2 to 3 minutes until stable.<br>• Monitor CVP and PAWP.<br>• Record urine output hourly. |
| • Do not mix with sodium bicarbonate.<br>• Do not use if your patient has a high-grade sinoatrial or AV block.<br>• Discontinue if PR interval or QRS complex widens, or if dysrhythmias worsen.<br>• Use cautiously in patients with severe renal or liver impairment.<br>• May lead to ventricular tachycardia if used to correct PVCs resulting from bradycardia.<br>• May lead to central nervous system (CNS) toxicity, especially in patients with heart failure. | • Titrate as ordered to control dysrhythmias.<br>• Observe your patient frequently for signs of CNS toxicity: numbness of lips, face, or tongue; tremors; paresthesia; blurred or double vision; dizziness; tinnitus; and seizures. If any occur, stop the infusion and treat the toxicity.<br>• Monitor cardiac rhythm constantly.<br>• Monitor blood pressure every 10 to 15 minutes until stable; slow infusion if hypotension occurs. |
| • Can cause precipitous hypotension; do not use for treating second- or third-degree heart block unless a pacemaker's been inserted.<br>• Can cause AV block and PVCs that may result in ventricular fibrillation. | • Monitor blood pressure continuously.<br>• Monitor EKG for widening QRS complexes.<br>• Maintain a slow administration rate to avoid serious hypotension.<br>• Always use an infusion pump. |
| • Can alter requirements for insulin and oral hypoglycemic drugs.<br>• Can cause excessive bradycardia.<br>• Use cautiously when administering with isoproterenol and aminophylline (exaggerates beta-blocking effect). | • Monitor EKG, heart rate, and rhythm frequently.<br>• Monitor for hypoglycemia.<br>• Ausculate for rales, gallop rhythm, and third or fourth heart sounds. |
| • Don't mix with epinephrine; causes epinephrine degradation.<br>• Don't mix with calcium salts; forms insoluble precipitates. | • After injection, thoroughly flush the line with I.V. fluid.<br>• Monitor arterial pH. |
| • Contraindicated in patients with hypotension, cardiogenic shock, severe CHF, and second- or third-degree AV block.<br>• High doses or overly rapid administration can cause a significant drop in blood pressure. | • Monitor cardiac rhythm for AV block and bradycardia.<br>• Monitor blood pressure. |

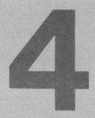

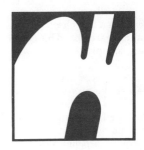

# Respiratory Emergencies

## Introduction

You're in the ED, assessing a patient's fractured arm, when ambulance attendants bring in Roy Hodges. He's a big man, about 40, sitting up in a wheelchair and showing no obvious signs of injury. But when you hear his gasping respirations across the room, you rush over to look at him. Roy's face is flushed and he's sweating heavily; he's also leaning forward in his chair, struggling to breathe. You note tachypnea and nasal flaring. Now you're really concerned. What's wrong with Roy? At this point, you don't know. What you *do* know is that Roy's respiratory distress is severe, and you must act quickly.

Would you know how to assess Roy's respiratory problem and intervene appropriately? Roy didn't have any other signs and symptoms requiring your attention, so you were able to focus on his respiratory distress immediately. But you won't always have patients like Roy. What if he'd been in a car accident and he'd had multiple serious wounds? Or what if he'd had another serious symptom, such as severe abdominal pain? You need to be aware that, no matter what else has happened to your patient, no matter how serious his other signs and symptoms, his airway and breathing emergencies take precedence over all others. Why? Because his life is directly threatened.

You need to act *fast* when a patient like Roy arrives in the ED. You may have only a few minutes to assess his respiratory problem and to intervene to avert hypoxemia, hypercapnia, respiratory acidosis, and death.

As you know, respiratory emergencies can arise on the medical-surgical unit, too. And you'll also see patients, recovering from respiratory emergencies, who relapse and again require emergency intervention. As a nurse, you must be prepared to manage any and all emergency situations.

When a patient has a respiratory emergency, in the ED or on the unit, you and members of the emergency team (usually a doctor and, perhaps, a respiratory therapist and another nurse) will have to act without delay. This means you need to thoroughly understand your role in an emergency *before* it happens.

Depending on how code teams and ED teams work in your hospital, and on whether medical-surgical nurses float to the ED, your role may be performing primary assessment, administering basic life support, assisting the doctor, or recording vital patient information. In fact, you may be called on to do all of these things almost simultaneously. Be sure you're prepared for what you may have to do during each critical minute.

## INITIAL CARE

## Prehospital Care: What's Been Done

If rescue personnel transported your patient to the hospital, they probably took steps to stabilize his airway, breathing, and circulation. If not, it's your *number-one* priority, no matter what else may be wrong with the patient. You may have to:

• use finger sweeps, back blows, or the abdominal thrust (Heimlich maneuver) to remove a foreign body obstructing the patient's airway

• insert airway adjuncts

• deliver moderate- to high-flow oxygen by nasal cannula, face mask, or Ambu bag

• assist with endotracheal intubation and then with esophageal obturator airway removal.

If the patient's condition is the result of chest trauma, rescue personnel (if qualified) may have started an I.V. They may also have performed other emergency interventions, such as covering an open pneumothorax with an occlusive dressing. You'll have to assess this as soon as the patient arrives, to make sure the dressing hasn't converted the open pneumothorax into a tension pneumothorax. If the patient showed signs and symptoms of a tension pneumothorax *before* he arrived at the hospital, rescue personnel may have performed an emergency needle thoracotomy. When you receive this patient, you'll see the needle in place. It's most commonly inserted in the interspace of the fourth and fifth ribs' midaxillary line or between the second and third intercostal space at the midclavicular line. (See *Understanding Needle Tho-*

*racotomy,* page 118.)

If the patient has a flail chest, rescue personnel may have stabilized his chest with sandbags or tape. Check the adequacy of the splinting and rearrange or add sandbags as necessary. Remember, splinting may be overdone. If the patient's chest wall has been taped, make sure the tape isn't so tight that it interferes with his breathing.

You may also find a penetrating object, such as a knife, bandaged in place to prevent the profuse bleeding that removal may cause. Leave the object bandaged in place until the doctor can remove it.

## What to Do First

For the patient with a respiratory emergency, your primary assessment and intervention should focus on his airway, breathing, and circulation. Your assessment and appropriate interventions must be *rapid*—if they're not, your patient may lose his life.

You'll have to perform repeated assessments throughout your patient's care, but your initial assessment gives you valuable baseline information to measure changes against.

### Airway
Start, as always, by making sure your patient's airway is open. If it isn't, you must act *immediately*. Whether the obstruction's mechanical (a foreign body) or physiologic (the result, for example, of laryngospasm or bronchospasm), you must immediately remove or bypass it, or the patient will suffer irreversible brain damage or die.

If the obstructing object is the patient's tongue, open his airway as described in the "Life Support" section in Chapter 3, page 98. If it's a foreign body, remove it if possible, using basic life-support techniques. Try finger sweeps first; if you're unsuccessful with these, use backblows and the abdominal

## NEW ADVANCES IN RESPIRATORY MONITORING—OXIMETRY

Until recently, you had to rely on arterial blood gas (ABG) measurements to sound the alarm when acute hypoxemia threatens your patient's life. But many hospitals now are using a new, improved version of an old procedure—oximetry—to provide continuous monitoring of arterial oxygenation in patients with cardiorespiratory disorders.

An oximeter monitors your patient's oxygen saturation continuously, so it rapidly (within 6 seconds) detects any trend in his oxygenation status—unlike ABGs, which you can measure only periodically. And, because oximetry's a simple, noninvasive procedure, you don't need to be specially trained to do it. Here's how these devices work.

An *ear oximeter* measures a patient's arterial oxygen saturation by monitoring the transmission of two light waves through his earlobe's vascular bed. Light emitters and sensors are contained in an ear probe that you clip to your patient's earlobe, as illustrated. A hearter in the hear probe's tip maintains the skin's surface temperature at 37° C, dilating the arterial vascular bed to enable more accurate readings. A cable conducts the ear probe's electrical signal to the oximeter, which calculates oxygen saturation and displays the values on a digital-readout front panel.

If low cardiac output causes insufficient arterial perfusion in your patient's earlobe—preventing an accurate determination of oxygen saturation with an ear oximeter—you can use a *pulse oximeter*. This instrument measures the wavelengths of light transmitted through a *pulsating* arterial vascular bed, such as in a fingertip. As the pulsating bed expands and relaxes, the light path length changes, producing a waveform. Because the waveform's produced solely from arterial blood, the pulse oximeter calculates the exact, beat-by-beat arterial oxygen saturation without interference from surrounding venous blood, skin, connective tissue, or bone. LED light emitters and a photodiode light receptor are mounted in a receptacle that you slip over your patient's fingertip (no heater is required). The receptacle is connected to a microprocessor that calculates and displays the saturation values.

You can't use the fingertip receptacle on a patient who has any condition that significantly reduces peripheral vascular pulsations (such as hypotherami or hypotension) or who's taking vasoactive drugs. Instead, you'll use a nasal probe that fits around your patient's septal anterior enthmoid artery, where vascular pulsations are less easily disrupted.

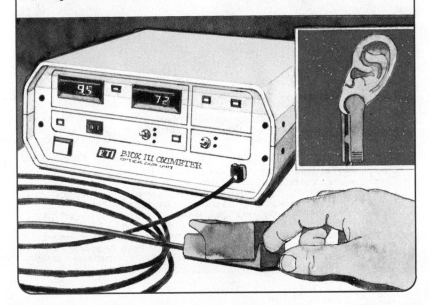

thrust (Heimlich maneuver), until the obstruction dislodges.

If your patient's airway is completely occluded as a result of trauma or laryngospasm, or if you or the doctor can't clear it using basic life-support techniques, prepare for an emergency cricothyroidotomy or tracheotomy. Assemble the necessary equipment.

Serious tracheobronchial injuries that completely disrupt the airway, such as a crushed larynx, may also require emergency cricothyroidotomy or tracheotomy. In these situations, you may assist the doctor in restoring a patent airway as he intubates the patient with an endotracheal tube that reaches beyond the level of the injury. (See *Assisting with Endotracheal Intubation,* pages 120 and 121.)

### Breathing

Once your patient's airway's patent (or if he doesn't need his airway opened), assess him for wheezing, gasping, cyanosis, and stridor. Your assessment of his breathing should also include external signs. Look at his bare chest to note any use of accessory muscles to assist breathing. Signs that his trachea's deviated from midline, or that his chest wall's asymmetrical, suggest a tension pneumothorax, which requires *immediate* intervention. Pre-

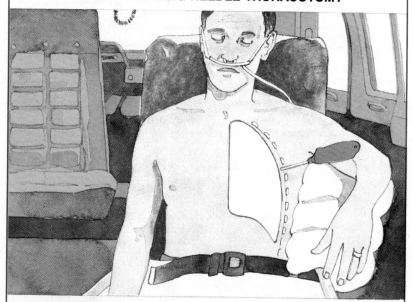

## UNDERSTANDING NEEDLE THORACOTOMY

If your patient's had a needle thoracotomy, he'll arrive in the ED with a large needle, topped by a flutter valve, protruding from his chest.

An emergency medical technician (EMT) or doctor usually performs this emergency procedure to temporarily relieve the perilous pressure of tension pneumothorax.

Here's how needle thoracotomy works: The EMT or doctor inserts the needle, with the flutter valve made from a perforated finger cot attached with a rubber band, into the affected pleural space. Trapped air escapes via the flutter valve instead of being retained under pressure. The flutter valve also prevents more air from entering the patient's lung.

In the ED, the doctor will remove the temporary needle and insert a chest tube to assist the patient's breathing.

pare the equipment and, if necessary, assist the doctor in performing a needle thoracotomy to release trapped air from the pleural space. (See *Understanding Needle Thoracotomy*.) If no doctor's present, you may have to perform this procedure if your state's nurse practice act and your hospital's protocols allow it.

If you see an open chest-wall wound, place your ear near it and listen for a characteristic sucking (or swishing) sound indicating an open pneumothorax (sucking chest wound). If you hear this, wait until the patient exhales fully and then cover the wound *immediately*. Use an occlusive petrolatum gauze dressing if possible. If you don't have one available, you'll have to improvise by using a dry dressing, plastic food wrap, or even the palm of your hand (see *Managing a Sucking Chest Wound*, page 122). Dress *any* chest-wall wound that may communicate with the lung, even if you *don't* hear a sucking sound. Watch this type of patient closely—he's at high risk for developing tension pneumothorax.

As you do for a patient with any type of open wound, ask him about tetanus immunization.

Is your patient's breathing adequate to supply the oxygen he needs? Assess his respirations for rate, depth, and pattern. If wheezing, gasping, cyanosis, or stridor is present, trauma or bronchopulmonary disease may be impairing his breathing. Is he *hypo*ventilating? Assess him for oversedation or the use of respiratory depressant drugs. If he's *hyper*ventilating, assess him for anxiety or metabolic changes. Remember, both these conditions impair ventilatory gas exchange.

While you're assessing your patient's breathing, double-check his chest-wall movements to assess for previously undetected flail chest or pneumothorax. Palpate for equal chest excursion. Asymmetrical movements suggest pneumothorax, whereas paradoxic movement suggests flail chest. If a portion of your patient's chest is drawing

PRIORITIES

## INITIAL ASSESSMENT CHECKLIST

**Assess the ABCs first and intervene appropriately.**

**Check for:**
• stridor or inability to talk, indicating airway obstruction
• cyanosis, indicating tissue hypoxia
• changes in mental status (apprehension, anxiety, agitation, confusion, restlessness, lethargy, or unconsciousness may indicate hypoxemia)
• severe chest pain and guarded posture, which restrict breathing and may indicate injury.

**Intervene by:**
• administering oxygen (respiratory emergencies cause poor gas exchange).

**Prepare for:**
• chest tube insertion
• assisted ventilation
• endotracheal intubation.

in when he *in*hales and puffing *out* when he *ex*hales, you need to stabilize this flail segment immediately, before the fractured ribs have a chance to puncture the lung. Use your hands for this until members of the emergency team can provide sandbags.

To relieve your patient's breathing difficulty, provide oxygen by face mask, nasal cannula, or Ambu bag. (If necessary, the doctor will insert an endotracheal tube.) If his condition allows you, assist him to a sitting position. This will make breathing easier for him. Remember, a patient in respiratory distress is extremely anxious, and this increases his breathing difficulty. Provide emotional support to help him relax, let him know what procedures he'll undergo, and explain that these procedures will make him more comfortable.

## Circulation

If the patient's suffered chest trauma or any kind of chest injury, start an I.V. *immediately*, if he doesn't already have one. Then, after taking his blood pressure and checking his pulse rate and amplitude, assess for:

• signs and symptoms of serious blood loss, which can lead to shock

• distortion in chest structures, which may impair circulation.

You know that respiratory emergencies commonly cause inadequate oxygenation of circulating blood; also remember that impaired circulation can compromise tissue perfusion even when ventilation is adequate.

## General appearance

Assess your patient's overall appearance for further clues to the cause of his respiratory distress. Check for changes in skin color, such as cyanosis or pallor. Is he sweating? Diaphoresis also can signal respiratory distress. If your patient's flushed, leaning forward, and sweating, position him so he's comfortable and administer oxygen to

---

PROCEDURES

 **YOUR ROLE IN AN EMERGENCY**

### ASSISTING WITH ENDOTRACHEAL INTUBATION

The doctor may insert an endotracheal tube in your patient for short-term mechanical ventilation or airway management. You'll assist by gathering the necessary equipment and preparing your patient for the procedure. Or—if you're specially trained to perform this emergency procedure and your hospital's protocol permits—you may insert the tube yourself.

#### Equipment
• Cuffed endotracheal tubes, assorted sizes
• Laryngoscope and blades
• Magill forceps
• Stylet
• 5- to 10-cc syringe
• Lubricant, water-soluble
• Xylocaine jelly or spray
• Ambu bag and mask
• Suction equipment—suction machine, suction catheters, sterile gloves, and sterile saline solution for irrigating and clearing the tubing
• Sedative and local anesthetic spray (for the conscious patient)

#### Procedure
• Set up the mechanical ventilator.
• Explain the procedure to your patient and sedate him if the doctor orders.
• Position the patient flat on his back with a small blanket or pillow under his head. This position brings the axis of the oropharynx, posterior pharynx, and the trachea into alignment.
• Check the cuff on the endotracheal tube for leaks.
• As soon as the doctor's intubated your patient by passing the tube alongside the laryngoscope blades, inflate the cuff using the minimal leak technique.
• Check tube placement by auscultating for bilateral breath sounds; observe the patient for chest expansion and feel for warm exhalations at the endotracheal tube's opening.
• Insert an oral airway or bite block.
• Secure the tube and airway with tape applied to skin treated with compound benzoin tincture.
• Suction secretions from the patient's mouth and endotracheal tube, as needed.
• Administer oxygen and/or initiate mechanical ventilation, as ordered.

#### Possible complications
• Broken teeth
• Vocal cord damage
• Improper tube placement resulting in *esophageal intubation,* causing stomach distention or rupture from forced air pressure; or *right mainstem bronchus* intubation, so only the right lung is ventilated
• Death from asphyxia due to aspiration

#### Nursing follow-up care
• Suction secretions as needed, at least every 1 or 2 hours, using aseptic technique.

help relieve his distress.

Look for external evidence of trauma, such as abrasions, contusions, or bruises on the chest or ribs: these may be signs of serious pulmonary damage. Both blunt trauma (such as a blow to the chest wall) and penetrating trauma (such as stabbings or wounds from flying debris) can produce blood loss leading to shock. Remember, *don't* remove any penetrating objects.

**Mental status**
Confusion, restlessness, and anxiety are indications of significant hypoxemia and hypercapnia in a patient with a respiratory emergency. (Of course, you'll consider other causes of confusion and disorientation, such as neurologic emergencies [see Chapter 6] and shock [see Chapter 14]). If your patient shows signs of hypoxemia, *administer oxygen* as necessary, while you and the rest of the emergency team work to correct the underlying cause. Draw blood for arterial blood gas analysis. Remember to do an Allen's test before you draw the blood. (See page 164.)

---

• Record the volume of air needed to inflate the cuff.
• *Caution*: Overinflation of the cuff can cause tracheal necrosis, so check the cuff pressure once each shift.
• Have a chest X-ray done to check tube placement.
• Restrain and reassure your patient as necessary.
• Check for adequate cuff inflation. Correct any air leaks, using the minimal leak

**WARNING: ACCIDENTAL EXTUBATION**

Any number of events may lead to endotracheal extubation. For example, a confused or disoriented patient may pull out the tube; saliva may loosen the tape anchoring the tube; or the tape may not stick well to a diaphoretic patient's skin.

Watch for the following signs and symptoms of extubation, then perform the appropriate nursing interventions. Remember that unless you intervene immediately, an extubated patient may develop progressive hypoxia, tissue damage, or acidosis—or die of asphyxiation.

**Early warning signs**
The tube may be extubating if:
• it appears much longer than it should.
• (for a patient attached to a ventilator) the low-pressure alarm and the exhaled volume alarm (spirometer alarm) sound.
• the patient shows signs and symptoms of hypoxia: tachypnea, tachycardia, diaphoresis, anxiety, agitation, dysrhythmias, bradycardia, or cyanosis.

**Nursing interventions**
• Remove any portion of the tube that's still in place.

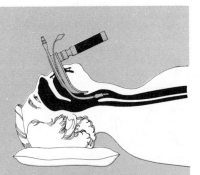

Tube passing alongside laryngoscope blades

• Ventilate the patient using mouth-to-mouth resuscitation or an Ambu (or anesthesia) bag.
• Send someone to notify the doctor to reintubate the patient.
• Restrain the patient if he's purposely extubated himself, to prevent it from happening again.
• Each time the patient's repositioned, check the tape holding the reinserted tube.
• To make the tube secure, anchor tape from the nape of his neck to and around the tube.

# What to Do Next

You've stabilized your patient's airway, breathing, and circulation. Now, you and the rest of the emergency team can assess him for other urgent respiratory problems and intervene appropriately. This includes stabilizing any obvious problems that *threaten* your patient's airway or breathing. Then, if time and the patient's condition permit, assess for his chief complaint by taking a quick history and performing an emergency physical examination.

If your patient has suffered a traumatic injury, ask him (or a family member or friend) where, when, and how the injury occurred. Ask if he has any pain, and determine its location and nature.

*Chest pain,* a frequent complaint of

---

PROCEDURES

## YOUR ROLE IN AN EMERGENCY

### MANAGING A SUCKING CHEST WOUND

If a sharp object or fragment from a missile injury penetrated your patient's chest wall, it may have created a sucking chest wound. Such a wound destroys the necessary pressure gradient between the pleural space and outside atmosphere. Unless you can restore this pressure gradient, the patient will quickly develop respiratory failure.

**Equipment**
• Nasal cannula, face masks, oxygen equipment
• Petrolatum gauze
• Wide tape
• Chest tube tray

**Procedure**
• Monitor your patient closely.
• Administer oxygen through a nasal cannula or a face mask.
• Don't remove any object protruding from your patient's chest—doing so will destroy the pressure gradient even faster and increase bleeding.
• Reassure the patient, then ask him to exhale forcefully. At the moment of maximum expiration, cover the wound with petrolatum gauze to seal it.
• Secure the gauze with wide tape.
• Monitor the patient closely for signs and symptoms of tension pneumothorax, and notify the doctor if this condition develops.
• If the doctor decides to insert a chest tube, get the equipment ready and be prepared to assist.
• If the doctor orders surgery, prepare your patient appropriately.

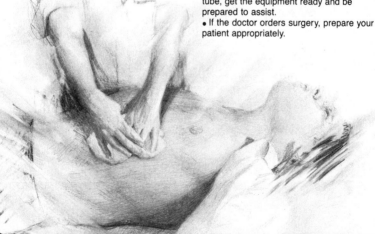

# CASE IN POINT: ADMINISTERING DRUGS

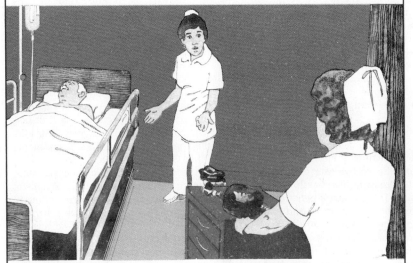

James Forbes, age 70, returned to your unit—following abdominal surgery—during the previous shift. Now he awakens, complaining of pain. On his chart, you find a p.r.n. order to give him morphine, 6 mg I.M., for pain. You check his vital signs (pulse, 90; blood pressure, 120/76; respirations, 18 and shallow), then administer morphine, as ordered. Later, you find that his respirations have dropped to 8. You immediately notify the doctor, who orders naloxone to counteract the morphine. But before you can administer the drug, James becomes apneic, goes into respiratory arrest, and dies, despite aggressive resuscitative efforts. His daughter later threatens to sue you for negligence.

Suppose this incident had really happened. Could you be held liable for the patient's death?

The court case *Brown v. State* (1977) involved a nurse who administered 200 mg of Thorazine, as ordered, but failed to reassess her patient afterward. A few hours later, the patient died.

The court found the nurse (and the other nurses on the unit) liable, because they failed to monitor the patient for complications after the drug was administered. The court reasoned that nurses should know about the drugs they give their patients, anticipate complications, and be aware of contraindications.

To reduce your risk of liability when you administer drugs, follow these guidelines:
• Be sure you understand the doctor's drug order. If it's illegible, confusing, or ambiguous, ask him for clarification.
• Know the drugs you're administering—particularly their potential side effects and possible adverse reactions.
• Assess your patient's condition before you administer *any* drug and soon after. Keep in mind possible complications from other medications or from surgery or diagnostic tests.
• Check your patient regularly. If you find adverse reactions, or other changes in his condition, immediately notify the doctor.
• Remember that legally, you can refuse to administer drugs you think will harm your patient. For example, your nursing judgment may tell you that the prescribed dosage is too high, a dangerous interaction with another drug may occur, or the drug is contraindicated in your patient's condition. If you do refuse to give a drug, notify your supervisor and the prescribing doctor immediately.

*Brown v. State,* 56 A.D. 2d 672; 391 N.Y.S. 2d 204 (1977).

the patient with respiratory difficulty, must be differentiated from cardiac pain. If your patient reports pleuritic pain (increasing with deep breaths, relieved when sitting up, exacerbated with chest-wall movement), suspect it's of pulmonary origin. A patient with pneumothorax may report:

• sharp pleuritic pain (sudden onset) associated with dyspnea

• dull chest pain (In a patient who's been on prolonged bed rest or who also complains of calf or leg pain, suspect a pulmonary embolism.)

• substernal pain similar to anginal pain

• nonspecific chest discomfort.

If he has a blunt injury, such as a blow against a steering wheel causes, look for ecchymoses on his chest wall that may indicate pulmonary contusion. If his injury's penetrating, locate the object's entrance (and exit, if it's a gunshot wound), and estimate the amount of bleeding. Try to determine the object's path through the patient's body—what organs may be affected? Continue to listen for the sucking sound that indicates an open pneumothorax. Observe him for distended neck veins, and monitor his pulse for rate and amplitude. Palpate his neck and upper chest for subcutaneous emphysema (a crackling, popping feeling), characteristic of pneumothorax and tracheobronchial injury.

Auscultate both sides of his chest for diminished or absent breath sounds, which may indicate pneumothorax or hemothorax. (See *Assessing Breath Sounds*.) If he has *dyspnea*, ask him whether it's acute or chronic. Chronic dyspnea may indicate cardiac failure or decompensating chronic obstructive pulmonary disease, whereas acute episodic dyspnea suggests asthma. Rapid onset of dyspnea (occurring spontaneously or following an injury) can accompany a number of respiratory disorders, including:

• pulmonary embolism

• pneumothorax

• hemothorax

• pulmonary contusion

• adult respiratory distress syndrome

• pulmonary edema

• chemical injury to the lung.

Or the patient may simply be hyperventilating and feeling anxious. (Of course, dyspnea may also indicate cardiac dysfunction. See Chapter 5.)

Also observe your patient for coughing, sputum production, and hemoptysis. *Hemoptysis* may occur following injury—pulmonary contusion, tracheobronchial injury, or hemothorax, for example—but it may also indicate a massive pulmonary embolism. Ask the patient whether this is a first occurrence or if it's recurrent. (Chronic hemoptysis may indicate a tumor in the lung.) Chronic productive *coughs* with mucoid *sputum* are associated with asthma or chronic bronchitis. You'll see an increase in sputum production if your patient is having an acute asthma attack, purulent sputum if he has an acute infection.

Listen for *wheezing*. Although almost any acute or chronic pulmonary disease causes some wheezing, this sign may indicate a serious respiratory disorder. Asthma is a common cause of wheezing, particularly in patients under age 40. If an adult patient reports wheezing of only a few months' duration, consider the possibility of a mechanical obstruction of the larynx, the trachea, or a mainstem bronchus—such as a neoplasm causes. Find out if the patient was hospitalized within the past 6 months. If he was, and he was intubated or had a tracheotomy, he may have stricture from the damage to his trachea. Transient wheezing may occur following a pulmonary embolism. In a longtime cigarette smoker, a long history of wheezing with progressive dyspnea on exertion and chronic sputum production suggests chronic bronchitis and emphysema.

If you suspect rib or sternal fractures, palpate the possible fracture sites for *point tenderness* and auscultate the sites for *crepitations*.

Be prepared to draw blood for a gen-

## ASSESSING BREATH SOUNDS

As part of your emergency assessment, percuss and auscultate your patient's chest. *Percussion* helps you identify compressed lung tissue or fluid or tissue that's replaced air in the alveoli. *Auscultation* helps you determine whether your patient has a bronchial obstruction or air or fluid in his lungs.

As you probably know, normal breath sounds are described as bronchial (tubular), bronchovesicular, and vesicular. Crackles (rales), wheezes (sibilant rhonchi), rhonchi (sonorous rhonchi), stridor, and pleural friction rub are adventitious (abnormal) breath sounds. You may hear abnormal breath sounds superimposed over normal ones.

The chart below will help you identify abnormal breath sounds associated with respiratory disorders, and their symbols.

| DISORDER | PERCUS-SION | CHANGES IN NORMAL BREATH SOUNDS | ADVENTITIOUS BREATH SOUNDS |
|---|---|---|---|
| **Consolidation** | Dull | High-pitched, bronchial 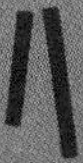 | Fine crackles early; coarse crackles later 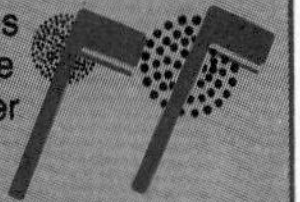 |
| **Atelectasis** | Dull | Diminished or absent; high-pitched, bronchial 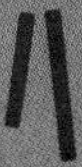 | Fine crackles early; coarse crackles later 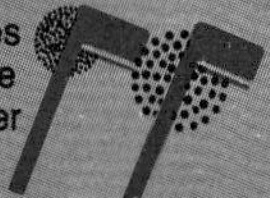 |
| **Pleural effusion or empyema** | Dull to absent | Diminished or absent; high-pitched, bronchial 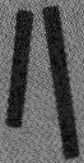 | Pleural friction rub 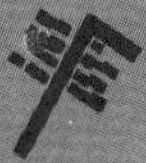 |
| **Pneumo-thorax** | Normal or hyperreso-nant | Diminished or absent; high-pitched, bronchial 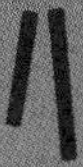 | Fine crackles when fluid present 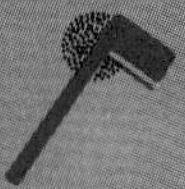 |
| **Acute or chronic bronchitis** | Normal | Vesicular with prolonged expiration 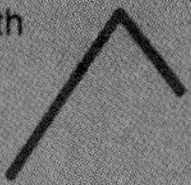 | Rhonchi; coarse crackles 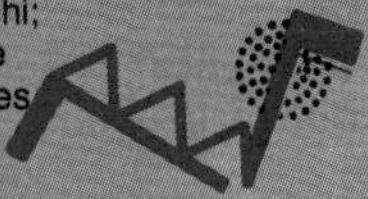 |
| **Bronchial asthma** | Normal or hyperreso-nant | Vesicular with prolonged expiration 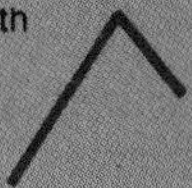 | Wheezes 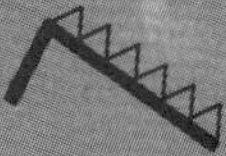 |
| **Pulmonary edema** | Normal or dull | Bronchial or vesicular 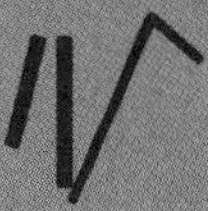 | Coarse crackles 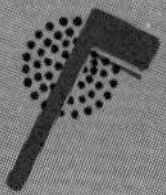 |

**Key:** Breath sounds

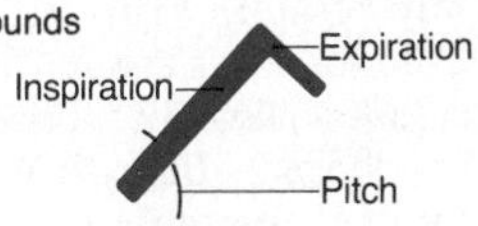

Inspiration — Expiration — Pitch

**Upstroke** represents inspiration
**Downstroke** represents expiration
**Length** of stroke represents duration
**Thickness** of stroke represents amplitude
**Angle** represents pitch

eral diagnostic workup: complete blood count, electrolytes, blood sugar, blood urea nitrogen, and creatinine.

# Special Considerations

## Pediatric

Pediatric patients with respiratory emergencies require your special attention. Be particularly alert to upper airway obstruction in infants and young children, who commonly aspirate small foreign objects, such as buttons and parts of toys. Remember, too, that a very young child's tongue occupies a proportionally larger space in his mouth and pharynx than in an adult's. So, to clear his airway when his tongue's blocking it, you'll need to use the jaw thrust maneuver or an oral airway. If you're assisting with endotracheal tube insertion, *don't* severely hyperextend the child's neck. Why? Because you may occlude his airway completely. Gentle extension (the "sniff" position) is all a pediatric patient requires. Another common problem is inadvertent placement of the tube into the right mainstem bronchus. This causes decreased breath sounds on the patient's left side. To check that the tube's placed correctly, auscultate the child's chest to be sure his breath sounds are equal on both sides.

With a young child, stridor occurring with fever and drooling may indicate *epiglottitis*—a life-threatening condition that can totally obstruct the airway (see *Nurse's Guide to Pediatric Emergencies* in the Appendix). If you or the doctor suspects epiglottitis, *don't* inspect the pharynx directly: this can cause laryngospasm, increasing edema, and asphyxiation. Instead, administer oxygen by face mask, and encourage the patient's parent to aid you in calming him. The doctor will confirm the diagnosis by lateral X-ray of the neck, and the child will usually go directly to the operating room for na-

sotracheal intubation. If the obstruction is severe, you may have to assist with emergency intubation.

Don't forget to consider that a child's injury may result from abuse (for example, a beating, fall, or near-drowning). If you suspect abuse, look for additional bruises and injuries. Ask the child and his parents about any you find. Remember, all 50 states and most Canadian provinces require healthcare professionals to report cases of suspected child abuse. (See the "When to Make a Report" entry in Chapter 2.) Be sure to document your findings completely.

## Geriatric

Chronic obstructive pulmonary disease is common in geriatric patients. When you administer oxygen to such a patient, provide it at a reduced flow rate (2 liters per minute), since hypoxemia is his main stimulus to breathe. If you give him too much oxygen, you may decrease his respiratory drive and cause apnea.

# CARE AFTER DIAGNOSIS

# Flail Chest

## Prediagnosis summary

Initial assessment revealed a history of blunt chest trauma and some combination of:

- paradoxic chest-wall movement
- palpable rib fractures
- bruising over the ribs
- decreased breath sounds
- respiratory distress.

The patient's unstable flail segment was temporarily splinted using hands, sandbags, or tape. He was given oxygen by nasal cannula or mask, and if his respiratory distress was severe, he was intubated. An I.V. was started, blood was drawn for ABGs, and he was connected to a cardiac monitor.

## Priorities

Your immediate priority is alleviating your patient's respiratory distress and controlling his pain. If his respiratory distress is mild to moderate, you'll continue oxygen administration via nasal cannula or mask to prevent hypoxemia. However, if he has severe respiratory distress, he'll need immediate mechanical ventilation to treat his hypoxemia and possible hypercapnia and to stabilize his flail segment.

Once you've taken your patient's vital signs, administer pain medication such as meperidine hydrochloride (Demerol) or morphine sulfate, as ordered. Even though narcotics may cause respiratory depression, the overriding concern is pain control. Why? Because pain may cause voluntary and involuntary splinting resulting in hypoventilation, which can lead to hypoxemia, hypercapnia, and atelectasis.

## Continuing assessment and intervention

Once you've given your patient pain medication and provided supplemental oxygen, perform a thorough nursing assessment. Before you start, make sure you're prepared for emergency chest tube insertion. Why? Because one of your patient's fractured ribs may perforate his pleural space and cause a pneumothorax.

Watch for paradoxic chest movement. Although this sign's commonly apparent immediately after injury, some patients don't develop it for several hours because the chest muscles are in spasm, effectively splinting the flail segment. If you observe this paradoxic movement, stabilize the segment immediately with your hands, tape, or a sandbag to prevent broken ribs from puncturing or bruising the lung.

Examine your patient's chest for palpable rib fractures and bruises. Circle the bruised areas so you can easily evaluate further bleeding.

Observe your patient frequently for tachypnea, cyanosis, dyspnea, confusion, or agitation, which may indicate hypoxemia. If at any time your patient shows signs and symptoms of inadequate ventilation, call the doctor. He may decide to intubate and mechanically ventilate the patient. Be prepared to assist with intubation, if necessary. You may need to give him sedatives after he's intubated to prevent him from resisting the ventilator.

Signs and symptoms of hypoxemia may also signal complications, such as hemothorax, closed pneumothorax, pulmonary contusion, or tension pneumothorax. For more information, see these entries in this chapter.) Auscultate his lungs for rales or decreased breath sounds. Rales may indicate fluid leakage into alveoli due to pulmonary contusion, whereas decreased breath sounds may be caused by splinting and hypoventilation or by developing hemothorax or pneumothorax.

If your patient's developing a *hemothorax*, you may also note hemoptysis and signs and symptoms of shock, such as increased respiratory rate, increased pulse rate, decreased blood pressure, and cyanosis. Report these findings to the doctor *immediately* and prepare for chest tube insertion and blood replacement.

If your patient's developing a *tension pneumothorax*, his respiratory distress will be severe, and you may note a deviated trachea. As you know, you must respond *immediately* to these signs because tension pneumothorax can rapidly become fatal. Call the doctor and prepare for emergency chest tube insertion. (See *Assisting with Chest Tube Insertion*, pages 144 and 145.)

If your assessment hasn't revealed complications so far, continue by taking your patient's history. Obtain a description of how his injury occurred, and find out if your patient's had any prior pulmonary disease. If your patient's on a mechanical ventilator, he won't be able to talk; try to get his history from his family or friends.

If your patient's on a ventilator, he may be given paralyzing agents, such as pancuronium bromide (Pavulon) or succinylcholine chloride (Anectine), to prevent him from breathing on his own and to allow the ventilator to control his chest-wall movement during the respiratory cycle. He may also need positive end-expiratory pressure (PEEP) to maintain positive pressure to prevent alveoli from collapsing. This treatment will:
• stabilize his flail segment
• treat his hypoxia and possible hypercapnia.

The doctor will determine ventilator settings (including percentage of oxygen, tidal volume, and rate), often in conjunction with a respiratory therapist. If your patient can assist the ven-

---

PATHOPHYSIOLOGY

# WHAT HAPPENS IN FLAIL CHEST

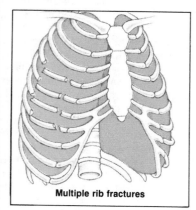

**Multiple rib fractures**

Flail chest—a disruption of the thorax due to multiple rib fractures, fractures of ribs and the sternum, or fractures of two or more adjacent ribs in more than one place—is caused most often by blunt trauma. A direct blow, such as occurs during assault or in a motor vehicle accident, causes the multiple fractures. These detach a segment of the chest wall so it's free to move inward during inspiration, rather than outward. As a result, the fractured bone ends may bruise or puncture a lung and cause pneumothorax, tension pneumothorax, or hemothorax.

Paradoxic breathing may signal flail chest, as illustrated below:

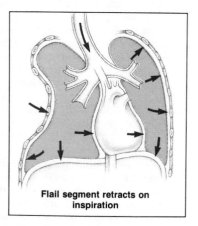

**Flail segment retracts on inspiration**

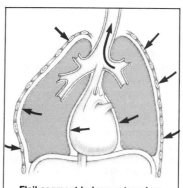

**Flail segment bulges outward on expiration**

tilator with his own respiratory effort, the doctor may set the ventilator to deliver intermittent mandatory ventilation. (See *Understanding Oxygen Therapy and Mechanical Ventilation Techniques,* pages 132 to 135.)

The patient may receive mininebulizer treatments, which administer a fine mist of water mixed with medications, without positive pressure, to help mobilize secretions and to aid in expectoration. Frequently suction your patient who's on a ventilator to remove secretions. Make sure your patient keeps his oxygen apparatus on. Give pain medications and prophylactic antibiotics, as ordered, to prevent pneumonia and infection. Encourage your patient to deep-breathe, and help him change his position frequently.

### Therapeutic care

Pain control will continue to be important. If your patient's receiving paralyzing agents, remember, these drugs *don't* reduce pain, so you'll need to give sedatives and analgesics on a regular schedule, as ordered. The doctor may give the patient an intercostal nerve block, particularly if he isn't intubated. Provide syringes and needles for this procedure—the doctor will request the appropriate sizes. He'll inject a long-acting local anesthetic, such as bupivacaine (Marcaine), into the affected area, often in combination with epinephrine to prolong the effect. Reassure your patient that the nerve block will make him much more comfortable and better able to tolerate the deep breathing and pulmonary care essential to his recovery.

If your patient's pulmonary dysfunction is minimal and he has few rib fractures, further care may include only oxygen administration, close observation, and good pulmonary care. While his rib fractures heal, he may be placed on intermittent positive-pressure breathing, which supplies air or oxygen under positive pressure during inspiration to improve alveolar ventilation and to prevent atelectasis; or he

may be placed on incentive spirometry, to encourage deep breathing and full lung inflation.

If your patient on a ventilator needs a chest tube, to allow air to escape and to prevent tension pneumothorax, assist with insertion and with underwater-seal chest drainage.

The patient may require surgery to stabilize the flail segment—for example, when the injury is severe or when the doctor wants to avoid prolonged mechanical ventilation. Prepare the patient for surgery and make sure his chest is stabilized during transport to the operating room.

Your patient's progress will be followed by serial chest X-rays and ABGs to monitor fracture healing and respiratory status. You'll continue pulmonary care, monitoring, and pain medications. If his flail segment requires stabilization with PEEP, he may be on a ventilator for weeks. You'll need to provide meticulous endotracheal tube care and proper suctioning to prevent infection. To prevent tracheal erosion or stenosis, the doctor may perform a tracheotomy 36 to 72 hours after the initial intubation.

As you're probably aware, long-term ventilation can make a patient psychologically or physically dependent on the ventilator. To prevent this, the doctor will start a program to wean him from the ventilator as soon as his respiratory status stabilizes and his chest X-rays show his ribs are healing. Of course, you'll continue aggressive pulmonary hygiene after the patient's extubated.

# Pulmonary Contusion

### Prediagnosis summary

Initial assessment findings included a history of blunt trauma to the patient's chest and some combination of:
- a cough with hemoptysis
- dyspnea
- signs and symptoms of hypoxemia

• decreased breath sounds or rales over the injured area.

Signs and symptoms of pulmonary contusion may not appear for several hours. Even if the patient had few or no signs and symptoms of pulmonary contusion initially, the doctor was careful not to underestimate the severity of the patient's injury and the possibility that pulmonary contusion might occur.

An I.V. and supplemental oxygen were started, and cardiac monitoring was established. The doctor ordered X-rays and arterial blood gases (ABGs) to estimate the severity of the contusion and the degree of hypoxemia. Although these tests may have been normal initially, the doctor admitted the patient for observation and further tests because he suspected pulmonary contusion might develop.

### Priorities
Make sure your patient's adequately oxygenated. If he doesn't have signs and symptoms of marked respiratory distress, give oxygen by nasal cannula or mask. Also encourage him to cough and deep-breathe to remove secretions, to prevent atelectasis, and to maintain good pulmonary hygiene. Assess his breath sounds and monitor ABGs for signs of developing hypoxemia.

If he has nasal flaring, accessory muscle use, extreme anxiety, or other signs or symptoms of respiratory distress, expect that he'll require intubation and mechanical ventilation, possibly with positive end-expiratory pressure. Assist the doctor with intubation as necessary. After intubation, auscultate your patient's breath sounds to check that the tube's placed correctly. The patient will also have another chest X-ray to verify that the tube's been placed correctly. Draw blood for ABGs to assess his respiratory status. The doctor will determine ventilator settings, including tidal volume, flow rate, and percentage of oxygen. Explain to your patient how the ventilator will help him breathe and that although he

won't be able to talk while he's intubated, he can communicate through notes.

### Continuing assessment and intervention
Your thorough nursing assessment follows stabilization of your patient's respiratory status. Because the signs and symptoms of pulmonary contusion may develop over several hours, your baseline data's especially important. Note the presence and degree of dyspnea, coughing, and tachypnea. Check his vital signs, watching closely for an increase in temperature (patients with pulmonary contusion are particularly susceptible to infection). Note his pulse rate and respiratory rate; any increase may be an early sign of respiratory difficulty.

Assess for signs and symptoms of shock, intervening as necessary:
• decreased blood pressure
• pallor
• diaphoresis
• increased pulse or respiratory rate.

If your findings are positive, notify the doctor—if the lung is severely damaged, he may perform an emergency thoracotomy and remove the contused area.

Listen to your patient's breath sounds, which may be decreased, with rales in the area of the contusion because of fluid leakage into the alveoli. Notify the doctor if you hear these sounds; he may want to start more aggressive oxygen therapy. If the patient isn't already on a ventilator, make sure you have artificial airways and intubation and suction equipment available in case his respiratory status deteriorates rapidly.

Assess your patient's fluid status. (If he has multiple injuries, he may have been given fluids initially for resuscitation.) Check his urine output and his blood pressure to determine if he's normovolemic. If he is, but he has signs of increased lung fluid—such as a productive cough, frothy sputum, tachycardia, or increased rales—the doctor may ask you to administer diuretics.

Take your patient's history. Find out how his chest injury occurred. Does the description of the incident suggest that he may have associated injuries? Determine whether he has any preexisting pulmonary disease, because this will impair healing of his contusion and affect the amount of oxygen you administer. If your patient's on a ventilator, preexisting pulmonary disease will also make weaning more difficult.

With a pediatric patient who's suffered a blunt chest injury, remember that a child's ribs are more resilient than an adult's. This means that even a severe blow causing pulmonary contusion or other lung injury may not fracture ribs. Be thorough in examining the child's chest wall for ecchymoses and contusions, locate the injury accurately, and get a careful history of the circumstances of the injury. Your high degree of suspicion may keep a seriously injured child from being discharged with apparently trivial chest-wall contusions.

## Therapeutic care

Your patient will need prophylactic pulmonary hygiene whether or not he's on a ventilator. He'll receive intermittent positive-pressure breathing (IPPB) or mini-nebulizer treatments to decrease bronchospasm and to increase secretion mobilization. (IPPB may also decrease a postoperative patient's atelectasis—if the patient can tolerate the treatment.) Monitor your patient's breathing before and after these treatments.

Continue to monitor your patient's vital signs. Give prophylactic antibiotics, as ordered, to minimize the risk of infection. Continue to check for an increase in temperature, which may indicate developing infection. If your patient's contusion is moderate to severe and he's had signs of severe respiratory distress, expect that he'll have daily chest X-rays to check contusion healing. Check his ABG results and his complete blood count daily to monitor

### WHAT HAPPENS IN PULMONARY CONTUSION

Characterized by damage to lung parenchyma, pulmonary contusion causes hemorrhage and edema in the affected area. Blood and colloid leak into the alveoli, making them unavailable for gas exchange. Impaired ventilation may cause systemic hypoxia. Potential problems depend on the extent of contusion:
- *minor* : damage to one segment or less
- *moderate*: damage extending from one segment up to an entire lobe
- *severe*: damage to more than one lobe.

Often accompanying flail chest, pulmonary contusion may also result from blunt trauma without rib fractures or from penetrating trauma.

his respiratory status and to detect signs of increased hemorrhage at the contusion site.

Pulmonary contusion usually heals without surgery. While your patient's recovering, continue to:
- maintain good pulmonary hygiene
- monitor his respiratory status and vital signs frequently
- check his ABG results routinely so you can detect developing hypoxemia and acidosis.

If you note hypoxemia and acidosis along with respiratory distress, tachycardia, fever, scattered rales, and pink, frothy sputum, your patient may be developing adult respiratory distress syndrome (ARDS). Remember—this is a very serious complication. (See the "Adult Respiratory Distress Syndrome" entry in this chapter.) Notify the doctor immediately. He will initiate aggressive ventilatory support, possibly including mechanical ventilation.

If your patient required mechanical ventilation, the doctor will begin a program to wean him from the ventilator when his respiratory status is stabilized. (Typical signs of this include improved breath sounds and ABGs.) Continue to assess his respiratory sta-

# UNDERSTANDING OXYGEN THERAPY AND MECHANICAL VENTILATION TECHNIQUES

If your patient's hypoxemic or can't breathe spontaneously, he'll need supplemental oxygen, mechanical ventilation, or both. The doctor orders the therapy, of course. But understanding how it works will help you reinforce your patient's breathing efforts, monitor the therapy's effectiveness, and do more effective patient teaching.

Here's a chart that explains some commonly used ventilation and supplemen-

| TECHNIQUE | USES | MECHANISM |
|-----------|------|-----------|
| **Nasal cannula** | • Delivers low-flow oxygen at 22% to 30% concentration<br>• Use restricted to spontaneously breathing patient | • Humidified oxygen is delivered through a two-pronged cannula in the patient's nose. |
| **Face mask** | • Delivers high concentrations of oxygen (45% to 90%)<br>• May be modified to allow partial rebreathing or nonrebreathing<br>• Use restricted to spontaneously breathing patient | • Humidified oxygen is delivered through the mask.<br>• Room air and exhaled air may be rebreathed. |
| **Venturi mask** | • Delivers exact oxygen concentrations between 24% and 40% despite patient's respiratory pattern<br>• Delivers humidity or aerosol therapy<br>• Treats chronic obstructive pulmonary disease (COPD)<br>• Use restricted to spontaneously breathing patient | • A precise concentration of oxygen is delivered through color-coded jet adapters that determine specific liter flow and oxygen concentration. |
| **Continuous positive airway pressure (CPAP)** | • Improves arterial oxygenation from ventilation-perfusion imbalances<br>• Opens alveoli and improves functional residual capacity<br>• Supplements oxygen therapy for patients not needing mechanical ventilation<br>• Helps treat adult respiratory distress syndrome (ARDS), acute respiratory failure (ARF), and reduced surfactant production | • The patient breathes while oxygen is delivered through an endotracheal tube or tight-fitting mask (with narrow opening to retard expiration) at constant pressure throughout the respiratory cycle. |
| **Intermittent positive-pressure breathing (IPPB)** | • Prevents or treats atelectasis<br>• Loosens secretions<br>• Delivers deep aerosol therapy<br>• Eases breathing and reduces panic in patients with pulmonary edema or COPD | • The patient initiates his breaths.<br>• The IPPB machine delivers a mixture of air and oxygen into the lungs under positive pressure.<br>• The patient exhales when a preset pressure is reached. |

tal oxygen techniques and gives you nursing tips for administering them. Remember, your patient's recovery—and maybe his life—depend on the equipment's smooth functioning. To ensure this, watch for equipment malfunctions and observe your patient for signs and symptoms of oxygen toxicity and carbon dioxide retention. Monitor his vital signs frequently.

## NURSING CONSIDERATIONS

- Tape the cannula in place.
- Apply gauze padding to the pressure areas under the patient's nose and over his ears.
- Moisten the patient's lips and nose with water-soluble jelly, but don't occlude the cannula.
- Remove the cannula every 8 hours and clean it with a wet cloth.
- Give meticulous mouth and nose care.
- Adjust the tubing so it doesn't pinch the patient's chin.
- Watch for cannula dislodgement.
- Monitor the patient for headache or dry mucous membranes.

- Make sure the mask fits snugly, so room air doesn't dilute the oxygen.
- Apply gauze pads under the elastic strap to prevent irritation of the patient's scalp and ears.
- Wash and dry the patient's face every 2 hours to reduce irritation.
- When a bag is used, avoid twisting it.
- Watch for signs and symptoms of oxygen toxicity.
- Remove the mask every 8 hours and clean it with a wet cloth.
- Be aware of hazards of using with patients who have COPD.

- Moisten the skin around the patient's mouth with petrolatum to prevent irritation.
- Fit the mask snugly and apply gauze pads under the elastic strap to prevent pressure sores.
- Check the patient's arterial blood gas (ABG) measurements frequently to anticipate changed oxygen concentration.
- Watch for altered $FIO_2$ concentration from a poorly fitted mask, kinked tubing, blocked oxygen intake ports, or incorrect liter flow.
- Make sure condensation doesn't collect and drain onto the patient.

- Make sure the patient's alert and able to communicate.
- Insert an endotracheal tube or apply a mask.
- Insert a nasogastric tube to decompress the stomach and to avoid distention and vomiting.
- Monitor the amount of positive pressure with an aneroid manometer.
- Watch for decreased cardiac output from high CPAP pressures.
- Watch for fatigue and carbon dioxide retention from increased work of breathing.

- Explain to the patient how to breathe using the mouthpiece.
- Monitor exhaled tidal volumes.
- Encourage the patient to cough.
- Maintain an airtight connection between the machine and the patient's airway.
- Adjust the gas flow pattern to achieve lung hyperventilation without patient discomfort.
- Watch for tension pneumothorax, decreased venous return, cardiac insufficiency, stomach distention, and systemic drug absorption.

*(continued)*

## UNDERSTANDING OXYGEN THERAPY AND MECHANICAL VENTILATION TECHNIQUES *(continued)*

| TECHNIQUE | USES | MECHANISM |
|---|---|---|
| **Positive end-expiratory pressure (PEEP)** | • Keeps airways and alveoli from collapsing<br>• Helps stabilize a flail chest and treat ARDS and ARF<br>• Increases functional residual capacity | • The ventilator keeps positive pressure in alveoli and airways through end expiration, reinflating collapsed alveoli.<br>• Low oxygen concentrations increase arterial oxygen pressure. |
| **Intermittent mandatory ventilation (IMV)** | • Lets the patient assist ventilation with his own breathing<br>• Weans him from the ventilator<br>• Reduces the chance of pneumothorax and decreased cardiac output | • The ventilator mandatorily delivers a preset number of breaths per minute.<br>• The patient breathes on his own between preset mandatory breaths, inspiring ventilator's set percentage of oxygen. |
| **High-frequency ventilation (HFV)** | • Supplements PEEP and CPAP<br>• Ventilates a patient under anesthesia for rigid bronchoscopy and direct laryngoscopy<br>• Helps treat bronchopleural fistulae and adult and infant respiratory distress syndromes<br>• Maintains cardiac output and improves gas exchange during mechanical ventilation | • The ventilator gives 60 to 3,000 breaths/minute (depending on the type of HFV) with low tidal volume, low airway pressure, and brief inspiratory time. |
| **Volume-cycled ventilator** | • Artificially controls or assists respiration or encourages spontaneous breathing, while guaranteeing minimum ventilation support<br>• Corrects serious gas exchange abnormalities in hypoxemia, hypercapnia, and labored breathing | • The ventilator delivers preset tidal volume and rate to a patient not breathing on his own (control).<br>• If the patient breathes slightly on his own, the ventilator senses his breath, then delivers full tidal volume (assist). |

tus and provide good pulmonary care. Expect that your patient will continue to have IPPB and mini-nebulizer treatments.

## Hemothorax

### Prediagnosis summary
The patient with a hemothorax probably had a history of blunt or penetrating trauma. He also had some or all of these signs and symptoms:

• chest pain
• tachypnea
• rapid-onset dyspnea
• tachycardia
• diaphoresis
• dusky skin color
• hemoptysis
• bloody, frothy sputum
• mild to severe hypotension, depending on how much blood he lost.

After his airway was cleared, he was given oxygen and placed on a cardiac monitor. He may have had few external signs of even a large blood loss, so his blood pressure, urine output, heart

## NURSING CONSIDERATIONS

- Prepare chest tubes, Pleur-evac, and thoracotomy tray in case tension pneumothorax develops.
- Watch for decreased cardiac output caused by increased intrathoracic pressure and low venous return.
- Watch for increased intracranial pressure.

- Take the patient's ABGs to monitor therapy.
- Reduce the frequency of assisted breaths as the patient weans himself from the ventilator
- Reassure the patient about fears of leaving the ventilator.

- Closely monitor the patient's vital signs.
- Adjust humidification infusion, as needed, to prevent secretions from becoming too viscous.

- Place the patient in a semi-Fowler position to encourage lung expansion.
- Monitor the patient's ABGs and blood pressure to assess oxygen and carbon dioxide levels, ventilation effectiveness, and oxygen toxicity.
- Administer several deep breaths hourly to prevent alveolar collapse and to stimulate coughing.
- Check for atelectasis from improper deep breathing, pneumothorax, or secretion retention.
- Beware of anxiety in the patient, which may cause him to hyperventilate or to fight the machine. He may need sedation.

rate, and cardiac status were assessed frequently.

An I.V. infusion—probably Ringer's lactate—was started to replace lost fluids. A central venous pressure (CVP) line may have been inserted for assessment of volume and for rapid fluid infusion.

He was placed in a semi-Fowler position (or assumed it on his own) to aid breathing. Breath sounds on his affected side were found to be diminished or absent on auscultation, and dullness was noted on percussion. The patient was examined for signs of blunt trauma (contusion or ecchymosis) or penetrating trauma (stab or gunshot wound).

The patient's chest X-ray showed that the hemothorax was either partial or total. The X-ray may also have shown a mediastinal shift. Arterial blood gas (ABG) studies may have shown hypoxemia. If his hemothorax was massive, his complete blood count (CBC) may have shown decreased hemoglobin and hematocrit levels.

### Priorities

Your first nursing priorities in caring

for a patient with a hemothorax are:
• to assist in the insertion of a chest tube to remove the blood from his pleural cavity
• to replace volume that the patient's lost due to bleeding.

Explain the chest tube insertion procedure to your patient and sedate him as ordered. Tell him that the doctor will use a local anesthetic at the tube insertion site; he'll feel pressure, but not pain. Of course, you'll also frequently check his CVP, urine output, blood pressure, and heart rate as guides to his fluid status.

After the tube's inserted, connect it to an underwater-seal chest drainage system and record the amount of initial drainage. Then record the type and amount of additional fluid drainage every 15 to 30 minutes. Auscultate breath sounds frequently to determine if the patient's improving.

If you find the following amounts of blood loss, tell the doctor immediately—he'll have to decide whether you should prepare the patient for blood transfusion, for immediate surgery (thoracotomy), or for autotransfusion:
• Initial drainage exceeds 1,000 ml.
• Drainage exceeds 200 ml/hour and isn't decreasing.
• Drainage exceeds 500 ml in the first 3 hours.

---

PATHOPHYSIOLOGY

## WHAT HAPPENS IN HEMOTHORAX

Blunt or penetrating chest trauma that lacerates the heart, lungs, great vessels, intercostal artery or veins, or blood vessels in the chest wall may cause hemothorax. Blood from these injuries accumulates in the pleural cavity. This causes partial or total lung collapse with impaired venous return to the heart—and potential mediastinal shift with problems such as decreased venous return and kinking of the great vessels and trachea.

---

If your patient needs a blood transfusion, draw blood for typing and cross matching, if this hasn't already been done. If immediate thoracotomy's ordered, make sure his preoperative blood work, chest X-ray, EKG (if ordered), and urinalysis results are on his chart. When you transport your patient to surgery, prevent backflow of fluid into the pleural cavity by making sure his chest drainage system doesn't tip over. Remember to bring rubber-tipped clamps so that you can clamp it if it becomes detached, keeping air from entering the chest cavity.

If you're going to start autotransfusion, explain the procedure to your patient. (See *Understanding Autotransfusion.*) Autotransfusion eliminates the disease transmission, transfusion reaction, isoimmunization, and incompatibility that can accompany blood transfusion. However, remember that autotransfusion may cause:
• clotting abnormalities from too little or too much anticoagulant
• platelet abnormalities
• microemboli
• sepsis
• air embolus (if connections aren't secure).

Following surgery or during blood transfusion or autotransfusion, you'll frequently monitor the patient's CVP, urine output, blood pressure, and heart rate to assess his fluid status for hypovolemia or fluid overload. If your patient had a mild hemothorax and doesn't immediately require these interventions, assess these parameters frequently for signs of increased blood loss or impending hypovolemic shock. If you see signs and symptoms of shock, you may have to apply medical antishock trousers (a MAST suit) as a short-term intervention until a blood transfusion or autotransfusion can begin. The doctor may also decide to take the patient to surgery at this time.

Monitor his ABGs frequently for the hypoxemia that often accompanies hemothorax. Watch your patient for changes in mental status, such as anx-

# UNDERSTANDING AUTOTRANSFUSION

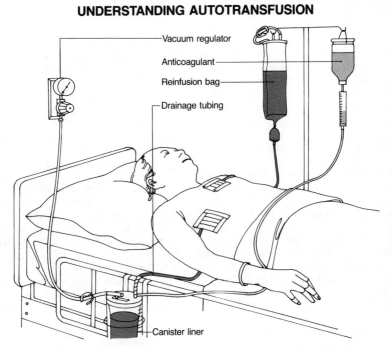

- Vacuum regulator
- Anticoagulant
- Reinfusion bag
- Drainage tubing
- Canister liner

You're assessing a boy's chest wound when you detect signs and symptoms of shock: blood loss, decreased blood pressure, and increased heart rate. The doctor examines the boy, tells you he has a hemothorax, and gives an order to prepare him for autotransfusion.

Using this procedure, the doctor will remove the blood that's filled the boy's pleural space. Then he'll reinfuse it into the boy's system—quickly—to treat the shock. Why not do a regular transfusion? Because the boy's shocky condition allows no time to type and cross match his blood.

Here's how autotransfusion works and what you need to know to assist with it.

## How it works

As you may know, autotransfusion collects, filtrates, and reinfuses the patient's own blood. It helps treat massive blood loss (1,000 ml or more) from hemothorax as well as heart or great vessel injuries. To use autotransfusion, the chest cavity can't be contaminated with gastrointestinal contents such as those from wounds of the esophagus, stomach, or bowel. The wound can't be more than 4 hours old, and the blood can't have been hemolyzed.

The procedure works as follows:

- The vacuum system sucks shed blood through the sterile chest tube and into the sterile canister liner.
- The canister contains citrate-phosphate-dextrose to prevent clotting of collected blood, and a fine-screen filter to remove microaggregated platelets, air bubbles, fat, and debris.
- The liner's removed from the canister when reinfusion is necessary or when 1,900 ml of blood have been collected.
- A microemboli filter's attached to the I.V. line. Blood is quickly reinfused through transfusion tubing, using gravity drip. Infusion pumps can be used for rapid infusion.

## Nursing interventions

- Before you assist with autotransfusion, be sure you're familiar with the procedure and the equipment.
- Maintain sterility of the equipment and the system during the procedure.
- Make sure all the connections on the equipment are secure.
- Change the microemboli filter after collecting 1,900 ml of blood.
- Carefully document all therapeutic measures, times, blood volumes lost and replaced, and serial assessments of the patient's condition.

iety, confusion, and restlessness, which may indicate decreased oxygen supply to the brain. Watch his cardiac monitor for dysrhythmias (for example, frequent premature ventricular contractions), which may also indicate hypoxemia. If you suspect hypoxemia, tell the doctor. He'll probably order ABGs. Check your patient's ABG results and reevaluate his respiratory status to substantiate your suspicions.

## Continuing assessment and intervention

Now that your patient with a hemothorax has been stabilized, you can do a thorough baseline nursing assessment. Keep in mind, however, that your patient may start to bleed excessively at any time and may require surgery or blood transfusion immediately. Be constantly on the alert for signs and symptoms of increased blood loss— tachycardia, hypotension, and decreased CVP. Auscultate his breath sounds and compare your findings with previous assessments. If his breath sounds are now diminished or absent on his affected side, be sure to check his chest tube for blood clots or kinks that may be obstructing it. The doctor may ask you to strip the tube if necessary, but be aware that mechanical strippers generate an extreme negative pressure, which may compromise lung integrity. Check to make sure the connections are secure. If the chest tube's already clear and you can find no other cause for your patient's decreased breath sounds, call the doctor, who'll probably order another chest X-ray. This will be evaluated for signs of increased bleeding and for the presence of a pneumothorax, which can accompany a hemothorax and may not have been evident before. (See the pneumothorax entries in this chapter.)

Take your patient's vital signs frequently, and continue to record the amount and type of drainage from his pleural cavity. Remember to monitor his ABGs for hypoxemia. Monitor his CVP intake and output frequently for signs and symptoms of blood loss or fluid depletion.

If your baseline assessment doesn't indicate the need for further interventions at this time, continue by taking your patient's history. Ask him (or whoever can give you the information) about the blunt or penetrating injury that caused his hemothorax—when, where, and how did it happen? Ask him if he has any preexisting lung disease, since this might affect the amount of oxygen he receives.

## Therapeutic care

After you've completed your baseline assessment, administer analgesics, such as meperidine (Demerol), as ordered for pain; but be sure to observe your patient for signs and symptoms of respiratory depression, which some of these drugs can cause.

Put your patient in a position that he feels is most comfortable. He may think he has to restrict his movements after the chest tube insertion; reassure him that he *can* change position (carefully) in bed—and that you'll be available to help him.

Continue to check and record the type and amount of drainage from his chest tube. Of course, keep checking and recording his fluid intake and output to make sure the amount of fluid he's getting is appropriate.

Do follow-up diagnostic studies, as ordered. Repeat the CBC (to check hemoglobin and hematocrit levels) and the ABG studies (to monitor oxygenation). He'll also need another chest X-ray to assess the extent of possible continued bleeding and the degree of lung reexpansion at this stage in his treatment.

If his hemothorax was mild, his condition will probably clear up within 10 to 14 days after the initial drainage. However, continue to observe him for signs and symptoms of increased or continued bleeding. When his chest tube drainage has decreased and his lungs have reexpanded sufficiently, the doctor will remove his chest tube. Continue to assess his respiratory status, and be alert for any signs and symptoms of respiratory distress that may indicate a recurrence of bleeding with subsequent collapse of the lung.

---

# Open Pneumothorax

## Prediagnosis summary
Initial assessment findings included a history of penetrating trauma, which produced an open wound in the upper torso, and signs and symptoms of acute respiratory distress:
- dyspnea
- tachypnea
- asymmetrical chest movement
- agitation
- sudden onset of pleuritic pain
- tachycardia
- diaphoresis
- hypotension.

On auscultation, a sucking or swishing sound and diminished or absent chest sounds on the injured side were noted. Oxygen was started, and an occlusive petrolatum gauze dressing was applied to prevent further flow of air into the pleural cavity. (If an occlusive petrolatum gauze dressing wasn't available, the wound may have been covered by a dry dressing, plastic wrap, or even the palm of someone's hand.)

An I.V. infusion was started, and blood was drawn for assessment of the patient's arterial blood gases (ABGs). A chest X-ray was taken to detect the extent of the pneumothorax and to determine whether mediastinal shift was present. The patient was placed on a cardiac monitor.

## Priorities
The first medical priority? Of course—to alleviate the patient's pneumothorax. You'll assist in the insertion of a chest tube to:
- drain the accumulated blood and air
- prevent (or alleviate) the development of a tension pneumothorax

(which can accompany open pneumothorax)
- restore the pressure gradient of the affected lung.

After the tube's inserted and attached to an underwater-seal drainage system, assess your patient's breath sounds to determine whether the pneumothorax is improving.

With the pressure gradient restored, you can clean and care for his open wound. Continue to administer supplemental oxygen by mask or nasal cannula.

Another chest X-ray will be done at this time to check for relief of the pneumothorax and for lung reexpansion. The patient's ABGs will be reassessed for hypoxemia. If his ABGs still indicate hypoxemia after chest tube insertion and partial or total lung reexpansion, the doctor may order the supplemental oxygen percentage increased.

With the pneumothorax alleviated, you can administer analgesics, as ordered, for pain. If your patient's wound was large, or if the penetrating object caused injury to underlying organs, you may have to prepare him for surgery.

## Continuing assessment and intervention
After you've stabilized your patient's respiratory status (or after he's had surgery), perform a complete baseline assessment. Continually assess his breath sounds to evaluate his respiratory status. If he shows any signs or symptoms of respiratory distress, check the chest tube for obstructions, kinks, or loose connections. (Remember, these can cause a tension pneumothorax. See the "Tension Pneumothorax" entry in this chapter.) Palpate his neck and chest for signs of subcutaneous emphysema—small air pockets under the skin, which may move around or pop if pressed.

Assess his cardiac output by checking his tissue perfusion indicators: urinary output, blood pressure, pulse quality, and mental status. Check the

PATHOPHYSIOLOGY

## WHAT HAPPENS IN OPEN PNEUMOTHORAX

Also called an open or sucking chest wound or penetrating pneumothorax, open pneumothorax results from an injury that creates an opening in the chest wall, allowing atmospheric air (positive pressure) to flow directly into the pleural cavity (negative pressure). As air pressure in the pleural cavity becomes positive, the lung collapses on the affected side. This causes impaired venous return and possible mediastinal shift—with the potential for tracheal deviation and kinking of the great vessels.

monitor, too, for dysrhythmias. Be alert for tachycardia, which may indicate beginning hypoxemia or compensation for a mediastinal shift.

Now check his chest and abdomen for signs of further organ injury that may not have been discovered during the rapid prestabilization assessment.

If you've found no signs or symptoms of complications, such as developing tension pneumothorax or hemothorax (see these entries in this chapter), continue assessing your patient by taking his history. Ask about the traumatic event that caused his injury. Does he have a preexisting pulmonary disease? This may affect his treatment.

### Therapeutic care
Auscultate your patient's chest for breath sounds frequently to determine if they're diminished or absent on the affected side, and check his ease of breathing (rate, rhythm, use of accessory muscles). Observe him for hypoxemia; the results of serial ABGs will help determine this. Check your patient's monitor often to keep track of his cardiac status. Assess and record the amount and type of the patient's chest tube drainage. Because hemothorax can accompany open pneumothorax, watch for increased bloody drainage.

Continue to administer analgesics as

needed for pain, such as meperidine (Demerol), but remember to watch for signs and symptoms of the respiratory depression these drugs can cause. To prevent an infection from developing in the patient's open wound, the doctor may order antibiotics.

Expect the doctor to order respiratory therapy to improve the patient's tidal volume and lung expansion. The patient may be given incentive spirometry; encourage him to use this frequently. He may also be given mini-nebulizer treatments; the respiratory therapist administers these.

Daily follow-up chest X-rays and ABGs will help you monitor your patient's recovery from open pneumothorax. His chest tube will be removed as soon as:
• a follow-up chest X-ray shows adequate lung reexpansion
• the amount of chest tube drainage has decreased sufficiently
• the wound site has healed satisfactorily
• ABGs show absence of hypoxemia.

After chest tube removal, continue meticulous pulmonary hygiene, encouraging the patient to cough and deep-breathe to remove any secretions. Continue giving the patient antibiotics, if ordered. He may continue to receive respiratory therapy—incentive spirometry and mini-nebulizer treatments—to further improve his tidal volume and lung function.

# Tension Pneumothorax

### Prediagnosis summary
Initial assessment of the patient revealed this picture of severe respiratory distress suggesting tension pneumothorax:
• tracheal deviation (the hallmark of tension pneumothorax)
• hypoxia
• sudden-onset dyspnea
• tachycardia

- agitation
- air hunger
- nasal flaring
- diaphoresis
- use of accessory muscles to breathe
- asymmetrical chest movements.

He may also have had:
- absent breath sounds on the affected side
- subcutaneous emphysema around his neck and upper chest
- severe pain on breathing
- distended neck veins
- hypotension.

(If the patient developed tension pneumothorax while in the hospital and on a ventilator, his signs and symptoms may have been difficult to recognize. This is why you should always monitor a patient on a ventilator very closely.)

Immediate initial treatment included supplemental oxygen to relieve his hypoxia; he may also have required needle thoracotomy to release trapped air from his pleural cavity. An I.V. infusion was started, and he was connected to a cardiac monitor.

Initial history findings revealed either blunt or penetrating trauma causing partial or total lung collapse; or preexisting chronic obstructive pulmonary disease (COPD) causing alveolar bleb rupture; *or* the patient may have developed tension pneumothorax while hospitalized and on a mechanical ventilator with increased positive end-expiratory pressure (>10 cm).

### Priorities

The *immediate* medical and nursing priority is to relieve the air pressure in the patient's pleural cavity. In this emergency situation, time won't allow for diagnostic tests, such as arterial blood gases (ABGs) and a chest X-ray. You must intervene as *quickly* as possible to keep the patient from dying. The doctor may immediately release the pressure in the patient's pleural cavity by performing a needle thoracotomy (this may have been done during transport to the hospital). As you know, nee-

dle thoracotomy is only a temporary measure. Prepare to assist with chest tube insertion to restore negative pressure which will relieve your patient's tension pneumothorax. Connect the chest tube to an underwater-seal drainage system (Pleur-evac).

After the chest tube's been inserted, the patient's respiratory status should improve dramatically—he should breathe more easily and slowly, his heart rate should decrease, and he should no longer be hypoxemic.

If your patient's tension pneumothorax was caused by a penetrating injury, his wound can now be cleaned and sutured.

### Continuing assessment and intervention

Now, with your patient's chest tube inserted and his respiratory status stabilized, you're ready to perform a thorough baseline assessment. Check his breath sounds on the affected side

PATHOPHYSIOLOGY

## WHAT HAPPENS IN TENSION PNEUMOTHORAX

Tension pneumothorax may be caused by penetrating chest wounds; puncture of the lung or airway by a fractured rib; post–chest-injury mechanical ventilation that forces air into the pleural space through damaged areas; high levels of positive end-expiratory pressure, causing rupture of an alveolar bleb; or chest tube occlusion or malfunction.

Air enters the pleural space either from within the lung (as the result of lung or airway damage) or from the outside atmosphere because of a sucking chest wound that creates a one-way valve effect. Whatever the cause, the air can't escape. Accumulating pressure causes partial or total lung collapse, usually with mediastinal shift and impaired venous return. The heart, trachea, esophagus, and great vessels are pushed to the unaffected side, compressing the heart and the contralateral lung. Without immediate intervention, tension pneumothorax is rapidly fatal.

to note improvement, and his respiratory status to mark his slower breathing rate and regular rhythm. Also check to see if he's still using accessory chest muscles to breathe. Are his respiratory movements symmetrical?

On palpation, you may feel subcutaneous emphysema in his neck and upper chest area.

Assess your patient's cardiac status, specifically his cardiac output and perfusion, by checking his monitor (for tachycardia or other dysrhythmias), his pulses, his urine output, and his mental status. Review the patient's ABGs (for hypoxemia) and chest X-ray (for lung reexpansion). If he develops signs and symptoms of increased respiratory distress, check the chest tube for kinks, obstructions, or loose connections that can allow air to enter the pleural cavity and cause *another* tension pneumothorax.

Frequently check the amount and type of drainage from your patient's chest tube. Don't be surprised to see a small amount of blood from the penetrating injury, but be alert for a larger amount of blood. This may indicate a hemothorax which can develop from a tension pnemothorax if the wound further injures a large blood vessel. (See the "Hemothorax" entry in this chapter.)

If you discover no complications, take your patient's history next. Ask about the traumatic event that caused his injury. (If he's very ill, or on a ventilator, obtain this information from his family.) Also find out if he has any preexisting pulmonary disease, such as COPD.

### Therapeutic care
Your continuing care will probably include giving the patient broad-spectrum antibiotics to prevent infection of his open wound. The doctor may also order analgesics, such as meperidine (Demerol), administered for pain. Remember to watch for signs and symptoms of respiratory depression—a potential side effect of these drugs.

Reassess your patient's respiratory status. Check his breath sounds and the rate, rhythm, and ease of his breathing. Compare this assessment with your earlier findings.

His follow-up chest X-ray should show further lung reexpansion, and his ABGs should show no hypoxemia. Continue to check the amount and type of chest tube drainage for excessive blood. If your patient's been on a ventilator, and his respiratory status has improved, he'll receive respiratory therapy to facilitate lung expansion. He'll receive intermittent positive-pressure breathing or mini-nebulizer treatments from the respiratory therapist, along with incentive spirometry, which you'll need to supervise. Encourage him to use this therapy frequently.

When your patient's follow-up chest X-rays show adequate lung reexpansion, and after his wound has begun to heal, his chest tube will be removed. Afterward, listen to his breath sounds again and assess his respirations for rate, rhythm, and ease of breathing. Continue to watch him for signs and symptoms of recurrent respiratory distress. Respiratory therapy should be continued during this phase of his treatment. Encourage him to cough and deep-breathe frequently to remove any secretions from the lungs.

# Closed Pneumothorax

### Prediagnosis summary
The typical patient with closed pneumothorax initially had:
• sudden chest pain that increased with deep inspiration but was unrelated to exertion
• decreased or absent breath sounds on the affected side.

He may also have had:
• a nonproductive cough related to his pleural irritation
• asymmetrical chest-wall movements
• dyspnea proportional to the amount

of his lung collapse. (Young adults may not complain of this even with 50% pneumothorax.)

Closed pneumothorax can result from blunt chest trauma as well as from rupture of an apical bleb—which occurs most often in a patient with chronic obstructive pulmonary disease (COPD) who's on mechanical ventilation. The doctor ordered a chest X-ray to visualize the extent of lung collapse, and arterial blood gases (ABGs) to estimate the severity of ventilation impairment. If he had dyspnea, the patient received oxygen by nasal cannula.

### Priorities

The size of your patient's pneumothorax determines the degree of his respiratory distress and the extent of your initial care. If his pneumothorax is minimal (less than 20%), he'll have only mild dyspnea and he may have little or no chest pain. Give oxygen by nasal cannula or mask, and keep him quiet and comfortable in bed.

If your patient has respiratory distress and his pneumothorax is moderate to severe (greater than 20%), he'll need a chest tube to remove air from his pleural space, in addition to oxygen by nasal cannula or mask. Have a chest tube tray and an underwater-seal drainage system ready, and assist the doctor with chest tube insertion. (See *Assisting with Chest Tube Insertion*, pages 144 and 145.) Administer pain medication (such as Demerol or morphine), and have a local anesthetic ready so the doctor can numb the area before he inserts the tube. Reassure the patient that he'll breathe easier when the chest tube's in place.

### Continuing assessment and intervention

Assess your patient for signs of respiratory distress. If he has a minimal pneumothorax that didn't require chest tube insertion initially, he'll still have decreased or absent breath sounds over the affected area, and he may have pain on inspiration. Continue to give him

PATHOPHYSIOLOGY

## WHAT HAPPENS IN CLOSED PNEUMOTHORAX

Closed pneumothorax is partial or complete lung collapse occurring when air enters the pleural space from within the lung and causes increased pleural pressure, which prevents lung expansion during normal inspiration. *Traumatic pneumothorax* occurs when blunt chest trauma causes the rupture of lung tissue and resulting air leakage. *Spontaneous pneumothorax* usually results from the rupture of a superficial apical bleb. More common in men than in women, it's often seen in older patients with chronic pulmonary disease, but it may occur in healthy young adults.

Both types of closed pneumothorax result in a collapsed lung with substantially decreased total lung capacity, vital capacity, and lung compliance. The resulting ventilation-perfusion imbalances lead to hypoxia.

oxygen, and encourage him to cough and deep-breathe. Respiratory therapy such as intermittent positive-pressure breathing, mini-nebulizer treatments, and incentive spirometry will also be given to promote good pulmonary hygiene. He should be breathing comfortably.

If your patient with closed pneumothorax has underlying pulmonary disease, such as COPD, or if he's on mechanical ventilation for another problem, he may develop increasing dyspnea, cyanosis, or other signs and symptoms of respiratory distress. *Call the doctor* if these signs and symptoms develop. He'll order a repeat chest X-ray to determine the size and extent of the pneumothorax. Prepare for chest tube insertion.

If your patient's had a chest tube inserted either initially or as a result of developing respiratory distress, you'll need to connect the chest tubes to an underwater-seal chest drainage system, such as a Pleur-evac. Once the drainage system's in place, check the connections for bubbling, signs of air

PROCEDURES

# YOUR ROLE IN AN EMERGENCY

## ASSISTING WITH CHEST TUBE INSERTION

The doctor places a chest tube in your patient's pleural space to:
- drain air, blood, fluid, or pus from his pleural space
- reestablish atmospheric and intrathoracic pressure gradients
- allow complete lung reexpansion.

You may assist by reassuring the patient, preparing him for the procedure, and monitoring his recovery.

### Indications
- Pneumothorax
- Hemothorax
- Empyema
- Pleural effusion
- Chylothorax

### Complications
- Bleeding from intercostal blood vessels at insertion site
- Pulmonary laceration
- Tube placed into lung instead of pleural space
- Tension pneumothorax

### Equipment
- Sterile gloves
- Betadine solution and prep sponges
- Sterile drapes
- Petrolatum gauze
- Dressing sponges and tape
- Local anesthetic, needles, syringes
- Chest tube tray that includes scalpel, assorted hemostats, curbed clamp (Kelly), trocar, chest tubes of assorted sizes
- Underwater-seal chest drainage system (Your hospital may use the disposable Pleur-evac system, its equivalent three-bottle drainage system, or a one- or two-bottle water-seal system.)

### Procedure
- Explain the procedure to the patient and that this procedure will help him breathe more easily.
- Sedate him as ordered.
- Assist in preparing his skin with povidone-iodine solution.
- Drape the area with sterile towels.
- The doctor will anesthetize the skin area where he plans to insert the tube.
- Help the patient hold still while the doctor makes a skin incision and inserts the tube.
- To relieve *pneumothorax,* the doctor will insert the chest tube in the second intercostal space along the midclavicular line. For *pleural effusion* or *hemothorax,* he'll insert it in the fourth to sixth intercostal space in the anterior or midaxillary line.
- Connect the tube to the Pleur-evac underwater-seal chest drainage system.
- The doctor will suture the tube in place and apply petrolatum gauze and a sterile dressing.
- Tape all tube connections securely and regulate suction as ordered.
- Secure the Pleur-evac system to the patient's bed.

### Nursing follow-up care
- Prepare the patient for a chest X-ray to check tube placement.
- Administer pain medication as ordered.
- Secure the tube to the draw sheet with a safety pin, allowing sufficient tubing for the patient to turn over. Don't leave dangling loops.
- Keep clamps and extra petrolatum gauze at the patient's bedside in case the tubing accidentally disconnects or pulls out.
- Watch for signs of chest tube occlusion from kinks, clots, or mucous plugs.
- Record hourly drainage on the collection chamber of the Pleur-evac.
- Observe the suction chamber for continuous bubbling. Lack of bubbling may indicate suction failure.

leakage, kinks, or obstructions. Watch your patient for cyanosis, distended neck veins, hypotension, subcutaneous emphysema, or increased respiratory distress—signs of developing tension pneumothorax. This may result from problems in the drainage system or from rupture of bilateral or emphysematous blebs, especially if the patient has COPD and is on a ventilator. (See the "Tension Pneumothorax" entry in this chapter.)

COPD also develop ruptured blebs more easily on mechanical ventilation, and they have a decreased tolerance for the hypoxemia and decreased cardiac output associated with pneumothorax.

### Therapeutic care

If your patient's pneumothorax is minimal and he didn't require a chest tube, expect his lung to reexpand spontaneously over several days. Watch him closely during this time—his breath sounds should return and his breathing should become easy and comfortable. Expect the doctor to order follow-up chest X-rays to make sure the lung has reinflated.

If your patient required a chest tube, he'll have it in place for several days while his lung reinflates—longer if he has underlying pulmonary disease. Expect that he'll have daily chest X-rays to check the progression of lung reinflation. Remember to check all connections in the underwater-seal chest drainage system frequently. Be sure no leak exists, and watch for kinks or occlusions in the chest tube. To facilitate his lung expansion, encourage the patient to cough and breathe deeply. Change the dressing around the chest tube insertion site as often as necessary. *Important:* If the chest tube dislodges accidentally, this will convert the *closed* pneumothorax to an *open* pneumothorax. To prevent lung collapse, cover the opening *immediately* with petrolatum gauze. (See the "Open Pneumothorax" entry in this chapter.)

Keep two padded hemostats and a package of petrolatum gauze taped to his bedside at all times while your patient has a chest tube in place. Use these if the chest tube drainage system becomes disconnected or the chest tube inadvertently falls out.

The doctor will remove your patient's chest tube when his lung has fully expanded. Have a petrolatum gauze dressing ready, and put it on as soon as the tube's removed. Continue to monitor the patient's vital signs, being especially alert to an increase in tem-

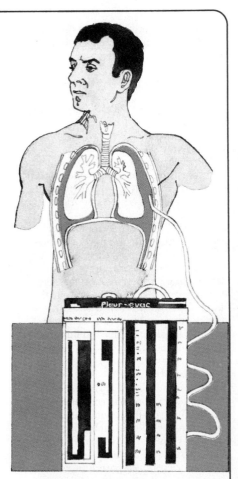

• Every 2 to 4 hours, check for fluctuation on respiration in water-seal chamber: turn off the suction and observe. Fluctuation will stop when the tubing is obstructed or the lung has reexpanded. If you observe air bubbles while the suction's turned off, check the tubing for an air leak.
• Report subcutaneous emphysema, chest pressure, cyanosis, or rapid, shallow breathing to the patient's doctor.

In an elderly patient with COPD, pneumothorax may further compromise his already decreased ventilatory capacity. Observe him closely for signs and symptoms of developing respiratory distress. Elderly patients with

perature. This may be a sign of infection resulting from the lack of ventilation in the affected area or from the chest tube itself.

# Tracheobronchial Injury

## Prediagnosis summary
Initial assessment findings for a patient with a tracheobronchial injury vary according to the injury's severity. For example, if his airways remain intact, he may complain only of hoarseness, sore throat, difficulty in swallowing, or neck pain. The doctor will determine whether this patient needs emergency care: He may need only supplemental oxygen, through a nasal cannula or a mask, and careful observation.

However, the typical patient with a severe tracheobronchial injury has suffered serious trauma to his airway. His initial assessment findings probably included:

- signs and symptoms of respiratory distress, including labored respiration, stridor, tachypnea, cyanosis, and accessory muscle use
- signs of hypoxemia, such as anxiety and restlessness
- some degree of subcutaneous emphysema
- hemoptysis
- hypotension.

The doctor inserted an endotracheal tube reaching beyond the site of the injury—if intubation wasn't possible, he performed an emergency tracheostomy. Because fractures of the cervical vertebrae frequently accompany tracheobronchial injuries, the doctor presumed a spinal injury existed; he was careful not to hyperextend the patient's neck during intubation. As soon as adequate oxygenation was ensured, the doctor ordered a cervical spine X-ray to rule out spinal fracture. The patient was placed on a cardiac monitor, and an I.V. was inserted.

## Priorities
Your *immediate* priority, of course, is stabilizing the patient's respiratory status. You'll typically provide initial oxygenation through an Ambu bag with 100% oxygen. If his tracheobronchial tree's perforated, he may require immediate surgery. Prepare him as necessary.

After surgery (or if surgery isn't necessary), the patient will be connected to a ventilator. Monitor his arterial blood gases (ABGs) to check whether his ventilation's adequate at the initial ventilator settings. The doctor will order a chest X-ray following the immediate crisis to check for free air and accurate endotracheal tube placement.

The doctor may use high-frequency ventilation to keep your patient's airway pressure low and to allow greater retention of oxygen in his lungs. (See *Understanding High-Frequency Ventilation*, pages 160 and 161.)

Remember that trauma sufficient to cause severe tracheobronchial injury

---

PATHOPHYSIOLOGY

## WHAT HAPPENS IN TRACHEO-BRONCHIAL INJURIES

Tracheobronchial injuries are rare, but they have a high mortality. Why? Because disruption of the tracheobronchial tree causes immediate and severe respiratory distress that, if not treated promptly, can lead to death within minutes. These injuries are most commonly caused by trauma with rapid deceleration—for example, from high-speed motor vehicle accidents or from falls or jumps from high places. Rapid deceleration causes flexible distal airways (trachea, mainstem bronchus, or both) to shear off from the relatively fixed central airways.

Blunt trauma may also cause these injuries when flexible distal airways are compressed against the cervical vertebrae or when direct blows to the larynx and cervical trachea cause contusions or fractures (usually mandibular fractures).

may also injure the esophagus, diaphragm, heart, or great vessels. Assess your patient carefully for signs and symptoms of other injuries.

### Continuing assessment and intervention

Once your patient's respiratory distress has subsided, begin your nursing assessment of his tracheobronchial injury. If he's in severe pain, administer medication, such as meperidine (Demerol) or morphine, as ordered, to make him comfortable. Obtain a history of how the injury occurred—it may lead you to suspect possible associated injuries, such as rib or facial fractures, that were overlooked during the initial assessment. Continue by taking his vital signs; pay particular attention to the rate and quality of his respirations. An increase in rate or depth may be an early indication of a developing respiratory problem.

Auscultate his lungs for signs of airway obstruction, such as decreased breath sounds or wheezing. Remember that a *partial* airway obstruction from a forceful injury can become *complete* within a few hours.

Gently palpate his chest and neck for signs of subcutaneous emphysema, which indicates air leakage.

### Therapeutic care

Administer medication for pain, as necessary, and continue to monitor your patient's respirations. Observe him closely for signs and symptoms of developing airway obstruction. (See the "Upper Airway Obstruction" entry in this chapter.) Monitor his ABGs carefully to ensure that his ventilation's adequate. Check his chest and neck for increasing subcutaneous emphysema from air leakage, and notify the doctor if you find any increase.

Once your patient's respiratory status has stabilized, as determined by improved ABGs, vital signs, and chest X-rays, he can be slowly weaned from the ventilator. Continue to monitor his ABGs throughout the weaning process.

Following weaning and extubation, he may require a high-humidity mask for about 24 hours. This will help reduce any swelling in the area of injury and relieve throat pain. Continue to observe your patient for signs and symptoms of recurrent respiratory distress from infection of the injured tracheobronchial or lung tissue. After you remove the high-humidity mask, reassess his ABGs to verify that he requires no further respiratory intervention.

# Upper Airway Obstruction

### Prediagnosis summary

If the patient's obstruction was *partial*, due to inflammation, thermal injury, hemoptysis, tumor, vomitus, or a foreign body, his initial signs and symptoms were:
- stridor
- wheezing
- intercostal muscle retraction
- nasal flaring
- indications of respiratory distress and developing hypoxia.

If the partial obstruction compromised his ventilation and oxygenation (for example, vocal cord edema), he was intubated and given oxygen to provide a temporary airway while his underlying problem was determined and treated. He was placed on a cardiac monitor to detect dysrhythmias arising from hypoxemia, and a chest X-ray was taken to identify the obstruction.

If his airway obstruction was *complete*, due to a foreign body or to a partial occlusion that progressed to a complete one, initial assessment revealed:
- inspiratory chest movement with no air movement heard on auscultation
- inability to talk
- diaphoresis
- tachycardia
- severe hypoxemia progressing rap-

idly so the patient became cyanotic, lethargic, and eventually unconscious.

Whether the obstruction was partial or total, the patient was treated *immediately*, to remove or bypass it and to reverse his hypoxemia. If the obstruction couldn't be cleared using finger sweeps, back blows, or the abdominal thrust (Heimlich maneuver), the patient was intubated, or the doctor performed a tracheostomy. (He may also have performed an emergency bronchoscopy to remove the object.) Obstruction-causing aspirated vomitus or blood was suctioned through the endotracheal tube or tracheostomy tube. Bypassing a tumor low in the trachea probably required intubation of a right mainstem bronchus.

### Priorities

If your patient's airway was obstructed by a smooth, regular object (such as a bead or a marble) that was successfully removed, he may not need postremoval care. However, if the object was sharp or irregular, you'll need to watch him closely after the object's removed. Why? Because an irritated or damaged airway may become edematous, *creating another obstruction.*

Assist with intubation (if neces-

sary), and provide oxygen. Watch the cardiac monitor for dysrhythmias, which may indicate the patient's becoming hypoxemic.

Administer humidified oxygen if your patient's obstruction resulted from inflammation (for example, from diphtheria, allergic reactions, croup, or epiglottitis) or edema (for example, from thermal injury). The cool mist will help decrease swelling, opening the airway.

You may be asked to administer intravenous corticosteroids, such as dexamethasone (Decadron) or methylprednisolone (Solu-Medrol), to further decrease edema and swelling. You may also give epinephrine to reduce swelling from an allergic reaction.

If massive hemoptysis was obstructing your patient's airway, initial endotracheal tube placement and suctioning may have removed clots and blood from his trachea. But if he's still bleeding, he'll need rigid bronchoscopy to locate the bleeding site and to clear the additional blood. Assist the doctor as necessary, and reassure the patient during the procedure.

### Continuing assessment and intervention

Perform your baseline nursing assessment when you've ensured that your patient has a patent airway. Listen for wheezing, and look for other signs and symptoms of increasing respiratory distress that may indicate edema or inflammation. *Notify the doctor* if you discover any.

Check your patient's vital signs. Increased temperature may indicate infection, which may have caused the inflammation and obstruction. Listen to your patient's breath sounds and note if they've decreased.

If he's aspirated a foreign body through his trachea and into a bronchus, the patient may suffer lung collapse, distal to the obstruction, and subacute infection. Remember, a patient who's aspirated a foreign object can develop atelectasis, pneumonitis, or edema distal to the affected area—

PATHOPHYSIOLOGY

## WHAT HAPPENS IN UPPER AIRWAY OBSTRUCTION

Causes of upper airway obstruction include:
• external compression
• trauma (including burns)
• laryngospasm (for example, from allergic reactions)
• vocal cord edema
• an infectious process, such as epiglottitis or retropharyngeal abscess
• a tumor
• a foreign object (for example, food or dentures).

If not treated promptly, complete airway obstruction leads—within minutes—from hypoxia to loss of consciousness to death.

# HOW RESPIRATORY DISORDERS AFFECT A.B.G.s

Arterial blood gas (ABG) tests help you assess your patient's respiratory status and monitor his therapy.

ABG tests evaluate gas exchange in your patient's lungs by measuring the partial pressures of oxygen ($PaO_2$), carbon dioxide ($PaCO_2$), and pH in arterial blood samples. For example, a low $PaO_2$ level indicates he's hypoxemic and may need oxygen. Subsequent $PaO_2$ measurements monitor the effectiveness of his oxygen therapy.

A rise in $PaCO_2$ indicates he's hypoventilating and retaining carbon dioxide, whereas a drop in $PaCO_2$ indicates he's hyperventilating and losing too much carbon dioxide. In both situations, he may need mechanical ventilation. You can monitor the mechanical ventilation's effectiveness by noting the patient's $PaCO_2$ levels on serial ABGs.

Here's a chart that shows you normal ABG values and how respiratory disorders affect them.

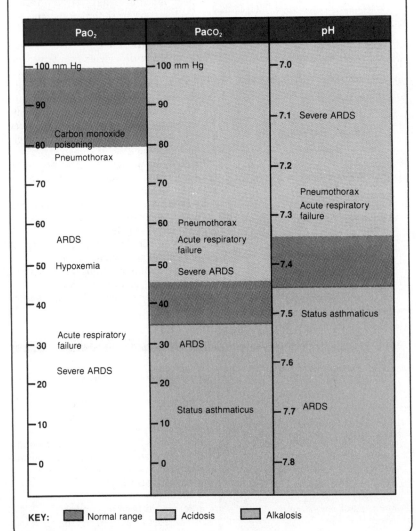

| $PaO_2$ | $PaCO_2$ | pH |
|---|---|---|
| 100 mm Hg | 100 mm Hg | 7.0 |
| 90 | 90 | 7.1  Severe ARDS |
| 80  Carbon monoxide poisoning  Pneumothorax | 80 | 7.2 |
| 70 | 70 | 7.3  Pneumothorax  Acute respiratory failure |
| 60 | 60  Pneumothorax  Acute respiratory failure | 7.4 |
| 50  ARDS  Hypoxemia | 50  Severe ARDS | 7.5  Status asthmaticus |
| 40 | 40 | 7.6 |
| 30  Acute respiratory failure  Severe ARDS | 30  ARDS | 7.7  ARDS |
| 20 | 20 | 7.8 |
| 10 | 10  Status asthmaticus | |
| 0 | 0 | |

KEY: ▨ Normal range   ▫ Acidosis   ▫ Alkalosis

## RESPIRATORY ACIDOSIS

Alveolar hypoventilation causes respiratory retention of $CO_2$, leading to carbonic acid excess and a decreased pH. Arterial $P_{CO_2}$ above 45 mm Hg and pH below 7.35 characterize respiratory acidosis.

### Predisposing factors

• Airway obstruction
• Chest-wall injury
• Neuromuscular disease
• Drug overdose (CNS depression)
• ARDS
• Pneumothorax
• Pneumonia
• Pulmonary edema

### Signs and symptoms

• Tachycardia
• Shallow, slow respirations
• Dyspnea
• Dysrhythmias
• Cyanosis
• Diaphoresis
• Lethargy
• Confusion
• $P_{CO_2} > 45$; pH < 7.35; but $HCO_3$ 22 to 26 (normal)

### Compensation

• In the presence of *increased* $P_{CO_2}$, the kidneys compensate by excreting hydrogen ions and reabsorbing $HCO_3$—to bring pH back to normal.

### Interventions

• Give $O_2$ (low concentrations in patients with chronic obstructive pulmonary disease).
• Give intravenous fluids.
• Give inhaled and/or intravenous bronchodilators.
• Start mechanical ventilation if hypoventilation can't be corrected immediately.
• Monitor ABGs and electrolytes.

within hours. Notify the doctor—he'll probably perform bronchoscopy to remove the object. *Early removal* is important, because the object may later become surrounded by granulation tissue. If this occurs, thoracotomy or bronchotomy may be necessary.

Obtain a history from the patient (or from his family if he's intubated). Does he have preexisting pulmonary disease? If his obstruction's caused by a tumor, find out if he's received treatment for this before. He'll probably need surgery or radiation therapy.

### Therapeutic care

Continue to provide oxygen until your patient's obstruction has been removed and the swelling and inflammation are reduced. He'll be extubated and weaned from the ventilator when the following indicators of his respiratory status show he can breathe adequately on his own:
• respiratory rate
• tidal volume (volume of air taken in with each breath)
• negative inspiratory force (amount of negative pressure required for the patient to breathe in)
• forced vital capacity (the deepest breath the patient can exhale).

Assess him carefully afterward to make sure his airway remains patent and no further edema or inflammation occurs.

## Pulmonary Embolism

### Prediagnosis summary

The patient may be hospitalized for another disorder, or he may have come into the hospital with signs and symptoms suggesting pulmonary embolism:
• sudden dyspnea and tachypnea
• severe pleuritic pain
• wheezing
• decreased breath sounds.

The doctor ordered diagnostic tests, blood studies, and a chest X-ray that may have shown atelectasis and pleural effusion. An EKG may have shown sinus tachycardia. Arterial blood gases (ABGs) probably revealed hypoxemia, hypocapnia, and respiratory alkalosis. A lung scan or pulmonary arteriogram confirmed the diagnosis.

The patient received supplemental oxygen by nasal cannula or mask, and an I.V. was inserted for medication access.

## Priorities

Your immediate priorities for a patient with a pulmonary embolism are to continue oxygen, to decrease his hypoxemia, and to relieve his pain, which will help reduce stress and decrease his hyperventilation. Take his vital signs, making sure to count his respirations for a full minute. This gives you time to assess his respiratory pattern as well, alerting you to early signs of respiratory distress. Then give pain medications, such as meperidine (Demerol) or morphine, as ordered.

You know that narcotics cause respiratory depression, reducing hyperventilation. In addition, the pain control they provide may encourage your patient to take deeper breaths, increasing his oxygen intake. Remember to monitor him closely, because he's already hypoxemic.

## Continuing assessment and intervention

Perform a thorough nursing assessment after you have medicated your patient for pain. Continue to observe the cardiac monitor for *dysrhythmias*, which may result from hypoxemia. If you observe serious dysrhythmias (such as frequent premature ventricular contractions) that may indicate hypoxemia, increase the oxygen flow rate and *call the doctor*. He'll order another ABG test to assess the degree of hypoxemia. Watch the patient for fainting or dizziness from hypoxemia or from decreased cerebral blood flow secondary to developing right heart failure. Watch for hemoptysis, too; this may indicate

## RESPIRATORY ALKALOSIS

Alveolar hyperventilation causes excess exhalation of $CO_2$, leading to carbonic acid deficit and an elevated pH. Arterial $P_{CO_2}$ below 35 mm Hg and pH above 7.45 characterize respiratory alkalosis.

### Predisposing factors

- Extreme anxiety
- CNS injury to respiratory center
- Fever
- Overventilation during mechanical ventilation
- Pulmonary embolism
- Congestive heart failure
- Salicylate intoxication (early)

### Signs and symptoms

- Tachycardia
- Deep, rapid breathing
- Light-headedness
- Numbness and tingling or arm and leg paresthesias
- Carpopedal spasm
- Tetany
- $P_{CO_2} < 35$; pH > 7.45; but $HCO_3$ 22 to 26 (normal)

### Compensation

- In the presence of *decreased* $P_{CO_2}$, the kidneys compensate by retaining hydrogen ions and *not* reabsorbing $HCO_3$—to bring pH back to normal.

### Interventions

- Have the patient breathe into a paper bag. (Rebreathing his $CO_2$ increases his $P_{CO_2}$.)
- Administer sedatives and give calm, reassuring support. (Hyperventilation is often triggered by "anxiety attacks.")
- Perform gastric lavage if salicylate overdose caused the alkalosis.
- Monitor ABGs and electrolytes.

congestive atelectasis or parenchymal damage.

When you auscultate your patient's lungs, you may hear wheezing resulting from spasm-induced bronchoconstriction. Listen for a pleural friction rub—this may indicate that your patient's pulmonary embolism has progressed to pulmonary infarction.

Be on the alert for development of congestive heart failure (see the "Congestive Heart Failure" entry in Chapter 5), a serious complication of pulmonary embolism. When you auscultate your patient's heart sounds, you may hear an increased pulmonary component of the second heart sound, a right ventricular $S_3$ gallop, and a tricuspid regurgitant murmur—signs of right ventricular dysfunction. Check your patient's jugular veins for distention, and be alert for a decrease in his blood pressure. These are also signs of right ventricular dysfunction and—along with altered heart sounds—may indicate that congestive heart failure's developing.

Congestive heart failure that results from pulmonary embolism worsens rapidly, so *stop your assessment and notify the doctor* if your patient has these signs. Expect to give vasopressor agents, such as dopamine, to increase blood pressure, along with drugs that increase heart contractility, such as digoxin. If these medications aren't effective, the doctor may order a pulmonary embolectomy to remove the clot. However, he'll do this only as a last resort, because it has an extremely high mortality.

If your patient doesn't have signs of developing congestive heart failure, continue your assessment by taking his history. Remember to take a thorough past medical history. If your patient has a history of heart disease, prior embolism, blood disorders, venous stasis, obesity, or neoplasms, he has an increased risk of developing recurrent pulmonary embolisms. Pregnancy, estrogen therapy, and the postpartum period also increase the risk of recurrent embolisms, so observe these patients closely.

### Therapeutic care

Anticoagulant therapy, using drugs such as heparin, is the standard medical treatment for a patient with a pulmonary embolism. To prevent extension of the embolism and further emboli, be prepared to administer this drug through an I.V. continuous infusion pump.

Keep protamine sulfate (a heparin antagonist) available whenever you're administering heparin by continuous infusion—1 mg of protamine sulfate will neutralize 78 to 95 units of heparin. You may be asked to give this if your patient's partial thromboplastin time (PTT) is grossly elevated or if you note signs of excessive bleeding.

Before you start the medication, draw blood for a PTT to determine your patient's baseline level. Then start continuous infusion of the anticoagulant. Check the patient's vital signs frequently. You'll need to draw blood at regular intervals to monitor ABGs and PTT. Your patient's PTT level is a reflection of the amount of anticoagulation achieved through heparin therapy—it should be 1½ to 2½ times the control level to be therapeutic. Check the test results when they return from the laboratory, and call the doctor if they're not within this range. If PTT levels are less than 1½ times control,

---

**SAVE THAT BEARD!**

The next time you tape an endotracheal tube to a patient with a beard, take the time to consider his self-image—he may value his beard more than you realize. Use umbilical tape to secure the tube in place. It'll hold the tube as securely as adhesive tape, but it won't hurt your patient when you remove it. And you *won't* have to shave his beard.

you know your patient isn't being anticoagulated sufficiently; if PTT levels are more than 2½ times control, you know he's being overmedicated and is at risk for hemorrhage.

Don't rely on laboratory tests alone. Monitor your patient for abnormal bleeding and unusual bruising. Inspect his gums and check his skin for petechiae and bruises. Note any nosebleeds, tarry stools, hematuria, or hematemesis. If your female patient's having her menstrual period, note whether her menstrual flow appears unduly heavy. As you know, any of these signs may indicate that excess anticoagulation is taking place. Call the doctor if you note these signs, and expect that your patient's anticoagulant levels will be reduced.

If your patient has a massive pulmonary embolism, you may also give thrombolytic drugs, such as I.V. streptokinase or urokinase, which break down the clot and prevent additional thrombus formation. Remember, the risk of excessive bleeding is higher with these drugs than with anticoagulants alone. If he doesn't respond to the drug therapy, the doctor may perform a pulmonary embolectomy.

If your patient continues to develop emboli, despite anticoagulant therapy, or if he develops bleeding or contraindications to anticoagulant therapy, he may require surgery. Make sure your patient has an EKG, chest X-rays, and blood studies prior to surgery, if time allows. Surgical procedures the doctor may use include ligation or partial occlusion of the inferior vena cava with clips or sutures to prevent the flow of emboli from the lower body to the lungs. If your patient can't tolerate major surgery, he may have an umbrella filter inserted through a small incision in the right internal jugular vein or femoral vein. The filter fixes itself to the walls of the inferior vena cava, preventing the flow of emboli from the lower body.

You'll continue to administer I.V. anticoagulant therapy whether your pa-

## KEEP IT CLEAN

When suctioning your patient through an endotracheal tube, what do you do with the ventilator tubing after you've disconnected it? If you're like most nurses, you simply lay it on the bed or the ventilator and forget about it until you're done suctioning. What's wrong with this? Well, although you've gone to great lengths to maintain sterility in your suctioning technique, the oxygen tube is left exposed and can become contaminated. Here's a better technique: Simply place the end of the oxygen tube in the suction kit or catheter's sterile wrapper before continuing with the procedure.

tient's had surgery or not. When his heart rate, blood pressure, breath sounds, and chest X-ray indicate that his cardiopulmonary status has stabilized and he has no signs or symptoms of hypoxemia, he will be started on oral anticoagulant therapy, using drugs such as Coumadin (warfarin sodium), while still on I.V. anticoagulants. Before you begin Coumadin therapy, draw blood for a baseline prothrombin (PT) level—this will help you determine when the medication reaches effective levels. When PT levels are in the therapeutic range, I.V. anticoagulants will be discontinued.

Keep AquaMephyton (vitamin $K_1$) available when you're administering Coumadin. You may need to give this if the patient's PT is grossly elevated or you see excessive bleeding.

Give Coumadin as ordered, explaining the drug therapy to your patient. Continue to monitor his ABGs and vital signs. Draw blood for PT levels at regular intervals, and check the laboratory test results when they return. Like PTT levels, PT levels should be 1½ to 2½ times the patient's control level. If the values are outside this range, notify the doctor. He may need to adjust the drug dosage appropriately.

# WHAT HAPPENS IN PULMONARY EMBOLISM

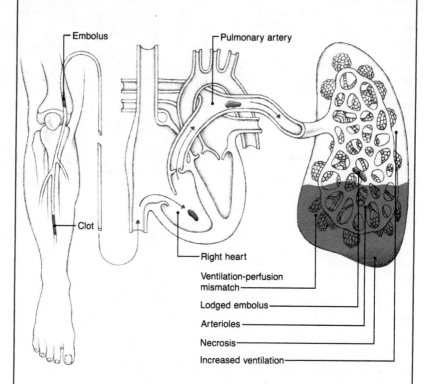

Embolus

Pulmonary artery

Clot

Right heart

Ventilation-perfusion mismatch

Lodged embolus

Arterioles

Necrosis

Increased ventilation

Pulmonary embolism—obstruction of the pulmonary arterial bed by a dislodged thrombus or foreign substance—is one of the most common acute respiratory problems seen in hospitalized patients.

Most pulmonary emboli result from dislodged thrombi, which commonly originate in the leg veins. (Other causes of pulmonary emboli include amniotic fluid and air.) If the thrombus breaks loose (becoming an embolus) and doesn't lodge in transit, it travels through the systemic circulation and passes through the right side of the heart into the pulmonary arterial system. It then lodges in a pulmonary artery or vessel too small to pass through, obstructing blood flow.

The result is a ventilation-perfusion mismatch: A portion of the lung is still being ventilated, but no blood is flowing to pick up oxygen and remove carbon dioxide. To maintain adequate gas exchange, ventilation then increases in the uninvolved lung areas. The airways distal to the embolus constrict and the alveoli shrink and collapse, shifting ventilation away from the poorly perfused area. Atelectasis may follow.

*Massive pulmonary embolism,* defined as occlusion of 50% or more of the pulmonary arterial circulation, can cause lethal hemodynamic changes, suddenly or within a few hours. Embolism of medium-sized vessels may cause pulmonary infarction.

Don't assume your patient's out of danger just because he's successfully had surgery or made the transition from I.V. anticoagulants to oral Coumadin. Pulmonary embolism frequently recurs, so watch your patient closely for signs of another embolus.

Your patient will be discharged on oral Coumadin, which he'll most likely need to take for 3 to 6 months. Remind him that he'll need regular follow-up blood studies to make sure his medication levels are within the effective range. And tell him to watch for bleeding gums, for blood in his stools or sputum, and for excessive bleeding if he cuts himself—for example, while shaving. He should report incidents like these to his doctor *immediately*.

# Status Asthmaticus

## Prediagnosis summary
The patient typically had most of the signs and symptoms of an acute asthma attack:
- shortness of breath
- wheezing
- use of accessory chest muscles to breathe
- tachycardia
- tachypnea
- restlessness.

He was treated with drugs, such as epinephrine or terbutaline, and with supplemental oxygen. Blood was drawn for arterial blood gases (ABGs), and an I.V. was established. When the patient didn't respond to the drugs, the doctor made a diagnosis of status asthmaticus—a severe asthma attack that's unresponsive to therapy.

## Priorities
If your patient's hypoxemia is severe, or he has a history of cardiac disease, connect him to a cardiac monitor. Continue to administer oxygen. Expect to give aminophylline I.V., first a loading dose and then a continuous drip, to "break" his attack. Aminophylline's mechanism of action differs from epinephrine's or terbutaline's, so it may work where initial drug therapy has failed. (See *Highlighting Aminophylline,* page 156.) Also expect to give corticosteroids to decrease inflammation.

Encourage your patient to drink fluids. Why? Because increased fluid intake will help to thin mucus. However, if his breathing's so labored that he's unable to drink, increase the I.V. fluid rate, as ordered. Your patient may also be started on respiratory therapy such as mini-nebulizer treatments. Encourage him to breathe deeply during this therapy. He'll receive additional bronchodilators, such as metaproterenol (Alupent) and isoetharine (Bronkosol), during this therapy. Expect these treatments to be repeated every 4 to 6 hours.

Because anxiety may increase bronchospasms, make sure your patient has a quiet room, and reassure him that the drugs you're administering will help relieve his breathing difficulty.

PATHOPHYSIOLOGY

## WHAT HAPPENS IN STATUS ASTHMATICUS

Status asthmaticus is a complication of asthma defined as an increasingly severe asthmatic attack that's unresponsive to bronchodilator therapy. With both nonallergic and allergic asthma, overreaction of the airways in response to irritation results in bronchoconstriction and increased mucus secretion. Simultaneous cholinergic stimulation causes the mast cells to produce the chemical mediators that lead to bronchospasm. Airway resistance and respiratory work increase, and expiratory flow decreases, trapping air and hyperinflating alveoli. Ventilation is impaired.

Although the patient is working harder to breathe, he can't improve his oxygen supply, so he becomes hypoxic and eventually hypercapnic. As he tires, his compensatory mechanisms become less and less effective. If this process isn't reversed promptly, the patient will die.

DRUGS

## HIGHLIGHTING AMINOPHYLLINE

A fine line exists between aminophylline's therapeutic value in a patient with status asthmaticus and its toxic effects. The following guidelines will help you to administer aminophylline—the I.V. form of theophylline—safely.
• Find out if your patient's been taking theophylline in any form. (Keep in mind that some over-the-counter bronchodilators, such as Bronkotabs and Primatene M and P, contain theophylline.) If he has, have a serum theophylline level taken to determine his exact blood level of the drug.
• Ask the patient if he smokes cigarettes. If he does, note his age. Why? Because the age of a person who smokes affects the rate at which he metabolizes theophylline. Young adult smokers, for example, need a larger maintenance dose. Older nonsmokers—particularly those with cor pulmonale, congestive heart failure, or liver disease—need a smaller maintenance dose.
• Because a fast infusion can cause convulsions, use an I.V. infusion pump or a minidripper to administer the drug.
• If you administer aminophylline by I.V.

piggyback, shut off the I.V. system already in place until the drug infuses.
• The usual loading dose is 5 to 6 mg/kg. This is followed by an infusion of 0.3 to 0.9 mg/kg/hr.
• Divide the daily dose into separate bags for infusion over 6-hour or 12-hour periods.
• Monitor the drug's effects carefully. Check your patient's pulse and blood pressure, and monitor his heartbeat for dysrhythmias. If you detect a dysrhythmia, *immediately* notify the doctor and stop the infusion.
• Aminophylline has a diuretic effect, so record your patient's intake and output to check for dehydration.
• Monitor the patient's serum theophylline levels after the first hour of administration, then after 12 and 24 hours. Therapeutic levels are between 10 and 20 mcg/ml.
• Watch for signs and symptoms of drug toxicity: anorexia, nausea, vomiting, abdominal pain, and nervousness. Notify the doctor if you detect any of these.
• Check the I.V. site frequently—the patient's breathing difficulty will make him very restless, so he may dislodge the I.V.

Don't let anyone smoke near the patient, and clear the room of anything he might be allergic to—such as flowers. Tell the patient what you're doing and why, and ask him what else you can do to make him more comfortable.

### Continuing assessment and intervention
Assess your patient's response to the drugs he's been given. *If he's responding,* this means his tachycardia, tachypnea, diaphoresis, wheezing, and accessory muscle use have decreased. As his breathing improves, he'll also be less restless and anxious.

*If he isn't responding,* you'll see increased respiratory distress—worsening of the above signs and symptoms or development of new signs and symptoms, such as cyanosis and lethargy. These signs and symptoms mean his

hypoxemia is severe, and you need to intervene *immediately.*

Auscultate your patient's lungs. You may hear hyperresonance (due to hyperinflation and trapping of air). You may or may *not* hear wheezing. Remember that a patient with status asthmaticus may not be able to wheeze because even his narrow airways are closed. So you may hear severely decreased breath sounds *without* wheezes. Consider this an ominous sign—when his condition improves, you'll hear wheezing.

Check your patient's cardiac monitor to see if he's developing dysrhythmias, such as frequent premature ventricular contractions or sinus tachycardia, that may be related to hypoxemia. Call the doctor if you see these. Check your patient's ABG results, too. You may see low $PCO_2$ and respiratory alkalosis due to hyperventilation. Or, you may see a normal or near normal $PCO_2$ with a normal pH—a *danger sign* indicating that your patient's tiring and no longer able to compensate for increasing hypoxemia.

If your patient's respiratory distress is increasing despite medication and oxygen therapy, notify the doctor, who may order immediate additional treatments with a mini-nebulizer. If this fails, the patient will be intubated and connected to a ventilator. ABG results will help determine the degree of the patient's respiratory failure and will assist the doctor in determining ventilator settings (flow rate, tidal volume, and percentage of oxygen).

Continue your assessment by taking your patient's history. Ask him if he knows what precipitated the status asthmaticus attack—he may have been exposed to an allergen or a chemical irritant, or he may have experienced acute emotional stress. Has he ever had an attack like this before? Is he taking antibiotics for an infection? An upper respiratory infection may have precipitated the attack. He may not have been treated for an existing upper respiratory infection, so obtain a sputum specimen and send it to the laboratory for Gram stain and culture and sensitivity tests. If he has an infection, the doctor will order antibiotics.

### Therapeutic care
Whether or not your patient's on a ventilator, continue to give I.V. aminophylline, corticosteroids, fluids, and antibiotics until his attack subsides. Suction a ventilated patient frequently. Monitor his ABGs. You'll know he's improving when his respiratory distress subsides, his lungs are free of wheezing, and his ABGs are returning to normal. This is the time to begin weaning him from the ventilator.

Once the attack has subsided, you'll discontinue the aminophylline and start your patient on oral bronchodilators, such as anhydrous theophylline (Theo-Dur or Slo-Phyllin). Remember,

encourage him to drink plenty of fluids to keep his secretions loose.

---

# Adult Respiratory Distress Syndrome (ARDS)

### Prediagnosis summary
On initial assessment, the patient showed the typical signs of acute respiratory distress:
- dyspnea
- tachypnea
- tachycardia
- diaphoresis.

As hypoxia developed, restlessness, anxiety, agitation, and alterations in consciousness became apparent. The patient also had pink and frothy sputum, together with rales and rhonchi, that characterizes ARDS.

He was placed on a cardiac monitor and given supplemental oxygen. An I.V. infusion was started to provide access for fluids and medications. A chest X-ray showed patchy, diffuse alveolar and interstitial infiltrates. The patient's arterial blood gases (ABGs) showed hypoxemia ($PO_2$ less than 50) without hypercapnia ($PCO_2$ less than 35).

### Priorities
Your first nursing priority is to improve your patient's oxygenation. For most patients with ARDS, expect to assist with endotracheal intubation and mechanical ventilation. But if the doctor chooses to give supplemental oxygen by mask, expect to use a tightly fitting mask with a narrow opening to retard expiration and to achieve continuous positive airway pressure (CPAP).

If the doctor chooses to use mechanical ventilation and you've already assisted with intubation, assess your patient's breath sounds for proper tube placement. (A chest X-ray will be done to confirm correct placement.) The doctor will make the initial ventilator settings, including tidal volume, oxy-

# WHAT HAPPENS IN ADULT RESPIRATORY DISTRESS SYNDROME

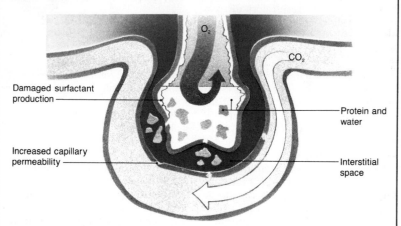

Damaged surfactant production

Increased capillary permeability

Protein and water

Interstitial space

$O_2$

$CO_2$

ARDS (adult respiratory distress syndrome) may be precipitated by trauma, shock, infection, embolism, drug overdose, and a wide variety of systemic diseases and insults to the lungs. Regardless of the initial precipitating factor, characteristics of ARDS include: hypoxemia (despite an increase in inspired oxygen), a progressive decrease in pulmonary compliance, and interstitial edema progressing to widespread areas of consolidation.

Initial damage to the alveolar-capillary membrane (possibly due to toxic agents, hypoxia, or other factors that aren't well understood) results in increased permeability, allowing protein and water to leak into the interstitial space. This produces interstitial edema that decreases:
• diffusion of oxygen and carbon dioxide across the alveolar-capillary membrane, producing hypoxia
• lung compliance, leading to decreased lung volume.

As edema increases, lung volume and compliance further decrease, and alveoli and small airways fill with fluid, causing microatelectasis and alveolar hemorrhage. Fluid accumulation and decreased blood flow impair alveolar production of surfactant—the substance that normally helps prevent alveolar collapse. Without surfactant, a hyaline membrane may form.

Now, with many of his alveoli either collapsed or filled with fluid, thus impairing gas exchange, the patient tries to compensate by hyperventilating. But although he's taking in more oxygen, it can't diffuse into the bloodstream through his damaged alveoli, so he remains hypoxemic. However, he loses carbon dioxide with each exhalation, because it crosses the alveolar-capillary membrane more easily than oxygen does. He thus becomes hypocapnic as well as hypoxemic. As his condition deteriorates, his respiratory alkalosis will be overcome by metabolic acidosis.

gen percentage, and rate. Approximately half an hour after mechanical ventilation's initiated, blood will be drawn for ABG tests, which will be reassessed for the degree of hypoxemia. Depending on the ABG results, the doctor may need to make a change in the ventilator settings. ABGs will be assessed half an hour after each setting change is made.

Techniques such as CPAP and positive end-expiratory pressure (PEEP) may be used with a mechanical ventilator. PEEP increases functional residual lung capacity, improves lung compliance, allows surfactant production, and decreases intrapulmonary arteriovenous shunt. PEEP also provides a higher degree of oxygenation while using a lower $FIO_2$. Remember that high levels of PEEP can cause rupture of a bleb or alveolus, resulting in air leakage and tension pneumothorax. (See the "Tension Pneumothorax" entry in this chapter.)

As you probably know, CPAP provides continual airway pressure, keeps the alveoli open, improves functional residual lung capacity, and allows for a high level of oxygenation with a reduced $FIO_2$.

High-frequency ventilation (HFV) may be used if your patient's condition is refractory to conventional means of mechanical ventilation. HFV delivers breaths at a high rate and with a low tidal volume. (See *Understanding High-Frequency Ventilation,* pages 160 and 161.)

If the patient can breathe on his own, intermittent mandatory ventilation may be used to provide the minimum amount of ventilation needed to achieve adequate oxygenation and easier weaning. (See *Understanding Oxygen Therapy and Mechanical Ventilation Techniques,* pages 132 to 135.)

## Continuing assessment and intervention

Before you begin assessing a patient with ARDS who isn't on a ventilator, have airway, intubation, and suction equipment available, because *his respiratory distress can become acute at any time.* (See *Recognizing the Stages of A.R.D.S.,* page 162.)

Begin your assessment by checking your patient's fluid status, because you must avoid overhydrating or underhydrating him. Be sure to keep accurate intake and output records. Overhydration can lead to increased pulmonary edema and eventual respiratory failure; underhydration can lead to hypovolemia, hypotension, and decreased cardiac output.

Although ARDS is a noncardiogenic form of pulmonary edema, it can still cause the patient's cardiac status to deteriorate because of the increase in ve-

nous and pulmonary pressures. This can progress to congestive heart failure. (See the "Congestive Heart Failure" entry in Chapter 5.) Watch for signs of decreased cardiac output:

• tachycardia
• decreased urinary output
• hypotension
• dyspnea on exertion (when not on a mechanical ventilator).

*Call the doctor* if you note any of these signs.

The patient may have a central venous line inserted in his internal jugular or subclavian vein to check central venous pressure (CVP). But, because CVP alone doesn't reliably indicate pulmonary pressures, expect that a Swan-Ganz catheter will be inserted to *measure* pulmonary artery pressures and pulmonary capillary wedge pressures. These pressure measurements also *reflect* left heart pressures and act as a guide to fluid volume needs. A Swan-Ganz catheter also provides access for blood to be drawn for ABGs and venous blood gas measurements and for I.V. fluid administration.

Pulmonary capillary wedge pressure combined with arterial and venous blood gas measurements provide information about the relationships among PEEP, intrapulmonary shunt, and cardiac output. The doctor will use this information to determine fluid administration and drug therapy. He may order diuretics for fluid overload. If your patient's normovolemic but continues to be hypotensive with poor car-

---

**BEDCHECK!**

Remember this: A patient being mechanically ventilated should *always* have an Ambu bag and suctioning equipment at his bedside. At the beginning of your shift, check to be sure you're prepared—if the ventilator fails, this equipment could save your patient's life.

## UNDERSTANDING HIGH-FREQUENCY VENTILATION

Don't be surprised if your hear the doctor order high-frequency ventilation (HFV) to treat a patient with respiratory failure. HFV is a recently developed mechanical ventilation technique that uses high ventilation rates (60 to 3,000 breaths/minute depending on the type of HFV), low tidal volumes, brief inspiratory time, and low peak airway pressures. HFV has three different delivery forms—high-frequency jet ventilation (HFJV), high-frequency positive-pressure ventilation (HFPPV), and high-frequency oscillation (HFO). You'll probably hear about HFJV most often. Here's a brief summary of how HFJV works:

### Mechanics of HFJV
• High pressure gas jet pulses through the narrow lumen gas jet valve on inspiration and accelerates as it flows through the port's narrow lumen and into the patient's endotracheal tube.
• The pressure and velocity of the jet stream cause a drag effect that entrains low pressure gases into the patient's airway.
• These gas flows combine to deliver 100 to 200 breaths per minute to the patient.
• The gas stream moves down the airway in a progressively broader wavefront of decreasing velocity.
• Tidal volume is delivered to airways under constant pressure.
• The gas stream creates turbulence, which causes the gas to vibrate in the airways.

Alveolar ventilation increases without raising mean airway pressure or peak inflation pressure.

### Uses
• Treatment of bronchopleural fistulae
• Rigid bronchoscopy
• Laryngeal surgery
• Thoracic surgical procedures
• Treatment of infant and adult respiratory distress syndrome (limited clinical experience)

### Benefits
• Improved venous return
• Decreased airway pressures and (possibly) improved pulmonary artery pressure
• Improved arterial gas exchange
• Decreased right ventricular afterload
• Reduced chance of pulmonary barotrauma and decreased cardiac output

### Nursing interventions
• Regularly check the mechanical setup, parameter alarms, and tubing connections.
• Assess breath sounds regularly.
• Suction the patient every 2 to 4 hours.
  During suctioning, disconnect the patient from the ventilator. Turn off the humidification system to prevent fluid from accumulating in the tubing and then being inspired when you restart ventilation. Assess airway secretions: if they're extremely viscous, you may need to increase humidification to prevent formation of mucous plugs.

diac output, he may require sympathomimetic agents, such as dopamine or dobutamine (Dobutrex), for hemodynamic support.

## Therapeutic care
Keep in mind that your patient's stabilized respiratory and cardiac status can deteriorate at any time; continue to watch for signs of respiratory distress and hypoxemia. The doctor will prescribe individual treatment for your patient according to the specific underlying condition causing his ARDS. However, regardless of the underlying condition, you need to follow certain *general* interventions to treat the patient with ARDS.

When the patient's receiving PEEP with mechanical ventilation, expect frequent adjustments of PEEP and $FIO_2$, because using PEEP allows for a higher degree of oxygenation with a lower oxygen percentage. Half an hour after each adjustment of ventilator setting, the patient's ABGs will be assessed and the PEEP settings readjusted. This pattern should continue in an effort to achieve the highest level of oxygenation using the smallest amounts of PEEP and $FIO_2$.

Assess your patient's fluid status carefully to avoid fluid overload, which can exacerbate pulmonary edema. Blood studies of the patient's total serum protein, hemoglobin, hematocrit, and albumin will determine the I.V. fluid to be used (intravenous crys-

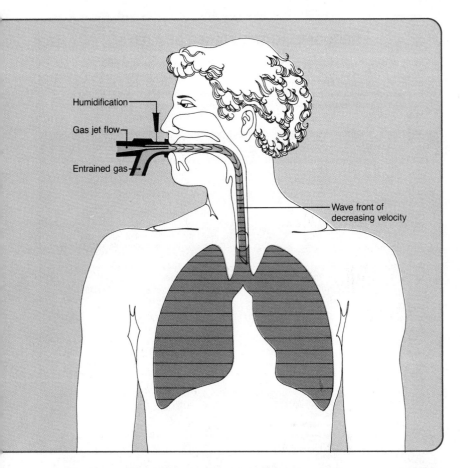

Humidification

Gas jet flow

Entrained gas

Wave front of
decreasing velocity

talloids or colloids) and whether protein replacement is needed. When you give colloids, such as normal serum albumin or low-molecular-weight dextran, the patient may require a diuretic as well, to prevent fluid overload.

To *increase* surfactant production and *decrease* inflammation, the doctor may order corticosteroids such as methylprednisolone (Solu-Medrol) or dexamethasone (Decadron). He may also order broad-spectrum antibiotics to prevent bacterial pneumonia resulting from microatelectasis and decreased pulmonary blood supply. If the patient has a high fever, a hypothermia blanket may help reduce it. If your patient's wheezing, or if he's coughing but doesn't need suctioning, he may re-

quire aminophylline or atropine to relieve bronchospasms. (Spasmolytic drugs can also act as bronchodilators.) The patient will require frequent chest physical therapy and postural drainage to loosen and facilitate removal of his secretions.

Now that your assessment is complete and your patient with ARDS is stable, give some attention to his family's needs. As you know, ARDS is a devastating disease with a high mortality. The patient's family is sure to need the same kind of reassurance and support you're giving the patient. Help them feel involved and necessary to his care. Let them see the patient, and explain what's been done for him.

His family can give you a more de-

## RECOGNIZING THE STAGES OF A.R.D.S.

Many emergency conditions (for example, lung contusion, drug overdose, or near-drowning) can cause ARDS—adult respiratory distress syndrome. In turn, ARDS can lead to acute respiratory failure, itself an emergency.

You probably know what ARDS is: noncardiogenic pulmonary edema. But can you recognize ARDS when it's developing? This chart will help you recognize the six developmental stages of ARDS and intervene appropriately.

| STAGES | SIGNS AND SYMPTOMS | NURSING INTERVENTIONS |
|---|---|---|
| **1** Inflamed and damaged alveolar-capillary membrane | • Depend on underlying cause of ARDS | • Do a brief assessment. <br> • Take the patient's vital signs. <br> • Auscultate for abnormal breath sounds. <br> • Prepare the patient for a chest X-ray. <br> • Begin treatment of underlying cause to prevent further ARDS development. |
| **2** Protein and water shift in the interstitial space | • Tachypnea, dyspnea, and tachycardia | • Draw blood for ABGs. <br> • Prepare the patient for oxygen therapy, intubation, and mechanical ventilation. <br> • Begin fluid management, avoiding fluid overload. |
| **3** Pulmonary edema | • Increased tachypnea, dyspnea, and cyanosis <br> • Hypoxemia (generally unresponsive to increased $FIO_2$) <br> • Decreased pulmonary compliance <br> • Rales and rhonchi | • Connect the patient to a mechanical ventilator with a positive end-expiratory pressure (PEEP) setting and a high oxygen concentration. <br> • Watch for complications from ventilation therapy. |
| **4** Collapsed alveoli and impaired gas exchange | • Thick, frothy, sticky sputum <br> • Marked hypoxemia with increased respiratory distress | • Anticipate that a Swan-Ganz catheter will be inserted to measure pulmonary capillary wedge pressure. |
| **5** Decreased oxygen and carbon dioxide levels in the blood | • Increased tachypnea <br> • Hypoxemia <br> • Hypocapnia | • Study ABGs, mixed venous blood gases, and pulmonary capillary wedge pressure to understand the relationship between PEEP, intrapulmonary shunt, and cardiac output. <br> • Monitor the patient's vital signs and urine output (hydration). |
| **6** Hypoxemia; metabolic acidosis | • Decreased serum pH <br> • Increased $PaCO_2$ level <br> • Decreased $PaO_2$ level <br> • Confusion <br> • Decreased $HCO_3$ level | • Watch for fluid restriction or overdiuresis that may cause hypovolemia, hypotension, and hypoperfusion. <br> • Check for shock, coma, respiratory failure, and neurologic complications secondary to metabolic alterations and respiratory failure. <br> • Reassure the patient and his family. |

tailed history of the illness or injury that precipitated the ARDS. Since the patient may have already been in the hospital, you should also review his complete chart to familiarize yourself with his previous care.

Your patient probably will continue to require mechanical ventilation. If he requires more than 36 hours on the ventilator, the doctor will probably do a tracheostomy to forestall tracheal erosion or stenosis. (The endotracheal and tracheostomy tubes require meticulous hygiene.) The patient will need frequent suctioning to free his lungs of secretions as much as possible. Continue to perform chest physical therapy and postural drainage to loosen the secretions and make suctioning easier.

Assess his breath sounds frequently, monitor his daily ABGs and chest X-rays, and expect that additional ABGs will be needed whenever he shows signs and symptoms of increased respiratory distress.

If the patient begins to produce a yellow, green, or brown sputum, send a specimen for a culture and sensitivity test. Depending on the results, he may need a change of antibiotic. You'll probably continue to give the patient aminophylline as long as he has bronchospasms.

Continue to monitor the patient's cardiac output and fluid status. Keep accurate records of:
• intake and output
• vital signs (especially blood pressure and quality of pulses)
• pulmonary capillary wedge pressures and pulmonary artery pressures.

Based on these indicators, the doctor will order frequent changes in fluid and drug administration.

Long-term ventilation and the deep psychological stress of extreme illness cause depression in most patients with ARDS. Besides continuing your emotional support, explain to your patient that recovery from ARDS is a painstakingly slow process. Reassure him that everything is being done to make him feel as comfortable as possible.

# Acute Respiratory Failure (ARF)

## Prediagnosis summary

On initial assessment, the patient had some combination of these signs and symptoms, reflecting *extreme* respiratory distress:
• dyspnea and tachypnea
• tachycardia
• hypertension or hypotension
• diaphoresis
• pale or cyanotic skin
• a cough with yellow or green sputum
• accessory muscle use and flaring of nostrils to ease breathing
• altered mental status progressing from alertness to confusion, lethargy, or combativeness
• sonorous rhonchi and decreased breath sounds.

He was connected to a cardiac monitor, which may have shown dysrhythmias—such as tachycardia and premature ventricular contraction—indicating hypoxemia. He was probably given pre-intubation ventilatory assistance from an Ambu bag.

A chest X-ray may have been normal. Blood was drawn for a complete blood count and for electrolytes, blood sugar, blood urea nitrogen, creatinine, and arterial blood gases (ABGs).

His ABG results showed $PaCO_2$ greater than 50, pH less than 7.35, and $PaO_2$ less than 50. These values indicate the inability of the lungs to clear carbon dioxide from the blood: this is the *major diagnostic indicator* of ARF, along with the patient's obvious severe respiratory distress with hypoxemia. Because ARF is characterized by this inability to clear carbon dioxide (*not* by insufficient oxygen), cyanosis is generally not a reliable indicator.

## Priorities

Your first nursing priority is to improve the patient's ventilation to increase oxygenation and clear carbon dioxide.

Usually, insertion of an endotracheal tube and use of a mechanical ventilator achieve this goal. If the doctor decides not to mechanically ventilate a patient with preexisting lung disease, such as chronic obstructive pulmonary disease (COPD)—because of the anticipated difficulty in weaning him from the ventilator—administer oxygen by mask or nasal cannula. Be especially alert for signs and symptoms of increasing respiratory distress. The rest of this patient's treatment will be the same as for a mechanically ventilated patient.

If the doctor does elect to use mechanical ventilation, he may order any of several techniques, including positive end-expiratory pressure (PEEP), continuous positive airway pressure, or high-frequency ventilation. He'll make the initial ventilator settings of tidal volume, oxygen percentage, and rate. If PEEP is used, the desired level of oxygen can be achieved using a lower oxygen percentage, facilitating patient weaning after long-term mechanical ventilation.

Assess his breath sounds to check for proper tube placement—a chest X-ray will confirm this. Once he has adequate ventilation, he should have a slower breathing rate and be less anxious and more comfortable.

Once the doctor makes the initial ventilator settings, the patient's ABGs will be assessed half an hour later for acidosis, hypercapnia, and hypoxemia. The doctor may then make adjustments in the settings, and the ABGs will be checked again in half an hour. The doctor may adjust the ventilator settings frequently so the ABGs will approach the desired range and the patient's condition will stabilize.

Explain to the patient that he won't be able to speak after intubation, so you'll provide other ways for him to communicate. (A "magic slate" or chalkboard, which can be erased readily, helps preserve the privacy of the patient's communications.)

## Continuing assessment and intervention

Now that your patient's oxygenation has improved, you'll be able to do a thorough baseline assessment. Reassess his breath sounds. Even if he's on a ventilator and his ABGs show improvement, you may still hear sonorous rhonchi and decreased breath sounds over the affected area. Remember, he can develop respiratory distress *at any time*. Watch for such signs as coughing and rapid breathing. If either occurs, check his ventilator tubing for any kinks, obstructions, or loose connections, and determine whether he needs suctioning. If you hear sibilant rhonchi (wheezing), suspect COPD—which may be the underlying cause of his ARF. If your patient's not on a ventilator, be especially alert for signs and symptoms of degenerating respiratory status. Check his ease of breathing by noting rate and rhythm. Compare his breath sounds, rate, and rhythm to earlier assessments, and record any differences.

Watch the patient's cardiac monitor to check for increasing heart rate and any other dysrhythmias. Notify the doctor of any such changes, which may

### ALLEN'S TEST... FIRST

Your patient needs an arterial line or arterial blood gases *now*. Despite the urgency, do the Allen's test first. Why? Because these procedures invade the radial artery and may damage it. Since the hand's only other main blood source is the ulnar artery, you need to make sure that's patent *before* the procedure. Here's how:

• Have your patient clench his fist. Next, compress his radial and ulnar arteries.

• Have him unclench his fist. His palm will blanch because you're stopping the blood flow.

• Release pressure from the ulnar artery *only*. If blood flow's adequate, his palm will flush within 5 seconds. If blood flow's inadequate, you'll have to find another insertion site.

# WHAT HAPPENS IN
# ACUTE RESPIRATORY FAILURE

Acute respiratory failure takes place when the patient's lungs can't maintain adequate arterial oxygenation or carbon dioxide elimination. This leads to hypoxemia—which, unless treated, leads to tissue hypoxia. Hypercapnia (inability to eliminate $CO_2$) will be present if hypoxia arises from hypoventilation or circulatory deficits.

Generally, you can recognize respiratory failure by $Po_2$ levels less than 50 mm Hg and $Pco_2$ levels greater than 50 mm Hg. In an acute crisis, $Pco_2$ levels usually rise suddenly, with a sharp drop in pH.

Three main mechanisms may cause hypoxemia that leads to acute respiratory failure: hypoventilation, ventilation-perfusion imbalances, and right-to-left shunting.

*Alveolar hypoventilation* commonly results from chronic airway obstruction that reduces alveolar minute ventilation. $Po_2$ levels and oxygen saturation decrease while $Pco_2$ levels increase, signaling hypercapnia.

*Ventilation-perfusion imbalances,* the most common cause of hypoxemia, occur when conditions such as massive pulmonary embolism or ARDS upset ventilation-perfusion in a specific region of the lung. Either too little ventilation with normal blood flow or too little blood flow with normal ventilation may cause an imbalance. Whichever happens, the result's the same: When the imbalance spreads over a large area, $Po_2$ levels become reduced throughout the lung.

If hypoventilation and ventilation-perfusion imbalances aren't treated, they may lead to *right-to-left shunting*. When this happens, a large amount of blood passes from the right to the left heart without being oxygenated.

Hypoxemia, along with hypercapnia, triggers several compensatory mechanisms in the body. Hypoxemia stimulates the sympathetic nervous system, which, in turn, produces tissue vasoconstriction, increases peripheral resistance, and increases the heart rate. Hypercapnia also works on local cellular and tissue function to cause cerebral depression, hypotension, and circulatory failure. Additionally, it stimulates the sympathetic nervous system to increase heartbeat and cardiac output. Eventually, it may lead to acute respiratory acidosis.

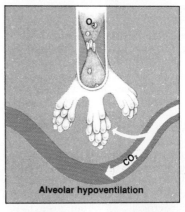

**Alveolar hypoventilation**

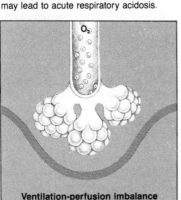

**Ventilation-perfusion imbalance**

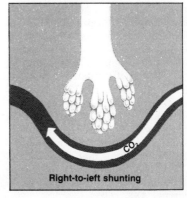

**Right-to-left shunting**

indicate the patient's still hypoxemic. Compare these results with the initial assessment.

Check your patient's ventilator settings, too. If adjustments are necessary, remember that his ABGs must be reassessed half an hour after any change is made.

Assess your patient's blood study results; be sure to check his hemoglobin and electrolyte levels. If his hemoglobin level's decreased, oxygenation efforts may be impaired. He may also have an electrolyte imbalance, which commonly accompanies respiratory acidosis due to hypercapnia. If you note either of these problems, call the doctor. He'll probably order diagnostic tests to determine the cause of the decreased hemoglobin level, but he may choose *not* to correct the electrolyte imbalance immediately. Why? Because ventilation will improve carbon dioxide clearance from the lungs and decrease acidosis so that the electrolyte imbalance will start to correct itself.

If you detect no complications during your assessment, if your patient's ventilation is adequate, and if he needs no further interventions, you're ready to take his history. Remember, if he has an endotracheal tube in place, he won't be able to speak. Get the information you need from his family. (This will also give you the opportunity to reassure his family that his condition is improving.) Ask about preexisting problems, such as acute bronchospasm, COPD, or prior ARF episodes. If the patient has preexisting COPD, be sure the doctor knows about it so he can act to forestall ventilator-weaning problems. Ask if the patient's had any recent pulmonary infections or traumas. Overwhelming pulmonary infection can cause ARF, especially in patients with preexisting pulmonary disease. Trauma can trigger neuromuscular problems that also can lead to ARF. Also ask about any prior neuromuscular diseases: these can cause recurring ARF episodes.

Finally, find out if the family's no- ticed any recent mental status changes in the patient (confusion, lethargy, agitation). This information will give you a clue to the duration of his present ARF episode.

### Therapeutic care

Expect the doctor to order a bronchodilator, which the patient will inhale either by intermittent positive-pressure breathing treatments or through the ventilator. Prepare to administer an I.V. bronchodilator, such as aminophylline. Whether or not your patient's on a ventilator, if he has episodic bronchospasms but no infection, expect to give him corticosteroids for their anti-inflammatory effect. If you detect signs and symptoms of infection—fever and yellow or green sputum—send a sputum sample for culture and sensitivity testing. According to the test results, the doctor will order antibiotics specific to the type of infection.

Avoid sedating your patient, because sedatives can further depress his respirations. If he's extremely anxious and restless, assess him for other signs and symptoms of hypoxemia, and check his ABGs. If he's not hypoxemic, and he's on a ventilator, he's probably just anxious from being on the ventilator. The doctor may order a *mild* sedative or antianxiety agent, such as diazepam (Valium), to improve his oxygenation by decreasing both his apprehension and his resistance to the ventilator.

Check the patient's ABGs at least once daily, in the morning, as well as any time you notice signs and symptoms of respiratory distress or any other change in your patient's condition. Continue to assess his other blood studies as well. A daily chest X-ray will also be done.

During this phase of his treatment, your patient will need aggressive chest physiotherapy and postural drainage, sometimes as often as every 1 to 2 hours, to remove secretions and improve pulmonary function.

While your patient's condition is improving, your serial ABG and respiratory assessments will follow his progress. If he continues to need mechanical ventilation, he may require a tracheostomy between 36 and 72 hours after initial intubation, to prevent such complications as tracheal erosion or stenosis. Perform meticulous endotracheal tube or tracheostomy care, and suction him periodically to prevent infection. As you know, long-term mechanical ventilation can render a patient psychologically and physically dependent on the ventilator, so he'll have to be weaned from it just as soon as his respiratory-status indicators—measured by the respiratory therapist—show he can breathe adequately on his own. These indicators include respiratory rate, tidal volume (volume of air taken in with each breath), negative inspiratory force (amount of negative pressure it takes for the patient to breathe in), and forced vital capacity (deepest breath the patient can exhale). Patients with a history of COPD are especially susceptible to ventilator dependence; this is why PEEP (which decreases $FIO_2$ below 50%) is often used for patients with ARF.

After extubation, continue aggressive pulmonary therapy and encourage your patient to breathe deeply and to cough as often as possible. These actions will improve his pulmonary function and clear away any secretions that collect after his endotracheal tube's removed.

Watch for signs and symptoms of recurring respiratory distress. If he begins to have tachypnea or dyspnea, call the doctor. Also have his ABGs reassessed. Give the patient any necessary ventilatory assistance, using an oxygen mask or Ambu bag as necessary. If these breathing aids prove inadequate, he may need to be intubated again.

# A FINAL WORD

As you know, severe respiratory illnesses and injuries have high morbidity and mortality. Adult respiratory distress syndrome, for example, has a mortality of over 40%—even with prompt, aggressive treatment. Thoracic injuries are the primary cause of about 25% of traffic-related deaths—and contributory in about another 50%.

These are gloomy statistics. However, today's advances in trauma transport and prehospital care offer hope that these statistics will improve. So do sophisticated management techniques, such as ventilatory support with positive end-expiratory pressure, continuous positive airway pressure, and high frequency ventilation. To help improve *your* patient's prospects of surviving a respiratory emergency, be sure your emergency care *and* respiratory care skills are as expert and practiced as you can make them.

## Selected References

Beth Israel Hospital, Boston. *Respiratory Intensive Care Nursing*, 2nd ed. Boston: Little, Brown & Co., 1979.

Glauser, Frederick L., ed. *Signs and Symptoms in Pulmonary Medicine*. Philadelphia: J.B. Lippincott Co., 1983.

Lance, Edward, and Sweetwood, Hannelore. "Chest Trauma: When Minutes Count," *Nursing78* 8:28-33, January 1978.

Moser, Kenneth M., and Spragg, Roger G. *Respiratory Emergencies*, 2nd ed. St. Louis: C.V. Mosby Co., 1982.

Shapiro, Barry A., et al. *Clinical Application of Respiratory Care*, 2nd ed. Chicago: Year Book Medical Pubs., 1979.

Stringer, L.W. *Emergency Treatment of Acute Respiratory Disease*, 3rd ed. Bowie, Md.: Robert J. Brady Co., 1981.

Traver, Gayle A. *Respiratory Nursing: The Science and the Art*. New York: John Wiley & Sons, 1982.

# 5

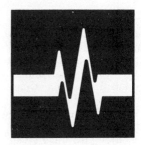

# Cardiovascular Emergencies

## Introduction

Just as you finish bandaging young Timothy Collier's toe laceration, a car pulls up and jerks to a stop in front of the ED door. A middle-aged woman leaps out and runs around to the passenger door. She's obviously upset and struggling to pull a man out of the car—at last she succeeds. But he's clearly unsteady on his feet, and she's having a lot of trouble steering him to the door of the ED. You rush to their aid and assist by placing the man in a wheelchair.

Richard Franklin is somewhat older than his wife Rose—he looks about 50. He's pale, short of breath, and appears apprehensive. His upper lip's beaded with sweat, and he's holding his hand to his chest. His wife, who's very upset, says that her husband's been complaining of pain and "indigestion" on and off all day, and now he's nauseous and has a backache and a headache. Angrily, she says she's been trying to bring her husband to the hospital since noon, but he's resisted her all day. He keeps repeating that his pain and nausea are nothing. "It's just heartburn," Mr. Franklin mutters, "It's just the pastrami I had for lunch. My wife's always fussing about nothing."

You're pretty sure you know better, just from looking at him. You don't know what's causing Mr. Franklin's signs and symptoms—they *could* be due to heartburn. But they could also be due to myocardial infarction (MI), hypertensive crisis, congestive heart failure with pulmonary edema, or a leaking, nondissecting aneurysm—among many possibilities. You know that Mrs. Franklin may have saved her husband's life. Now, Mr. Franklin needs prompt emergency assessment and care.

As you know, cardiac emergencies can arise from chest trauma or from preexisting disorders, such as coronary artery disease and hypertension. Many of these disorders can appear in patients on your unit. Like respiratory emergencies, they require particularly quick assessment and intervention because they disrupt your patient's basic life processes. You must be prepared to perform basic and advanced life-support measures instantly—you may have only 2 to 5 minutes to restore an adequate flow of oxygenated blood to your patient's brain before brain damage or death results.

When emergency problems evolve this quickly, your response must be almost reflexive—you have to *know* what to do without taking time to stop and ponder. Remember, part of knowing what to do is knowing your role as part of the emergency team—whether you're in an ED or on the unit—when a patient has a cardiovascular emergency.

## INITIAL CARE

## Prehospital Care: What's Been Done

When you receive a patient with a cardiac emergency in the ED, the care he's had will depend on several things:
• what type of rescue personnel responded (emergency medical technicians or paramedics)
• what equipment was available to treat him
• whether he's suffered chest trauma
• whether he's gone into cardiac arrest
• how seriously the emergency has af-

fected his overall condition.

The rescue team checked the patient's airway, breathing, and circulation, clearing his airway if necessary and providing oxygen by nasal cannula or mask. If paramedics responded, they may have started an I.V. of dextrose 5% in water ($D_5W$) at a keep-vein-open rate and placed the patient on a cardiac monitor. They may also have given morphine I.V. on doctor's orders if the patient had chest pain and the doctor suspected a myocardial infarction or congestive heart failure.

If chest trauma or a dissecting aortic aneurysm caused the patient's cardiovascular emergency, he probably had signs and symptoms of shock. Rescue personnel may have applied medical antishock trousers (a MAST suit), if available, and started Ringer's lactate solution I.V. in addition to initiating cardiac monitoring. If the patient's venous pressure was elevated, they will have hung the I.V. bag extra high to avoid blood backflow. (Maintain the position of the I.V. when you receive the patient.)

Rescue personnel gave CPR in the transport vehicle if the patient arrested. When they arrive at the ED, one rescuer will be ventilating the patient with an Ambu bag, another will be riding on the stretcher rail while giving the patient continuous chest compressions, and the third will be pushing the stretcher. You and a co-worker should take over CPR without interrupting the rhythm (see the "Life Support" section in Chapter 3). If another ED team member takes over one of the CPR roles, your job may be to transfer the patient from the ambulance cardiac monitor to the ED monitor. Make sure you connect the leads and start the monitor *before* you disconnect the patient from the ambulance monitor. This way, you won't risk losing vital monitoring information during the transfer.

Ask rescue personnel what drugs, if any, they've given the patient. In addition to morphine, they may have given furosemide (Lasix) on doctor's

PRIORITIES

## INITIAL ASSESSMENT CHECKLIST

**Assess the ABCs first and intervene appropriately.**

**Check for:**
• changes in skin color and temperature, decreased or absent pulses, or pain, possibly indicating vascular compromise
• hypotension, oliguria, or changes in level of consciousness, indicating decreased cardiac output.

**Intervene by:**
• starting an I.V.
• initiating cardiac monitoring.

**Prepare for:**
• defibrillation
• emergency drug administration
• taking a 12-lead EKG
• temporary pacemaker insertion
• pericardiocentesis.

# NEW ADVANCES IN CARDIOVASCULAR TECHNOLOGY

Would you know how to handle a patient who came into the ED with an automatic implantable defibrillator (AID) in place? You might assume you shouldn't externally defibrillate such a patient, and you'd be right up to a point—his AID monitors his heart continuously and *automatically* defibrillates it within 20 seconds of a dysrhythmia's onset. If necessary, it can refire three times at 15-second intervals, delivering extra energy for the fourth shock. But if that fourth shock doesn't work, you'll need to call a code and prepare for emergency external defibrillation.

Luckily, this situation's rare. AIDs are used to treat patients with recurrent life-threatening dysrhythmias, and they're usually very effective. A small lithium-powered pulse generator is subcutaneously implanted in the patient's abdomen; three electrodes lead from it to the right ventricle (to sense heart rate), the right atrium (to sense morphology and, hence, rhythm and to defibrillate), and the apical pericardium (to defibrillate). Each device is factory-programmed to respond to the patient's needs, and uses far less energy than an external defibrillator—around 25 joules (with an increase to 30 on the fourth shock) as compared with up to 400 joules.

Bateries last about 3 years, or about 100 defibrillations.

The AID's few—and rare—complications (infection, bleeding, and thrombosis) are mostly related to surgical implantation. Occasionally, the device misreads a supra-ventricular tachycardia, discharges, and causes a more severe ventricular fibrillation; but the next shock—in 15 seconds—usually corrects this. Repeated shocks may cause myocardial damage, yet even this potential complication seems minor compared to the risk involved in *not* having an internal defibrillator.

Another similar device—the implantable cardioverter—is on the horizon. Now being tested, it holds great promise for patients with recurrent life-threatening dysrhythmias. It has several advantages:
• smaller size
• a single lead, requiring no chest surgery
• the ability to be reprogrammed after insertion
• low energy requirement
• a back-up pacemaker effect.

Just a few years ago, patients with recurrent life-threatening dysrhythmias almost always died. Now, these advances in cardiovascular technology may save their lives.

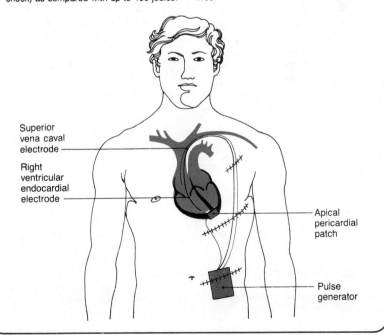

Superior vena caval electrode

Right ventricular endocardial electrode

Apical pericardial patch

Pulse generator

# ELECTROCARDIOGRAMS: MEASURING THE HEART'S ELECTRICAL CURRENT

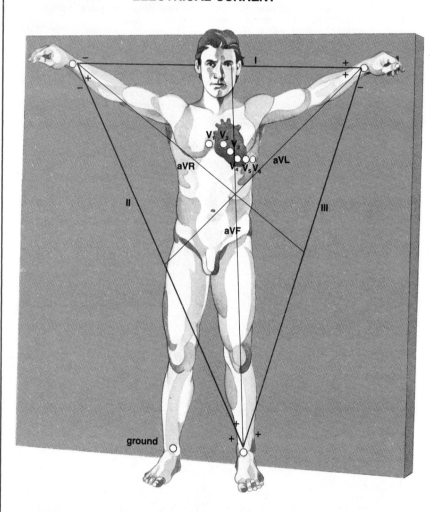

**Limb leads**

$V_1$: Fourth intercostal space to right of sternum

$V_2$: Fourth intercostal space to left of sternum

$V_3$: Halfway between $V_2$ and $V_4$

$V_4$: Fifth intercostal space at midclavicular line

$V_5$: Anterior axillary line (halfway between $V_4$ and $V_6$)

$V_6$: Midaxillary line, level with $V_4$

A 12-lead electrocardiogram (EKG) is one of the first diagnostic procedures the doctor may do for your cardiac emergency patient.

As you probably know, an EKG measures electrical potential—the force of the heart's electrical current—from 12 different leads. By studying these 12 electrical patterns, you can accurately assess your patient's myocardial function. For example, an EKG determines the presence of acute or past myocardial infarction, myocardial ischemia, or injury. It may also help detect dysrhythmias, drug toxicity, and electrolyte imbalances.

Standard EKG machines have 5 electrodes—1 on each limb and 1 movable chest electrode—to record the 12 different views. Newer machines use 10 electrodes—4 on the patient's limbs plus 6 individual chest electrodes—to record the 12 views. Some machines record up to 15 views, using 12 electrodes.

Three of the electrodes represent standard bipolar limb leads (I, II, III) and augmented unipolar limb leads (aVR, aVL, and aVF). The *a* means *augmented; V, voltage; R, right; L, left; F, foot.* The fourth electrode serves as the electrical "ground."

Standard bipolar limb leads measure variations in the heart's electrical potential at two points (negative and positive poles) and record the difference. Unipolar augmented limb leads measure between one augmented limb lead and the electrical midpoint of the remaining two leads.

The six chest leads ($V_1$ through $V_6$) view electrical potential from a horizontal plane and help locate abnormalities in the heart's anterior, lateral, and posterior walls.

The illustration below shows you how to place the electrodes correctly. While you're doing this, explain the EKG's purpose to your patient and reassure him that the procedure's painless.

orders if congestive heart failure is suspected or cardiac-arrest drugs, such as epinephrine, lidocaine, or atropine. Make sure to determine the dosage, the time given, and the patient's response so the ED doctor can decide whether to continue this treatment.

# What to Do First

Rapid assessment, recognition of acute and potential cardiac problems, and initiation of lifesaving measures are the keys to providing proper care for a patient with a traumatic or nontraumatic cardiovascular emergency. Your initial priorities are to stabilize his airway and to ensure that his breathing and circulation are adequate. Your quick primary assessment should provide essential information about the patient's present condition. Don't waste valuable time gathering other information if the patient's present condition is unstable. The most important thing for you to do now is *recognize danger signals* and intervene as necessary or notify the doctor before you proceed with a more detailed assessment.

### Airway

Airway assessment is always your first priority, even though rescue personnel may previously have checked and cleared your patient's airway. Check to see if air is moving in and out of his upper airway. Watch the patient for labored breathing, excessive respiratory effort with accessory muscle use, and intercostal, supraclavicular, and sternal retractions. Look for cyanosis, which indicates hypoxemia.

Although a patient's cardiovascular emergency condition may not directly compromise his airway, its precipitating event(s) or subsequent complications may. For example, if the patient's suffered a traumatic injury, his airway may be compromised by blunt or penetrating trauma to his face, neck, or mouth. If he's unconscious or has suffered a myocardial infarction that results in cardiac arrest, his tongue may fall back to occlude his airway when he's supine.

Clear your patient's airway, if necessary, with a mouth sweep; open his airway with a jaw thrust, a chin-lift maneuver, or hyperextension. (If your patient has traumatic injuries, assume his cervical spine's injured and manage him accordingly. See the "What to Do First" entry in Chapter 6.) If you can't open his airway with these steps, insert an oral or nasal airway and suction the patient. Prepare to assist with endotracheal tube insertion if the patient has respiratory insufficiency.

## Breathing

Assess your patient for the presence and adequacy of his respirations. Look for chest expansion, and place your ear over the patient's nose and mouth to listen and feel for exhaled air. Remember that deficient oxygen transport resulting from cardiovascular emergencies may easily compromise breathing. An insult to the heart—for example, myocardial contusion, myocardial infarction, or cardiac tamponade—may result in decreased contractility so that pumping is ineffective. Cardiac output and oxygen transport are reduced accordingly. As oxygen transport decreases and carbon dioxide accumulates in the blood, the patient's respiratory rate increases in an effort to blow off carbon dioxide.

If your patient has a sudden loss of blood volume (such as occurs in a ruptured aortic aneurysm), extreme hypoxemia leading to anoxia will affect his brain's respiratory center. The result may be respiratory arrest. Of course, cardiac arrest from *any* cause results in immediate loss of blood flow and oxygen delivery to the brain's respiratory center and in consequent respiratory arrest.

Be alert for significant changes in the rate and depth of your patient's respirations, as these may signal respiratory fatigue and decompensation. Such conditions as congestive heart failure may cause pulmonary edema with resulting rapid, shallow, labored respirations. Draw blood for arterial blood gases to help determine your patient's respiratory status.

Give your patient oxygen by nasal cannula or mask, and anticipate the need for intubation and assisted ventilation. *Your patient may arrest at any moment,* so make sure you have intubation supplies and appropriate oxygen administration equipment available.

## Circulation

Assess the adequacy of your patient's cardiac output by evaluating his pulses and blood pressure and by checking his capillary refill time. *If you can't detect a pulse,* start CPR (see the "Life Support" section in Chapter 3). If a pulse is present, check it at different sites for quality, rate, and regularity of rhythm. Palpate for a radial pulse first—if this is palpable, you know that your patient's systolic blood pressure is greater than 80 mm Hg and that some measure of cardiac output and perfusion pressure is assured. If you can't palpate a radial pulse, check for a femoral or carotid pulse. A palpable femoral pulse indicates systolic pressure greater than 70 mm Hg, whereas a palpable carotid pulse indicates systolic pressure greater than 60 mm Hg. Note the rate and rhythm. Weak, thready, irregular, extremely rapid, or profoundly slow pulses are danger signs.

Once you've established the presence of a pulse, assess your patient's blood pressure in both arms. Of course, any extremes in range (elevated or low blood pressure) warn you that alterations in hemodynamics may be occurring. Watch for *extremely* high blood pressure readings, which may indicate hypertensive crisis. Place the patient in the semi-Fowler position, and expect to administer an intravenous diuretic, such as furosemide (Lasix), and antihypertensive medications, such as diazoxide (Hyperstat), sodium nitroprusside (Nipride), and hydralazine hydrochloride (Apresoline).

Because the catecholamine response to stress can initially elevate a patient's blood pressure, evaluate this data carefully. Serial blood pressure readings are generally more valuable than your initial reading, which serves as a baseline.

Also watch your patient for Beck's triad (decreased systolic pressure, increased venous filling, and distant heart sounds) and pulsus paradoxus (systolic pressure decrease of greater than 15 mm Hg with inspiration), which may indicate cardiac tamponade.

If your patient doesn't already have one, establish an I.V. (usually $D_5W$) at a keep-vein-open rate to provide access for fluids and drugs that may be necessary to support your patient's circulation. If his circulation's been compromised by an injury, such as aortic rupture or a dissecting aortic aneurysm, he's losing blood rapidly and needs immediate fluid infusion and a blood transfusion. Insert two large-bore peripheral I.V. lines for maximum access, and type and cross-match his blood for transfusion. Be prepared to assist the doctor with central venous pressure (CVP) line insertion to monitor the effectiveness of fluid replacement, and with pericardiocentesis if the patient's suffered trauma and the doc-

## POSITIONING ELECTRODES FOR HARDWIRE MONITORING

Hardwire monitoring lets you continuously monitor your patient's dysrhythmias. You place electrodes directly on his chest—the way you would for an EKG. They pick up his heart's electrical activity, and the monitor displays it as heartbeat and rhythm.

Here's an illustration that shows you electrode placement for common hardwire monitoring leads.

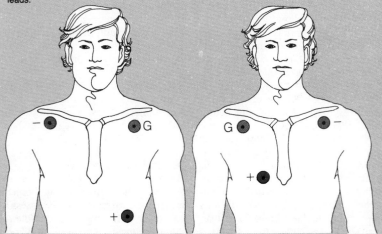

### THREE-ELECTRODE MONITOR

**Lead II**
Positive ( + ): left side of chest, lowest palpable rib, midclavicular line
Negative ( − ): right shoulder, below clavicular hollow
Ground (G): left shoulder, below clavicular hollow

**MCL₁**
Positive ( + ): right sternal border, lowest palpable rib
Negative ( − ): left shoulder, below clavicular hollow
Ground (G): right shoulder, below clavicular hollow

## MONITORING YOUR PATIENT DURING EMERGENCY PERICARDIOCENTESIS

If the doctor suspects your patient has cardiac tamponade, he may do emergency pericardiocentesis. (This procedure is also used to diagnose pericardial effusion.) Pericardiocentesis involves inserting a 16G to 18G intracardiac needle into the pericardial sac to aspirate fluid and to relieve intrapericardial pressure.

Pericardiocentesis may cause life-threatening complications, such as ventricular dysrhythmias, bleeding from the myocardium, and coronary artery laceration. A precordial lead, attached to the needle's hub, lets the EKG monitor reflect needle position. If the needle contacts the patient's myocardium inadvertently, causing bleeding and ventricular irritability, you'll see abnormal waveforms—large and erratic QRS complexes. Elevated ST segments indicate that the needle's contacted the ventricle; prolonged PR intervals indicate that it's touched the atrium.

Monitor your patient's EKG, blood pressure, and central venous pressure (CVP) constantly. Make sure, too, that emergency resuscitation equipment's on hand.

Following the procedure, monitor your patient's vital signs every 5 to 10 minutes. His blood pressure should rise as the tamponade's relieved.

Be alert for signs and symptoms of recurring tamponade (which may require repeated pericardiocentesis):
• decreased blood pressure
• narrowing pulse pressure
• increased CVP
• distended neck veins
• tachycardia
• tachypnea
• muffled heart sounds
• friction rub
• anxiety
• chest pain.

tor suspects pericardial tamponade. (See *Monitoring Your Patient During Emergency Pericardiocentesis*.)

Next, connect your patient to a cardiac monitor to assess his heart rate and rhythm. (See *Electrocardiograms: Measuring the Heart's Electrical Current*, pages 172 and 173.) You may use a 12-lead EKG machine or hardwire monitoring, depending on the equipment available and your hospital's policy. (See *Positioning Electrodes for Hardwire Monitoring*, page 175.) If monitoring reveals a serious cardiac dysrhythmia, such as ventricular fibrillation, the doctor may order I.V. antiarrhythmic drugs, such as lidocaine or epinephrine. (See *Identifying Life-Threatening EKG Waveforms*, pages 192 to 194.) Remember that digitalis toxicity may cause atrioventricular block. Make sure you have a defibrillator on hand. Remember, ventricular fibrillation, ventricular asystole, ventricular tachycardia, electromechanical dissociation, and third-degree heart block are *life-threatening dysrhythmias* that must be treated immediately.

Remember, too, that adequate tissue perfusion is essential to life, so any cardiovascular emergency that compromises cardiac output and circulation is a threat. (Of course, cardiac arrest is the ultimate compromise of cardiac output.)

Be prepared to draw blood for laboratory tests, including cardiac enzymes, electrolytes, a clotting profile, and a complete blood count (CBC), and arrange for a portable chest X-ray.

### General appearance
Check your patient for signs of trauma, such as open wounds, impaled objects, or disrupted chest structure. Assess his skin color and temperature. Note any pallor, cyanosis, coolness, and moisture. Skin color, temperature, and hydration are important indicators of your patient's peripheral perfusion. If his skin is cold and sweaty, he may be suffering from the massive peripheral vasoconstriction that accompanies myocardial infarction.

Note any expressions of anxiety or impending doom: these should alert you to the seriousness of your patient's situation.

## Mental status

Your patient's level of consciousness and mental status will help you determine the adequacy of his brain perfusion and provide a baseline for subsequent assessments. For example, a patient's stupor or confusion may indicate poor cerebral perfusion resulting from decreased cardiac output secondary to myocardial damage or dysrhythmias. Alterations in level of consciousness may be secondary to changes in oxygen delivery to the brain. Watch for restlessness and uncooperative behavior, often seen in patients with hypoxemia.

# What to Do Next

When you've assessed your patient's airway, breathing, and circulation and intervened as necessary, you're ready to use your emergency assessment skills to identify his most serious cardiovascular problems. Start by determining his chief complaints; then focus the rest of your emergency assessment around them. That way, you won't have to perform all assessment steps for every patient.

Monitor your patient's vital signs frequently while you're performing your assessment, and be alert to any changes. Be prepared to intervene *immediately* if your patient's condition deteriorates suddenly. Remember, this can happen at any time during your assessment.

Start your assessment by asking if your patient has *chest pain*—an indicator of many serious cardiovascular problems (see *"How Bad Is It?"* page 68). If your patient reports chest pain, quickly determine its:

• *quality*—For example, "tearing" chest pain may suggest dissecting aortic aneurysm; pressure-like pain may suggest myocardial ischemia.

• *severity*—For example, mild pain may suggest dysrhythmias or myocardial contusion; severe pain may suggest myocardial infarction or dissecting aortic aneurysms.

• *location*—For example, substernal pain that radiates to the precordium and left arm may indicate angina, myocardial infarction, pericarditis, pulmonary embolus, or dissecting aortic aneurysm. Back pain may indicate pericarditis or aortic dissection distal to the left subclavian artery.

• *onset*—For example, pain from aortic dissection, angina, myocardial infarction, or pulmonary embolus can be sudden and severe; pain from pericarditis or a musculoskeletal problem usually evolves more slowly.

• *aggravating factors*—For example, typical angina pain is induced by exertion or exposure to heat or cold; pain from a myocardial infarction may arise spontaneously.

• *alleviating factors*—For example, pain relieved by rest or nitroglycerin suggests angina; pain relieved by antacids suggests gastrointestinal distress.

Ask if your patient's ever experienced similar pain. If so, when and what happened? Document your findings.

Quickly inspect the patient's chest for signs of trauma that may have caused his pain. Look for bruises, contusions, or reddened areas that you may have missed earlier. Ask your patient if he's been in an accident and, if he has, whether he suffered a blow to his chest, such as by banging against a steering wheel. Find out whether his pain has increased or decreased since then. Note his position—he may be splinting if broken ribs or bruised areas cause painful respirations.

The doctor will probably order medications to relieve your patient's pain and to reduce his anxiety. Be prepared to give medications, such as nitroglycerin (sublingual, oral, or topical), morphine sulfate, or meperidine (Demerol), because reducing pain and anxiety reduces stress on your patient's heart. Of course, before you give any medications, ask your patient specifically about medication allergies.

Ask your patient if he has *extremity pain,* which may be related to peripheral arterial occlusion or to myocardial infarction or angina (left arm pain). If he has pain in an arm or leg, ask about the same factors as you did for chest pain (quality, severity, location, onset, aggravating factors, alleviating factors). Note skin color and temperature changes that may be associated with the pain, and ask the patient if he's had recent trauma, surgery, or a history of vascular disease. Palpate peripheral pulses methodically in his arms (brachial, radial, ulnar) and his legs (femoral, popliteal, posterior, tibial, pedal).

An absent pulse in a cool, pale, cyanotic limb indicates a real emergency—an acute arterial occlusion that may require immediate surgery. Call the doctor immediately, and expect to give pain medications, such as meperidine (Demerol) or morphine sulfate. *Don't* elevate the affected limb—this will only decrease blood supply to the area.

If your patient doesn't have signs of an acute arterial occlusion, continue your assessment by asking him if he's had episodes of *dyspnea.* If he has, ask him when it started and how long he's had it; also ask if any body position makes his dyspnea better or worse—dyspnea from pulmonary edema is usually worst when the patient lies

---

## RECOGNIZING DIGITALIS TOXICITY

Digitalis' therapeutic range is narrow—in some patients even a therapeutic dose may be toxic. Of course, this is why toxicity from digitalis glycosides is relatively common in patients taking the drug.

Patients taking digitalis preparations who are also taking certain other drugs, or who have certain disorders, are at particularly high risk for developing toxicity.

**Examples include:**
• the patient with reduced renal function, who's taking digoxin
• the patient with reduced hepatic function, who's taking digitoxin
• the patient with electrolyte imbalances, myocardial infarction, pulmonary disease, or hypothyroidism
• the patient on quinidine or verapamil therapy.

If you suspect your patient's developing toxicity, discontinue digitalis and notify the doctor. He may order antiarrhythmic drugs and a temporary pacemaker. Also, he may discontinue diuretics, which contribute to potassium loss (hypokalemia), and take action to correct electrolyte imbalances.

Expect the doctor to discontinue the digitalis or to readjust the dosage. If you suspect an intentional overdose, assess the patient's mental status—his disease may be causing suicidal depression.

Watch your patient for signs and symptoms of digitalis toxicity, listed at right.

*Note:* Digitalis toxicity affects the cardiovascular system and other body systems. So nausea, vomiting, and anorexia commonly accompany toxicity—especially in geriatric patients. But digitalis-induced dysrhythmias may occur *without* any other signs and symptoms.

### SIGNS AND SYMPTOMS

**Most common:**
• Anorexia
• Nausea, vomiting
• Malaise
• Headache
• Ventricular ectopic beats
• Premature ventricular contractions (bigeminy)
• Bradycardia

**Less common:**
• Blurred vision
• Headache
• Yellow cast to vision or halos around lights
• Disorientation
• Diarrhea
• Ventricular tachycardia
• Sinoatrial and atrioventricular block
• Ventricular fibrillation

down. If he's had dyspnea for some time, find out whether it's precipitated by exercise or activity—dyspnea on exertion is one of the earliest signs of congestive heart failure (CHF). Inspect his jugular veins for distention (another indication of CHF), and note if the patient is sitting upright and leaning forward to breathe. Quickly palpate your patient's liver, and note any enlargement or tenderness—a characteristic of CHF that results from excessive venous congestion. Check his arms and legs for edema, which may indicate venous pooling due to pump failure. Record the degree and extent of the edema, to provide an accurate baseline. Tell the doctor if you note these signs, because he may want you to adjust the I.V. infusion rate to avoid fluid overload. He may also ask you to provide additional supplemental oxygen.

Ask your patient if he's had episodes of *syncope* or *dizziness*, which commonly occur when cardiac output and, consequently, brain perfusion are reduced. Ask the patient what he was doing at the time of the episode and whether he had any warning signs. He may report palpitations or a feeling that his heart "skipped a beat" just prior to the episode—a signal that underlying dysrhythmias may be the cause. Of course, you'll be watching your patient's cardiac monitor all during your assessment for any dysrhythmias, but you'll be particularly watchful if your patient has these signs and symptoms. If your patient has certain dysrhythmias, the doctor may ask you to give I.V. lidocaine.

Auscultate his carotid arteries for bruits, which may indicate carotid stenosis or atherosclerotic narrowing—another factor that may interfere with brain perfusion and cause syncope. As you may know, if he has carotid stenosis, there's a good chance he also has atherosclerotic disease affecting other vessels, which could produce angina or even a myocardial infarction (MI). Note your findings carefully—your patient could be suffering from transient ischemic attacks and may be at risk for a cerebrovascular accident (see the "Ischemic Cerebrovascular Accident" entry in Chapter 6). Ask your patient if he's had these episodes before.

When you've assessed your patient's chief complaints, perform a quick auscultation of his heart sounds to detect any abnormalities and to provide a baseline. Palpate your patient's precordium to determine the point of maximal impulse, and use that to guide your auscultation. Listen for muffled heart sounds (possibly indicating cardiac tamponade) or abnormal sounds, such as $S_3$ (ventricular gallop—an important early sign of heart failure) or $S_4$ (atrial gallop—an indication of hypertension, aortic stenosis, or a recent MI). You may hear both together (summation gallop) if your patient has severe myocardial disease and tachycardia. Document your findings carefully and, particularly if you hear muffled heart sounds, notify the doctor immediately. You may need to assist with emergency pericardiocentesis if your patient has developed cardiac tamponade that was not discovered initially. (See *Monitoring Your Patient During Emergency Pericardiocentesis,* page 176.)

Ask your patient if he has any *chronic diseases,* such as hypertension, diabetes, congestive heart failure, or lung disease, and ask if he's ever had an episode similar to the one he's experiencing now. Don't forget to ask if anyone in his family has a history of these diseases, because a positive family history will alert you to your patient's increased risk factors. Find out if he's had surgery to correct a congenital defect, coronary artery bypass surgery, valve replacement, or vascular surgery.

Complete your assessment by finding out what *medications* your patient takes. Ask especially about cardiovascular medications, such as nitrates, diuretics, or antiarrhythmics, such as beta blockers, calcium channel blockers, and digitalis—your patient's signs and symptoms may be the result of drug toxicity (especially with digitalis) or of failure to take medication as prescribed. Document current medication use to provide a baseline and to help the doctor determine any underlying disease.

Remember that your patient may be very anxious during your assessment, because of the pain (often severe) and sense of doom that often accompany cardiovascular emergencies. Reassure him frequently, and ask your patient's family for information if he's too sick to respond.

# Special Considerations

### Pediatric
Congenital problems, such as septal defects or tetralogy of Fallot, cause most cardiovascular emergencies in children. You generally won't see MIs or dysrhythmias in children, but you may see CHF caused by underlying congenital defects or by an acute pulmonary infection. Be particularly alert for tachycardia, tachypnea, and hepatomegaly—edema and cyanosis may not be present. Ask the child's parents about a history of lethargy, poor growth, difficulty in feeding, and upper respiratory infections. Find out if he has labored breathing during bowel movements and if he often assumes a squatting position. Ask an older child if he has trouble keeping up with his friends during active play. Does athletic exercise quickly tire him?

Remember this: As a nurse, you may be the first person to see these signs of your pediatric patient's underlying cardiac defect. If you do see any of these signs, be suspicious—more obvious signs and symptoms may not appear for some time, and early identification's important.

### Geriatric
Elderly patients have an increased risk of developing CHF, hypertensive crisis,

MI, and arterial occlusion. When you assess an older patient, remember that his cardiac rate and stroke volume may be diminished and that his heart contractions may be considerably slowed. Cardiac output at rest is decreased up to 35% in many patients age 70 and older. Atherosclerotic deposits result in diminished blood flow to various organs, and systolic and diastolic blood pressure is often elevated. Fibrotic and sclerotic valve changes may cause heart murmurs.

Expect that your elderly patient's normal EKG will be somewhat different from that of a young adult. Changes include an increase in PR, QRS, and QT intervals and a decrease in QRS complex amplitude.

Don't forget that many older patients may be on digitalis therapy for preexisting cardiac disease, so they're prone to digitalis toxicity. For example, if an older person comes in with dysrhythmias, ask if he's had diarrhea over the past 2 to 3 days. Why? Because diarrhea causes potassium loss, which makes a patient on digitalis more susceptible to digitalis toxicity.

# CARE AFTER DIAGNOSIS

# Myocardial Infarction

### Prediagnosis summary
The patient's initial findings included:
- chest pain
- diaphoresis
- pallor
- dyspnea
- nausea.

An I.V. was inserted, and he received oxygen and was placed on a cardiac monitor. Blood was drawn for cardiac enzymes, electrolytes, a clotting profile, and a CBC. He was given medi-

# UNDERSTANDING HOW AN INTRAAORTIC BALLOON PUMP WORKS

### SYSTOLE

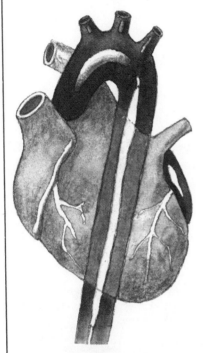

### DIASTOLE

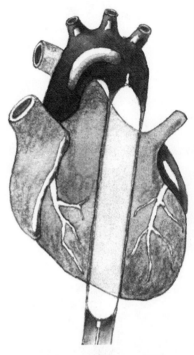

The intraaortic balloon pump (IABP) is a key therapy for treating complications of myocardial infarction. Once it's positioned in the patient's aortic artery, the balloon's timed inflation-deflation cycle causes counterpulsation. This extra boost to the heart's pumping action causes increased coronary artery perfusion and left ventricular ejection—both helpful in treating left ventricular failure and cardiogenic shock.

After he inserts the IABP, the doctor may ask you to monitor the patient. Here's what you need to know about the procedure and aftercare.

To insert the IABP, the doctor transfers the patient to a cardiac-care unit, operating room, or cardiac catheterization laboratory. There, he inserts the balloon catheter through the patient's femoral artery and threads it up the descending thoracic aorta. He positions it distal to the left subclavian artery, then connects the catheter to

the external pump. The R wave of the patient's EKG triggers the pump's inflation-deflation (counterpulsation) mechanism. Helium or carbon dioxide inflates the balloon during early diastole. Inflation displaces blood so aortic blood pressure's increased—and blood flow's enhanced.

The balloon rapidly deflates as the heart prepares for left ventricular ejection at systole. This decreases aortic pressure, making ejection easier and decreasing the left ventricle's work load.

Once the balloon's in place, monitor the patient's circulatory status. Check his arterial pulses and temperature as well as the skin color of the leg with the insertion site to make sure the catheter isn't occluding the artery. Check his vital signs every 15 minutes to 1 hour. Hourly, assess his cardiac and urine output, cardiac rhythm, and pulmonary artery pressure.

# WHAT HAPPENS IN MYOCARDIAL INFARCTION

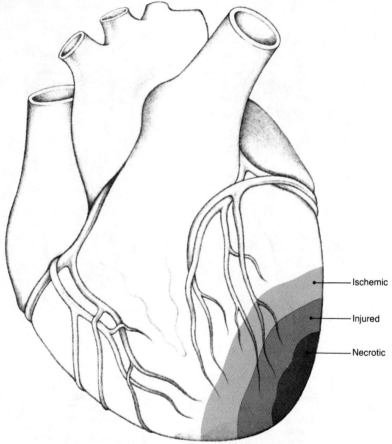

— Ischemic

— Injured

— Necrotic

Understanding the causes and pathophysiology of myocardial infarction (MI) will help you care for your patient more confidently. As you probably know, MI occurs when a portion of the cardiac muscle (myocardium) is deprived of oxygenated coronary blood flow, resulting in cellular ischemia, tissue injury, and then necrosis; irreversible myocardial damage ensues. Causes include:
• a buildup of atherosclerotic plaque

(the major cause)
• coronary artery emboli
• coronary thrombosis
• hypertension
• massive hemorrhage
• coronary artery spasm.

When coronary artery blood flow is diminished, the heart pumps harder, increasing heart rate and blood pressure to meet increasing myocardial oxygen demands. Pulmonary circulation may back up

**Some common causes of occlusion**

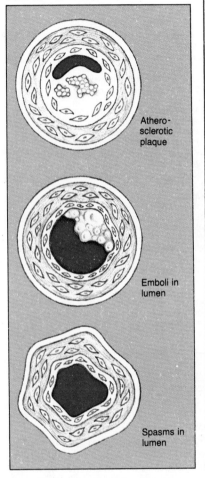

Athero-
sclerotic
plaque

Emboli in
lumen

Spasms in
lumen

in response to increased cardiac output,
increasing the pressure needed to fill
the atria. Dyspnea and fatigue result, further
diminishing the heart's oxygen supply.
The infarcted area alters the heart's contractile properties; this interferes with
the ventricular relaxation period and the
normal conduction system, creating irritable
foci in the myocardium with a resulting
decrease in cardiac output. The result may
be heart failure, dysrhythmias, or cardiogenic shock (see Chapter 14, SHOCK).

cation, such as morphine sulfate, for
his chest pain.

(Note: A patient may have an acute
*clinically silent* MI with no chest pain
or associated signs or symptoms. If your
patient on the unit has sudden dyspnea
or worsening CHF, particularly if he's
diabetic, hypotensive, or elderly, suspect MI and take a 12-lead EKG—the
only conclusive way to show that an MI
has occurred.)

### Priorities

Now, your nursing priority is continued pain control. You'll give sublingual
nitroglycerin or sublingual isosorbide
dinitrate (Isordil) to dilate his coronary arteries and to improve coronary
blood flow. Also, expect to administer
medication—usually I.V. morphine
sulfate, meperidine (Demerol), or hydromorphone (Dilaudid). *Don't give
these medications I.M.,* because I.M.
administration causes creatine phosphokinase (CPK) and serum glutamic-
oxaloacetic transaminase (SGOT) elevation, invalidating enzyme test results. Also, the absorption of I.M.
medications from muscle is unpredictable due to decreased cardiac output and decreased peripheral perfusion.

If these medications don't control the
patient's pain immediately, expect to
give I.V. nitroglycerin by continuous
drip. You may also give verapamil (Isoptin, Calan) I.V. or nifedipine (Procardia) orally to reduce coronary artery
spasm and to decrease his pain (see
*Highlighting Calcium Channel Block-
ers,* page 187). Expect to give lidocaine
as an I.V. bolus followed by a continuous drip to prevent ventricular dysrhythmias.

### Continuing assessment and intervention

Now that your patient's pain has been
relieved and he's on oxygen and a monitor, you'll have time for a thorough
nursing assessment to compare with
initial findings and to provide a baseline for future assessments.

DRUGS

## HIGHLIGHTING STREPTOKINASE

If streptokinase is administered to a patient with an acute myocardial infarction, his chances of survival and recovery may improve. Here's why:

Streptokinase is a thrombolytic, so it dissolves the clot occluding the artery. This improves myocardial perfusion and, if the drug's given within 3 to 4 hours of the onset of the patient's chest pain, it limits the infarction's size.

Administering streptokinase directly into the occluded coronary artery, using angiography in a cardiac catheterization laboratory, is the most effective treatment. (You may also give streptokinase by continuous I.V. for such disorders as pulmonary emboli and deep-vein thrombosis.)

Remember these important points about administering streptokinase:
• Always establish a perfusion baseline of peripheral pulses.
• Before infusion, double-check all doses and infusion rates with another nurse.
• Don't give intramuscular or intravenous injections during infusion or for 24 hours afterward.
• Establish two I.V. lines before infusion. Use one for streptokinase, the second for any other drugs you need to give.
• Align and immobilize the affected limb.
• Inspect the infusion site hourly for signs of bleeding. After infusion, inspect the site every 15 minutes the first hour, every 30 minutes for 2 to 8 hours, then once per shift.
• Monitor and document the following every hour, before and after infusion: the patient's pulses and color, and the sensitivity of his affected and unaffected limbs.
• Keep a laboratory flow sheet so you can monitor the following during and after infusion: partial thromboplastin time, prothrombin time, hemoglobin, and hematocrit.
• Monitor carefully, for dysrhythmias, any patient receiving intracoronary streptokinase for lysis of coronary artery thrombi.
• Test all the patient's nasogastric aspirate and his stools and urine for blood, during and after infusion.
• Apply direct pressure to the infusion site for at least 30 minutes after the catheter's removed.
• Watch the patient for flushing, itching, urticaria, headaches and muscle aches, and nausea. These may indicate a mild allergic and febrile reaction.

Look at your patient's skin. Is it cool, pale, clammy, cyanotic? When you take his vital signs, he may have a low-grade fever as a result of the inflammatory response. Check his sedimentation rate and his white blood cell count—they may be elevated as well. When you take his blood pressure, most commonly you'll see *hypo*tension, due to decreased cardiac output. However, you may first see *hyper*tension, an initial response to stress-induced catecholamine release from the adrenals and the sympathetic nervous system.

If pulmonary edema or CHF is developing, you'll note distended jugular veins, tachypnea, and edema of the extremities, and you'll hear rales and a moist cough when you auscultate his lungs. (See the "Congestive Heart Failure" entry in this chapter.) When you

report these signs and symptoms, expect the doctor to order further treatment, such as diuretics.

When you auscultate your patient's heart, you may hear ventricular gallop ($S_4$), common in the first 24 hours after an MI. However, if you hear an atrial gallop ($S_3$) or a blowing systolic murmur, this may indicate complications of MI, such as left ventricular failure and mitral valve involvement. Further treatment may include diuretics and vasodilators. You may also hear a friction rub, possibly indicating pericarditis. Watch the monitor for any dysrhythmias; expect to administer antiarrhythmics or to defibrillate if necessary. (See the "Cardiac Dysrhythmias" entry in this chapter.)

Compare your assessment findings with those noted in the ED, and notify the doctor about any changes. If your findings don't suggest any further complications, continue your assessment by taking the patient's history.

Ask your patient to describe the pain that caused him to come to the hospital—he may use such terms as burning, pressure, heaviness, constriction, tightness, aching, or indigestion. If he's had a history of angina, he may tell you that his pain is similar to what he had before but more severe and unremitting, that it didn't subside with rest or nitrates, and that it's increased over several days. He may also tell you he's had numbness or weakness in one or both arms, shortness of breath, fainting, sweating, fatigue, nausea, vomiting, and severe anxiety with a sense of impending doom.

Determine if your patient has a history of diabetes, hypertension, angina, or vascular insufficiency (cerebral or peripheral). As you know, these are risk factors that may affect patient care. Also ask about a family history of these diseases: a positive family history increases your patient's risk of developing them. Find out if your patient's been under stress lately; if he smokes and, if so, how much; how much alcohol, if any, he consumes; and what his dietary habits are. This information will help you plan his continuing care.

Your patient may be taking diuretics, digoxin, antiarrhythmics, or antihypertensives for preexisting conditions. Determine whether he's taking these or any other medications, his dosage schedule, and his response—you may find that the medication wasn't effective or that the patient's been noncompliant.

**Therapeutic care**

Now you're ready to review the patient's chart and continue his care. This will probably include giving sedatives or antianxiety agents to help reduce stress. Also, the doctor may order heparin I.V. or subcutaneously to prevent thrombus and embolus formation and a beta-blocking agent, such as pro-

## A PATIENT PRECAUTION

Just as diabetics and hemophiliacs should wear Medic Alert bracelets, your patient who's had a cardiovascular emergency should carry a copy of his EKG and his medications list (with dosages).

So, provide your patient with copies of these documents before he goes home. This will speed diagnosis and help ensure accurate treatment if he has to go to an ED again.

pranolol hydrochloride (Inderal), to decrease contractility and heart rate, thus reducing myocardial oxygen consumption.

Your patient will be on bed rest for 24 to 48 hours. Encourage him to do range-of-motion exercises to prevent venous stasis. Apply antiembolism stockings (such as TEDS) to promote venous return to the heart and to avoid thrombus and embolus formation—which may cause pulmonary embolism or ischemic cerebrovascular accident. (See these entries in Chapters 4 and 6.) Give stool softeners to prevent straining and Valsalva's maneuver, and a clear liquid diet to reduce his heart's work load and to prevent nausea and vomiting due to decreased peristalsis. Begin cardiac teaching to help your patient understand his condition.

Hemodynamic monitoring may be used. For example, an arterial line may be inserted to allow continuous blood pressure monitoring and to provide easy access to blood for laboratory analysis and oxygen content. A Swan-Ganz catheter may also be inserted for measuring pulmonary pressures, which reflect left ventricular function. Pulmonary capillary wedge pressure and pulmonary artery diastolic pressure reflect left ventricular filling pressure; these measurements also provide a guide to volume status, medication response, and development of complications, such as CHF and cardiogenic shock. If a thermodilution catheter is selected, cardiac output can also be measured.

If the patient has severely decreased cardiac output or signs and symptoms of cardiogenic shock (such as hypertension, decreased blood pressure, and decreased urinary output), the doctor may insert an intraaortic balloon pump to improve ejection of blood from the left ventricle and to increase coronary artery perfusion. (See *Understanding How an Intraaortic Balloon Pump Works,* page 181.)

The doctor may also start intracoronary infusion of streptokinase if your patient's condition meets certain criteria:
• arrival at the hospital within 3 hours of initial chest pain
• EKG evidence of progressing infarction
• age less than 70
• no contraindications to thrombolytic agents.

Streptokinase is a thrombolytic drug used to dissolve formed clots, thereby restoring normal circulation, reducing infarct size, and improving left ventricular function (see *Highlighting Streptokinase,* page 184).

Diagnostic studies used to measure the patient's progress will include serial 12-lead EKGs and enzyme analysis, begun in the ED. EKG changes reflect the site of coronary artery occlusion, myocardial ischemia, or necrosis. Watch for:
• pathologic Q waves (wider and deeper than normal), caused by complete and lengthy oxygen deprivation leading to tissue death and necrosis. Q waves indicate *permanent* damage and don't appear immediately—expect to see them 1 to 6 hours after the onset of symptoms. Remember, however, that your patient may have Q waves from an earlier MI.
• ST segment elevation, caused by less severe oxygen deprivation leading to tissue injury that may be reversed if adequate circulation is restored. A *de-crease* in ST segment elevation indicates improving oxygenation of the damaged area; an *increase* indicates increasing ischemia that may further damage the heart.
• T-wave inversion, caused by the brief oxygen deprivation that leaves the tissue viable if adequate circulation is restored. Sudden T-wave inversion indicates mild ischemia that may lead to injury; it may be seen anytime.

You'll see these changes in leads oriented to the damaged area; expect reciprocal changes in leads opposite the damaged area. Evaluate serial EKGs carefully and notify the doctor if you see any of the changes discussed above. And remember—in the early stages of acute MI the patient's EKG may be normal.

Note changes in cardiac enzyme levels (SGOT, lactate dehydrogenase [LDH], and CPK), which elevate with myocardial damage. Because these are nonspecific, you'll also watch myocardial specific isoenzymes (CPK-MB, $LDH_1$, and $LDH_2$). CPK-MB rises within 4 to 8 hours after the infarction and usually peaks after 20 hours; $LDH_1$ and $LDH_2$ rise within 8 to 12 hours and peak around 24 to 48 hours. If your patient's had an MI, his $LDH_1$ will usually exceed his $LDH_2$. Make sure you report enzyme and isoenzyme changes to the doctor—they'll help him gauge the patient's progress.

Your patient may be considered stable when his serial EKGs and enzyme levels are returning to normal, his pain is controlled, and he has no dysrhythmias (usually within 3 to 5 days for uncomplicated MI).

Expect to administer sublingual, oral, or topical nitrates to dilate your patient's coronary arteries and to prevent further damage and chest discomfort. If he develops increased chest pain despite medication, stay with him, have someone call the doctor immediately, and arrange for an EKG.

Continue to watch him closely for signs and symptoms of fluid retention, which may indicate impending heart

# HIGHLIGHTING CALCIUM CHANNEL BLOCKERS

You've probably cared for patients taking nifedipine (Procardia, Adalat), diltiazem (Cardizem), or verapamil (Isoptin, Calan). Or perhaps you've seen verapamil I.V. given in a cardiac emergency. All these drugs are calcium channel blockers.

Do you understand how these drugs work, when you may administer them, and what you need to watch for in a patient taking them?

**Mechanism of action**
Calcium channel blockers work by:
• decreasing myocardial oxygen demand by reducing myocardial contractility and dilating peripheral arterioles
• improving myocardial perfusion by dilating coronary arteries
• reducing electrical excitation.

In the normal cell, calcium ions trigger a chemical reaction inside each myocardial cell, causing it to contract; but before this can happen, the cell must take in additional calcium ions from the extracellular space. It does this by changing its membrane, opening channels to receive outside calcium ions.

Calcium channel blockers close off some channels, limiting calcium's passage into the cell during depolarization. So fewer calcium ions are present to trigger the reaction. The muscle cell contracts, but not as forcefully.

**Uses**
Nifedipine, diltiazem, and oral verapamil all treat typical and variant (Prinzmetal's) angina. They also reduce coronary artery spasms in patients with Prinzmetal's angina.

Verapamil I.V. inhibits calcium influx into myocardial conduction fibers of sinoatrial and atrioventricular nodes. Because of this, it's used to treat supraventricular tachydysrhythmias, such as atrial fibrillation, atrial flutter, and paroxysmal supraventricular tachycardia. Diltiazem has similar, but less extensive, electrophysiologic effects. So far, the Food and Drug Administration hasn't approved it for treating supraventricular tachycardia dysrhythmias.

**Nursing considerations**
Be alert for:
• hypotension, especially if your patient's also taking antihypertensive drugs
• signs and symptoms of congestive heart failure, especially if your patient's also taking a beta-blocker
• bradycardia, heart blocks, and sinus arrest when Verapamil I.V. is given (always connect him to a cardiac monitor)
• increased severity of anginal pain until the drug reaches therapeutic levels when Nefedipine is given
• signs and symptoms of digitalis toxicity if your patient's also taking digoxin.

---

failure. Monitor his daily weight and intake and output.

# Cardiac Dysrhythmias

## Prediagnosis summary
The patient may have initially complained of:
• palpitations, experienced as a rapid, skipping, fluttering, or jumping heartbeat
• chest discomfort or dull chest pain.

He may have had pale, cool, clammy skin; dizziness; fainting; dyspnea; tachypnea; and decreased alertness (stupor or confusion) progressing to other signs and symptoms of hypoxemia. He may also have had hypotension and a rapid, slow, or absent pulse—depending on the specific type of dysrhythmia.

If the patient's dysrhythmia produced cardiac arrest and he was unresponsive and apneic with no pulse or blood pressure, CPR was started with defibrillation, cardioversion, and appropriate drug therapy as indicated (see the "Life Support" section in Chapter 3).

He was given supplemental oxygen, an I.V. infusion was started, and he was connected to a cardiac monitor. Blood was drawn for a complete blood count, electrolytes, blood urea nitrogen (BUN), blood sugar, cardiac enzymes, and creatinine, to help identify the cause of the patient's dysrhythmia. An EKG was done to determine the type of dysrhythmia.

### Priorities

Your first priority is to provide definitive treatment for your patient's specific type of dysrhythmia. He may be asymptomatic or have signs and symptoms of decreased cardiac output, such as decreased blood pressure, weak transient pulses, and deteriorating mental status. Your patient's EKG may show abnormal heart rate or rhythm or specific disturbances in the P waves, PR interval, and QRS complexes, depending on his specific type of dysrhythmia. (See *Identifying Life-Threatening EKG Waveforms,* pages 192 to 194, for some examples.) Use lead MCL$_1$ on the monitor to allow the best visualization of your patient's P wave; this helps distinguish between his supraventricular and ventricular rhythms. P waves are present in supraventricular tachycardia, but they may be superimposed in the QRS complex, ST segment, or T wave. They're absent in ventricular tachycardia and ventricular fibrillation.

Monitor your patient's vital signs constantly while he's on the cardiac monitor. Why? Because even if a regular rhythm appears on the monitor, it may not produce effective heart muscle contractions. So if you note a sudden drop in your patient's blood pressure or pulse, suspect a further reduction in cardiac output. Remember that his dysrhythmia can worsen and his condition can deteriorate rapidly at any time during his care, so always keep emergency drugs and intubation equipment available.

If your patient has *frequent premature ventricular contractions (PVCs)* or *multifocal PVCs,* he'll receive lidocaine, which increases the ventricular stimulation threshold, as an I.V. bolus first, followed by a continuous drip.

If he has *supraventricular tachycardia* (SVT)—such as atrial flutter or fibrillation, multifocal atrial tachycardia, or paroxysmal atrial tachycardia with rapid ventricular rates—the doctor may try one of two procedures to slow the rate before initiating drug therapy. Either he'll ask your patient to take a deep breath and bear down (Valsalva's maneuver), or he'll use carotid sinus pressure. Run a strip on the cardiac monitor as the doctor does this, and mark the areas where Valsalva's maneuver or carotid sinus pressure started and stopped. If these procedures fail, expect to give I.V. verapamil (Isoptin), propranolol hydrochloride (Inderal), or digoxin.

For a patient with *complete heart block,* I.V. atropine or isoproterenol (Isuprel) may be ordered. If drug therapy doesn't produce an effective rhythm and the patient still has signs and symptoms of decreased cardiac output, the doctor may insert a temporary transvenous pacemaker. (See *Assisting with Temporary Pacemaker Insertion,* page 191.) After insertion, attach the external pacemaker unit to the patient's gown or an arm board so it's safe and comfortable. Wrap the insertion site securely in a dry dressing. Why? Because if you don't do this, aberrant current sources can conduct through a damp dressing and cause ventricular tachycardia.

If your patient has *symptomatic bradycardia* producing reduced cardiac output, expect to give him I.V. atropine to block vagal stimulation and to speed conduction through the atrioventricular junction.

### Continuing assessment and intervention

When your patient's dysrhythmia is no longer life-threatening, perform a complete baseline assessment while watching his monitor. If your assessment findings reveal that his specific dysrhythmia isn't responding to initial drug therapy, intervene as necessary. For example, if the patient with PVCs

# WHAT HAPPENS IN CARDIAC DYSRHYTHMIAS

Cardiac dysrhythmias are irregularities in heart rate, rhythm, or conduction produced by automaticity (cell-firing) abnormalities or by electrical or mechanical conduction disturbances. When automaticity fails or is disturbed, electrical conduction disturbances alter specific conduction pathways—the ones that normally conduct impulses at 60 to 100 beats/minute to produce muscle fiber contraction and pumping of the heart: normal sinus rhythm.

Causes of cardiac dysrhythmias include:
• cardiac disorders that strain the myocardium and cause myocardial hypoxia—for example, coronary artery disease, myocardial infarction, congestive heart failure, hypertension, or valvular defects
• other organic disorders—for example, pulmonary embolism, aortic aneurysm, thyrotoxicosis, pheochromocytoma, systemic infection, or heart or lung cancer
• electrolyte imbalances—for example, from dieting, profuse sweating, excessive vomiting, renal failure, or diuretic overuse
• toxicity or side effects from drugs—for example, digoxin, depressants, anesthetics, alcohol, nicotine, and caffeine
• hypoxemia
• congenital heart defects.

Dysrhythmias are classified by rate (tachycardias or bradycardias), by rhythm (regular or irregular), and by site (ventricular or atrial). Their effect on cardiac output depends on the type of dysrhythmia and on the patient's underlying cardiac status.

*Tachycardias* can interfere with normal cardiac output by decreasing ventricular filling time between contractions and by increasing myocardial oxygen demands. Potentially serious or life-threatening tachycardias include ventricular tachycardia, ventricular fibrillation, and supraventricular tachycardias—atrial fibrillation, atrial flutter, paroxysmal atrial tachycardia, and multifocal atrial tachycardia with rapid ventricular rates. *Bradycardias* can interfere with normal cardiac output by decreasing the rate of ventricular ejection and so increasing cardiac output. Serious bradycardias include asystole, partial heart block, and third-degree heart block.

*Irregular heart rhythms* potentially threaten cardiac output but aren't life-threatening themselves. A frequently encountered irregular rhythm is atrial fibrillation with a normal ventricular rate (60 to 120).

*Atrial dysrhythmias* or *dysrhythmias where the atria are nonfunctioning* (for example, ventricular tachycardia and complete heart block) compromise cardiac output because 10% to 20% of cardiac output is obtained through atrial contraction, which completes ventricular filling (atrial kick). *Ventricular dysrhythmias* directly compromise cardiac output because they directly affect ventricular ejection.

---

is unresponsive to lidocaine, expect to administer I.V. bretylium (Bretylol) or procainamide hydrochloride (Pronestyl).

Or if his dysrhythmia is SVT, and he's not responding to his initial drug treatment, cardioversion may be required. Expect to give him diazepam (Valium) before the procedure to relax him. The doctor will use a current of 50 to 100 watt-seconds for cardioversion; he'll also synchronize the current so it's delivered to the heart on the R wave of the QRS complex. If the patient with symptomatic bradycardia doesn't respond to the atropine he was given, he'll probably need isoproterenol hydrochloride (Isuprel), or a transvenous temporary pacemaker may need to be inserted.

Assess your patient's hydration and perfusion levels. Keep accurate records of his fluid intake and output. Check his blood pressure and pulses frequently for signs of hypoperfusion. (Remember, a dysrhythmia causing decreased cardiac output can lead to CHF. See the "Congestive Heart Failure" entry in this chapter.) Compare these assessment findings to any noted earlier. Check your patient for deteriorating mental status (confusion, anxiety, lethargy).

Assess your patient's heart sounds.

**STATIC STOPPER**

The next time you attach a temporary pacemaker, remember this—to avoid static interference, place the pacemaker in a rubber surgical glove before strapping it to your patient's limb. The glove will insulate the pacemaker to prevent free-floating static electricity from disrupting pacemaker function.

On auscultation, you'll hear rate and rhythm disturbances that correspond to those you found when you assessed his pulse quality. You may also hear gallops and murmurs if your patient has heart failure or valvular defects.

Auscultate his lungs; you may hear rales, wheezes, and decreased breath sounds if your patient also has underlying cardiopulmonary disease. Watch for signs and symptoms of hypoxemia. As you may know, tissue hypoxia can result from the dysrhythmia and the decrease in cardiac output. You may have to increase the percentage of supplemental oxygen you're patient's receiving. Remember that hypoxemia can cause further dysrhythmias.

The doctor may insert a CVP line to administer drugs and to determine the patient's CVP—reflecting the relation between heart function and total circulating volume.

Now that you've assessed your patient and intervened as necessary and you're continuing to watch his cardiac monitor, you can take his history. Ask him if he's had a recent MI, CHF, or chronic obstructive pulmonary disease (COPD); dysrhythmias may accompany these conditions. Also ask if he's had a dysrhythmia before and if he's taking any antiarrhythmics. If so, find out the dosage and number of times per day he takes the medication. If he's taking digoxin, make sure blood was drawn for a digoxin level, because digitalis toxicity can cause dysrhythmias, such as heart blocks. Ask if he's taking diuretics; hypokalemia, which often results, may cause ventricular tachycardia. Ask about his diet and whether he takes in large amounts of alcohol, nicotine, or caffeine, which can also cause dysrhythmias. Find out if he's experienced sudden stress or had vigorous exercise recently; these can cause heart rate and rhythm changes.

## Therapeutic care

Now that your patient's condition is stabilized, continue to monitor his cardiac output, perfusion, and hydration levels. Reassess his heart and lung sounds and his respirations.

If the patient's dysrhythmia has an underlying cause, expect to treat it at this time. If he has underlying coronary artery disease, he'll probably be given nitrates, such as isosorbide dinitrate, to dilate his coronary arteries. If his underlying condition is hypertension, he'll probably need antihypertensives with other appropriate drug therapy, such as diuretics. A patient with an electrolyte imbalance will need to have it corrected. Hypokalemia from diuretic use is common; you may have to replace potassium. If digitalis toxicity caused his dysrhythmia, expect digoxin to be discontinued.

If your patient's dysrhythmia is under control and he's still receiving I.V. continuous drip medication, such as lidocaine or procainamide, or I.V. individual doses of medication, such as digoxin or verapamil, expect to discontinue the I.V. medication and to start him on oral antiarrhythmics.

Continue monitoring your patient's vital signs and heart sounds even after his dysrhythmia is under control, his cardiac output and hydration are adequate, and he's off the cardiac monitor, because he may develop recurrent dysrhythmias and may go into cardiac arrest at any time. If this happens, secure his airway immediately and *start CPR*. Remember, you may be the first person to recognize the physical signs of recurrent dysrhythmias.

Evaluate your patient's heart sounds

# YOUR ROLE IN AN EMERGENCY

## ASSISTING WITH TEMPORARY PACEMAKER INSERTION

Suppose a patient comes into the ED with acute dysrhythmias from a myocardial infarction. First you may administer antiar-rhythmic drugs, as ordered. But if the drugs don't work, the doctor may insert a temporary pacemaker. It electrically stimulates the heart muscle to maintain adequate cardiac rate and rhythm. Here's how a pacemaker works and what you need to know to assist with its insertion.

### Pacemaker mechanics
Temporary pacemakers may be inserted for either atrial or ventricular pacing (more common in an emergency).

To insert a pacemaker, the doctor threads a pacing catheter through the patient's subclavian, femoral, jugular, or antecubital vein. Once the catheter's in place, resting at the apex of the right heart, he connects it to an external pacemaker that's set on either a fixed or a demand mode. The patient's stimulation threshold determines the pacemaker's milliamp setting.

Doctors select demand mode more often than fixed mode. This is because fixed mode interferes with a patient's intrinsic heart rate and may cause ventricular tachycardia or ventricular fibrillation.

### Equipment
• Skin-preparation supplies

• Sterile gloves, towels
• 5-ml syringe and needle
• Introducer wire
• Sterile suture tray
• Antiseptic ointment, sterile gauze dressing, nonallergenic tape
• Temporary pacer and pacing catheter

### Nursing considerations
• Make sure a signed consent form has been obtained before the procedure.
• Gather the necessary equipment, and assist the doctor with inserting and setting the pacemaker.
• Watch the EKG monitor for premature ventricular contractions, ventricular tachycardia, or ventricular fibrillation caused by electrode irritation of the ventricle. Have lidocaine and a defibrillator ready.
• Record the pacemaker's mode, rate, and stimulation threshold on your patient's chart and nursing-care plan.
• Make sure the pacing spike is in the correct position on the EKG waveform—just before the QRS complex (see illustration).
• Continuously monitor the patient's EKG. Notify the doctor if you see ventricular ectopic beats.
• Check the patient's vital signs and level of consciousness hourly.
• Auscultate the patient's lungs and heart for rales, decreased breath sounds, or friction rubs every 2 to 4 hours.
• If you move the patient, elevate the affected limb to immobilize it and to ensure adequate circulation. Use a drawsheet to reposition the patient in bed.
• Change the dressings using sterile technique, and apply antibiotic ointment.
• Check the insertion site for signs of infection and for bleeding.

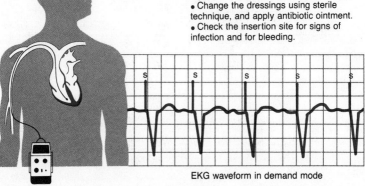

EKG waveform in demand mode

# IDENTIFYING LIFE-THREATENING EKG WAVEFORMS

As you monitor your patient on a cardiac monitor or 12-lead EKG, watch for any of the waveforms below. They indicate that your patient faces an immediate life-threatening situation. Notify the doctor; then prepare to perform the nursing interventions described.

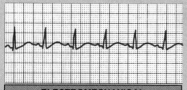

### ELECTROMECHANICAL DISSOCIATION (EMD)
### (Electrical conduction but no pulse)

### Characteristics
• Organized electrical activity without any evidence of effective myocardial contraction
• Possible failure in the calcium transport system (can cause EMD)
• Possible association with profound hypovolemia, cardiac tamponade, myocardial rupture, massive myocardial infarction, or tension pneumothorax

### Interventions
• Give CPR with optimal ventilation, as needed. Continue CPR if no palpable pulse is present. (Do this despite presence of rhythm.)
• Prepare to give epinephrine, sodium bicarbonate, and possibly calcium chloride, as ordered.
• Prepare to start an I.V. infusion of isoproterenol, as ordered.

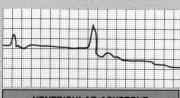

### VENTRICULAR ASYSTOLE
### (Cardiac standstill)

### Characteristics
• Totally absent ventricular electrical activity
• Possible P waves
• Possibly the main event in cardiac arrest (may also occur after ventricular fibrillation)
• May occur in a patient with complete heart block and no pacemaker
• Possible severe metabolic deficit or extensive myocardial damage

### Interventions
• Begin CPR.
• Assist with endotracheal intubation.
• Start an I.V.
• Prepare to give epinephrine, sodium bicarbonate, atropine, calcium chloride, and isoproterenol, as ordered.
• Prepare to assist with temporary pacemaker insertion and defibrillation.

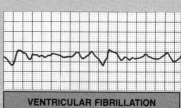

### VENTRICULAR FIBRILLATION

### Characteristics
• Possible ventricular fibrillation arising spontaneously or triggered by premature ventricular contractions or ventricular tachycardia
• Ventricular rhythm rapid and chaotic, indicating varying degrees of depolarization and repolarization; QRS complexes not identifiable
• Patient unconscious at onset
• Absent pulses, heart sounds, and blood pressure
• Dilated pupils, rapid development of cyanosis
• Possible convulsions
• Possible death of patient within minutes, depending on his age (ventricular fibrillation is the most common cause of sudden death in patients with coronary heart disease)

### Interventions
• Give precordial thump if ventricular fibrillation appears on the monitor.
• Defibrillate the patient.
• Begin CPR.
• Administer bretylium, epinephrine, and sodium bicarbonate, as ordered. (Sodium bicarbonate is given according to the patient's arterial blood gas levels, after dysrhythmia terminates, to treat lactic acidosis.)
• Prepare to give lidocaine to treat myocardial irritability and to prevent recurring dysrhythmias.

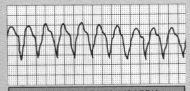

## VENTRICULAR TACHYCARDIA

### Characteristics
• Dangerously low cardiac output that may produce hypotension, chest pain, palpitations, dyspnea, anxiety, shock, coma, and sudden death resulting from ventricular fibrillation

### Interventions
• Perform precordial thump if the patient's pulseless and on a monitor.
• Prepare to give lidocaine to treat the dysrhythmia.
• Prepare to give cardioversion immediately if lidocaine's ineffective.
• Administer lidocaine drip, procainamide, and bretylium, as ordered.
• Suspect hypokalemia if the patient's tachycardia returns despite antiarrhythmic drugs.
• Prepare to give potassium chloride for hypokalemia.
• Suspect lactic acidosis if the patient's tachycardia persists for more than 5 minutes, and prepare to give sodium bicarbonate.
• Prepare to assist with temporary pacemaker insertion for recurrent tachycardia.

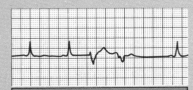

## PREMATURE VENTRICULAR CONTRACTIONS (PVCs)

### Characteristics
• Common form of dysrhythmia
• Longer-than-normal pause occurring immediately after premature beats (compensatory pause)
• Indicator of myocardial irritability
• May initiate ventricular tachycardia, then ventricular fibrillation when they occur

frequently (six or more times/minute), strike on the T wave of preceding complex (R on T pattern), have more than one configuration (multiple form PVCs), occur sequentially for two or three beats (coupling or short runs of PVCs), or when every second beat is a PVC (bigeminy)
• Trigeminy: pattern of two normal beats followed by a PVC
• Increased risk of sudden death if occurring with angina

### Interventions
• Prepare to give lidocaine (sometimes procainamide or later potassium) as ordered to suppress the irritable ventricular focus.
• Be aware that digitalis or diuretic therapy can pause PVCs, and anticipate continuing the drug or giving the patient potassium to restore electrolyte balance and to correct drug-induced ectopic beats.
• Watch the patient for signs and symptoms of lidocaine overdose—such as seizures.
• With procainamide, watch the patient for hypotension.

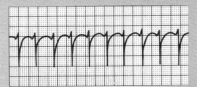

## SYMPTOMATIC SUPRAVENTRICULAR TACHYCARDIA (SVT)

### Characteristics
• Unusually rapid rhythms arising in sinus, atrial, or atrioventricular junctional tissue
• Dysrhythmias adversely affecting hemodynamics due to rapid ventricular response rate, ineffective atrial contraction, or lost normal atrial and ventricular contraction sequence
• Possible reentrant atrial tachycardia, ectopic atrial tachycardia, multifocal atrial tachycardia, atrial fibrillation and atrial flutter with rapid ventricular response, paroxysmal atrial tachycardia, nonparoxysmal junctional tachycardia

### Interventions
• Prepare to give I.V. verapamil, Inderal, and digoxin as ordered.
• Prepare to give cardioversion.

*(continued)*

## IDENTIFYING LIFE-THREATENING EKG WAVEFORMS (continued)

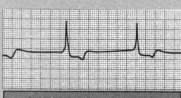

### SYMPTOMATIC BRADYCARDIA

**Characteristics**
• Bradydysrhythmias possibly including sinus bradycardia, junctional rhythm, idioventricular rhythm, heart block
• Reentry facilitated, possible ectopic rhythms when ventricular rate is low
• Reduced threshold for ventricular fibrillation, possible decreased cardiac output

**Interventions**
• Start an I.V. and prepare to give atropine, then isoproterenol, as ordered.
• Assist with temporary pacemaker insertion, as ordered, if the patient's heartbeat doesn't respond to drugs.
• Restore volume status if the patient's hypotensive. (If hypotension persists, you may be ordered to start an infusion of dopamine or norepinephrine.)

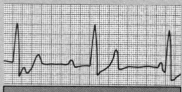

### COMPLETE HEART BLOCK
(Third-degree AV block)

**Characteristics**
• Slow, regular, steady heartbeat (less than 40 beats/minute)—no fluctuations
• Possible episodes of syncope and convulsions, left ventricular failure
• Cardiac output insufficient to meet circulatory demands
• Potential cessation of ventricular impulse or replacement by irritable ventricular foci

**Interventions**
• Prepare to assist with temporary pacemaker insertion.
• Prepare to give atropine, as ordered.
• Prepare to give an infusion of isoproterenol, as ordered.
• Bring a defibrillator to the patient's bedside, and be ready to use it.

and listen for a long pause between the two heart sounds ($S_1$ "lub" and $S_2$ "dub") that may indicate some type of conduction defect. You may hear the first heart sound faintly or not at all, but you may hear the second with no difficulty—possibly indicating atrial fibrillation or flutter. Or you may hear the two heart sounds very close together on some beats—possibly indicating premature atrial contractions. You may also hear many other variations in your patient's rate or rhythm that indicate dysrhythmia. Call the doctor if you do—he may ask you to reestablish cardiac monitoring or obtain an EKG.

Take apical and radial pulses at the same time you listen for heart sounds. In some dysrhythmias, such as PVCs, you may hear the beat with your stethoscope but not feel it at the radial pulse. This indicates that the contraction was ineffective and did not produce peripheral perfusion. Count the patient's apical pulse for 60 seconds, especially if his heart rate is too slow or too fast for an accurate radial pulse count.

If you detect an abnormal apical pulse or your patient exhibits signs and symptoms of hypoperfusion, indicating decreased cardiac output, call the doctor to examine the patient. Stay with the patient, reassure him, and take his vital signs frequently to detect any changes.

# Congestive Heart Failure

### Prediagnosis summary
At initial assessment, the patient had these signs and symptoms of acute respiratory distress:
• air hunger
• labored breathing
• tachypnea
• cyanosis
• lethargy
• diaphoresis

# CASE IN POINT: FAILING TO GIVE THE CORRECT DOSE

Suppose everything's going well for you, so far, in the unfamiliar environment of the ED. You've been floated here from your usual duty on your small community hospital's medical-surgical unit. But now Nelson Williams, an electrical engineer, age 52, comes in complaining of chest pains. The doctor orders cardiac monitoring for Nelson. Another nurse helps you connect him to the monitor—and as soon as the connection's complete, the monitor tells you he's in ventricular tachycardia.

The other nurse calls the doctor, who writes an order for a 50-mg bolus of lidocaine to be given by I.V. and followed by a 4-mg/minute lidocaine drip. While the other nurse is setting up the defibrillator to be ready if the drug doesn't work, you set up the I.V. and prepare to give the lidocaine. Looking at the doctor's written order for the first time, you see his handwriting isn't very clear—and you decide his order's for *500* mg. That seems OK; you've given large doses of lidocaine to patients on the obstetrics unit.

You give Nelson a 500-mg bolus of lidocaine. To your horror, he quickly becomes unresponsive, goes into cardiac arrest, and dies despite vigorous resuscitative efforts.

If this really happened and Nelson's family decided to sue, would you be liable? You may think, "No, because the doctor's handwriting wasn't clear." Or you may think, "Possibly, because I shouldn't have assumed that the dose for this patient could be that high."

In a similar real-life situation that did result in a lawsuit (*Dessauer v. Memorial General Hospital*, 1981), the court found the hospital liable for the nurse's negligence (under the doctrine of respondeat superior). The court reasoned that a certain standard of care must apply when a drug is administered—and that these standards weren't met in this case.

In cardiovascular emergencies, where drugs play a routine part in stabilizing your patient, administration errors may be particularly critical. Avoid them by following these precautions:
• Clarify every unclear written drug order with the doctor who wrote it.
• Know the proper drug dose, administration route, and procedures connected with giving *any* drug. If you're not sure, check your department's drug reference book. The few seconds you spend reading about a drug may prevent your patient's injury or death—*and* a lawsuit.
• Remember, the courts will not permit substandard care that harms a patient. If you're sued for negligence, your care will be compared in court with a reasonable standard of care established to ensure that patients are protected.

*Dessauer v. Memorial General Hospital*, 96 N.M. 92; 628 P 2d 337 (N.M. Ct. App. 1981)

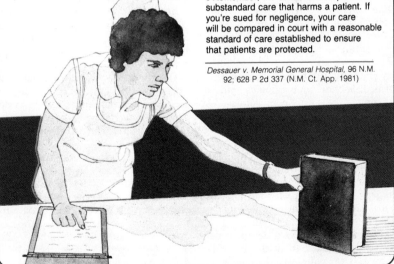

• accessory muscle use.

His other signs and symptoms may have included:

• anxiety, combativeness, and restlessness

• coughed-up sputum that was foamy and blood-tinged.

The patient was given oxygen to decrease his respiratory distress. If his respiratory distress was severe, he may have been intubated. An I.V. was started, and he was connected to a cardiac monitor. A 12-lead EKG and a chest X-ray were done and blood was drawn for arterial blood gases (ABGs), electrolytes, and a CBC. The chest X-ray may have shown pulmonary vascular congestion, interstitial edema, and cardiomegaly. The 12-lead EKG may have shown changes indicative of the underlying cause of CHF, such as left ventricular hypertrophy or an MI (see the "Myocardial Infarction" entry in this chapter).

## Priorities

Your initial priorities for the patient with CHF are to improve oxygenation and to reduce venous blood return to the heart, reducing left ventricular work load. Continue to provide high-flow oxygen by mask. (If the doctor suspects COPD, give 24% oxygen, since higher percentages may cause respiratory arrest.) If your patient's respiratory status deteriorates, anticipate intubation, and provide assisted ventilation with an Ambu bag and 100% oxygen until intubation can be performed. Suction your patient's trachea if his air passages are compromised by foamy or blood-tinged sputum bubbling through the upper airway.

Place your patient in a sitting position with his feet dangling (if possible). This promotes optimal lung expansion, because increased venous pooling in his legs reduces venous return to his heart. The patient may assume this position himself—it's most comfortable.

Give medications, as ordered, to decrease the work load of the patient's heart and to maintain adequate oxy-

genation. Expect to administer a rapid-acting diuretic, such as furosemide (Lasix), to promote excretion of fluid from the lungs and to decrease pulmonary edema. Insert an indwelling (Foley) catheter to measure urine output. You may also administer morphine sulfate to increase venous capacitance, to pool blood peripherally, and to decrease venous return. Morphine also reduces systemic vascular resistance at the arteriolar level (reducing afterload) and relieves anxiety, which can interfere with respirations. However, you'll need to check the patient's respirations and blood pressure before and after each dose, because morphine causes respiratory and circulatory depression.

Other medications you may immediately give your patient with CHF include digoxin, nitrates, and bronchodilators:

• *Digoxin* promotes contractility by slowing the conduction rate and increasing the refractory period of the cardiac cycle, increasing the force of contraction. If your patient had an MI, the doctor may not use digoxin. Why? Because the ischemic myocardium is sensitive to digoxin's cardiotonic effects.

• *Nitrates* cause vasodilatation and decreased preload and afterload.

• *Bronchodilators* (such as aminophylline) decrease respiratory distress and augment myocardial contractility and renal blood flow, promoting sodium and water excretion.

Occasionally, you may be asked to apply rotating tourniquets to the extremities of a patient with CHF to decrease venous return to the heart. Some doctors now rely exclusively on diuretic therapy; however, others use rotating tourniquets in conjunction with medications. (See *Applying Rotating Tourniquets,* page 202.) Monitor the patient's blood pressure frequently during this procedure, and make sure the tourniquets are inflated properly. Check your patient's pulses below the tourniquets to make sure arterial circulation is maintained.

# UNDERSTANDING PULMONARY ARTERY CATHETERIZATION

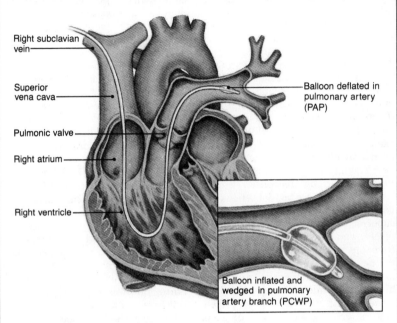

Right subclavian vein

Superior vena cava

Pulmonic valve

Right atrium

Right ventricle

Balloon deflated in pulmonary artery (PAP)

Balloon inflated and wedged in pulmonary artery branch (PCWP)

When your patient's hemodynamic status needs constant monitoring, the doctor may order pulmonary artery (Swan-Ganz) catheterization. A common invasive procedure, it lets you monitor your patient's pulmonary artery pressure (PAP), pulmonary capillary wedge pressure (PCWP), cardiac output, and mixed venous oxygen saturations. PAP and PCWP are particularly helpful in assessing cardiac status in a patient with myocardial infarction (MI), congestive heart failure, pulmonary edema, or bundle-branch block.

**PAP and PCWP reflect:**
• left ventricular capacity to receive and eject blood
• pulmonary vascular status.
   They also:
• help detect MI complications
• evaluate the effectiveness of drug and volume replacement therapy.
   To perform catheterization, the doctor may transfer your emergency patient to the intensive care unit or cardiac catheterization laboratory. There, he inserts a balloon-tipped catheter into a major vein—internal jugular, subclavian superior, or basilic. He threads it through the superior vena cava and the right atrium, where he inflates

the catheter balloon. The balloon, along with the heart's blood flow, carries the catheter through the right ventricle, the pulmonary artery, and into a distal pulmonary artery branch. There, it wedges in place, and PCWP measurements may be taken. When the doctor deflates the balloon, the catheter drifts back into the pulmonary artery, where it normally stays. Here, PAP measurements may be taken.

   Blood pressures may be taken during and after insertion. Pressure recorded as the catheter passes through the right atrium, right ventricle, and pulmonary artery may later help diagnose cardiac dysfunction. For example, comparing right atrial pressure and PCWP yields important information:
• Acute left ventricular dysfunction raises left ventricular filling pressure but only slightly changes right atrial pressure.
• Cardiac tamponade, pericardial constriction, right ventricular infarction, septal defects, restrictive cardiomyopathy, or severe biventricular congestive failure may occur when right and left side filling pressures are about equal.
• Blood samples drawn as the catheter passes through the patient's heart may be analyzed for oxygen content.

## Continuing assessment and intervention

By now, the medications you initially administered should have reduced your patient's pulmonary and systemic congestion. You'll continue administering medications during your assessment. The doctor may insert a Swan-Ganz catheter for continuing fluid and medication administration and evaluation of the patient's cardiac status. (See *Understanding Pulmonary Artery Catheterization,* page 197.) When you examine your patient, look for pitting edema in his extremities and dependent edema in his sacrum and shoulders, caused by decreased venous return. You may see jugular venous distention from increased pressure in the superior vena cava. If his congestion's severe, you may find ascites as fluid from the portal circulation leaks into the peritoneum, and you may be able to palpate his liver easily. Auscultate his lungs for rales. You may also hear wheezes and rhonchi if your patient has underlying pulmonary disease. When you auscultate his heart, you may find tachycardia (the body's first compensatory mechanism for left-sided heart failure) and abnormal heart sounds. Listen for $S_3$ and $S_4$ gallops, which reflect ventricular decompensation. Watch the cardiac monitor for dysrhythmias; these may have precipitated the heart failure—or they may result from hypoxemia or drug therapy.

Monitor your patient's vital signs. He may be hypotensive after diuretic therapy, because diuretics can decrease circulatory blood volume as well as edema. His blood pressure may also drop after his initial dose of morphine. If his blood pressure drops below 100 mm Hg systolic, decrease I.V. nitrate administration; or hold oral, sublingual, or topical nitrates and call the doctor. If his blood pressure doesn't increase after withdrawal of nitrates, the doctor may order a sympathomimetic, such as dopamine.

During diuretic therapy, monitor your patient's electrolyte levels. Be aware that hypokalemia often develops because of increased potassium excretion, and be prepared to administer supplemental potassium I.V.

Assess your patient's mental status. He may be lethargic, confused, or disoriented because of developing hypoxia. Call the doctor *immediately* if you note these signs—the patient may need intubation and mechanical ventilation if his hypoxia is severe. Check his ABGs—if they're normal, they may indicate that his altered mental status is the result of cerebral hypoperfusion rather than hypoxia.

Remember that fluid balance is very unstable in the patient with CHF—any extra fluid volume can increase the strain on the decompensated heart. Careful monitoring of I.V. fluids and maintenance of fluid restriction are *imperative.* Monitor your patient's heart rate, blood pressure, and respirations every 5 to 10 minutes to assess for worsening pulmonary edema. Note the presence of dark, concentrated urine, which may signal decreased urine output resulting from decreased renal perfusion.

Assess your patient for calf tenderness, which can indicate thromboembolism due to venous stasis. Notify the doctor, and expect to apply antiembolism stockings (TEDS) and to administer anticoagulants.

Take your patient's history. He may complain of increasing fatigue (related to the increased work load of the heart) and difficulty in walking (related to accumulating fluid in his feet and legs). He may report a steady weight gain (the result of fluid retention) and nocturnal diuresis. Ask about a persistent cough, paroxysmal nocturnal dyspnea, dyspnea on exertion, and orthopnea requiring two or more pillows—the patient may have had these symptoms for some time.

Your patient's past medical history may include an MI, COPD, hypertension, rheumatic fever, or other conditions that precipitate a decrease in cardiac output. His family history may be positive for heart disease or hypertension.

Ask your patient if he's been taking cardiovascular drugs, such as diuretics, antiarrhythmics, antihypertensives, or cardiotonics. If he has, this may be an indication of the seriousness of his underlying condition. Ask him what specific drugs he's taking, the dosage, and how frequently he takes them. Also ask him if he's experienced any adverse reactions and whether he's had any recent dosage adjustments.

### Therapeutic care

Accurate monitoring of your patient's fluid balance is essential, so continue intake and output records. The doctor may order further EKGs to determine the underlying causes of your patient's CHF. Look for EKG findings characteristic of an MI or for multifocal atrial tachydysrhythmias, which are associated with COPD. Echocardiography may show left ventricular dilatation, chamber-wall-motion abnormalities, and valve-motion abnormalities. Most likely, your patient will have a Swan-Ganz catheter in place. If he has left-sided heart failure, expect to see elevated pulmonary capillary wedge pressure (PCWP) and pulmonary artery pressure (PAP). CVP or right atrium pressure may also be elevated, but only if the left-sided heart failure has already affected the right side of his heart. If your patient has cor pulmonale, his CVP (a measure of right-sided pressure) and PAP will be elevated; his PCWP will usually be normal (PAP and PCWP are measures of left-sided pressure). If the doctor orders liver function tests, expect that they'll be altered—reflecting hepatic dysfunction.

If your patient's pulmonary edema persists despite drug therapy, the doctor may perform a phlebotomy, drawing off 100 to 500 ml of blood to decrease the heart's work load. Assist the doctor as necessary during the procedure and monitor your patient's blood pressure carefully. Why? Because the reduction in blood volume

---

## CLARIFYING HEMODYNAMIC CONCEPTS

Understanding the following terms will help you assess and manage your cardiac patient's condition more effectively.

**afterload** • The tension in the ventricular muscle during contraction. The amount of force needed to overcome pressure in the aorta determines afterload in the left ventricle. Also known as *intraventricular systolic pressure*. (In the right ventricle, *afterload* may be used to describe the amount of force needed to overcome pressure in the pulmonary artery.)

**cardiac output** • Probably the most important circulatory measurement of left ventricular function. It describes the volume of blood ejected by the left ventricle in a given period, usually 1 minute. Normal cardiac output ranges from 4 to 8 liters/minute. *Cardiac output* may also refer to blood ejected by the right ventricle. (You can calculate this for either ventricle by multiplying stroke volume times heart rate.)

**ejection fraction** • The ratio of the amount of blood expelled from each ventricle in one contraction (systolic volume) to the ventricle's total capacity (end-diastolic volume). A healthy heart at rest has an ejection fraction of 60% to 70%. The 30%-to-40% reserve contributes to the next stroke volume.

**preload** • The force exerted on the ventricular muscle at end diastole that determines the degree of muscle fiber stretch. Preload is a key factor in the heart's contractility—the more cardiac muscles are stretched during diastole, the more powerfully they contract in systole. Also known as *ventricular end-diastolic pressure*.

**stroke volume** • The output of each ventricle in one contraction, normally 60 to 70 ml/beat. Also known as *systolic volume*.

---

may cause hypotension.

Perform frequent lung assessments. Your patient's congestion and rales should decrease with medication therapy. If you note an *increase* in these signs, call the doctor: your patient may be lapsing back into CHF and may need intubation and mechanical ventilation or additional drug therapy.

If he's taking digoxin, watch for signs and symptoms of digitalis toxicity, in-

PATHOPHYSIOLOGY

# WHAT HAPPENS IN CONGESTIVE HEART FAILURE

Congestive heart failure (CHF) occurs when cardiac output is inadequate to meet the body's needs. Disease states (such as dysrhythmias, atherosclerosis, or renal failure) or trauma can impair the heart's pumping ability. The resulting inadequate cardiac output, venous pressure increase, and arterial pressure decrease trigger a series of compensatory mechanisms (shown graphically at right) designed to ensure perfusion of vital organs. These mechanisms may not prevent CHF, however, because they:
• may not totally compensate for radical changes in hemodynamics
• can't sustain perfusion for a prolonged period (because the reserve capacity will be depleted)
• further stress the patient's already overworked heart.

When compensation efforts fail, heart failure typically occurs in the left ventricle first (causing pulmonary congestion) and then progresses to the right ventricle (causing visceral and tissue congestion). The right ventricle may fail first, however, because of conditions that create resistance to right ventricular ejection (for example, pulmonary embolism or chronic obstructive pulmonary disease). Right- and left-sided heart failure can also occur simultaneously—particularly in elderly patients.

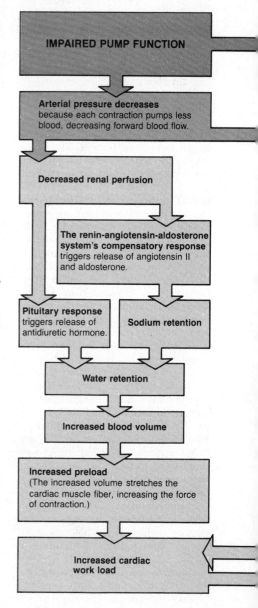

IMPAIRED PUMP FUNCTION

**Arterial pressure decreases**
because each contraction pumps less blood, decreasing forward blood flow.

**Decreased renal perfusion**

**The renin-angiotensin-aldosterone system's compensatory response** triggers release of angiotensin II and aldosterone.

**Pituitary response** triggers release of antidiuretic hormone.

**Sodium retention**

**Water retention**

**Increased blood volume**

**Increased preload**
(The increased volume stretches the cardiac muscle fiber, increasing the force of contraction.)

**Increased cardiac work load**

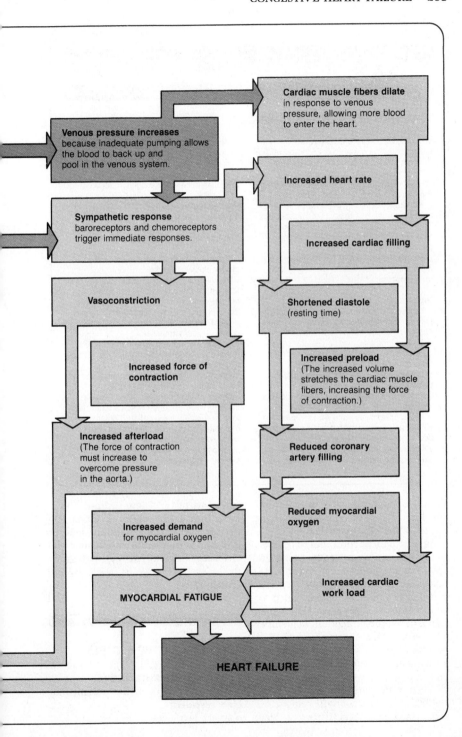

PROCEDURES

## YOUR ROLE IN AN EMERGENCY

### APPLYING ROTATING TOURNIQUETS

You may be asked to apply rotating tourniquets to a patient with congestive heart failure or acute pulmonary edema. Rotating tourniquets help treat these conditions by impeding venous return from the patient's arms and legs to his heart.

Although not widely used today, rotating tourniquets are still used in some hospitals. The doctor may order them in conjunction with potent diuretic or digitalis therapy or after a phlebotomy fails.

Here's the procedure for connecting and monitoring a patient on a rotating tourniquet machine:

**Procedure**
• Explain the procedure to your patient. Tell him the tourniquets may be uncomfortable and could cause temporary limb swelling and discoloration.
• Place him in the Fowler position. Then record his blood pressure, heart and respiratory rates, and radial and pedal pulse rates.
• Apply the tourniquets snugly over towels and around the patient's legs and arms, 4″ (10 cm) from his groin and armpits. (Snugness means you should be able to fit two fingers between tourniquet and skin.)
• *Make sure the machine's turned off.* Connect the tourniquet hoses to their color-coded mates on the machine.
• Close the tourniquet inflation valves, then turn on the machine and set its pressure dial, as the doctor ordered. Also set the inflation timing mechanism, as ordered.
• Open the tourniquet valves. Three of the four tourniquets will inflate. About every 15 minutes, one of the tourniquets will deflate while a deflated tourniquet inflates. The four tourniquets never inflate at the same time.
• Make sure the tourniquets inflate in proper clockwise order.
• Regularly assess your patient's arms and legs below the tourniquets for color, temperature, and pulse. Check his heart and lung sounds, and measure his blood pressure often. Notify the doctor if you detect any abnormalities.
• To stop the therapy, when ordered, remove the tourniquets one by one. (Gradually stopping the therapy prevents a sudden venous blood volume increase that could cause circulatory overload.) As each tourniquet deflates, first close its inflation valve and then remove it until all four tourniquets have deflated. Assess the patient's limbs for changes in arterial pulse rate and character and for skin color and temperature. Monitor his vital signs during weaning.

cluding nausea, vomiting, palpitations, and loss of appetite. (See *Recognizing Digitalis Toxicity,* page 178.)

As your patient continues to recover, weigh him daily—a steady weight increase may indicate recurring CHF. Continue intake and output records, and monitor his vital signs. Watch for an increase in temperature, which may signal developing infection. Remember that, even when the cycle of CHF is broken, your patient may be left with permanently compromised heart and lung function.

When your patient's condition has stabilized, the doctor will remove his Swan-Ganz and Foley catheters. Start your patient on a low-sodium diet to keep him from retaining fluids. Diuretics will cause potassium loss, so give him a potassium supplement and encourage him to eat high-potassium foods, such as bananas, apricots, and orange juice.

# Hypertensive Crisis

### Prediagnosis summary
Initial assessment of the patient may have revealed:
• severe headache

- blurred vision
- confusion
- nausea
- vomiting
- chest pain
- stupor
- convulsions
- characteristic hemorrhage, exudates, and papilledema seen on examination of his optic fundi.

The patient's blood pressure in both arms was grossly elevated—especially the diastolic, which may have been as high as 140 mm Hg.

Supplemental oxygen was given by nasal cannula, and an I.V. for medication access was started with dextrose 5% in water ($D_5W$) at a keep-vein-open rate. The patient probably was given an I.V. diuretic, such as furosemide (Lasix) to lower his arterial pressure and enhance the effect of other antihypertensive drugs. A chest X-ray was taken to determine the presence of cardiomegaly or left ventricular prominence, an EKG was done to detect possible left ventricular hypertrophy and ischemia, and he was connected to a cardiac monitor.

## Priorities

Your immediate concern is to lower your patient's blood pressure. Expect to administer a parenteral antihypertensive agent, such as diazoxide (Hyperstat) or nitroprusside sodium (Nipride). (See *Highlighting Vasodilators Used in Hypertensive Crisis*, page 205.) These drugs, which lower the blood pressure by causing vasodilation, take effect within minutes but have short durations. Usually you'll give either repeat boluses of diazoxide or a continuous I.V. drip of nitroprusside sodium. You'll also give him a sedative to decrease his anxiety. Valium is often used for this, because it decreases blood pressure as well.

Evaluate your patient *constantly* when he receives these medications. Check his pulse and cardiac activity every 5 to 10 minutes. Monitor his blood pressure continuously. You may use an

---

### YOUR PATIENT'S FEAR OF ELECTROCUTION

When you prepare to bathe a patient who's attached to a cardiac monitor, anticipate his fear of electrocution. Reassure him that the electrodes stuck to his chest won't electrocute him if they get wet. Then explain why: cardiac monitor electrodes only pick up electrical activity of the heart—they don't conduct electricity. During a time when your patient feels anxious about his condition, fear of electrocution is one concern you can easily relieve.

---

external monitoring device (Dynamap), or the doctor may insert an arterial line. Lowering his blood pressure rapidly is important, but it shouldn't be lowered to normointensive levels at this time. Why? Because normal pressure in arterial walls that are thickened from chronic hypertension can compromise perfusion of vital organs. You'll insert a Foley catheter to permit measurement of your patient's output; this will help identify impaired renal function, either as an underlying cause of the hypertensive crisis or as a response to it.

## Continuing assessment and intervention

Once antihypertensives are given, expect to see a rapid decrease in your patient's blood pressure. Place him in semi-Fowler's position to maximize his hemodynamic stability; then perform a thorough physical assessment. When checking his vital signs, be alert for tachycardia and tachypnea. Look for signs of CHF, such as jugular venous distention, peripheral edema, dysrhythmias, or abnormal heart sounds. Auscultate his lungs for rales and rhonchi, which may indicate respiratory complications, such as pulmonary edema. (See the "Congestive Heart Failure" entry in this chapter.)

Assess your patient's mental status. Changes in level of consciousness, such as confusion, disorientation, or lethargy, may be a sign of decreased cerebral blood flow leading to hypoxia. Other possible causes include a cerebrovascular accident or a transient ischemic attack due to rupture of a cerebral blood vessel or a severe decrease in cerebral perfusion. If you note any change in your patient's mental status, notify the doctor *immediately*.

Obtain urine and blood samples from the patient for analysis. *Urinalysis* may show microscopic or gross hematuria and proteinuria as well as casts. *Blood analysis* may show elevated BUN and serum creatinine levels, depending on the degree of renal involvement. If your patient's renal failure is advanced, the CBC findings may indicate anemia. Other findings may include hypokalemia (when primary aldosteronism is the cause of the hypertension), thrombocytopenia, and fragmented blood cells on peripheral smears, indicating microangiopathic hemolytic anemia.

Obtain a detailed patient history. Ask your patient if his doctor has found fluctuations in his blood pressure during prior medical care. If so, has your patient been treated for hyper- or hypotension? He may report a history of elevated blood pressure prior to the crisis and a family history of primary hypertension.

Find out if your patient's taking oral contraceptives or monoamine oxidase inhibitors. Why? Because these may precipitate hypertension. Ask him if he's on any antihypertensive drugs and whether he's been taking them as prescribed. (Antihypertensive medication withdrawal can also cause hypertensive crisis.) Determine if he's taking any other medications. This may give you insight into possible predisposing disease states.

Always find out what your patient's antihypertensive medication dosage schedule is and when he remembers taking his medication last. This is important because hypertensive crisis may be caused by abrupt discontinuation of antihypertensive medication. If your patient's elderly and lives alone and his mental function's decreased secondary to atherosclerosis, he may have forgotten to take his medication. If your patient's mobility is impaired, he may be dependent on others to refill his presciptions. If no one's available, he may have waited a few days after his medication ran out, thinking nothing serious would happen.

A detailed review of systems will help you determine your patient's underlying disease. He may report a history of dizziness, fainting, or transient ischemic attack—implying cerebrovascular involvement. Flank pain, frequent urinary tract infections, or flank trauma point to renal involvement. Complaints of past chest pain, palpitations, dyspnea on exertion, or orthopnea indicate cardiac involvement. A history of weight loss may indicate pheochromocytoma; a history of weight gain may indicate Cushing's syndrome.

## Therapeutic care

Once your patient's blood pressure is lowered to an acceptable level, continue to monitor it closely for any changes. A slow, steady increase may indicate a need for a change in drug therapy; notify the doctor. Carefully monitor your patient's fluid intake and output also to assess renal function. If his urine output falls below 30 ml/hour, notify the doctor. Weigh the patient daily; an increase in body weight may indicate fluid retention and possible renal disease.

You'll continue to administer antihypertensive drugs I.V., as ordered. If your patient's receiving nitroprusside sodium, remember to be alert for signs and symptoms of cyanide toxicity, such as diaphoresis, palpitations, substernal pain, headache, and nausea. Note that an acutely hypertensive patient with renal or liver impairment will be especially sensitive to cyanide toxicity, because nitroprusside sodium is me-

DRUGS

# HIGHLIGHTING VASODILATORS USED IN HYPERTENSIVE CRISIS

| DRUGS | | |
|---|---|---|
| **nitroprusside sodium** (Nipride*) | **diazoxide** (Hyperstat*) | **hydralazine hydrochloride** (Apresoline*) |
| **INITIAL DOSE** | | |
| Dilute 50-mg vial with 2 to 3 ml of dextrose 5% in water (D₅W). Then add this to 250, 500, or 1,000 ml of D₅W. Infuse at 0.5 to 10 mcg/kg/minute. | Administer 300 mg I.V. bolus push; administer in 30 seconds or less into peripheral vein. Repeat at intervals of 4 to 24 hours p.r.n. | Give 20 to 40 mg slowly I.V. and repeat as ordered, usually q 4 to 6 hours. |

| NURSING CONSIDERATIONS | | |
|---|---|---|
| • Obtain baseline vital signs on your patient before giving the drug, and find out what the doctor wants to achieve by giving it.<br>• Check the patient's blood pressure every 5 minutes at the start of the infusion and every 15 minutes thereafter. If severe hypotension occurs, turn off the I.V. (the effects of the drug reverse quickly). Notify the doctor.<br>• Run the drug piggyback through a peripheral line, *with no other drug.* Don't adjust the rate of the main I.V. line while the drug is running. Remember, even a small bolus of nitroprusside can cause severe hypotension.<br>• Prepare the solution right before administration. Don't keep it or infuse it for more than 24 hours. Watch for color changes in the solution—from brown to blue, green, or dark red—an indication for replacing it.<br>• Protect the solution from light by wrapping the I.V. bottle with aluminum foil.<br>• Use cautiously in patients with hypothyroidism or hepatic or renal disease and in patients receiving other antihypertensives. | • Monitor the patient's blood pressure frequently. Notify the doctor immediately if severe hypotension develops. Keep norepinephrine available.<br>• Monitor the patient's intake and output carefully. If fluid or sodium retention develops, the doctor may order furosemide.<br>• Tell the patient that he can minimize orthostatic hypotension by rising slowly and avoiding sudden position changes. Instruct him to remain supine for 30 minutes after the injection.<br>• Use cautiously in patients with impaired cerebral or cardiac function, diabetes, or uremia, and in patients taking other antihypertensives. | • Monitor the patient's blood pressure and pulse rate frequently. Remember, hydralazine is a potent cardiac stimulator.<br>• Tell the patient that he can minimize orthostatic hypotension by rising slowly and avoiding sudden position changes.<br>• Use cautiously in patients with cardiac disease and in patients taking other antihypertensives. |

*Also available in Canada

# WHAT HAPPENS IN HYPERTENSIVE CRISIS

**Causes of hypertensive crisis include:**

- abnormal renal function
- hypertensive encephalopathy
- intracerebral hemorrhage
- acute left-sided heart failure
- clonidine hydrochloride (Catapres) withdrawal
- myocardial ischemia
- eclampsia
- pheochromocytoma
- monoamine oxidase inhibitor interactions.

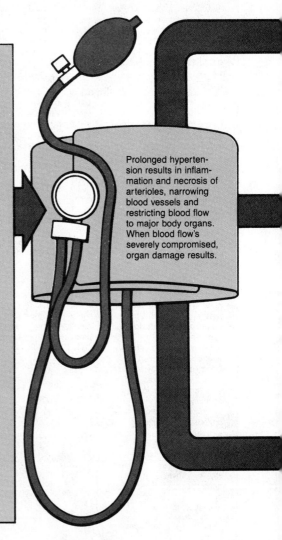

Hypertensive crisis is a severe rise in arterial blood pressure caused by a disturbance in one or more of three blood pressure–regulating mechanisms:
- *Arterial baroreceptors*—sensors that monitor arterial pressure—respond to adrenergic stimulation of the central nervous system by causing arteriole constriction and elevating blood pressure. If pressure remains elevated, the baroreceptors reset at the higher levels, sustaining the hypertension.
- *Fluid volume regulation* is the body's response to fluid underload or overload. Changes in fluid volume alter venous system distention and venous return to the heart, affecting cardiac output and tissue perfusion. Changes in tissue perfusion lead to changes in vascular resistance, resulting in changes in blood pressure.
- The *renin-angiotensin system* responds to the decreased renal perfusion of kidney disease by releasing renin. This results in production of angiotensin II, which causes venous constriction and peripheral arteriole constriction. Aldosterone release also occurs, increasing sodium reabsorption and causing increased fluid volume.

Prolonged hypertension results in inflammation and necrosis of arterioles, narrowing blood vessels and restricting blood flow to major body organs. When blood flow's severely compromised, organ damage results.

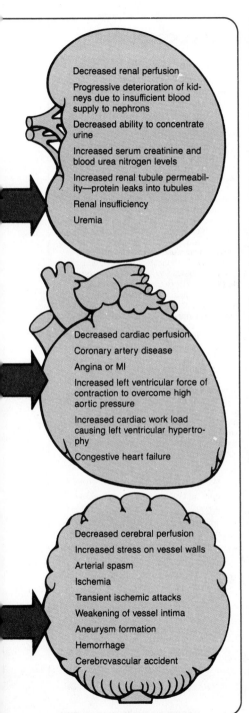

Decreased renal perfusion

Progressive deterioration of kidneys due to insufficient blood supply to nephrons

Decreased ability to concentrate urine

Increased serum creatinine and blood urea nitrogen levels

Increased renal tubule permeability—protein leaks into tubules

Renal insufficiency

Uremia

Decreased cardiac perfusion

Coronary artery disease

Angina or MI

Increased left ventricular force of contraction to overcome high aortic pressure

Increased cardiac work load causing left ventricular hypertrophy

Congestive heart failure

Decreased cerebral perfusion

Increased stress on vessel walls

Arterial spasm

Ischemia

Transient ischemic attacks

Weakening of vessel intima

Aneurysm formation

Hemorrhage

Cerebrovascular accident

tabolized in the liver and excreted by the kidneys. A patient receiving this drug for an extended period of time should have blood drawn often to check thiocyanate levels.

When your patient's condition has stabilized, I.V. medications will be discontinued and he'll be started on oral antihypertensives, such as methyldopa (Aldomet) or clonidine hydrochloride (Catapres). Continue to monitor his blood pressure, and watch for side effects. Teach him the importance of taking his medication regularly.

Encourage a change in your patient's dietary habits if he's obese or if his diet's high in sodium. Provide him with an appropriate exercise plan, and help him to reduce his stress levels.

If your patient's hypertensive crisis was secondary to a condition such as renal or heart disease, he'll also require continuing care specific to his underlying problem.

# Acute Peripheral Arterial Occlusion

### Prediagnosis summary
Initial assessment findings included:
• pain (severe and sudden or aching and aggravated by extension and flexion) in an arm or leg—or in both legs in a patient with a saddle embolus (see *Assessing for Acute Arterial Occlusions*, page 208)
• numbness, tingling, paresis, or a sensation of cold in the affected area
• coolness, pallor, and cyanosis
• diminished or absent arterial pulses (when checked by Doppler) and decreased or absent capillary refill and cutaneous sensation.

The patient was given supplemental oxygen and placed on a cardiac monitor. An I.V. infusion was started in an unaffected extremity.

If the diagnosis of severe arterial occlusion was made (based on the af-

## ASSESSING FOR ACUTE ARTERIAL OCCLUSIONS

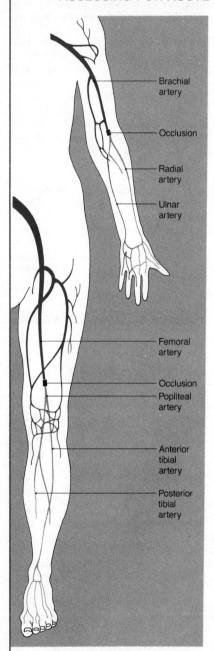

Brachial artery

Occlusion

Radial artery

Ulnar artery

Femoral artery

Occlusion

Popliteal artery

Anterior tibial artery

Posterior tibial artery

If your patient has an acute arterial occlusion, the cause may be:
- trauma
- embolism
- acute arterial thrombosis
- thrombosis within an aneurysm
- chronic arterial occlusive (usually atherosclerotic) disease.

Whatever the cause, you'll have only a few hours to restore blood flow to the affected area before irreversible ischemia sets in.

When the occlusion's onset has been gradual—as in arteriosclerosis—collateral circulation networks have developed, so blood can flow around the occlusion. But with sudden onset, no collateral circulation exists. Blood flow stops at the occlusion site, causing muscle ischemia that can eventually lead to loss of the affected limb.

The occlusion's location also affects its severity. For example, an occlusion of the brachial artery at the elbow may be tolerated, but a popliteal artery occlusion may cause muscle ischemia and irreversible tissue damage within 4 hours. Why? Because the knee doesn't have adequate naturally occurring collateral circulation, and the elbow does. Arterial occlusions occurring at major-vessel bifurcations are potentially dangerous because blood flow to two arteries may be cut off.

The signs and symptoms listed below tell you what to watch for in a patient you're assessing for an occlusion. The illustration shows how the presence or absence of naturally occurring collateral circulation affects the limb's viability.

### Signs and symptoms of occlusion

- Pain may be sudden and severe (embolic) or may occur gradually over several hours (thrombotic).
- Muscle weakness may progress to paralysis.
- The limb may be pale and cool with mottling proximal to the occlusion and cyanosis distal to it.
- Peripheral pulses may be absent.
- Hypalgesia, anesthesia and paresis, or paralysis of ischemic muscles may be present. (Muscle tenderness indicates profound ischemia; rigor indicates muscle death.)

fected area's being cold, numb, pale, and pulseless), the patient was taken to surgery immediately without further testing or assessment. If his occlusion was less severe, the doctor may have ordered arteriography to determine the exact site and degree of the occlusion.

## Priorities

Your first nursing priority is to maintain viability and to prevent further tissue damage in the involved extremity, whether or not the patient has surgery. During the first few hours after the occlusion occurs, watch for signs and symptoms of subcutaneous hemorrhage and gangrene. (Note that arteriosclerotic vessel damage in patients over age 60 makes them prone to gangrene after an acute arterial occlusion.) Staining of the skin may be due to tissue necrosis, which can occur if the occlusion isn't treated immediately.

Draw blood for diagnostic studies— prothrombin time (PT), partial thromboplastin time (PTT), CBC, electrolytes, BUN, creatinine, and blood sugar. This is done in anticipation of surgery and to establish a baseline before anticoagulant therapy is started. After the patient's blood studies are done, expect to administer an I.V. anticoagulant—usually heparin by continuous drip—to prevent further emboli formation. Monitor the infusion carefully to ensure proper dosage, and watch for signs of bleeding (I.V. site oozing, nosebleed, hematuria, bruising, and gum bleeding) that may develop from heparin overdose.

To keep your patient comfortable, expect to give him pain-relief medication, such as meperidine hydrochloride (Demerol) or morphine sulfate, possibly intravenously to achieve adequate pain relief.

Take a quick history and prepare your patient if surgery is now indicated. (The history can be delayed if the patient's occlusion is only partial and the doctor gives medical treatment only.) Ask if he's taking any medication and has any allergies. Make sure that all blood studies, urinalysis, EKG, and chest X-ray results are on his chart. Keep his affected extremity warm to promote vasodilation, and place it in a dependent position.

Surgery is most effective if performed within 6 to 12 hours of the occlusion. Embolectomy may be done under local anesthesia using a balloon-tipped Fo-

PATHOPHYSIOLOGY

## WHAT HAPPENS IN ACUTE PERIPHERAL ARTERIAL OCCLUSION

Embolism, thrombosis, or trauma may cause acute arterial occlusion in healthy arteries and in arteries affected with progressive atherosclerosis. Thrombi from the heart (occurring because of vegetative plaque formation in rheumatic heart disease or endocarditis or because of stagnation of blood in the heart secondary to myocardial infarction, atrial flutter, or valvular stenosis) may embolize and eventually obstruct a healthy distal artery. Emboli and thrombi can also develop within the peripheral arterial tree because of progressive atherosclerosis, aortic or popliteal aneurysm, disseminated intravascular coagulation, or trauma to the arteries. Arterial occlusion occurs most often at bifurcation of vessels partially obstructed by atherosclerotic plaque.

Plaque formation in atherosclerosis may cause progressive narrowing of the lumen, or the plaque may break off to form emboli. With advanced atherosclerosis, the lumen narrows so much that even small emboli cause obstruction. If blood pressure is low, platelets may aggregate to become occlusions. Mechanical obstruction of the artery prevents sufficient blood flow distal to the affected part. The resulting ischemia may cause necrosis, gangrene, and limb loss if circulation is not restored quickly.

DRUGS

## A PROMISING ALTERNATIVE TO VASODILATORS

You now expect to see a vasodilator ordered for a patient with a cerebral or peripheral vascular disorder. But soon you may be administering a new drug for these disorders—pentoxifylline (Trental). Why? Because, although vasodilators are effective in treating such coronary disorders as angina, they have limited clinical value for patients with obstructive vascular disease. Pentoxifylline shows real promise for such patients. Unlike vasodilators, which act on the blood vessels, pentoxifylline improves microcirculation by acting directly on the blood. Here's how it works:
• It reduces red blood cell aggregation by stimulating prostacyclin (a prostaglandin) production.
• It increases fibrinolysis, thereby decreasing fibrinogen concentration.
  The result? Increased blood flow and better circulation, particularly in the smaller capillaries.

garty catheter; thromboendarterectomy—direct incision of the artery and removal of the obstruction—and patch or bypass grafting may also be done.

## Continuing assessment and intervention

If your patient's occlusion was *total*, you won't have a chance to assess him thoroughly until he returns from surgery. Perform a baseline assessment, observing and recording his blood pressure, pulses, respirations, and cardiac rhythm every 30 minutes. Pay particular attention to his respiratory rate and effort: his chances of developing pulmonary emboli increase with any disease process that causes thrombus formation. Notify the doctor *immediately* if you note any signs or symptoms of respiratory distress.

Remember also that embolic cerebrovascular accident can develop from the underlying disease that caused the occlusion. So check your patient's mental status frequently. Assess and record his neurovascular status (including

pulses and sensation) every 15 to 30 minutes.

During your assessment, keep the patient's bed covers away from the affected extremity and keep it warm—but don't apply heat. You can cushion it with pillows, but don't elevate it. Inspect his skin color and temperature, and check the distal pulses of the affected limb. Document your findings so you can detect improvement or deterioration in the affected extremity. Watch for signs and symptoms of hemorrhage. Expect to give medication for pain as needed. Monitor fluid intake and urine output for signs of renal failure from decreased kidney perfusion.

Watch for *swelling* in a revascularized extremity, because this may compromise the arterial blood flow. If swelling is present, call the doctor; he may decide to perform a fasciotomy.

Once your patient's condition has been stabilized, take a complete history. Ask if he's had prior intermittent claudication, which suggests longstanding atherosclerotic occlusive disease. Find out if he or any member of his family has hypertension, diabetes mellitus, hyperlipidemia, MI, or chronic dysrhythmias, which are predisposing factors to emboli or thrombi formation. Ask if your patient is taking medication that may be associated with thrombus and embolus formation—such as oral contraceptives.

Find out if he has any dysrhythmias, such as atrial fibrillation or flutter, that predispose him to emboli formation. If his history reveals a preexisting embolus or thrombus-forming condition, heparin therapy may be continued after his surgery. Blood will be drawn frequently to check PTT, which should be kept at 1½ to 2½ times control for therapeutic results. His electrolytes will also be checked frequently. Because blood trapped in the occluded vessel is hypoxemic and acidotic and is released into circulation during surgery, electrolyte imbalance can result.

If your patient's occlusion was only *partial* and he's being treated with medical therapy instead of surgery, continue giving the heparin that was started initially. Assess his blood pressure, pulses, sensation, respirations, and cardiac rhythm as you would if he'd had surgery.

### Therapeutic care

If your patient's occlusion was *total* and he had surgery, continue to check his pulses, capillary refill, and the temperature and skin color of the affected extremity to monitor improvement. Watch for any signs and symptoms of bleeding, clotting, or infection at the surgery site. If he's still receiving heparin therapy, the doctor will discontinue the drug as soon as he feels that the danger of reembolization is over. Watch for signs and symptoms of infection (such as fever) that may occur after surgery. Because ischemic toxins in the blood from the occlusion can cause renal failure and hypertension, be alert for decreased urine output, increased BUN and creatinine, and rising blood pressure. When your patient's vital signs are stable and he has no signs of infection or renal involvement, begin active range-of-motion exercises.

If the reconstructive surgery wasn't successful, amputation of the extremity may be necessary. If this occurs, explain the procedure and provide emotional and psychological support. Discuss the rehabilitative care that'll be provided and, if possible, show the patient and his family the variety of prostheses that are available.

If the patient's occlusion was *partial* and he didn't require immediate surgery, continue to assess his neurovascular status by checking his pulses and sensation. Call the doctor if you note signs of deterioration in his affected extremity; the patient may need immediate surgery. If his neurovascular status is adequate, expect to continue heparin therapy, with frequent PTT assessments to ensure proper heparin dosage, until the doctor no longer feels that the patient's circulation is threatened and he discontinues it. After hep-

arin's discontinued, start the patient on an activity program to further improve his circulatory status.

# Dissecting Aortic Aneurysm

### Prediagnosis summary

Initial assessment of the patient revealed:
- sudden, severe chest pain—described as having a tearing quality and as being greatest at onset—with or without pain in the neck, throat, shoulders, lumbar region, viscera, or lower extremities
- signs of shock, such as pallor, diaphoresis, and cool, clammy skin.

He was given oxygen and placed on a cardiac monitor, and a large-bore I.V. was started in case he'd need blood. Blood was drawn for CBC, electrolytes, type and cross matching, and other laboratory work. The doctor may have applied a MAST suit to reduce the patient's shock, even though the MAST suit increases pressure and can expand the dissection. The doctor may have taken this risk if the patient's death from shock was imminent.

The doctor ordered an EKG to rule out MI, an abdominal plate and lateral abdominal X-ray to detect any visible mass, and a chest X-ray to detect widened aortic and mediastinal shadows. If the patient's condition permitted, the doctor ordered aortography to demonstrate the origin and extent of the dissection.

### Priorities

Dissecting aortic aneurysm is a *life-threatening emergency* that may be rapidly fatal without immediate intervention. As the dissection advances, it may cause cardiac tamponade (from rupture into the pericardium), aortocoronary fistula (from rupture into a cardiac chamber), or exsanguination.

The dissection must be repaired surgically.

Your immediate priorities are to stabilize your patient's hemodynamic status and to prepare him for surgery.

Assist the doctor in placing a CVP line or a Swan-Ganz catheter, as necessary. A CVP line reflects heart function and total blood volume and allows you to administer fluids; a Swan-Ganz catheter also allows you to give fluids—and to measure the patient's pulmonary pressures and assess his left ventricular function. You may also need to assist in placing an arterial line in your patient for continuous blood pressure monitoring.

Continue to give your patient oxygen; monitor his blood pressure, pulses, and respirations; and take his CVP or Swan-Ganz catheter readings every 5 to 10 minutes. Check for variations in blood pressure and pulse quality between the patient's arms and legs—these variations are common. For example, your patient's left arm systolic pressure may be significantly lower than his right arm systolic pressure if the dissection is in the aortic arch near the origin of the left subclavian artery. Make sure to assess *all* his peripheral pulses.

Expect to give medications to immediately reduce your patient's blood pressure and left ventricle ejection force, limiting further dissection. As ordered, you may give trimethaphan (Arfonad) as an I.V. drip to maintain systolic blood pressure below 120 mm Hg, or you may give nitroprusside sodium (Nipride) or I.V. nitroglycerin (Tridil). (Nitroprusside may cause increased cardiac output, which is not desirable.) Also give pain medications, such as morphine sulfate I.V., as ordered.

Before your patient goes to surgery, insert a Foley catheter and check his chart to make sure all blood tests, urinalysis, EKG, and X-ray results are included. Explain the surgical procedure (which will usually include graft and resection) to the patient and his family. Remember, the patient will be on a cardiopulmonary bypass machine during surgery, so obtain a quick history (including allergies and medication history).

## Continuing assessment and intervention

When your patient returns from surgery, you'll need to maintain (and eventually improve) his hemodynamic status. Frequently assess your patient's blood pressure, CVP, PCWP, and urinary output; monitor his hemodynamic status and quickly note any decreases in cardiac output. If your patient's cardiac output decreases, he may not be receiving enough fluid; the doctor may increase I.V. fluids. His decreased cardiac output may also be caused by bleeding at the graft site. Look for drainage from the mediastinal chest tube inserted during surgery—this may indicate increased bleeding at the graft site. *Notify the doctor*, who may order blood replacement or further surgery.

Administer antihypertensives, as ordered, to control your patient's blood pressure and reduce stress on the graft site. You may give I.V. propranolol (Inderal) in small doses (1 mg) to keep his mean arterial blood pressure at approximately 80 mm Hg. You may also administer morphine sulfate or hydromorphone (Dilaudid) to control your patient's pain.

If your patient was on antihypertensives and was noncompliant, this may have precipitated his dissecting aneurysm. After surgery, explain why he should take his medication regularly.

If, during surgery, your patient had a blood transfusion to replace lost blood, check his hemoglobin and hematocrit levels. Call the doctor if they've *decreased*; you may need to give a blood transfusion. Check the patient's clotting factors and platelets frequently (every 6 hours), and check for hematuria, petechiae, or other signs of increased bleeding. Your patient received heparin during surgery and was given protamine sulfate to reverse the heparinization. If his PT and PTT are still

# WHAT HAPPENS IN DISSECTING AORTIC ANEURYSM

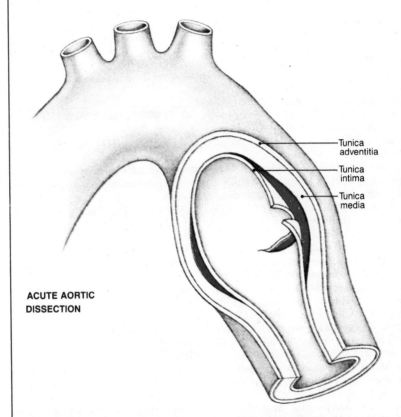

Tunica adventitia

Tunica intima

Tunica media

**ACUTE AORTIC DISSECTION**

Dissecting aortic aneurysm occurs when disorders that increase hemodynamic stress on the aorta (such as hypertension, arteriosclerosis, infection, coarctation, or Marfan's syndrome) damage its middle layer (media), causing separation of the intima from the media. Trauma that partially ruptures the aorta can also cause dissecting aortic aneurysm.

With weakening of the vessel and loss of its elasticity, the media and adventitia of the aorta are stretched outward. Blood flow pressure on the weakened wall ultimately causes a tear in the intima, with hemorrhagic separation of the aortic wall. Blood enters the media, forming a hematoma.

Stress from the resulting turbulent blood flow then dissects the layers of the media, forming a false channel between it and the intima. The heart's contractile force extends the dissection distally and proximally.

Dissection occurs most often in the ascending aorta (60% to 70%) (see the illustration) and in the descending aorta just below the left subclavian artery (30% to 40%). It may extend toward the heart, involving coronary artery circulation. Or it may extend distally to the abdominal aorta, involving circulation to the GI tract, the kidneys, the spinal cord, and the legs. In most untreated patients, dissecting aortic aneurysm is rapidly fatal.

elevated, he may need platelets or more protamine sulfate. Also, monitor his electrolytes every 6 hours, especially potassium. Remember, multiple blood transfusions and the use of the bypass machine frequently cause potassium imbalance.

Your patient may be on a ventilator for 24 hours after surgery to improve his lung function and to assist him while he's recovering from his initial crisis. If he's on a ventilator, obtain a history from an available family member. If he isn't, obtain his history from him. Ask about a history of atherosclerosis, heart disease, or hypertension. Also ask if your patient has structural defects, such as coarctation of the aorta or a bicuspid aortic valve. Determine his medication history, and ask particularly about use of antihypertensive vasodilators or cardiac medication, which may identify his underlying disorder.

### Therapeutic care

Continue to administer antihypertensives and to monitor your patient's hemodynamic status. As the patient's incisional pain decreases, you may give I.M. meperidine hydrochloride (Demerol), as ordered for pain relief, rather than morphine sulfate. Look for an improvement in blood pressure, pulse quality, and other assessment parameters as compared with the patient's condition immediately after surgery. Watch for fever, which may indicate infection, and check your patient's dressings for purulent drainage.

Your patient's mediastinal chest tube will be removed when drainage subsides; provide wound care as needed. If your patient was on a ventilator immediately after surgery, he'll be weaned as his condition improves. Usually this isn't a problem unless your patient has underlying chronic obstructive pulmonary disease. The patient may be started on incentive spirometry and other forms of respiratory therapy; encourage him to cough, to turn frequently, and to deep-breathe.

Help your patient perform range-of-motion exercises with his legs to prevent thrombus formation.

Your patient's Swan-Ganz catheter or CVP line will be removed when his hemodynamic status is stable. Continue assessing your patient's vital signs and urine output to monitor hemodynamic status. Start him on graduated activity; but remember that a sharp rise in blood pressure, from a sudden increase in activity, may put excessive stress on the graft site.

# Cardiac Tamponade

### Prediagnosis summary

Initial assessment of the patient revealed:
- diminished or muffled heart sounds
- jugular vein distention
- low blood pressure.

(Together, these findings comprise Beck's triad—a classic finding in cardiac tamponade.)

Other assessment findings included:
- tachycardia
- diaphoresis
- pallor or cyanosis
- anxiety
- dyspnea
- the body position characteristic of cardiac tamponade, with the patient sitting upright and leaning forward.

The patient was immediately given supplemental oxygen. An I.V. was started with normal saline or Ringer's lactate, and he was connected to a cardiac monitor. A chest X-ray was taken to check for an enlarged cardiac silhouette, and an EKG was done to look for electrical alternans and for decreased QRS complex amplitude. The doctor may have inserted a CVP line to monitor right-heart filling pressure.

### Priorities

Your immediate concern is to maintain the patient's cardiac output until the intrapericardial pressure can be relieved. Continue to give your patient supplemental oxygen to enhance tissue perfusion. Continue cardiac monitoring, too, and check blood pressure, pulse, and respirations every 5 to 10 minutes. Constant monitoring of blood pressure and pulse is *vital* in determining cardiac output. *Don't* rely totally on the cardiac monitor—it may show normal heart rhythm and electrical conduction even when his heart's contractions and output are being impaired by increasing pressure in the pericardial sac (electromechanical dissociation). If this occurs, the patient will become pulseless, and he'll require CPR (see the "Life Support" section in Chapter 3).

If a CVP was inserted, take an initial CVP reading to establish a baseline. Expect it to be very elevated—(as high as 20 mmH$_2$O) because of the increased extrapericardial pressure. The doctor will perform an emergency pericardiocentesis to relieve pressure in the pericardial sac. This procedure restores the effective pumping action of the myocardium and restores hemodynamic stability—improvement can be seen with removal of as little as 20 to 30 ml of fluid. (See *Monitoring Your Patient During Emergency Pericardiocentesis,* page 176.) Assist the doctor at the bedside or, if time permits, prepare your patient and transfer him to a special procedures lab.

### Continuing assessment and intervention
Once your patient's cardiac function has been stabilized by the pericardiocentesis, you can begin your nursing assessment. Start by obtaining a detailed patient history. If trauma caused the tamponade, ask your patient how the injury occurred. If your patient hasn't sustained an injury, ask if he's had cardiac surgery within the past 30 days. Why? Because occult bleeding sites and anticoagulant therapy often cause blood leakage into the pericardium. Make sure you determine whether he's taking anticoagulants.

Also ask if he has a history of cancer, recent MI, or infection—all these are conditions predisposing to tamponade.

Continue to monitor your patient's vital signs. When checking his blood pressure, be alert for pulsus paradoxus—a drop in systolic blood pressure greater than 10 mm Hg on inspiration. You can also detect pulsus paradoxus by palpating your patient's radial pulse over several cycles of slow inspiration and expiration. Marked pulse diminution during inspiration is evidence of pulsus paradoxus. Monitor fluid administration carefully: decreased cardiac output is a result of ineffective pumping action, and overhydration in a compressed heart can compromise cardiac status. Use your patient's CVP and vital signs as guidelines for fluid administration.

Distended neck veins in your patient are a result of increased CVP caused by reduced heart filling. Auscultate his heart for diminished or distant heart sounds, which are muffled by the fluid accumulating in the pericardium. For example, rising CVP can indicate a reaccumulation of fluid in the pericardial sac. Carefully record your patient's total intake and output, and notify the doctor if *signs of overhydration* occur.

Be alert for signs of decreased cardiac output, such as tachycardia, hypotension, and urinary output of less than 30 ml/hour. These can be warning signs of recurring pericardial effusion.

In most patients with cardiac tamponade, you won't hear a third heart sound, which helps distinguish tamponade from MI. You may hear a pericardial friction rub in your patient and, when you percuss his anterior chest, you may hear a widening of the area of flatness. An echocardiogram will show an abnormal echo-free space in the pericardium and changes in cardiac motion.

When you auscultate your patient's lungs, be alert for decreased or absent breath sounds. Either of these signs may indicate a pneumothorax. Notify the doctor *immediately.* He will prob-

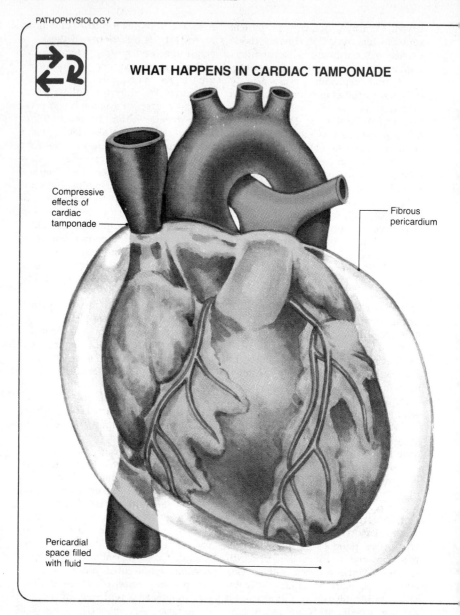

## WHAT HAPPENS IN CARDIAC TAMPONADE

Compressive effects of cardiac tamponade

Fibrous pericardium

Pericardial space filled with fluid

ably order a repeat chest X-ray. If the X-ray results confirm pneumothorax, expect to assist with chest tube insertion.

Although the emergency pericardiocentesis will have provided immediate temporary relief, it probably didn't correct the underlying defect. You may

have to prepare the patient for surgery as soon as the definitive diagnosis is made, so the underlying injury can be corrected. Draw blood for routine laboratory work and for type and cross matching for transfusion. Take a urine sample for urinalysis. Explain the procedures to the patient and his family,

**CROSS SECTION OF HEART WALL**

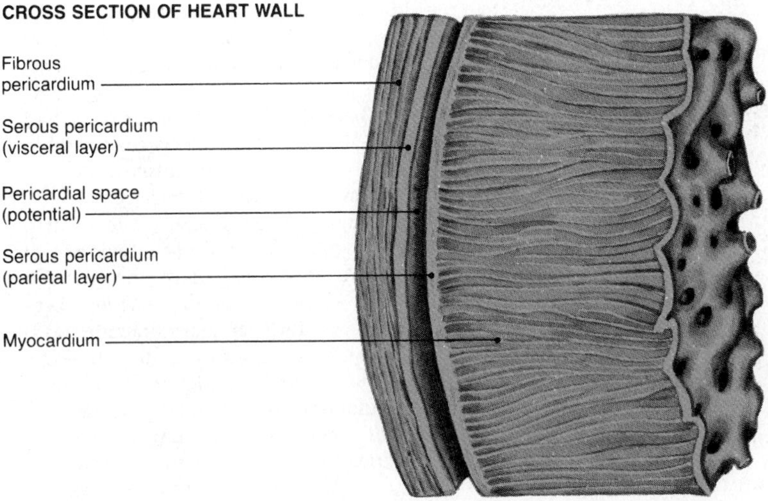

Fibrous
pericardium ——————————————

Serous pericardium
(visceral layer) ——————————

Pericardial space
(potential) ———————————————

Serous pericardium
(parietal layer) ——————————

Myocardium ——————————————

Cardiac tamponade results when excessive amounts of fluid accumulate within the pericardial space.

The pericardial sac is a fibroserous membrane with limited distensibility. The pericardial space is a potential space between the parietal and visceral layers of the serous pericardium. When excess fluid (as little as 150 to 250 ml) accumulates in the pericardial space, it compresses the heart, increasing intrapericardial pressure and obstructing venous return. The result is increased central venous filling pressure and seriously diminished right-sided cardiac filling. This causes a low-flow state in the heart, with a consequent reduction in stroke volume and cardiac output from the left ventricle despite increased heart rate and vasoconstriction. The amount of fluid required to cause tamponade is variable, mainly depending on the rate of fluid accumulation.

The most common causes of cardiac tamponade are bleeding into the pericardial cavity (hemopericardium), neoplasm, and infection.

*Hemopericardium* most commonly results from penetrating trauma, but it may also result from an aortic aneurysm that dissects into the pericardium or from iatrogenic causes, such as anticoagulant therapy after cardiac surgery, use of epicardial pacing wires, diagnostic pericardiocentesis, cardiopulmonary resuscitation, or cardiac catheterization.

*Neoplasm* can cause rapid accumulation of serous or serosanguinous fluid in the pericardial space.

*Pericarditis* from any cause can result in the production of a pericardial effusion that leads to tamponade.

and answer any questions they may have.

**Therapeutic care**

After your patient's injury has been surgically corrected, continue to monitor his hemodynamic status closely, watching for increased heart rate, decreased urine output, or any of the signs in Beck's triad.

Be aware that tamponade may recur after pericardiocentesis or cardiac surgery. If your patient develops repeated pericardial effusions, he may be taken to the operating room for a pericardiectomy ("pericardial window").

## WHAT HAPPENS IN MYOCARDIAL CONTUSION

Myocardial contusion results from blunt trauma to the chest—for example, from a direct blow or a fall that results in sternal or anterior thoracic compression. The most frequent cause? Steering-wheel impact to the chest when the patient's been in a motor vehicle accident.

In myocardial contusions, the heart is compressed between the sternum and the spinal column, resulting in capillary hemorrhage varying in size from petechial to hemorrhagic involvement of the full thickness of the myocardium. Extravasation of blood and fluid disrupts and separates the myocardial fibers, causing ischemic changes and early necrosis. The patient's clinical picture may resemble myocardial infarction.

This surgical procedure involves creating an opening in the pericardial sac to allow constant fluid drainage into the pleural space, where it's reabsorbed. Explain the procedure to your patient, and prepare him as necessary.

After surgery, continue monitoring his cardiac status. Periodically check his cardiac monitor, vital signs, and CVP readings.

Your patient can be considered stabilized when a repeat chest X-ray shows no signs of mediastinal widening. Observe the surgical site for proper healing. If you see signs of infection, call the doctor. Increase the patient's activity gradually.

# Myocardial Contusion

## Prediagnosis summary

On initial assessment, the patient had a history of recent blunt anterior chest trauma and may have had:
• some degree of angina-like substernal chest pain—refractory to nitroglycerin but responsive to oxygen—unassociated with movement or respiration
• palpitations
• no prior cardiovascular disease or risk factors for MI
• ecchymoses over the sternum
• a rapid heartbeat or an abnormal heart sound, such as an early pericardial friction rub.

The patient was given oxygen, had an I.V. inserted, and was connected to a cardiac monitor because of the suspicion of myocardial damage.

Diagnostic tests were done to help distinguish myocardial contusion from MI. An EKG may have shown ST-T wave elevations or depressions. Less common EKG changes include widened QRS complex or acute pathologic Q waves. Atrial flutter or fibrillation, conduction disturbances, and ventricular irritability may have occurred—depending on the area of injury. Creatine phosphokinase (CPK) enzyme levels (especially the MB fraction)—sensitive to myocardial damage—showed the extent of the contusion. Radionuclide scanning (myocardial imaging) may have been positive if myocardial damage was extensive.

(Note: the presence of myocardial contusion is sometimes missed in patients with multiple severe injuries who have no obvious thoracic trauma. Keep this in mind whenever you assess such a patient.)

## Priorities

Your first nursing priorities are pain relief and close observation of your patient to detect consequences of myocardial contusion and to intervene if they occur. Life-threatening conditions may develop, including cardiac dysrhythmias—such as heart block—and cardiac tamponade, which can follow a myocardial contusion. (See the "Cardiac Dysrhythmias" and "Cardiac Tamponade" entries in this chapter.) Watch for their signs and symptoms—jugular vein distention, lowered blood pressure, and muffled heart sounds. Also check for signs and symptoms of reduced cardiac output, because the ischemic areas of the myocardium resulting from myocardial contusion cause a pathophysiologic state similar to that of an MI, ranging from microscopic interstitial hemorrhage to transmural necrosis.

Continue giving your patient supplemental oxygen by nasal cannula at 2 to 6 liters/minute to decrease pain, to reduce myocardial irritability, and to prevent hypoxia. To further reduce your patient's pain—if it's severe—you may be asked to give analgesics, such as meperidine hydrochloride (Demerol) or morphine sulfate, as ordered, because myocardial contusions don't usually respond to nitroglycerin. However, *don't* give these medicines intramuscularly. Intramuscular administration elevates the patient's CPK levels (mimicking the elevation caused by contusion), and intramuscular absorption is unpredictable when cardiac output is reduced.

Monitor the patient's electrolytes for any imbalance, and watch for signs and symptoms of respiratory distress, which can cause hypoxia and hypercapnia—and possible subsequent acidosis. These can increase his chances of developing dysrhythmias.

## Continuing assessment and intervention

After you've relieved your patient's chest pain, you're ready to do a complete nursing assessment. Continue to observe him closely for signs and symptoms of complications that may arise from his contusion. And keep the appropriate drugs available in case the patient develops a cardiac dysrhythmia. For example, you may need to give digitalis or verapamil if he has atrial fibrillation or supraventricular tachycardia with a rapid ventricular response (see the "Cardiac Dysrhythmias" entry in this chapter). Ventricular irritability or ventricular fibrillation also may follow a contusion and may require you to give the patient lidocaine as ordered. Keep temporary transvenous pacemaker equipment and atropine nearby, too, because conduction defects are also common.

Continue to watch for the signs and symptoms of cardiac tamponade, which can occur at any time during this phase of the patient's care. (See the "Cardiac Tamponade" entry in this chapter.)

Auscultate your patient's heart and breath sounds. If you hear rales in his lungs and an $S_3$ heart sound, he may be developing congestive heart failure. (See the "Congestive Heart Failure" entry in this chapter.) *Call the doctor* and expect to give the patient diuretics.

Continuously watch his cardiac monitor for any other irregularities; these can develop as rapidly as in MI. The doctor may insert a CVP line to monitor the patient's CVP, which reflects his heart function and total circulating volume. Or he may insert a Swan-Ganz catheter to measure the patient's pulmonary pressures if his cardiac output is severely reduced with inadequate peripheral perfusion. Monitor his cardiac output by checking his vital signs, urine output, CVP or Swan-Ganz pressures, mental status, and skin temperature and color at least every 30 minutes. Keep accurate intake and output records, too.

If your patient shows no evidence of developing complications at this time, you can complete your baseline assessment by taking his history. Ask him about the trauma that caused his contusion. Find out whether he has any preexisting heart disease or MI risk factors. This will help you determine what complications, if any, may occur following his contusion.

Also ask about any antiarrhythmics the patient may be taking. If he's taking an antiarrhythmic, and therefore has an underlying heart problem, you'll have to watch him especially closely for signs and symptoms of reduced cardiac output and dysrhythmias. Remember that the ischemia in the myocardium, caused by his contusion, may exacerbate the problem he already has.

## Therapeutic care

When you've completed your assessment, continue to observe him for signs and symptoms of the complications discussed earlier. Monitor his serial cardiac enzymes and EKG daily. Assess his CVP or Swan-Ganz catheter readings frequently to monitor his hemodynamic status. If your patient has severely reduced cardiac output, the doctor may give anticoagulant therapy with heparin to prevent embolus formation. Continue the patient's pain medication, as ordered and if needed. If he needed verapamil or digoxin I.V. to control atrial dysrhythmias with rapid ventricular responses, expect to change this to quinidine orally to maintain sinus rhythm. If your patient has a ventricular dysrhythmia that is refractory to lidocaine, expect to administer procainamide hydrochloride (Pronestyl) or bretylium tosylate (Bretylol).

When your patient no longer has evidence of reduced cardiac output or dysrhythmias, the doctor will take him off the monitor and remove his CVP or Swan-Ganz catheter. But the patient may still have an I.V. infusion of $D_5W$ or a heparin lock to keep a vein open as a means of access if emergency medications must be given.

Try to reduce the work load on your patient's heart, because the ischemic areas of the myocardium (caused by his contusion) need time to heal. Measures for reducing the heart's work load include keeping the patient's environment quiet, decreasing his stress, and planning frequent rest periods with a gradually increasing activity program.

## A FINAL WORD

Although cardiovascular diseases are still the leading cause of death in the United States, sophisticated precare, rapid transport, and improved emergency treatment methods have significantly reduced mortality from acute cardiovascular insults. New technology, including sensitive monitors and specially designed critical care and telemetry units, also helps keep acutely ill patients alive. In fact, these improvements can make the difference, for these patients, between life and death.

You may feel that the "important" part of your patient's care is completed by the time he reaches your unit. After all, he's received dramatic, high-technology care in the ED, followed by intensive monitoring and, maybe, sophisticated surgery. He reaches your unit only when he's stable. But he still needs your help even though his acute emergency has been stabilized. As you know, recovery and rehabilitation from a cardiovascular emergency is a long process. Your patient may be exhausted, depressed, and emotionally worn out from days or weeks of invasive procedures and monitoring. Now is when he needs your *personalized* nursing care.

Reassurance and emotional support are particularly important for these patients. Stress—never helpful in any illness—is particularly harmful to patients recovering from cardiovascular emergencies. Your goals should be to:
• help your patient relax
• help him understand his illness
• prepare him for reentry into active life.

But what about patients who aren't acutely ill yet but who have underlying cardiovascular disorders that could one day take their lives? Here's where your nursing care can help avert or delay life-threatening cardiovascular emergencies. Here's where *you*, not technology, can make the all-important difference. Through active teaching and participation in rehabilitation programs, you can help your patients control such disorders as hypertension and coronary artery disease.

The American Heart Association reports that nearly *one quarter* of all Americans have hypertension, a contributing factor to such cardiovascular emergencies as MI, hypertensive crisis, congestive heart failure, and dissecting aortic aneurysm. Coronary artery disease is also prevalent in our society, particularly among older Americans. Heredity may play a part in the development of these chronic conditions, but so do life-style factors, such as smoking, obesity, stress, lack of exercise, and a diet high in saturated fats and sodium.

As you work with a patient who's recovering from a cardiovascular emergency, help him identify life-style factors that contribute to his coronary disease and work out a plan to alter or eliminate them. By treating your patient like a *person*, not just a heart attached to a monitor, you'll enhance his recovery and help him prevent recurrent cardiovascular emergencies.

## Selected References

Andreoli, Kathleen G. "Complications of Coronary Artery Disease" and "Coronary Artery Disease," in *Comprehensive Cardiac Care: A Text for Nurses, Physicians and Other Health Practitioners,* 4th ed. St. Louis: C.V. Mosby Co., 1979.

Bitran, D., et al. "Intra-aortic Balloon Counter Pulsation in Acute Myocardial Infarction," *Heart & Lung* 10(6):1021-7, November/December 1981.

Coakley, L.D., and Capasso, V.C. "Trauma to the Heart," *Journal of Emergency Nursing* 7(6):255-61, November/December 1981.

Collicott, Paul E. "Acute Cardiac Tamponade: Early Recognition and Treatment," *Current Concepts in Trauma Care* 15:5-14, Fall 1981.

Cook, R.L. "Psychosocial Responses to Myocardial Infarction," *Heart & Lung* 8:130-5, January/February 1979.

Finnerty, F.A., Jr. "Symposium: Treatment of Hypertensive Emergencies," *Heart & Lung* 10(2):275-84, March/April 1981.

Hoffman, J.R. "Hypertension: A Pharmacologic Approach," *Journal of Emer-* gency *Nursing* 8(1):17-22, January/February 1982.

Jodice, J. "Management of Acute Pulmonary Edema," *Journal of Emergency Nursing* 4:19-22, March/April 1978.

Perdue, P. "Stab and Crush Wounds to the Heart," Part 2. *RN* 44:26-33, April 1981.

Petersdorf, Robert G., et al, eds. *Harrison's Principles of Internal Medicine,* 10th ed. New York: McGraw-Hill Book Co., 1983.

Schwartz, Seymour I. "Peripheral Arterial Disease," in *Principles of Surgery,* 3rd ed. New York: McGraw-Hill Book Co., 1979.

Sladen, A., et al. "Advanced Cardiac Life Support," in *American Heart Association Manual,* 1975.

Werner, W., and Chrzanowski, A. "Streptokinase Intracoronary Thrombolysis in Acute Myocardial Infarction," *Journal of Emergency Nursing* 8(6):277-84, November/December 1982.

Young, L.C. "Streptokinase Therapy," *Focus on Critical Care* 10(2):20-3, April 1983.

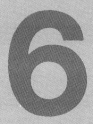

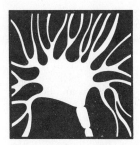

# Neurologic Emergencies

## Introduction

At midnight, on the Fourth of July, you're in the ED. Throughout the afternoon and early evening you've cared for patients who've come in with a variety of cuts, bruises, and fractures resulting from minor accidents. Now the ED's quiet. You're about to go out for coffee with another nurse when you hear not one, but *two* ambulances arriving at the ED. Within seconds, two patients are wheeled in—23-year-old Roger Swift, on a stretcher, and 68-year-old Marcia Baker, in a wheelchair.

At first glance, Roger's condition seems much more serious. He's unconscious and bleeding profusely from the scalp; clear fluid is leaking from his nose. The ambulance attendants tell you that Roger's car crashed head-on into a bridge abutment and that they suspect head and cervical spine injury. You know you've got a real emergency on your hands.

But Mrs. Baker demands your attention, too. An elderly woman, she's sitting up in her wheelchair and doesn't look obviously sick. However, she's confused and keeps calling you by her daughter's name, and she's complaining of a severe headache. Ambulance attendants tell you that Mrs. Baker has a blood pressure of 200/120 and that they were called when she fainted in her kitchen. Mrs. Baker's daughter,

who followed her to the hospital, tells you that her mother has had several episodes of confusion over the past 2 weeks and has complained of numbness and tingling in her right arm for several days. You suspect that Mrs. Baker may have had a series of transient ischemic attacks (TIAs) and that she may be on the verge of having a serious stroke. So you realize that you can't afford to let her wait while you attend to Roger's obvious trauma. As a nurse, you know that the probable effects of her impending stroke may be as life-threatening as the effects of Roger's head injury.

Would you know how to respond effectively to both these patients' emergency needs? Caring for a patient with a neurologic emergency involves assessing his level of consciousness, performing a quick neurologic examination, stabilizing any spinal injuries, and, possibly, managing seizures. This isn't all, however. You may have to do all this while coping with your patient's confusion, restlessness, and even combativeness.

Roger Swift and Marcia Baker are examples of two of the most common neurologic emergencies—head trauma and stroke. Less common, but equally deadly, are spinal cord injuries, status epilepticus, myasthenia gravis crisis, and acute brain infection. You must act quickly to manage patients with these life-threatening emergencies. And remember, serious neurologic disorders compromise not only the neurologic system but also the respiratory, cardiovascular, and other vital systems.

Patients who've suffered head trauma, spinal cord trauma, cerebrovascular accident, or acute brain infection require hospitalization, often for long periods. Here, too, your emergency assessment and intervention skills play an important role. Your patient's chances for recovery may depend on your ability to assess him continuously and to recognize when his condition's deteriorating.

As you can see, neurologic emergencies can involve complex pathologic and systemic interactions. In this chapter, you'll find the information you need to manage these patients effectively—and with increased confidence.

## INITIAL CARE

# Prehospital Care: What's Been Done

Prehospital care of a patient with a neurologic emergency depends not only on available ambulance equipment and personnel but also on the accident or illness that caused the emergency. This means that rescue personnel will start different care procedures depending on whether the patient's primary problem is neck or spine trauma, head trauma, or an altered level of consciousness.

If the patient has any trauma, especially above the shoulders, rescue personnel will assume he has a *cervical spine fracture* until an X-ray rules this out. They'll *maintain alignment* and *immobilize the patient's head* by ap-

plying a cervical collar and strapping him to a short backboard (wood, aluminum, plastic, or canvas over an aluminum frame).

If the patient's fallen from a height or the rescue personnel have any other reason to suspect he has an additional spine injury, they'll immobilize him and strap him to a full-length backboard, positioned in a neutral anatomical position. They'll usually also administer oxygen and start an I.V.—Ringer's lactate if they note hemorrhage, dextrose 5% in 0.45% normal saline ($D_5\frac{1}{2}NS$) at a keep-vein-open rate if they suspect neurologic injury. When you receive the patient, check that he's truly immobilized. Soft cervical collars are inadequate; you may need to tape the patient's head to the backboard and use sandbags or, preferably, a Philadelphia (hard) collar for firmer support.

If the patient has *head trauma* in addition to neck or spine trauma, ambulance personnel will also do a basic neurologic examination after they clear his airway and check his vital signs. They'll assess for:
• decreased level of consciousness
• pupillary changes
• pulse, blood pressure, and respiration changes
• other signs and symptoms that may indicate injury to the brain—for example, vomiting, blurred vision, dizziness, or confusion.

Make sure you get a full report of their findings, including the time and degree of any changes.

Although fluids are usually limited for patients with head injuries, if the patient's obviously hemorrhaging, rescue personnel may insert a large-bore I.V. catheter and give Ringer's lactate to prevent shock. They may also give corticosteroids (believed to prevent cerebral edema and shock). If the patient's vital signs don't reflect hemorrhage and he isn't obviously bleeding, but neurologic damage is suspected, they may start $D_5\frac{1}{2}NS$ at a keep-vein-open rate, as in spinal in-

# A SKIING ACCIDENT

What would you do if you were skiing and saw someone slam into a tree at high speed, falling unconscious to the ground? Would you know how to assess his injuries and intervene appropriately without further harming him? Here's how:

Quickly assess his overall appearance. Suspect spinal injury *automatically*, because he hit the tree hard. And, of course, suspect head injury as the cause of his unconsciousness. Note any blood draining from his ears, mouth, or nose—this may indicate skull or facial fracture. Check his pulse and respirations, but be careful *not* to move him. If they're adequate, pack clothing (such as a ski jacket) around his head and neck to immobilize them.

Now, try to arouse the victim. Since you suspect head and spine injury, don't shake him—shout at him instead. If he doesn't respond, press a fingernail bed and see if he moans, winces, or otherwise responds to the pain. If he doesn't respond, try a deep form of painful stimuli, such as a sternal rub.

Check his pupils, noting if they're equal in size and responsive to light—this will provide baseline information that will help with hospital care later. Look for other injuries, such as a broken arm or leg. If you suspect a fracture, use a ski pole, tree branch, or other rigid object to splint the injury—tie the splint in place with a belt, suspenders, or article of clothing. If nothing's available, secure a fractured leg to the other leg as a temporary splint,

or secure a fractured arm to his torso.

Continue to check the victim's respirations—he may develop apneustic breathing, signaling brain stem injury. If his respirations and pulse deteriorate, you'll have to start CPR—but make sure you open his airway using the jaw-thrust method rather than the head-tilt method, since you suspect spinal injury.

When the ski patrol or other rescuers arrive, make sure you immobilize his head while you help them logroll him onto a board for transport. If you're in the wilderness (cross-country skiing, for example), and there's no ski patrol or help in sight, you'll have to transport him yourself. Improvise a sled by sliding the victim's skis under him and securing them and supporting the patient's back and neck with articles of clothing. Then, ease the sled carefully along the trail to help.

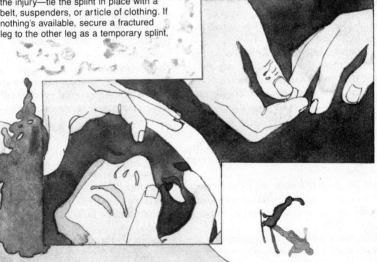

jury. They'll usually give oxygen at 10 liters/minute to assist maximal support of the patient's brain cells. If the patient has seizures as a result of his injury, ambulance personnel will take steps to prevent further injury by placing a bite block or padded tongue depressor between his teeth, if possible. They'll also use suction, as necessary, to keep the patient from aspirating secretions or vomit.

If the patient's primary problem is a *decreased level of consciousness* or *unconsciousness,* rescue personnel will try to obtain a history from the patient, his family, or his friends to determine the precipitating cause. Again, make sure you record this vital information.

If the patient's unconscious and the cause is unknown, rescue personnel will start an I.V., usually dextrose 5% in water ($D_5W$) at a keep-vein-open rate, and test the patient's blood glucose with Dextrostix or Clinistix (if available). A qualified paramedic may give dextrose 50% as an I.V. push and naloxone (Narcan) to reverse a possible narcotic overdose. The dextrose won't hurt an already hyperglycemic patient—his blood glucose level is already grossly elevated. However, it may save a hypoglycemic patient's life. Rescue personnel will also give the patient oxygen at 10 liters/minute, monitor his vital signs, and assess his pupil size and reaction.

If stroke is a possibility, rescue personnel may give the patient oxygen at 4 to 10 liters/minute—depending on the patient's level of consciousness—and they may initiate cardiac monitoring. They'll start an I.V. if the patient's general condition is poor.

When you receive the patient at the hospital, remember these important points:
• If the patient's suffered head or neck trauma, make sure his spine—especially his cervical spine—is adequately immobilized.
• Obtain all vital sign readings and the results of any neurologic assessment from the ambulance personnel.
• Determine what the patient's been given by I.V. (if anything) and the results of his blood glucose test, if one was done.
• Get a detailed history of the patient's accident or illness. You may not be able to get this from the patient, so be prepared to ask anyone who may know— a friend or family member or someone who was present at the scene. You'll need this information to establish the cause and seriousness of the patient's condition.

---

# What to Do First

Primary assessment of a patient with a neurologic emergency and timely intervention require that you assess his airway, breathing, circulation, *and:*
• his cervical spine
• his level of consciousness.

You'll need to assess *all* these parameters rapidly. Compromised breathing and circulation make neurologic injuries worse; cervical spine injury and decreased level of consciousness require immediate care. Patients with neurologic emergencies also require close *continuing* assessment. Your initial findings may not always tell you what's happening with your patient, but they do provide absolutely vital baseline information to measure any change against. In neurologic emergencies more than in others, *changes* in your patient's condition may tell you more than static assessments do.

### Airway
Airway obstruction is common in patients with neurologic emergencies. Airway occlusion in a head-injured patient may be from debris—such as secretions, blood, or dentures—or from direct damage to his mouth, pharynx, or trachea. Listen for stridor or gurgling in his throat and for moist breath sounds. Suction any debris from his mouth, using a large-bore suction cath-

eter or a tonsil tip. If the patient has facial injuries, you may need to insert an artificial airway to maintain patency. You may have to use a nasopharyngeal airway if the patient has severe trauma to the jaws or mouth—but *don't do this* if you see clear fluid or thin, bloody secretions coming from his nose. This may be cerebrospinal fluid (CSF) leakage—indicating a possible skull fracture and a tear in the patient's dura mater. In this situation, a nasopharyngeal airway could contaminate the dura mater, causing brain infection. Tell the doctor about the CSF leakage; he'll decide which airway to use.

The flaccid tongue of an unconscious patient may fall backward, occluding his oropharynx. If your patient's gag reflex is absent, secretions may accumulate in his posterior pharynx and cause occlusion. *Be alert* for the possibility of seizures. If these occur, suction the patient as necessary (to prevent aspiration of secretions), and turn him on his side to aid in secretion drainage.

Remember to *suspect cervical spine injury in every patient with head or neck trauma,* and *don't* hyperextend his neck while opening his airway. You may be able to open his airway using a modified jaw thrust or chin lift; if not, expect that he'll be intubated.

Intubating a cervical spine–injured patient can be very difficult. To intubate the patient using minimal neck motion, an experienced anesthesiologist may be required.

You may be asked to apply axial traction to maintain alignment of the patient's head while the doctor intubates him. The doctor may choose to intubate the patient nasally to avoid hyperextending his neck.

### Breathing
Observe your patient for the presence or absence of respirations. Assess their character if the patient's breathing (if he isn't, *begin CPR* at once). Watch for diaphragmatic or abdominal breathing, which may indicate cervical spine

---

---

injury. Respiratory alterations are common in patients who are unconscious or have head injuries. Rising intracranial pressure (ICP), spinal injury, or myasthenia gravis crisis may cause grossly inadequate respirations. (Of course, if the patient has suffered trauma, don't forget to consider direct chest or airway injury.) Notify the doctor of any respiratory difficulty *at once*, and prepare for intubation and mechanical ventilation.

Remember, hypoxia is particularly significant in neurologically injured patients. In fact, it's a primary cause of neurologic decline. Why? Because the brain uses—and *must have*—approximately 18% of all body oxygen. Brain cells have no capacity for anaerobic metabolism, so poor oxygenation of the brain, whether from airway occlusion, ineffective ventilation, or poor perfusion, results in massive brain damage. Hypoxia can also contribute to increased cerebral edema, which increases ICP. Administer oxygen, as necessary.

## Circulation (C₁)

Check the patient's pulses and blood pressure. As you probably know, brain injury alone rarely causes hypotension and rapid pulse. If your patient shows these signs of shock, look for some other cause, such as obvious hemorrhage or occult blood loss elsewhere in the body (see Chapter 14, SHOCK). Shock must be treated *promptly*.

As a nurse, you know that the brain receives about 20% of all cardiac output and that adequate perfusion is *essential* to brain function. If your patient has borderline or frank *hypotension*, report this to the doctor and *intervene immediately* to prevent decreased cerebral blood flow (due to poor cardiac output) from extending his primary brain insult or spinal injury. If his systemic mean blood pressure drops below 60 mm Hg, your patient's brain autoregulatory mechanism will become less effective. His brain will initially attempt to compensate by extracting more oxygen from the available blood, but if his blood pressure continues to drop, cerebral ischemia may appear. If your patient has low systolic blood pressure and a rapid pulse, start an I.V. of Ringer's lactate

---

### HANDLE WITH CARE

*Always* assume cervical spine injury in *any* patient who's sustained trauma. Remember, improper handling can cause damage to the spinal cord.
So be sure to keep his head and neck immobilized with a Philadelphia (hard) collar or sandbags until X-rays rule out spinal injury.

---

solution. Expect to type and cross-match blood, and prepare for a possible transfusion.

You may also see *bradycardia* (40 to 60 beats/minute) and systolic *hypertension* with a widening pulse pressure. These are late signs of severe brain damage with ICP. Report these findings *immediately:* they require the doctor's immediate intervention.

The doctor may ask you to administer an osmotic diuretic, such as mannitol, to your patient. (Be sure to insert an indwelling [Foley] catheter when administering mannitol, to prevent bladder distention from rapid diuresis. The catheter also permits accurate measurement of urine output and evaluation of the drug's effectiveness.) The doctor may also order corticosteroids and an I.V. of $D_5\frac{1}{2}NS$ at a keep-vein-open rate. (Usually the doctor *won't* order $D_5W$, because it may lead to water intoxication and cerebral edema in a head-injured patient.) If your patient has a spinal cord injury, you may see bradycardia and hypotension as a result of sympathetic loss. (See the "Neurogenic Shock" entry in Chapter 14.) Again, report these findings to the doctor *immediately*.

## Cervical spine (C₂)

*Always* suspect spine injury when your patient's suffered head or neck trauma, whether as the result of a motor vehicle accident or a fall causing loss of consciousness. *Don't* hyperextend or flex the patient's neck. Always keep this in mind, even as you rush to correct a life-threatening airway, breathing, or circulation problem. Maintain the patient's neck in a neutral position and immobilize it with a hard cervical collar as soon as possible. Be sure you immobilize his chest *before* you immobilize his head so his body can't act as a lever. (You may also use sandbags if you don't have a collar, or in addition to a collar.) Apply a backboard if rescue personnel didn't do this. Keep in mind that some spine fractures are not associated with spinal cord injury, so

# ASSESSING YOUR PATIENT'S LEVEL OF CONSCIOUSNESS USING THE GLASGOW COMA SCALE

To assess a patient's level of consciousness quickly in an emergency, use the Glasgow Coma Scale. Below you'll find an expanded version of this useful—though not comprehensive—assessment technique. (A patient scoring 7 or less is comatose and probably has severe neurologic damage.)

| TEST | SCORE | PATIENT'S RESPONSE |
|---|---|---|
| **Verbal response (when you ask, "What year is this?")** | | |
| Oriented | 5 | He tells you the current year. |
| Confused | 4 | He tells you an incorrect year. |
| Inappropriate words | 3 | He replies randomly: "tomorrow" or "roses." |
| Incomprehensible | 2 | He moans or screams. |
| None | 1 | He gives no response. |
| **Eye opening response** | | |
| Spontaneously | 4 | He opens his eyes spontaneously. |
| To speech | 3 | He opens his eyes when you tell him to. |
| To pain | 2 | He opens his eyes only on painful stimulus (for example, application of pressure to bony ridge under eyebrow). |
| None | 1 | He doesn't open his eyes in response to any stimulus. |
| **Motor response** | | |
| Obeys | 6 | He shows you two fingers when you ask him to. |
| Localizes | 5 | He reaches toward the painful stimulus and tries to remove it. |
| Withdraws | 4 | He moves away from a painful stimulus. |
| Abnormal flexion | 3 | He assumes a decorticate posture (below). |

| | | |
|---|---|---|
| Abnormal extension | 2 | He assumes a decerebrate posture (below). |

| | | |
|---|---|---|
| None | 1 | He doesn't respond at all, just lies flaccid—an *ominous sign.* |

# UNDERSTANDING PUPILLARY CHANGES

Along with assessing your patient's level of consciousness in an emergency, you'll also need to check his pupils for size and reaction to light. By doing so, you may be able to identify the possible cause of his neurologic problem. Use this chart as a guide to what your patient's pupillary changes may signify.

| PUPIL DESCRIPTION | POSSIBLE CAUSES |
|---|---|
| 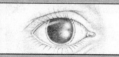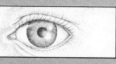<br>Dilated, unilateral, fixed, no reaction to light | • Uncal herniation with oculomotor nerve damage<br>• Brain stem compression due to an expanding mass lesion or an aneurysm<br>• Increased intracranial pressure<br>• Tentorial herniation<br>• Head trauma with subsequent subdural or epidural hematoma |
| 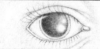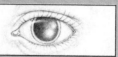<br>Dilated, bilateral, fixed, no reaction to light | • Severe midbrain damage<br>• Cardiopulmonary arrest (hypoxia)<br>• Anticholinergic poisoning |
| 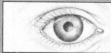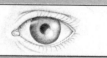<br>Midsized, bilateral, fixed, no reaction to light | • Midbrain involvement due to edema, hemorrhage, infarctions, lacerations, contusions |
| 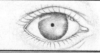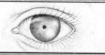<br>Pinpoint, usually bilateral, no reaction to light | • Lesion of pons, usually after hemorrhage, leading to blocked sympathetic impulses<br>• Opiates (morphine)—pupils may be reactive |
| 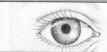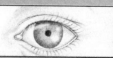<br>Small, unilateral, no reaction to light | • Disruption of sympathetic nerve supply to head due to spinal cord lesion above T1 |

the patient may have normal motion and feeling in his extremities even though his spine isn't stable. The doctor will order a cross-table lateral X-ray and an anteroposterior view of the seven cervical vertebrae. You may be asked to assist by pulling on the patient's arms to obtain the best view of the seven vertebrae.

### Consciousness ($C_3$)

You'll begin to obtain information about your patient's level of consciousness at the moment you begin your emergency assessment and intervention. Note, for instance, how the patient responds to such procedures as intubation and I.V. placement. His level of consciousness during this primary period is a sensitive indicator of whether increased ICP, an expanding mass lesion (such as subdural hematoma), or metabolic or environmental toxicity is present. These conditions may demand immediate intervention.

When you're finished assessing your patient's airway, breathing, circulation, and cervical spine, test his level of consciousness on two levels—arousal and cognition. Arousal is determined by the patient's wakeful state and cognition by his level of thinking, memory, and intellectual skill.

Use the Glasgow Coma Scale to quickly determine your patient's level of consciousness. (See *Assessing Your Patient's Level of Consciousness Using the Glasgow Coma Scale*, page 229.) The best score, 15/15, doesn't determine the patient's exact level of cognition; however, the scoring system does provide an easy way for you to describe the patient's basic level of consciousness.

Begin your examination by testing the patient's ability to respond to verbal stimulation. Does he turn his head toward you when you speak? Does he recognize his name and follow simple commands? Use simple commands, such as "Hold up two fingers" or "Stick out your tongue." Be careful not to use commands that can elicit reflex actions. (For example, eye blinking can be a response to the command or a reflex response.) Similarly, hand squeezing can be a reflex, particularly in deeper levels of coma. If you use hand squeez-

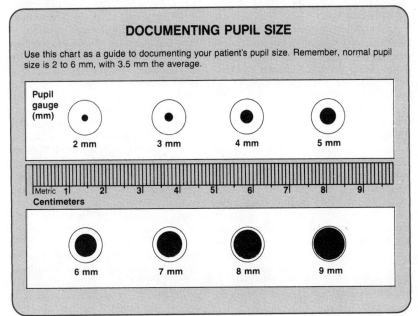

## DOCUMENTING PUPIL SIZE

Use this chart as a guide to documenting your patient's pupil size. Remember, normal pupil size is 2 to 6 mm, with 3.5 mm the average.

Pupil gauge (mm)

| 2 mm | 3 mm | 4 mm | 5 mm |

Metric Centimeters: 1 2 3 4 5 6 7 8 9

| 6 mm | 7 mm | 8 mm | 9 mm |

ing, be sure you always ask the patient to release the action.

If your patient can talk to you, assess him for orientation to person, place, and time. Is your patient's conversation relevant, or does he respond randomly to your efforts to make conversation? Does he have difficulty naming objects or finding appropriate words? These indicators reflect different types of aphasia. If the patient has trouble speaking, ask him to write his responses. Some aphasic patients will be able to do this.

Test your patient's memory. Ask him questions to which there is only one answer, such as "What is your name?" "Where do you live?" "Do you have children?" To see if he can learn new information, tell him your name, and then ask him to repeat it 10 or 15 minutes later.

Remember that your assessment of your patient's level of consciousness isn't complete until you've obtained his *best* response. Don't be timid when you're performing this assessment. Determining his maximum response now gives you an accurate baseline to compare with any subsequent deterioration in his condition.

If the patient doesn't respond to your normal voice, shout. If he doesn't respond when you shout, try shaking him. (Don't do this if there's any possibility that he has a cervical spine injury.) If he still doesn't respond, you'll have to test his reaction to painful stimulation. Use sternal rub, orbital notch pressure, or trapezius muscle squeeze. (Although it's often used, a fingernail squeeze isn't the best test because the spinal cord, not the brain, mediates the response.) Whichever test you use, don't be afraid to apply strong pressure. Remember, you're trying to get the best response your patient is capable of giving. Apply pressure for at least 30 seconds (time it on your watch).

Purposeful responses to pain are:
• *localization* (the patient moves his hand toward the painful area and eventually touches it)

• *flexion withdrawal* (the patient flexes either arm but doesn't find and touch the painful area).

Nonpurposeful responses include:
• *abnormal flexion* (decorticate posturing), in which the patient adducts his shoulder, flexes and pronates his arm, flexes his wrist, and makes a fist
• *abnormal extension* (decerebrate posturing), in which the patient adducts his shoulder and rotates it internally, extends his forearm, flexes his wrist, and makes a fist
• *flaccidity* (no response).

Describe the patient's best response when you talk to the doctor—this will help him determine further treatment.

In a patient with head trauma, altered level of consciousness may indicate increased ICP. Your patient may be restless, confused, or unconscious. If you suspect increased ICP and if the patient's spine is stable, you can position his head in a neutral position and maintain it with a firm cervical collar (Philadelphia collar) to decrease jugular venous compression, which prevents venous blood flow from the head. You can also elevate the patient's head 15° to 30° to promote venous drainage. *Don't* place the patient in the prone or Trendelenburg's position.

If the patient's unconscious, draw blood for blood glucose levels and for a toxicologic screen to test for hypo- or hyperglycemia and for drug toxicity. At the same time, draw additional blood for a complete blood count (CBC) and for electrolytes, serum osmolality, serum creatinine, serum ammonia, and blood urea nitrogen (BUN) to determine other causes of the patient's unconsciousness. Draw arterial blood for arterial blood gases (ABGs). Establish an I.V., if the patient doesn't already have one. The doctor may order an I.V. push of dextrose 50% to prevent brain damage from hypoglycemia; he may also order an I.V. push of naloxone to reverse possible narcotic overdose.

Don't forget, the unconscious patient also needs your support. He may be able to hear even if he can't respond, so talk to him. Explain what you're doing and why, and encourage family members to talk to him, too. (In addition to helping him, you'll make the family members feel useful and needed.)

Remember to check an unconscious patient's body alignment when you change his position—he can't tell you if he's uncomfortable or if a body part is positioned awkwardly. And always respect your patient's privacy: keep him properly draped and covered as you would any awake patient.

### General appearance
Note if your patient has hemiparesis of the face, arm, or leg; this may indicate stroke. Also note any bilateral paresis or paresthesias, which may indicate spinal injury. If your patient's suffered trauma, look for scalp lacerations, which require immediate debridement and suturing and may indicate underlying skull fracture or brain damage. If rescue personnel dressed the wound, leave the dressing on until the doctor's available—removing it may disturb the clot. If the wound's open, cleanse it with a broad-spectrum germicide, such as povidone-iodine, then shave around the laceration area. Apply sterile saline gauze, dry gauze, or a pressure wrap to the wound until the doctor arrives to suture it. Expect to call a plastic surgeon if the wound extends into the patient's face. (Don't shave the patient's eyebrows; the doctor will use them as a guide to the patient's natural face contour and markings.) As with any open wound, remember to ask the patient about tetanus immunization (follow the protocol on pages 66 and 67).

Examine the patient's ears and nose for escaping CSF. *Notify the doctor* if you detect fluid, and elevate the patient's head 30°. Instruct him not to change his position. You can test the fluid with a Dextrostix or Clinistix—CSF tests positive for sugar, but mucus does not. If the fluid's bloody, test it by allowing a drop to fall onto a piece of filter paper or bed linen. If CSF is mixed with the blood, it will form a clear ring, or "halo," around a central blood-tinged spot.

Observe the patient's skull for any disruption in normal contour or any obviously depressed areas that may indicate skull fracture. Be sure to tell the doctor if you note any suspicious findings.

Your patient may experience seizures as a result of his head injury or an underlying neurologic disorder. Turn the patient on his side, protect him from further injury, and maintain a patent airway. If the seizure doesn't terminate, the doctor may order diazepam (Valium) or phenytoin (Dilantin) by slow I.V. push—never more than 50 mg/minute. Be prepared to start an I.V. and to draw blood for laboratory work to aid in identifying the cause of the seizure.

Complete your assessment with an overall examination of the patient. Check his skin for needle marks: a diabetic may have these on his abdomen or thighs, whereas a drug abuser may have them on his arms. Smell the patient's breath for alcohol or a fruity odor (acetone), which may signal diabetic ketoacidosis. Note any yellowing of his skin or sclera, which may suggest liver failure.

Check his tongue for lacerations or contusions that may have occurred during a seizure. Your patient may be unconscious because of an unobserved generalized convulsion. Bowel or bladder incontinence may indicate a seizure, an intracranial hemorrhage, or a long period of unconsciousness.

---

# What to Do Next

You've assessed your patient's airway, breathing, circulation, cervical spine, and level of consciousness, intervening as necessary. Now you'll continue your emergency assessment, looking for:
• further clues to the cause of his neu-

rologic emergency
• signs and symptoms of additional emergency problems.

This information will expand your baseline data. Remember that your patient's family and friends are important information sources—particularly if the patient's unconscious or otherwise unable to communicate. Don't ignore them: asking them questions not only helps you assess your patient—it also makes them feel needed.

You'll want to organize your emergency assessment around the signs you see and the symptoms your patient, his family, or his friends tell you about. Depending on the seriousness of his condition, you may see various levels of consciousness—from slight confusion to coma. If you noted *confusion* during your initial assessment, ask your patient's family if they've noticed this before and, if so, how long ago they first noticed it. Sudden confusion can indicate stroke, head injury, or an acute infection producing a high fever. Chronic or recurrent episodic confusion, however, may indicate TIAs, brain tumor or other lesion, or hepatic dysfunction.

You assessed your patient's respirations during your initial assessment; now take a few seconds to look for *altered respiratory patterns*. The types of respiratory pattern alterations you see will provide clues to your patient's emergency problem.

If your patient's breathing is stertorous and labored, he may have a severe brain injury. For example, if he has Cheyne-Stokes respirations, he may have deep cerebral or cerebellar lesions or a metabolic brain dysfunction. If his breathing is sustained, rapid, and regular with forced inspiration and expiration (central neurogenic hyperventilation), suspect lesions, anoxia, or hypoglycemia affecting the low midbrain or pons area of the brain stem. If your patient's breathing completely irregularly—ataxic breathing—it may indicate a medulla lesion and impending *respiratory arrest*.

If you note *any* of these signs of altered respiratory patterns, *call the doctor immediately* and prepare to use life-support techniques. (See *Abnormal Breathing Patterns Associated with Brain Injury,* page 241.)

Check your patient's pupil responses to further assess his level of consciousness. (See *Understanding Pupillary Changes,* page 230.) Don't forget to consider the possibility that your patient might have an artificial eye. Remember, too, that some people have pupils that are normally somewhat unequal in size. Neurologic causes of abnormal pupil responses include:
• optic nerve injury
• oculomotor nerve injury
• increasing ICP
• mass lesion
• tentorial herniation.

An epidural hemorrhage will cause a dilated, fixed pupil, usually on the side of the patient's brain where the hemorrhage occurred. Report *all* pupil response changes to the doctor immediately, *especially* this one. Epidural hemorrhage can be rapidly fatal if the hematoma isn't removed quickly. (If it's removed in time, the patient's prognosis is usually excellent.)

If your patient's unconscious, watch him for any unusual movements, such as reflex sucking, grasping, rigidity, gegenhalten (an involuntary resistance to passive movement), or focal seizures. Check for Babinski's sign—normally seen only in infants. Also check his corneal and gag reflexes and his extraocular movements (see *Assessing Extraocular Muscle Function,* page 69). If he doesn't blink and if his eyes don't stay closed, provide meticulous eye care. If his gag reflex is absent, suction him as needed.

After you've assessed his level of consciousness, ask your patient (if he's conscious) if he has a *headache*. If so, ask when it started and how severe it is. You may want to have him rate his pain from 0 (no pain) to 10 (the worst pain he's ever felt). If he has a headache, ask also about nausea, vomiting,

dizziness, or visual disturbances. Headache with various combinations of these other symptoms can indicate:
- increased ICP
- stroke
- meningitis
- bleeding (an acute epidural, subdural, or subarachnoid hemorrhage)
- concussion
- cerebral contusion.

A patient's complaint of *neck and back pain* following injury is potentially extremely serious. Why? Because neck and back pain may signal spinal fracture. Vertebral fractures produce pain at the midline of the spine, at the fracture site. Remember, vertebral pain associated with *muscle weakness* or *paralysis* is a reliable indicator of spinal cord injury. Get as much information as you can about the pain and about when the weakness or paralysis first occurred. Is it as bad, the same, or worse since the initial injury? If he can move his arms and legs without assistance, test your patient's strength. Ask him to push against your hand with his hands, then his feet. Check his facial muscles by asking him to smile, to "make a face," to move his tongue from side to side while keeping his mouth open, and to squeeze his eyes shut. Note any asymmetry (such as a drooping eyelid or a turned-down corner of his mouth) when he does this.

Back muscles strained during acceleration-deceleration injuries may cause cervical and thoracolumbar pain. If ligaments are stretched, too, the patient's spine may be unstable. If you suspect this, you'll have to take steps to immobilize the patient.

Remember, neck pain may also indicate meningeal irritation from infection or bleeding. If your patient has neck pain, be sure to ask if he knows what caused it, when it started, and if he has associated symptoms—such as pain radiating down the arm, extremity weakness, or sensation loss.

Of course, an emergency patient who *hasn't* suffered spinal cord trauma may also report muscle weakness. In the ab-

sence of spinal trauma, this symptom may indicate myasthenia gravis, stroke, TIAs, or a head injury. Ask if this weakness is a chronic problem, now acutely exacerbated, or a first occurrence. If his weakness is chronic, find out if he's unable to take deep breaths—this may further indicate myasthenia gravis. Check his motor strength, as described earlier, by having him push against your hand with his hands and feet.

As a nurse, you're aware that a *high temperature* (102° F. [38.9° C.] orally or 103° F. [39.4° C.] rectally, or greater) in a patient with a neurologic emergency may indicate a viral or bacterial brain infection, such as meningitis or an abscess. If your patient has a high temperature, he may be unable to respond to your questions; if necessary, ask an available family member if the patient's had a recent infection, respiratory illness, head trauma, or brain tumor or if he's recently had neurosurgery.

As you know, fever causes increased cerebral blood flow, which in turn increases ICP and acutely exacerbates existing brain injury. If your patient's temperature is elevated, the doctor may order antibiotics for infection or antipyretics, such as acetaminophen or aspirin. Your intervention will depend on the degree and rapidity of the temperature change. If necessary, you may also use a tepid sponge bath, alcohol sponge bath, ice bags applied to the patient's groin and axillae, or a hypothermia blanket.

An *extreme* drop in your patient's temperature also requires your quick intervention. Why? Because it may cause decreases in level of consciousness, in pupillary response, and in cardiac output. Expect to give your patient chlorpromazine (Thorazine) or diazepam (Valium) to control shivering, because shivering increases the metabolic rate, thus increasing his ICP. Also expect to keep him warm with blankets or to place him on a hyperthermia blanket.

# Special Considerations

## Pediatric

Always consider the possibility of poisoning in an unconscious infant or young child (see Chapter 17). If the child's very ill, with lethargy, high fever, irritability, or vomiting, be alert to the possibility of meningitis—more common in children than in adults. Remember, in an infant, the only signs of infection may be fretfulness, lack of appetite, and vomiting. Watch for these signs and, if you suspect *any* viral infection in a child of any age, don't give the child aspirin. Give him acetaminophen instead. Aspirin ingestion during viral illness has been linked to the development of Reye's syndrome, a very serious sequela of acute viral infection in children.

If your pediatric patient has signs of minor head trauma, such as bruises or lacerations, without serious skull or scalp damage, don't rule out the possibility that he has severe brain injury. The most common causes of head trauma in children are physical abuse and motor vehicle accidents when the child wasn't properly restrained. (Remember, you're responsible for reporting instances of suspected child abuse—see the "When to Make a Report" entry in Chapter 2.) As you know, any head trauma may cause increased ICP. In an infant or a very young child, early signs of increased ICP are usually subtle. Assess an infant for a tense, bulging anterior fontanel (normally, it's slightly depressed and pulsatile). Assess an older child for nausea, vomiting, irritability, fatigue, and headache.

## Geriatric

Because cerebral blood flow's decreased in many older patients, they have an increased incidence of stroke. Arteriosclerosis of the cerebral arteries is commonly the cause of a geriatric patient's confusion; particularly in an emergency, be careful to distinguish between this and an increased or acute level of confusion from stroke, recurrent TIAs, or head trauma. Ask your patient's family for a detailed history of his mental status over the past few weeks or months.

Remember that your geriatric patient's neurologic signs and symptoms may have *preceded*—even *precipitated*—his injury. For example, if an elderly patient comes in with injuries from a fall, find out the details of how he was injured. If he answers you by saying something like, "I was just standing at the sink, and the next thing I knew I was lying on the floor," a TIA may have caused his fall.

# CARE AFTER DIAGNOSIS

# Coma

## Prediagnosis summary

On initial assessment, the patient was:
- unconscious
- unresponsive to even the strongest stimuli.

An airway was established, and he was suctioned, if necessary. He received supplemental oxygen. If his respirations were impaired, he was intubated and started on mechanical ventilation. To determine the cause of the patient's unconsciousness, the doctor ordered a computerized tomography (CT) scan and blood tests. The patient was put on a cardiac monitor and started on an I.V. infusion of $D_5\frac{1}{2}NS$, followed by a bolus of dextrose 50% and naloxone (Narcan). His vital signs and his pupil size and reaction time were assessed; the Glasgow Coma Scale was used to assess the depth of his unconsciousness. He was examined for internal and external bleeding and

## CASE IN POINT: WHEN THE PATIENT'S CONDITION DETERIORATES

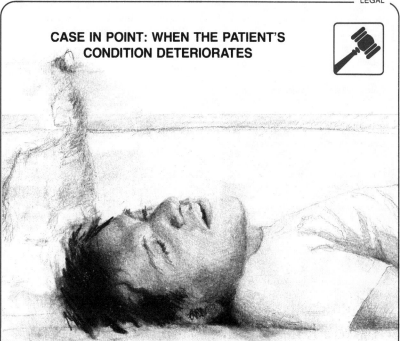

Roger Johnson, age 45, arrives in the ED at 1 p.m. while you're working a very busy shift. Involved in a construction-site accident, he was brought to the ED along with two seriously injured co-workers. You observe he has a scalp abrasion and other minor injuries. You telephone the doctor on call and relate Roger's signs and symptoms, his vital signs, and his history. Then, because Roger's two co-workers have more serious injuries and the ED's crowded, you place him in the hall to await the doctor.

At 2 p.m., you check on Roger. His blood pressure is 72/50, his pulse is 128, and his respirations are 44. He's pale, cool, and diaphoretic. You note these findings on his chart. The doctor still hasn't seen him.

When you check on Roger again, at 2:45 p.m., he has Cheyne-Stokes respirations, and you can't find a pulse. Aggressive cardiopulmonary resuscitation is unsuccessful.

Mrs. Johnson and her children later file suit against you, the doctor, and the hospital for negligence contributory to Roger's death. Are you liable for any damages? (After all, the doctor's the one who didn't attend to the patient.)

In a court case based on a similar incident (*Thomas v. Corso,* 1972) involving a nurse's alleged negligence, the doctor and the hospital were found liable. The nurse performed her initial assessment and reporting duties promptly, but she failed to notify the doctor of a change in the patient's vital signs when she checked him a few hours later. The court reasoned that if the nurse had called the doctor again, after finding a change in the patient's vital signs, and the doctor had performed his duty to attend to the patient, the patient might have survived.

What can you do to protect yourself from liability in emergency situations like this? Following these tips will help:
- Be sure you know the clinical signs and symptoms that indicate when a patient's condition is deteriorating.
- Assess your patient frequently to identify problems promptly.
- Call the doctor immediately if you find *any* change in the patient's condition.
- Promptly document all signs and symptoms that you report to the doctor, and document his reply.
- Follow your hospital's policy for notifying management if the doctor's not responsive.

*Thomas v. Corso,* 288 A. 2d 379 (Md., 1972).

## WHAT HAPPENS IN COMA

Coma isn't just unconsciousness, but unconsciousness from which the patient can't be aroused by even strong stimulation. The brain's reticular activating system (RAS)—an intricate network of connections extending from a brain stem center to the hypothalamus, thalamus, and cerebral cortex—is disturbed, preventing the intercommunication that makes consciousness and active motor function possible. Because the RAS is centered in the brain stem core and then fans out over the cortex, insult or injury to different areas of the brain affects consciousness in different ways.

Consciousness is altered by two pathologic mechanisms broadly classified as those that widely depress cerebral hemisphere function and those that specifically depress or destroy areas of the brain stem RAS. For example, significant bilateral cerebral hemisphere damage may produce the same effect on consciousness as a pinhead-sized brain stem injury.

Coma-producing processes are further classified by the regions they affect:
- *Supratentorial*—for example, intracerebral, epidural, or subdural hematoma; arterial (thrombotic or embolic) or venous occlusions; tumors; abscesses
- *Subtentorial*—for example, cerebellar hemorrhage, infarct, or abscess; brain stem infarct or aneurysm; pons hemorrhage
- *Metabolic or diffuse brain dysfunction*—for example, anoxia (see Chapter 4); hypoglycemia, uremia, electrolyte imbalance, liver failure, or endocrine disorders (see Chapter 10); drug toxicity (see Chapter 11); cardiogenic or hypovolemic shock (see Chapter 14).

Some severe psychiatric disorders can also produce a coma-like state (psychogenic unresponsiveness).

for signs of seizures (for example, tongue lacerations and bladder and bowel incontinence).

The patient's family or friends or the rescue personnel who brought him to the hospital supplied information about the onset and duration of his unconsciousness. So if the patient had any recent trauma, infection, or behavior changes, if he was ever treated for a psychiatric disorder, if he was taking any drugs, or if he had any preexisting illness, this information should now be on his chart.

### Priorities

Your first nursing priority is to ensure adequate perfusion and oxygenation of the patient's brain and other vital organs. You can do this while you perform a thorough assessment and evaluate the results of his laboratory studies.

Although the patient's airway and respirations were stabilized initially, remember that his respiratory status can deteriorate suddenly at any time while he's unconscious. If his respiratory status worsens and if he was given oxygen earlier, he may need to be given a higher percentage of oxygen now. Or, if he wasn't intubated and placed on a ventilator earlier, this may have to be done now. Observe your patient carefully, and always keep airways and intubation equipment on hand. To prevent aspiration of vomitus, a nasogastric tube will be inserted.

Continue to check your comatose patient for signs and symptoms of internal or external bleeding. A central venous pressure line may be inserted for accurate evaluation of the patient's hemodynamic status and for fluid infusion. You'll insert an indwelling (Foley) catheter to help you evaluate his output.

### Continuing assessment and intervention

The comprehensive assessment you'll do now will give you further clues to the cause of his coma. You'll also use your assessment findings as a baseline for evaluating subsequent changes in his condition.

Before you begin to assess your patient, take a few moments just to watch him. Note every movement he makes, no matter how random. You may see signs of changes in his level of consciousness—changes such as focal seizures or random limb movement.

Start your complete baseline assessment by checking all the patient's vital signs. If he was previously hospitalized and his chart from that hospitalization is available, ask someone to get it for you. It will broaden your assessment baseline.

If your comatose patient's blood pressure is low, causes may include:
• low circulating volume—which may result from hemorrhagic or traumatic shock or fluid depletion or from low cardiac output due to heart problems, such as myocardial infarction (MI).
• low peripheral resistance—for example, from a drug overdose
• sepsis.

Assess your patient's pulse rate. Tachycardia can be a sign of reduced cardiac output from a dysrhythmia, such as supraventricular tachycardia (SVT). Bradycardia (also a sign of reduced cardiac output) can be due to other types of dysrhythmias (such as heart block), to increased ICP, to Adams-Stokes syndrome, or to an MI. You know, of course, that severely reduced cardiac output can cause extreme hypoxia, leading to coma.

Observe your comatose patient's respirations, too—evaluating their rate, pattern, and depth. You may see Cheyne-Stokes, apneustic, cluster, or ataxic breathing or central neurogenic hyperventilation; your findings may point to the cause of his coma. (See *Abnormal Breathing Patterns Associated with Brain Injury,* page 241.) Auscultate his lungs and listen for wheezes, which may suggest advanced pulmonary disease and carbon dioxide narcosis as a cause of his coma.

If your patient's temperature is elevated, suspect infection, inflammation, or a neoplasm. If his temperature is below normal, this may be the result of sepsis, hypoglycemia, atropine or glutethimide ingestion or overdose, or brain stem injury—all possible causes of coma.

Check his pupil size and reaction. Normal pupil size and reaction may indicate psychogenic unresponsiveness

or a toxic or metabolic cause of his coma. (Exceptions include atropine and glutethimide ingestion or overdose, which causes fixed and widely dilated pupils, and narcotic overdose, which causes fixed and severely constricted pupils.) Abnormal pupil size and reaction may help pinpoint the location of a coma-causing brain injury. (See *Understanding Pupillary Changes,* page 230.) If your patient's pupils are very constricted (1 to 2 mm), they may not respond noticeably to light. To check for a reaction, use a bright light and a magnifying lens.

If cervical spine injury has been ruled out for your patient, perform the "doll's eye" maneuver to check his oculocephalic reflex. To do this, hold his eyelids open and quickly (but gently) rotate his head to one side. Normally, the patient's eyes will move toward the side opposite the direction you turned his head. Absence or asymmetry of eye movement may indicate brain stem dysfunction. Remember, however, that some drugs (such as barbiturates) can abolish this reflex. The psychogenically unresponsive patient won't have the doll's eye reflex, either. Why? Because awake patients don't show this reflex.

If your comatose patient does have an abnormal oculocephalic reflex, the doctor may perform cold caloric testing

## NOW HEAR THIS!

Just because your patient's comatose doesn't mean he can't hear.
Remember to:
*Treat him with dignity.*
• Don't discuss his condition when standing by his bedside.
• Don't perform a procedure without telling him first.
*Keep him stimulated.*
• Talk to him, and encourage his family and other staff members to do so.
• Suggest to his family that they tape-record messages at home and play them at his bedside.

to determine if the oculovestibular reflex is intact. An absent response suggests brain stem dysfunction.

Next, assess your patient's motor response. Does he react to a painful stimulus with a purposeful response (such as localization or flexion withdrawal) or with a nonpurposeful response (such as abnormal flexion, abnormal extension, or flaccidity)? Test both sides of his body and compare the results. An asymmetrical response suggests a structural brain dysfunction. If he's in a light coma, he'll respond by withdrawing from a painful stimulus. Normal motor response may indicate psychogenic unresponsiveness.

If your patient's in a deep coma, he may respond with *abnormal flexion* (decorticate posturing), which reflects intact brain stem function, or *abnormal extension* (decerebrate posturing), which suggests brain stem involvement. In the deepest stages of coma, your patient may show no response at all to stimuli. Be sure to document all your findings and report them to the doctor.

To continue your assessment, examine your patient's skin for *petechiae*, which may result from such coma-causing diseases as meningococcemia or bacterial endocarditis. Observe him also for *jaundice,* which may indicate underlying liver disease.

Palpate your patient's abdomen, checking for liver or spleen enlargement. Liver enlargement may indicate advanced underlying liver disease and hepatic coma. Spleen enlargement may indicate blood dyscrasias or infectious mononucleosis: both can cause an encephalitis-like illness and coma.

Be sure to document all your findings so you can keep track of whether your patient's condition is improving or deteriorating. Continue to watch his monitor for dysrhythmias and to monitor his fluid intake and output and his electrolyte status. Every 15 minutes (if he's unstable) or as ordered, reassess his vital signs, level of consciousness, and pupil and motor responses.

## Therapeutic care

After you've completely assessed your patient, review his blood studies and CT scan report before you begin to implement his medical treatment. You'll need to monitor these studies and assess his vital signs and level of consciousness frequently during this phase. Each time, compare your findings with earlier ones.

Make sure the patient's receiving the correct I.V. fluids, too. The doctor usually *won't* order plain dextrose solutions because they enhance brain swelling. Instead, he may order a solution of $D_5\frac{1}{2}NS$, administered at a rate of 75 ml/hour or less. (High infusion rates will increase cerebral blood flow, worsening the ICP that may be associated with coma.)

The results of the blood studies done during your comatose patient's initial assessment provide valuable baseline information as you monitor his condition. Now, the doctor will review the patient's laboratory tests, as follows:

● *blood glucose level* test, to detect hypo- or hyperglycemia. Expect to give dextrose if your patient's hypoglycemic; insulin if he's hyperglycemic.

● *toxicologic screen,* to detect the presence of drugs or poisons. If the patient does have a drug or poison in his system, the doctor may order dialysis or an antagonistic drug. For example, for an anticholinergic overdose, expect to give physostigmine; for phenothiazines, benztropine mesylate (Cogentin) or diphenhydramine hydrochloride (Benadryl). You may also give mannitol, which promotes diuresis, to eliminate the drug.

● *CBC,* to obtain clues to hypo- or hypervolemia and infection. For hypovolemia, expect to give fluids or blood as needed; for hypervolemia, expect to give diuretics. If the patient has an infection, more blood will be drawn for culture-and-sensitivity tests so the doctor can order specific antibiotics.

● *electrolyte* tests, to detect any imbalance in the patient's sodium, potassium, or chloride levels.

# ABNORMAL BREATHING PATTERNS ASSOCIATED WITH BRAIN INJURY

If your patient has a brain injury, his breathing pattern will change as the injury affects certain vital brain areas. Use the chart below to learn how abnormal breathing patterns indicate the location of brain injuries.

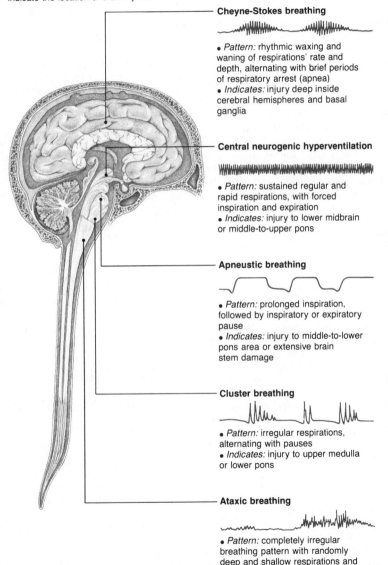

**Cheyne-Stokes breathing**

- *Pattern:* rhythmic waxing and waning of respirations' rate and depth, alternating with brief periods of respiratory arrest (apnea)
- *Indicates:* injury deep inside cerebral hemispheres and basal ganglia

**Central neurogenic hyperventilation**

- *Pattern:* sustained regular and rapid respirations, with forced inspiration and expiration
- *Indicates:* injury to lower midbrain or middle-to-upper pons

**Apneustic breathing**

- *Pattern:* prolonged inspiration, followed by inspiratory or expiratory pause
- *Indicates:* injury to middle-to-lower pons area or extensive brain stem damage

**Cluster breathing**

- *Pattern:* irregular respirations, alternating with pauses
- *Indicates:* injury to upper medulla or lower pons

**Ataxic breathing**

- *Pattern:* completely irregular breathing pattern with randomly deep and shallow respirations and pauses
- *Indicates:* injury to medulla

• *serum creatinine and BUN* tests, to detect kidney disease and dehydration. If kidney disease caused the patient's coma, he may require dialysis. If he's dehydrated, administer fluids as needed.

• *serum ammonia* test, to detect the presence of liver disease. If the patient's serum ammonia level is elevated, expect to give ammonia-leaching agents, such as lactulose.

• *serum osmolality* test, to detect severe dehydration, water intoxication, hyperosmolarity, or the presence of alcohol. Expect to give fluids if the patient's dehydrated or hyperosmolar, diuretics if he's overhydrated.

• *ABG analysis,* to assess the patient's acid-base balance and respiratory status. Expect to correct any imbalance in acidity or alkalinity and to intubate and ventilate the patient if his acid-base balance can't be maintained.

• *clotting profile,* to detect clotting factor defects and to provide a baseline for the use of heparin therapy if the patient's coma is due to embolic or thrombotic stroke.

If your patient's CT scan shows evidence of a hematoma or brain tumor, he may need immediate surgery. (See the hematoma entries in this chapter).

Your careful assessment and interventions up to this point may have helped to reverse the patient's coma. But remember, even the most conscientious care and treatment may not improve his condition; he may be comatose for an extended time. So as you continue to care for him, do all you can to keep him oriented and comfortable and to preserve his dignity and privacy:

• Watch for complications associated with total parenteral nutrition if your patient's receiving intravenous hyperalimentation.

• Give meticulous eye and mouth care. Corneal irritation and abrasion can occur within 4 to 6 hours if your patient's eyes remain open. Instill artificial tears every 2 to 3 hours. Cleanse his mouth several times a day, and coat his lips with petrolatum to prevent dryness.

• Bathe your patient and inspect his skin integrity regularly. Use therapeutic touching as a way of letting your patient know you care. Dry his skin thoroughly after bathing, and turn him frequently to prevent pressure sores. Perform passive range-of-motion exercises four times daily to prevent contracture deformities.

• Remember to check your patient's body alignment when you change his position—he can't report the discomfort that would indicate inappropriate positioning.

• Respect his privacy by keeping him properly covered.

• Provide the patient with as much communication and stimulation as possible. Talk to your comatose patient. Always introduce yourself to him, addressing him by name. Establish a day and night schedule in your care, as much as possible. Each time you perform a procedure, explain what you're doing. Encourage family members to communicate with the patient, too, and involve them in the patient's care as much as you can. Ask them to bring in familiar objects, such as a favorite pillow or afghan. If hospital policy permits, turn on a radio to stimulate the patient.

# Increased Intracranial Pressure

## Prediagnosis summary

Following head trauma or head surgery, the patient developed:

• alterations in his level of consciousness (restlessness, confusion, irritability, lethargy, personality changes, or even coma)

• headache

• visual disturbances (blurred or double vision, photophobia)

• widened pulse pressure

• respiratory pattern changes.

# NURSE'S GUIDE TO BRAIN HERNIATIONS

Cerebral edema or a space-occupying lesion (such as a tumor or hematoma) causes pressure within the patient's cranium to increase in the affected area. This uneven pressure shifts his brain mass toward areas of less pressure, depressing vital structures and causing herniation above or below the tentorium. Here's what you need to know about brain herniations.

## CENTRAL HERNIATION

Pressure causes downward displacement of cerebral hemispheres, basal ganglia, diencephalon, and midbrain through the tentorial notch. This process occurs in orderly, progressive sequence, from front to back, in four stages.

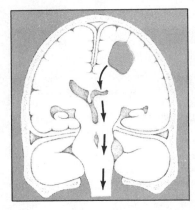

**Signs and symptoms**
*Diencephalon stage* (treatable stage):
• possible decreased consciousness
• normal pupillary reactions
• normal extraocular movement (EOM)
• appropriate or abnormal flexion (decorticate posture) motor response
• normal or Cheyne-Stokes breathing
*Midbrain stage:*
• coma
• no pupillary reaction
• normal or abnormal EOM
• abnormal flexion (decorticate posture) or abnormal extension (decerebrate posture)
• normal or central neurogenic hyperventilation
*Pons stage:*
• deep coma
• no pupillary reaction
• abnormal extension
• flaccid motor response
• apneustic breathing
*Medullar stage:*
• deep coma
• no pupillary reaction
• abnormal EOM
• flaccid motor response
• cluster, ataxic, or apneustic breathing

## UNCAL HERNIATION

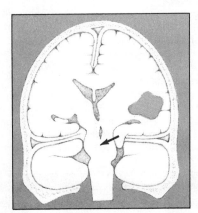

Uncal herniation occurs suddenly, in two stages. Pressure causes lateral displacement of the temporal lobe's medial portion through the tentorium into the posterior fossa.

**Signs and symptoms**
*Early stage* (treatable stage):
• lethargic or fully awake level of consciousness
• sluggish and unequal pupillary reaction
• normal or asymmetrical EOM
• appropriate or asymmetrical motor response
• normal breathing
*Late stage:*
• coma
• unequal or fixed pupillary reaction
• asymmetrical or absent EOM
• abnormal extension or flexion
• Cheyne-Stokes breathing or central neurogenic hyperventilation

# WHAT HAPPENS IN INCREASED INTRACRANIAL PRESSURE

Increased intracranial pressure (ICP) is the pressure exerted within the intact skull by the intracranial volume—about 10% blood, 10% cerebrospinal fluid (CSF), and 80% brain-tissue water. The rigid skull allows very little space for expansion of these substances. When ICP increases to pathologic levels, brain damage can result.

The brain compensates for increases by regulating the three substances' volume by:
• limiting blood flow to the head
• displacing CSF into the spinal canal
• increasing absorption or decreasing production of CSF—pulling water out of brain tissue into the blood and excreting it through the kidneys. When compensatory mechanisms become overworked, small changes in volume lead to very large changes in pressure.

Here's a flowchart to help you understand increased ICP's pathophysiology.

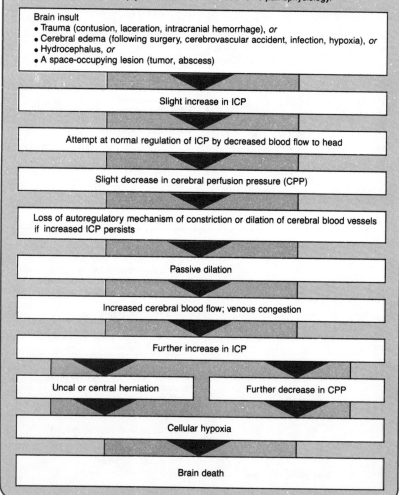

Brain insult
• Trauma (contusion, laceration, intracranial hemorrhage), *or*
• Cerebral edema (following surgery, cerebrovascular accident, infection, hypoxia), *or*
• Hydrocephalus, *or*
• A space-occupying lesion (tumor, abscess)

Slight increase in ICP

Attempt at normal regulation of ICP by decreased blood flow to head

Slight decrease in cerebral perfusion pressure (CPP)

Loss of autoregulatory mechanism of constriction or dilation of cerebral blood vessels if increased ICP persists

Passive dilation

Increased cerebral blood flow; venous congestion

Further increase in ICP

Uncal or central herniation | Further decrease in CPP

Cellular hypoxia

Brain death

A neurologic exam was done to evaluate the patient's response to verbal and painful stimuli and to assess his pupillary reactions, reflexes, and muscle tone. The doctor ordered blood tests—ABGs, electrolytes, blood glucose, CBC, and BUN—skull X-rays, and a CT scan. The patient was placed on a cardiac monitor and started on supplemental oxygen.

### Priorities, assessment, and intervention

Your first priority in caring for a patient with increased intracranial pressure (ICP) is to perform a complete neurologic assessment; then you'll have the accurate baseline data you need to assess subsequent changes. Remember, *changes* in your patient's condition, rather than any one sign or symptom, signal increasing ICP. Make sure you keep artificial airways, intubation equipment, an Ambu bag, and suction equipment on hand: your patient's condition may deteriorate suddenly.

Keep the head of your patient's bed elevated 30° to 60° to promote venous drainage. (*Don't* put him in a jackknife position—this increases intraabdominal and intrathoracic pressure.) Place the patient's head in a neutral position, and use a cervical collar or neck rolls to maintain it. Now perform a complete nursing assessment.

Assess your patient's level of consciousness frequently. Why? Because alterations in level of consciousness are the earliest and most sensitive indicator that your patient's ICP is increasing. Watch for restlessness, confusion, unresponsiveness, or decreased level of consciousness. Compare your findings carefully. His respiratory status may deteriorate as his level of consciousness deteriorates; be prepared to assist with intubation and mechanical ventilation. If he's unconscious, expect to insert a nasogastric tube to prevent him from aspirating vomit and secretions.

Check your patient for pupillary changes. Note if his pupils are equal, constricted, or dilated and if they react

## HIGHLIGHTING MANNITOL

Mannitol is an osmotic diuretic often used to decrease intracranial pressure in patients with neurologic disorders. Remember these important points when using mannitol:
• It may crystallize out of solution at concentrations of 15% or greater, especially when exposed to low temperatures. If this happens, you can warm the solution in hot water and shake it vigorously, or you can autoclave it. Be sure it's cooled to body temperature before you administer it to your patient.
• Don't use mannitol if it's not completely dissolved.
• Always administer mannitol solutions intravenously, through an in-line filter.
• Adding electrolytes to a 20% or greater solution of mannitol may cause precipitation.
• Don't infuse mannitol in the same line as whole blood; precipitation will result.

to light briskly, sluggishly, or not at all. Watch particularly for *pupil constriction,* which appears just prior to herniation. *Call the doctor immediately if you see this sign.* Constriction may last only a few minutes, but if your patient's increased ICP remains untreated, herniation will follow quickly and his pupils will become fixed and dilated (see *Nurse's Guide to Brain Herniations,* page 243).

Assess your patient's motor and sensory function. You may find impairment or even complete loss of function when increasing ICP exerts pressure on motor or sensory nerve tracts.

Monitor your patient's vital signs at least every hour. In a patient with increased ICP, *altered vital signs* appear *after* his level of consciousness changes. You may see Cushing's triad: bradycardia, hypertension, and respiratory pattern change. Increased ICP will at first *stimulate* the patient's respiratory and circulatory centers and then *depress* them. Watch for a widening pulse pressure (systolic pressure increasing

# UNDERSTANDING INTRACRANIAL PRESSURE MONITORS

As you probably know, intracranial pressure (ICP) monitors can detect elevated ICP early, before your patient shows signs and symptoms of a worsening neurologic condition. Are you familiar with the different types of ICP monitoring systems? All three give you a choice between digital readout or strip-chart recording—but otherwise they differ in important ways. And, as you'll see, each one has a drawback. Here's a comparison of three types of ICP monitors.

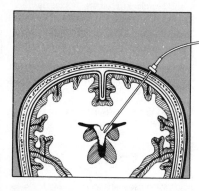

## INTRAVENTRICULAR

Small polyethylene catheter inserted into patient's ventricle; gives most accurate ICP measurement and allows for draining excess cerebrospinal fluid (CSF); *may permit CSF leakage and promote brain infection.*

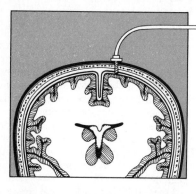

## SUBARACHNOID

Small hollow screw and transducer wick implanted into subarachnoid space; allows for accurate ICP monitoring and for draining excess CSF; *may promote brain infection.*

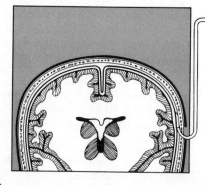

## EPIDURAL

Fiber-optic sensor implanted into epidural space; allows direct invasive monitoring, therefore least risk of infection; *monitor doesn't allow for CSF drainage.*

while diastolic pressure remains normal).

Monitor your patient's intake and output closely. You may need to insert an indwelling (Foley) catheter to obtain accurate measurements if he's unresponsive or incontinent. Total fluids are usually restricted to 1,200 to 1,500 ml/day to reduce total fluid volume and intracerebral swelling. A central venous pressure line or Swan-Ganz catheter may be inserted to aid in fluid management; an arterial line may be inserted to monitor his blood pressure continuously.

Expect to administer diuretic therapy to further reduce fluid volume. Most often, you'll give an osmotic diuretic such as mannitol as an I.V. bolus through a filtered administration set. (See *Highlighting Mannitol*, page 245.) Make sure you've inserted a Foley catheter *before* you give mannitol, because this rapid-acting diuretic can cause bladder distention. You may also give corticosteroid therapy, which may decrease cerebral edema, and I.V. lidocaine, a new treatment that seems to lower ICP in some patients.

Small increases in ICP may be difficult to detect. So the doctor may start ICP monitoring to detect subtle changes before the patient's condition deteriorates. (See *Understanding Intracranial Pressure Monitors*.) Prepare the equipment and calibrate the monitor. The doctor will insert a sensor through your patient's skull and into the subarachnoid or epidural space or ventricle to measure the patient's CSF pressure. The pressure on the sensor, screw or catheter generates mechanical impulses that a transducer converts into electrical energy and transmits to an amplifier, where visible waveforms appear on an oscilloscope or chart recorder. Record the results hourly, and be alert for sudden increases in pressure.

If you note a sudden increase, call the doctor *immediately*. He may order any (or a combination) of several methods of reducing ICP:
- *controlled hyperventilation with me-*

*chanical ventilation,* to help the patient blow off $CO_2$ (Decreased $CO_2$ constricts cerebral blood vessels and reduces cerebral blood flow, thus reducing ICP.)
- *an additional dose of diuretics,* to reduce fluid volume
- *barbiturates* (usually pentobarbital or phenobarbital) I.V., to the point of unresponsiveness or coma, to decrease the patient's metabolic rate, cerebral blood flow, and ICP
- *CSF withdrawal,* using a ventricular catheter. (The reduction in CSF pressure reduces ICP as well—however, the sudden pressure drop can *cause* the brain herniation it's planned to prevent.)

Assess your patient carefully to detect improvement or deterioration in his condition. Remember to take precautions against seizures for any patient with increased ICP. Pad the side rails of his bed, and keep an airway nearby.

## Therapeutic care

Continue to assess your patient frequently, watching for changes in his neurologic status that may indicate a recurrence of increasing ICP—for example:
- slowing pulse rate (bradycardia)
- widening pulse pressure
- abnormal respiratory patterns, such as Cheyne-Stokes respirations. (See *Abnormal Breathing Patterns Associated with Brain Injury*, page 241.)

When the underlying cause of your patient's increased ICP has been detected (possibly by blood tests, skull X-ray, CT scan), definitive treatment can begin. If *infection* is the primary cause, expect to administer antibiotics, ·as ordered. If your patient has a *brain tumor,* he may require surgical intervention to remove as much of it as possible, followed by radiation or chemotherapy. CT scan may have revealed a *hematoma,* which may need to be evacuated (see the "Subdural Hematoma," "Intracerebral Hematoma," and "Epidural Hematoma" entries in this chapter). A *penetrating wound* may also require surgery. If *hydro-*

*cephalus* (an increase in CSF fluid production) is causing your patient's increased ICP, a shunt tube with a one-way valve may be inserted surgically. This will shunt CSF from the patient's brain directly into his bloodstream or into a body cavity, thereby reducing volume and CSF pressure within the ventricles.

Take measures to prevent your patient's ICP from increasing further:

• Keep his environment quiet.

• Administer stool softeners and avoid giving enemas to prevent straining and Valsalva's maneuver.

• Instruct him to exhale while he's turning or moving in bed.

• Prevent straining due to isometric muscular contractions: help your patient if he needs to sit up, and instruct him not to push against the footboard of the bed.

• Monitor his blood gases frequently.

• Give him oxygen before you suction him, and don't suction him for more than 15 seconds at a time.

If your patient has an ICP monitor in place, watch for signs of infection at the insertion site. Periodically check his white blood cell (WBC) count and temperature, and call the doctor if either is elevated.

When your patient's neurologic status has stabilized, the ICP monitoring will be discontinued, and the doctor will remove the bolt. Continue your neurologic assessments, and maintain accurate intake and output records.

If the patient required mechanical ventilation, the doctor will begin weaning him from the ventilator once his respiratory status has stabilized.

Your patient will require prolonged bed rest while he's being treated. Turn and reposition him frequently; this will help prevent sores and other complications.

Assess the patient for epigastric pain, hematemesis, or tarry bowel movements—these may indicate he's developing a stress ulcer. Check his CBC routinely for decreased hematocrit and hemoglobin levels.

# Skull Fractures

## Prediagnosis summary

In a patient with a history of severe head trauma, initial assessment may have revealed:

• scalp lacerations or contusions, or disruption of his skull contour

• a swollen, tender, ecchymotic area on his scalp

• altered level of consciousness.

An I.V. may have been started for medication access, and blood may have been drawn for routine laboratory tests. He had a skull X-ray and, possibly, a CT scan.

## Priorities

If your patient has scalp lacerations, control any bleeding with temporary, sterile dressings. Reassure your patient that the bleeding, isn't life-threatening. (Make sure he's aware that the blood is coming from his scalp, not from his brain.) Question him about what caused his injury—the details may help you determine the area of the fracture.

Once the patient's scalp bleeding is under control, alert the radiologist and prepare the patient for a skull X-ray or CT scan. Suturing, if necessary, will usually be done after a skull X-ray. Vigorously irrigate the laceration, as ordered, with an antimicrobial agent (such as povidone-iodine) to decrease the patient's susceptibility to meningitis.

As you're probably aware, even a skull X-ray may not show the fracture. *Depressed fractures* and *linear fractures* are usually—but not always—visible on X-ray; *basilar fractures*, however, may not be visible at all. So your thorough assessment can help identify the type and extent of the fracture.

## Continuing assessment and intervention

Begin your assessment by carefully in-

## "THEY'RE GOING TO CUT OPEN MY HEAD?"

Many neurologic emergencies, such as depressed skull fracture or hematoma, require the doctor to perform a craniotomy or to drill burr holes. A patient who needs a craniotomy may be conscious and fearful; his fear and anxiety are likely to reach a peak when he learns he has to have surgery that involves opening his skull. He needs support and reassurance. Use these tips to help your patient understand and accept the brain or cranial surgery he needs:

• Encourage him to ask questions. He probably has a lot of them, but he may not ask them unless you indicate your willingness to talk.

• As needed, clarify what the doctor has told him about the type of surgery he'll be having.

• If you have to shave his head, make sure you tell him his hair will grow back. He may otherwise fear he'll be permanently bald.

• Let him know what to expect after the surgery. Will he go to the intensive care unit? What monitors, tubes, or other special equipment can he expect to wake up with?

• Explain that his personality won't change. Many patients fear that brain surgery will have this effect.

• Let him see his family. He needs their support, and they need to see him. Don't forget to answer their questions as well as you can.

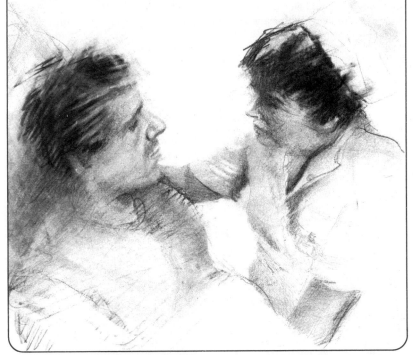

specting your patient's head and scalp for lacerations, contusions, and areas of swelling. Gently palpate his skull—if you feel an indentation, your patient may have a *depressed fracture*. Report this finding to the doctor *immediately*, and *don't probe any further*. This is the doctor's responsibility. He must be very careful, during his examination, to avoid depressing bone fragments farther into the patient's brain.

Once your patient's depressed skull fracture has been confirmed by X-ray (showing fragments of bone pressing in toward the brain), he'll require immediate surgery to elevate the depressed fragments and to repair any laceration. Prepare him for surgery and make sure the results of all ordered tests are on his chart. Take the time to tell your patient why he's having surgery, and explain how it will help him. Remember, cranial surgery is a mysterious and frightening concept for most people. (See *"They're Going To Cut Open My Head?"*, page 249.)

You probably won't be able to feel a *linear fracture*, but you may see a swollen, ecchymotic area on the skull that's tender on palpation. A linear fracture requires no treatment other than bed rest and close observation. Your patient will be admitted for observation for at least 24 hours. Monitor him hourly for any changes in vital signs, level of consciousness, or general appearance, and report any *significant change* to the doctor. It may indicate further brain injury, such as a contusion or hematoma. Linear fractures that cross the vascular grooves are the most common cause of epidural hematoma. (See the "Cerebral Concussion and Contusion" and "Epidural Hematoma" entries in this chapter.)

CSF leaking from the patient's nose or ear indicates a tear in his dura ma-

ter—which, in turn, indicates a possible *basilar fracture* of either the anterior or the middle fossa.

A patient with a basilar fracture of the anterior fossa may have:
• CSF drainage from the nose
• bilateral periorbital ecchymoses ("raccoon's eyes") from bleeding into the sinuses
• altered sense of smell due to olfactory nerve damage
• epistaxis.

If he has a basilar fracture of the middle fossa, you'll note:
• ecchymosis over the mastoid bone (Battle's sign) from bleeding into the area
• hearing loss from CSF buildup behind the intact tympanic membrane and (on otoscopic examination) a bulging tympanic membrane
• CSF drainage from the ear (if the tympanic membrane isn't intact).

Basilar fractures are inoperable. Keep your patient on complete bed rest, with the head of his bed elevated 15° to 30°. Perform a neurologic assessment every hour, using the Glasgow Coma Scale to assess his level of consciousness. (See *Assessing Your Patient's Level of Consciousness Using the Glasgow*

PATHOPHYSIOLOGY

## WHAT HAPPENS IN SKULL FRACTURES

As you know, any head trauma can cause a skull fracture. Classified as *linear, depressed,* or *basilar,* skull fractures are further classified as *simple/closed* (where the tissues overlying the fracture are intact) or *compound/open* (where the bone protrudes through the scalp).

Linear fractures extend lengthwise in the bone and are most common, accounting for about 70% of all skull fractures. If a linear fracture interrupts a major vascular channel, it may cause an intracranial hemorrhage (commonly an epidural hematoma).

A depressed fracture involves an inward depression of bone fragments. This can lacerate the dura (which may result in

central nervous system infection) or compress and lacerate the brain tissue (which may cause an intracerebral hemorrhage).

A basilar fracture involves the base of the skull and can have serious consequences. Not only can it result in cerebrospinal fluid leakage, but it can also injure the internal carotid artery at the point where it enters the skull through the foramen at the skull's base. This may produce severe hemorrhage or an aneurysm. Compression of the cavernous sinus may damage the oculomotor, trochlear, and abducent cranial nerves.

Serious brain damage can accompany any skull fracture.

*Coma Scale,* page 229.) Also check his vital signs hourly. If you note any changes—such as decreased heart rate, increased blood pressure, increased temperature, or decreased respirations—*notify the doctor immediately.*

To prevent further tearing of the dura, tell your patient with a basilar fracture *not* to blow his nose, cough vigorously, or strain. To help prevent infection, tell him *not* to insert anything (such as a tissue or a cotton swab) into his nose or ears, even if fluid is dripping from them. Stress the importance of allowing the fluid to drain freely. To increase your patient's comfort, place a folded gauze pad on his upper lip to catch fluid draining from the nose. For fluid draining from his ear, tape a pad loosely below his ear or on his neck. Make sure you don't obstruct the flow.

Remember, don't insert a nasogastric tube or suction the patient nasally if CSF is draining from his nose—the tube could go through the fracture and the torn dura and into the brain. Administer prophylactic antibiotics, as ordered. If your patient needs surgery to repair his torn dura, that won't be done until the swelling or infection has subsided.

Remember that, in infants, devastating brain injuries may be present with even minor skull injuries. Why? Because an infant's flexible skull resists fracture but provides less protection for cranial contents.

In an *elderly patient,* an open fracture is more apt to lacerate the dura, which adheres more closely to his skull than it does in someone younger.

### Therapeutic care
If your patient had surgery or a basilar skull fracture, watch him closely for signs of infection, ranging from fever, chills, and malaise to signs of meningeal irritation, such as restlessness, headache, stiff neck, or nuchal rigidity. (See the "Meningitis" entry in this chapter.) If he's had surgery, keep his head dressings clean and dry; if they become soiled with blood or drainage, reinforce them, as necessary, to prevent bacterial growth. Check his WBC count for elevated levels. If he suspects infection, the doctor may ask you to administer a systemic antibiotic—penicillin, which crosses the blood-brain barrier, is usually the drug of choice.

The doctor will avoid ordering sedatives or barbiturates if possible—these drugs alter your patient's level of consciousness and so may confuse your assessment of his condition. If your patient's brain integrity has been disrupted, the doctor may ask you to administer anticonvulsant drugs such as diazepam (Valium) or phenytoin (Dilantin). Keep your patient on bed rest, and continue prophylactic drug therapy, as ordered. Continue frequent neurologic assessments, too, until his condition has stabilized and he's ready for discharge.

# Cerebral Concussion and Contusion

### Prediagnosis summary
On initial assessment, the patient had head trauma that may have been followed by a brief period of unconsciousness. He may also have had some combination of the following signs or symptoms:
- blurred or double vision
- headache
- general neurologic deficit
- pallor
- diaphoresis
- fever
- altered respirations
- tachycardia
- disoriented, confused, bizarre, irrational, immature, or socially unrestrained behavior
- expressive or receptive aphasia
- prolonged unconsciousness, with impaired brain stem reflexes and abnormal flexion or extension.

PATHOPHYSIOLOGY

## WHAT HAPPENS IN CEREBRAL CONCUSSION AND CONTUSION

*Cerebral concussion* is a jarring of the brain, usually the result of a direct blow to the patient's head.

A cerebral concussion causes no permanent damage; loss of consciousness is brief (seconds to minutes), and rapid recovery usually follows.

*Cerebral contusion* is a bruising of the brain caused by a direct blow, a contrecoup injury, or acceleration/deceleration forces (for example, when a fast-moving car stops suddenly, hurling the occupant's brain backward against his skull and then forward). Either direct force or rotational and shearing forces tear small blood vessels, causing small hemorrhages and possible edema, and may bruise the brain surface against bony skull ridges.

Loss of consciousness following contusion is prolonged, ranging from many hours to days or weeks. Damage from a contusion can range from mild neurologic deficits to irreversible coma. Cerebral contusion may even cause death.

If his signs and symptoms were severe, he received an I.V. infusion and supplemental oxygen, and he was connected to a cardiac monitor. The doctor ordered a skull X-ray to determine the extent and type of injury.

The doctor diagnosed *cerebral concussion* based on a *brief* period of:
- loss of consciousness
- blurred or double vision
- headache
- disorientation or confusion
- general neurologic deficit
- pallor.

The doctor diagnosed *cerebral contusion* based on finding the same signs and symptoms as for concussion, as well as:
- diaphoresis
- fever
- altered respirations
- tachycardia
- inappropriate behavior
- aphasia
- prolonged unconsciousness.

## Priorities

First, perform a baseline assessment of your patient with a contusion or concussion to help you define the extent of his injury and to let you evaluate changes in his condition. (You'll be performing frequent assessments throughout his treatment, measuring your findings against this baseline.) Remember, if your patient's condition deteriorates, suspect hematoma or cerebral edema, which causes increased ICP.

If your patient has a *contusion*, the doctor will order further tests, such as a CT scan, to visualize the contusion and to determine the extent of cerebral edema. If the patient's breathing is inadequate, expect to assist with intubating and mechanically ventilating him. Remember, if he's also extremely agitated, you may have to use mild sedation before the doctor can proceed with mechanical ventilation. To prevent mistaking drowsiness from the sedation for a deterioration in his status, perform a thorough neurologic assessment *after* he's sedated.

## Continuing assessment and intervention

Frequently assess your patient's level of consciousness, his pupils, and his orientation to time, place, and person. Compare these findings with earlier ones. If he has a *concussion,* he may be disoriented. (A young child with a concussion may also have a generalized seizure. If he does, reassure his parents that his seizure's due to the injury and probably won't recur.)

If you find other mental status abnormalities in your patient, he may have a cerebral *contusion.* For example, if he behaves in a bizarre, irrational, or immature manner and has expressive aphasia, he may have a *frontal lobe* contusion. Remember, your patient can't control his behavior; he needs your support and understanding. If he exhibits receptive aphasia, he may have a *temporal lobe* contusion. If your unconscious patient with a contusion has abnormal flexion (decorticate posturing) or abnormal extension (decerebrate posturing), suspect a *brain stem* contusion. Contusion-caused focal or generalized neurologic deficits may be permanent.

While you assess your patient, take his history. Ask if the patient recalls the trauma that caused his injury. A patient with a concussion may report a period of amnesia extending from just before the injury to the end of his brief unconscious period. If anyone was with the patient when he was injured, ask that person how long the patient was unconscious. Find out if your patient has any preexisting medical problems that may affect his treatment or recovery. Ask if he's ever had a neurologic disorder. For example, if he's confused, this may be due to progressive atherosclerosis rather than to his injury. Of course, if the patient's unconscious, a friend or family member will have to answer your questions.

### Therapeutic care

Your patient with an uncomplicated concussion may be discharged in the care of a responsible family member if you've found no further abnormalities. The doctor may ask the family member to awaken the patient briefly every hour throughout the first night he's home. Why? Because in this way, the family member can quickly check the patient's mental status for any changes. Before you discharge the patient, teach the family member how to assess the patient's consciousness level, motor response, and pupil size. Instruct him to watch for:
• vomiting
• double vision
• weakness
• headache
• convulsions
• blood or fluid draining from the nose or ears
• personality changes
• altered level of consciousness.

Be sure to have the family member return the patient to the hospital if these or other changes occur. Be aware that postconcussion syndrome—headache, personality changes, dizziness, tinnitus, diplopia, ataxia, irritability, and poor concentration and memory—can last for years after the injury.

If the patient had a *cerebral contusion*, expect to give him corticosteroids, such as dexamethasone (Decadron). Corticosteroids may decrease cerebral edema, which can follow a cerebral contusion, and prevent severely increased ICP as well. Expect to restrict the patient's fluid intake—this helps decrease cerebral edema, too. Always watch for signs and symptoms of increased ICP; these include altered level of consciousness, headache, and disturbances in vision.

The patient with a large cerebral contusion and severe cerebral edema with increased ICP may become unconscious. If unconsciousness occurs, expect to use ICP monitoring, to give him osmotic diuretics, and, possibly, to ventilate him mechanically for controlled hyperventilation (see the "Increased Intracranial Pressure" entry in this chapter). If a ventricular shift accompanies this pressure effect, the doctor may need to remove the contused lobe to prevent further deterioration. Expect to prepare the patient for surgery if this operation is needed.

If your patient had surgery, watch for signs and symptoms of infection:
• Check the surgical dressing and the area around the surgery site for signs of a local infection—oozing, purulent or bloody drainage, and redness.
• Check for signs and symptoms of meningeal irritation or inflammation—for example, nuchal rigidity or fever. (See the "Meningitis" entry in this chapter.) If you suspect infection, expect to draw blood for a CBC, and check the results for an increased WBC count. The doctor will treat the infection with an appropriate antibiotic.

In your patient with cerebral edema and increased ICP, monitoring will be discontinued as soon as his ICP and neurologic status are normal. He'll be weaned from the ventilator when his status is stable. Continue to assess his neurologic status, just as a precaution. Keep an accurate fluid intake and output record to ensure proper hydration.

If the patient's treatment involved long-term hospitalization, watch for signs and symptoms of a developing stress ulcer, including:
• epigastric pain
• hematemesis
• tarry stools (melena).

If you suspect an ulcer, expect to draw blood for a CBC. Check the laboratory results—bleeding will cause decreased hemoglobin and hematocrit levels.

# Epidural Hematoma

## Prediagnosis summary
The patient had a history of head trauma and brief unconsciousness, followed by a lucid interval. During the lucid interval, the patient may have had any or all of the following signs and symptoms:
• severe headache
• nausea
• vomiting
• bladder distention
• decreased level of consciousness, progressing from drowsiness to deep coma
• unilateral hemiparesis or hemiplegia
• jacksonian seizures
• unilateral or ipsilateral fixed and/or dilated pupils
• high fever, bradycardia, hypertension
• abnormal extension (decerebrate posturing).

An I.V. was started to keep his vein open and to provide access for medications. The doctor inserted a bladder catheter to relieve distention and to provide for accurate measurements of urine output. If he suspected increased ICP, the doctor may have given the patient osmotic diuretics and corticoste-

roids. If the patient was vomiting, the doctor may have inserted a nasogastric tube to prevent aspiration. The patient received supplemental oxygen or was intubated and mechanically ventilated, depending on his respiratory status. He was connected to a cardiac monitor, and an EKG was taken. Blood was drawn for ABGs, electrolytes, CBC, clotting profile, and typing and cross matching.

The doctor may have ordered one or more of these diagnostic studies:
• a CT scan and—if time permitted—an arteriogram or echoencephalogram to determine the extent and location of the injury
• a lumbar puncture—if no signs of increased ICP were present—which showed increased CSF pressure
• a skull X-ray, which most likely revealed a linear fracture crossing over the middle meningeal artery.

## Priorities
The first priority for the patient with an epidural hematoma is *prompt* removal of the hematoma and ligation of the bleeding site. Before surgery, make sure that the patient's preoperative laboratory results and his drug allergies are recorded on his chart. Because of the urgency of the patient's condition, the operating room staff will shave him and prepare him for surgery.

*Never* leave your patient alone during procedures or further diagnostic tests, such as CT scans, X-rays, or echoencephalograms. Stay with him to watch for sudden signs of deterioration, which can develop rapidly at any time.

Remember to provide emotional support to your patient before he has surgery to remove the hematoma. If your patient's conscious, his severe headache may make him very anxious, which may increase his ICP.

## Continuing assessment and intervention
After your patient's surgery, perform a thorough neurologic assessment to establish a baseline to measure subse-

quent changes against. Watch for signs and symptoms of increasing ICP (see the "Increased Intracranial Pressure" entry in this chapter). These include altered respirations, deteriorating level of consciousness, and disturbances in vision.

Evaluate your patient's respiratory status and use his ABG results to assess him for hypoxia and hypercapnia, which can cause cerebral edema. Monitor his fluid status closely, too, by accurately measuring and recording his intake and output. Expect to keep your patient slightly dehydrated by restricting his fluid intake. Why? Because this precaution helps reduce cerebral edema.

Record his temperature frequently— at least every 4 hours. If he's febrile, notify the doctor. A significant rise in body temperature may suggest neurologic damage or an infection. It also increases the metabolic demands of the brain (which can increase ICP).

Keep the head of the bed elevated 30° to enhance venous drainage from the patient's brain. Check the surgical dressing and the area around it for signs of excessive bleeding or drainage. Reinforce the dressings if they become stained with blood or secretions.

### Therapeutic care
You may expect to give your patient an analgesic, such as codeine, to control his pain. But remember to avoid giving any strong narcotic medication, because this may affect the patient's level of consciousness and falsify your neurologic assessments. The doctor may ask you to give corticosteroids to reduce the cerebral edema that may develop after surgery. Expect to give antibiotics to prevent infection and anticonvulsants to prevent seizures.

Be sure to monitor your patient's electrolytes for any sodium, potassium, or chloride imbalances. Uncorrected electrolyte imbalances can cause an altered level of consciousness (ranging from lethargy to stupor) that you may mistake for a neurologic deficit.

# Subdural Hematoma

### Prediagnosis summary
On initial assessment, the patient had a history of head trauma and may have had:
- headache
- fever
- unilateral pupil dilation
- papilledema
- hemiparesis or hemiplegia.

He may also have had signs and symptoms of increased ICP, such as changed breathing patterns and marked systolic hypertension (see the "Increased Intracranial Pressure" entry in this chapter). As his brain compression increased, the patient may have become increasingly dull and lethargic and may have exhibited focal neurologic changes. His signs and symptoms may have been confusingly similar to those of stroke, tumor, or even senility.

The doctor ordered a CT scan and may also have ordered a magnetic resonance imaging (MRI) or a digital subtraction angiography (DSA) scan if the equipment was available (see *What Are D.S.A. and M.R.I.?*, pages 260 and 261). He may have done a lumbar puncture to check for blood in the CSF *unless* he noted signs and symptoms of increased ICP, a contraindication for this procedure.

The emergency team quickly assessed the patient's respiratory status. Depending on the severity of his respiratory inadequacy, he was given supplemental oxygen by nasal cannula or was intubated and connected to a mechanical ventilator. An I.V. line and a bladder catheter were inserted, and he was connected to a cardiac monitor.

### Priorities
The first priority is immediate removal of the subdural hematoma. Prepare your patient for surgery. Obtain a brief patient history to determine medica-

PATHOPHYSIOLOGY

# WHAT HAPPENS IN INTRACRANIAL HEMATOMA

### Epidural hematoma

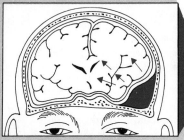

Bleeding between the skull and dura mater into the epidural space

Laceration of middle meningeal artery and/or vein, often resulting from a fracture, is the most common source of bleeding. But bleeding may also result from a tear in a dural sinus.

### Intracerebral hematoma

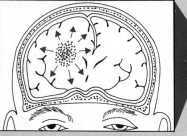

Bleeding deep within the cerebral hemispheres

Cerebral contusion or concussion is a common cause.

### Subdural hematoma

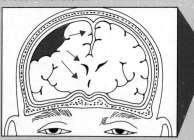

Bleeding between the arachnoid membrane and the dura mater in the subdural space
*Acute* within 48 hours
*Subacute* from 2 days to 2 weeks
*Chronic* over 2 weeks

Bleeding usually occurs from a torn bridging vein or cortical vessel or (less commonly) from a ruptured saccular aneurysm or an intracerebral hemorrhage.

As you may know, three types of intracranial hematomas can result from head trauma: epidural, intracerebral, and subdural. (Subdural hematomas are classified as acute, subacute, or chronic, depending on how much time passes between the injury and the appearance of your patient's signs and symptoms.) Epidural hematomas have the highest mortality; however, any intracranial hematoma that's left untreated is life-threatening. This flowchart explains the pathophysiology of intracranial hematomas.

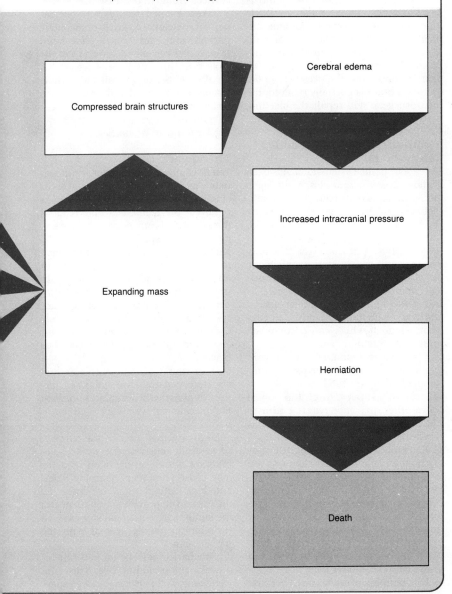

tion use and allergies and any current or recent illness or surgery. Expect to draw blood for preoperative laboratory studies, including type and cross matching.

The neurosurgeon will remove your patient's subdural hematoma by evacuating the clot, either through a *burr hole* (if the clot is *fluid*) or by *intracranial surgery* (if the clot is *solid*). He may order the surgery to be done immediately—without a CT scan or skull X-ray—if the patient's condition is deteriorating rapidly. After enough of the clot is removed so the pressure on the patient's brain is partially relieved, the neurosurgeon will repair the bleeding vessel and remove any remaining clot.

## Continuing assessment and intervention

After your patient's hematoma has been removed, watch him closely for signs and symptoms of its recurrence. Establish a complete neurologic baseline by assessing his level of consciousness, mental status, motor function, pupillary reaction, and vital signs. The doctor may ask you to start prophylactic antibiotic therapy, using a broad-spectrum antibiotic. You also may be asked to administer an anticonvulsant, such as phenytoin (Dilantin), to prevent seizures, which can occur when brain tissue is irritated.

Continue to monitor your patient's respiratory status. If your patient's intubated, maintain good pulmonary hygiene by supervising his chest physiotherapy, encouraging him to deep breathe, and suctioning, as needed.

Remember that increasing ICP may accompany subdural hematoma, so you should take precautions to avoid increasing it *further*. Keep in mind that the patient who's had a burr hole drilled is at higher risk for developing increased ICP than one who's had intracranial surgery. Here are some measures for preventing increased ICP in a patient with a burr hole:

• Tell your patient *not* to cough because

this can increase ICP.
• Elevate his head 30° to 60°—if his condition permits—to promote venous drainage from his brain.
• Avoid placing him in a jackknife position, which further increases ICP.
• Expect to administer osmotic diuretics, such as mannitol, and perhaps corticosteroids to decrease ICP.

Take a detailed history from your patient, if you can. An elderly or alcoholic patient may not recall past head trauma, so you might have to get the facts from his family or a friend. (A family member may recall a seemingly minor head injury that the patient has forgotten.) Ask if the patient's had mental status changes, psychomotor slowing, or frequent headaches.

## Therapeutic care

You'll continue to monitor your patient's neurologic status and vital signs closely. If a large subdural clot was removed, the hematoma may recur if the patient's brain doesn't fully reexpand to fill the space where the original hematoma was. This is most common in elderly patients because of brain atrophy. The doctor may ask you to help prevent this by placing the elderly patient in the head-down position after surgery and by keeping him generously hydrated. Provide scrupulous care for any subdural drains the doctor has placed.

Once your patient's neurologic and respiratory status have stabilized, expect to assist with weaning him from the mechanical ventilator and extubating him.

Be aware that, even if the surgeon successfully removes your patient's hematoma, other severe head injuries may cause permanent neurologic deficit, long-lasting coma, or death. So make sure you provide your patient and his family with emotional support and time for the family to visit with the patient alone.

Your patient will be on bed rest for a prolonged period of time. Turn him frequently, and perform passive range-of-motion exercises to prevent formation of pressure sores and to enhance circulation.

# Intracerebral Hematoma

## Prediagnosis summary

Initial assessment findings may have included:
- recent or weeks-old head trauma
- headache
- dizziness
- nausea and vomiting
- seizures
- hemiparesis or hemiplegia
- altered level of consciousness or gradually deteriorating mental status
- cranial nerve dysfunction
- pupillary changes—dilation, constriction, abnormal light response (see *Understanding Pupillary Changes,* page 230)
- bradycardia
- hypertension
- altered breathing patterns
- abnormal flexion (decorticate posturing) or abnormal extension (decerebrate posturing).

If the patient's respirations were inadequate, he received supplemental oxygen by nasal cannula or by intubation and mechanical ventilation, depending on the severity of his respiratory deficiency. He had a CT scan to determine the location and extent of the injury. The doctor may have done a lumbar puncture to look for bloody CSF unless he found signs of increased ICP, which contraindicates this procedure.

## Priorities

The first medical priority, ideally, is removal of the hematoma—but surgery may not be feasible. The doctor will evaluate the results of the patient's CT scan, or he may order a cerebral angiogram to make this determination. If he *can* operate, prepare your patient for surgery. If the CT scan showed blood in the ventricular system, the doctor may insert an intraventricular cerebral drain before he operates.

If the doctor *can't* operate, your first priority is to watch your patient closely for evidence of increased ICP, which often accompanies intracerebral hematoma (see the "Increased Intracranial Pressure" entry in this chapter). Signs and symptoms include altered level of consciousness, disturbances in vision, altered respirations, and pupillary changes. The doctor will probably insert an arterial line for continuous blood pressure monitoring. Expect to assist with placement of an ICP monitoring sensor (see *Understanding Intracranial Pressure Monitors,* page 246). Check his ICP frequently by watching the monitor. Insert an indwelling (Foley) catheter to accurately measure urine output. Carefully document all your measurements.

## Continuing assessment and intervention

Perform a thorough assessment of your patient. You'll use your findings as a baseline for evaluating improvement or deterioration in his condition. Take his vital signs and note any increased bradycardia, increased hypertension, or respiratory pattern changes. Watch for signs of decreased level of consciousness, which accompanies a deterioration of the patient's condition. Continue to check pupil size and reaction. If his deterioration is extreme, you may see abnormal flexion (decorticate posturing) or abnormal extension (decerebrate posturing). (See the "Coma" entry in this chapter.)

Remember this: No matter what your patient's diagnosis is or how stable his condition seems, if he has a history of recent head injury, he can develop an intracerebral hematoma even weeks after the injury. So watch this type of patient carefully for signs of increased ICP. An elderly or alcoholic patient may develop a hematoma but have no recollection of a head injury. Elderly peo-

# WHAT ARE D.S.A. AND M.R.I.?

When the doctor examines your patient with a neurologic emergency, his tentative diagnosis is epidural hematoma. He turns to you and says, "Let's get a DSA on him."
   Would you know what to do? What if the doctor ordered "an MRI" instead?
   As you probably know, the computerized tomography (CT) scan is the most widely used

## WHAT IT IS

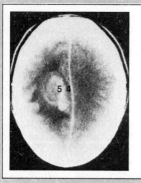

### DSA: Digital subtraction angiography

DSA is a type of intravenous arteriography. It combines X-ray methods and a computerized subtraction technique with fluoroscopy for visualization without interference from adjacent structures, such as bone or soft tissue.

1   Edema

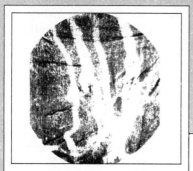

### MRI: Magnetic resonance imaging

A noninvasive imaging technique that detects structural and biochemical abnormalities by directing magnetic and radio waves at body tissues to determine the nuclear response of a test element—hydrogen.

2   Hematoma mass (left parietal lobe)
3   L internal carotid blockage

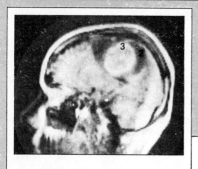

### CT: Computerized tomography
(Note: Some health-care professionals still refer to this procedure as computerized axial tomography [CAT].)

A noninvasive X-ray technique that produces a series of tomograms, translated by a computer and displayed on an oscilloscope screen, representing cross-sectional images of various tissue layers.

4   Edema
5   Hyperdense mass (left parietal lobe)

diagnostic tool for locating an area of injury such as a hematoma. But two new computerized diagnostic tests, in addition to the CT scan, are available: digital subtraction angiography (DSA) and magnetic resonance imaging (MRI)—formerly referred to as nuclear magnetic resonance, or NMR. These tests also produce detailed images of body tissue for evaluating areas of injury or disease. Here's information about DSA and MRI plus comparative information on the CT scan.

## HOW IT WORKS

## BENEFITS

A contrast dye's injected through a catheter threaded into a large vein. As the contrast dye circulates through the arteries, X-rays are taken. The computer then projects the image onto a screen, automatically "subtracting" structures that block a clear view of the arteries and leaving only the vessels being studied.

DSA can be performed quickly, even on an outpatient basis, and is an excellent tool for visualizing cerebral blood flow and detecting vascular abnormalities or disruptions, such as aneurysms, tumors, and hematomas. Because the dye's injected into a vein, risk of arterial bleeding is eliminated.

MRI uses a resistive magnet that creates a magnetic field via electricity. (*Note:* This magnet can affect pacemaker function.) This magnet causes the body's hydrogen protons to align themselves in its field. They're then bombarded with radio frequency signals, causing them to move out of alignment. When the radio signal stops, these energized protons emit a return signal. A computer analyzes both this signal and the time it takes the protons to return to their original alignment. (The time and signal vary with each tissue type.) Eventually, the hydrogen pattern's converted into an image of body tissue.

MRI doesn't use ionizing radiation (X-rays), so it's safer than CT scanning or DSA. It doesn't use contrast dye, either, as DSA (and sometimes CT) does, so fluid balance problems are eliminated. It provides greater tissue discrimination than CT scanning and allows serial studies to be done safely, especially in children and pregnant women. In the future, it may allow visualization of blood flow.

CT scanners use a large circular X-ray beam in a full circle around the patient's body or the area being studied. The computer then puts the information into cross-sectional pictures, eliminating the obstructive shadows that appear in single X-rays. Contrast dye can be injected I.V. to enhance tissue density.

CT scanners are widely available as a diagnostic tool; many hospitals have their own. By discriminating among minute tissue density variations, this procedure can help confirm a diagnosis such as hematoma or tumor. It may eliminate the need for more hazardous and painful invasive procedures.

ple often fall during TIAs; alcoholics, during seizures or blackouts. Ask a family member if he can recall the head trauma that may have led to the patient's hematoma.

Continue to check your patient's ICP often by watching his ICP monitor. Also measure his fluid intake and output carefully, and keep an accurate record of your measurements. Expect to give osmotic diuretics, corticosteroids, barbiturates, or anticonvulsants to control his increased ICP. You may also expect to assist with controlled hyperventilation using a mechanical ventilator.

If your patient has had surgery, continue to monitor his ICP, neurologic status, and vital signs frequently. Inspect the dressing for any signs of increased bleeding or drainage at the surgical site. Because hematoma causes too much brain hemorrhage and cell damage for successful surgical repair, the surgery usually has poor results.

### Therapeutic care

Continue to assess your patient's vital signs and neurologic status and to monitor his intake and output and his ICP. (Maintaining your patient's fluid restriction will help reduce increased ICP.) He'll probably be unconscious and require prolonged hospitalization while the intracerebral bleeding stops and the clot is absorbed. So familiarize yourself with the prolonged-care measures you'll have to provide:

• If his eyes are open, you will have to instill artificial tears to prevent corneal irritation.

• Turn the patient and change his position every 2 hours to prevent pressure sores.

• Frequently perform passive range-of-motion exercises for all his extremities.

• Provide meticulous mouth care at least once every 8 hours.

• The patient will probably be fed via nasogastric tube or total parenteral nutrition.

• Perform chest physiotherapy and postural drainage to loosen secretions and facilitate their removal.

• Suction him as often as necessary to keep his endotracheal tube clear and to prevent pulmonary complications.

Give the patient's family emotional support. Explain the poor prognosis and the need for prolonged hospitalization. To help family members feel needed, let them care for and visit with the patient as much as hospital policy permits.

# Spinal Cord Injury

## Prediagnosis summary

The patient's signs and symptoms may have included:

• neck or back pain
• vertebral tenderness or deformity
• extremity numbness or tingling
• muscle weakness or paralysis
• reflex asymmetry or absence of reflexes
• bowel and bladder incontinence
• hypotension
• bradycardia
• respiratory insufficiency.

If the patient's spine wasn't immobilized before his arrival, he was placed on a long backboard and a Philadelphia collar was applied in the ED to prevent further spinal cord damage. The patient had an I.V. line established for medication access and fluid administration, and he was placed on a cardiac monitor. If he had respiratory insufficiency, he was given oxygen by Ambu bag until X-ray results identified the injury site (intubation may have required a specialist if the cervical spine was injured). If his respirations were sufficient, he was given supplemental oxygen by nasal cannula or mask.

The doctor immediately evaluated all seven of the patient's cervical vertebrae by examining these X-ray film views:

• cross-table lateral view with downward arm traction
• anteroposterior view
• odontoid view.

## Priorities

Your initial priorities are to control the patient's respirations, blood pressure, heart rate, and temperature, which may all be affected by sympathetic nervous system loss from spinal cord injury. Of course, you'll need to use extreme caution when handling the patient, to avoid injuring him further.

If his cord injury is between *C1 and C4*, he'll be completely unable to breathe, so you'll continue to ventilate him with an Ambu bag until he can be intubated and mechanically ventilated. Usually, a doctor highly skilled in intubation (such as an anesthesiologist) will perform the procedure, because it's difficult to do without hyperextending the patient's neck and causing further damage. The doctor may intubate nasally or orally, using a fiberoptic scope to aid in placement. The patient with this type of cord injury will require lifelong ventilation and supportive care.

If the patient's injury is in the *C4 to C8* area, he'll be breathing diaphragmatically and probably won't need immediate intubation. But keep intubation and tracheostomy supplies on hand, because he may tire quickly. He'll have a paralytic ileus, which can lead to abdominal distention. Anticipate inserting a nasogastric tube to prevent aspiration of vomit and to help secure his airway.

Cord injury may cause sympathetic nervous system loss below the level of injury, resulting in neurogenic shock (see Chapter 14, SHOCK). The patient will have low systolic blood pressure (100 mm Hg or less), bradycardia (60 beats/minute or less), and a loss of overall vascular tone. If you suspect spinal shock, place the patient in a supine position and administer fluids, as necessary. Monitor flow rate carefully—fluid overload may be dangerous for the patient in spinal shock. If his hypotension and bradycardia are severe, the doctor will order vasopressors, such as dopamine and dobutamine (Dobutrex). Expect to assist in insertion of an arterial line and, possibly, a Swan-Ganz catheter, which will help you evaluate your patient's blood pressure and volume status, and titrate his drug infusion.

You may find blood pressure control difficult because of your patient's sympathetic nervous system loss. In addition, severe muscle spasms or bladder distention can cause hypertension. Expect to give diazepam (Valium) to reduce muscle spasm and to help reduce his hypertension. You may give trimethaphan camsylate (Arfonad), phentolamine hydrochloride (Regitine), or hydralazine hydrochloride (Apresoline) if the patient's hypertension is severe.

Insert an indwelling (Foley) catheter to monitor your patient's fluid intake and output. The catheter will also prevent bladder distention, which can cause severe hypertension, diaphoresis, shivering, and bradycardia due to abnormal sympathetic nervous system reflexes.

The patient may rapidly develop hypothermia or hyperthermia. Even the patient's room temperature may affect his body temperature. Monitor his body temperature by rectal probe: he'll probably become *hypothermic*. If he does, place him in a warm area and cover him with blankets. If his hypothermia is severe, use a warming mattress and administer heated aerosol oxygen by mask or ventilator. Remember that hypothermia and hypoxemia aggravate bradycardia.

If he becomes *hyperthermic,* place him in a cool area with good ventilation. If he's severely hyperthermic, provide a hypothermia blanket or give him a tepid bath.

If your patient needs suctioning, oxygenate him first. Watch his cardiac monitor while suctioning—the vasovagal reflex can cause cardiac arrest during this procedure.

## Continuing assessment and intervention

Before you begin a thorough assess-

## UNDERSTANDING SPINAL CORD SYNDROMES

### CENTRAL CORD SYNDROME

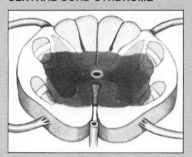

- Results from hyperextension or flexion injuries
- Causes greater loss of motor function in the patient's arms than in his legs
- Causes slight sensory loss

### ANTERIOR CORD SYNDROME

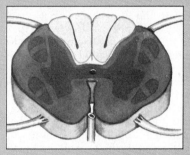

- Usually results from flexion injuries
- Causes loss of upper and lower motor neuron function (voluntary and reflex motor activity)
- Causes loss of temperature and pain sensation
- Causes *no* loss of patient's ability to sense light touch, vibration, and pressure

ment, the doctor will provide more permanent stabilization of your patient's spine. If the patient has a stable minor fracture, he may require only a firm cervical collar. (Soft cervical collars don't give adequate support for fracture healing—they're more appropriate for providing comfortable head support for patients with whiplash injuries.)

If, however, your patient has a fracture of the cervical vertebrae (especially if he also has a dislocation), he'll require external skull traction by skull tongs or a halo traction device (see *Using Traction to Immobilize a Spinal Cord–Injured Patient*, page 271). Assist the doctor in applying skull traction. He may ask you to administer muscle relaxants, such as diazepam (Valium), to keep spasms in the patient's neck from interfering with alignment. Items to have ready include:
- sterilized trays
- appropriate torque wrenches
- traction ropes and weights
- local anesthetics.

During the procedure, support the patient emotionally—he'll feel some pain and pressure, and you may not be able to administer narcotic agents because of their respiratory depressant effect. Let him know that his pain will decrease once the traction device is applied and the fracture is stabilized.

After your patient's spine is stabilized, perform a thorough assessment and take his history. This will help you determine the mechanism of injury and the probable extent of his dysfunction (see *Understanding Spinal Cord Syndromes*, above, and *Nurse's Guide to Understanding Motor and Sensory Impairment in Complete Cord Injury*, pages 268 and 269).

(Remember that an elderly patient's spinal cord is tightly encased in vertebrae that may be studded with bony spurs or shrunken around the cord.

If your patient's spinal cord is only partially severed, his clinical picture may reflect all or some of the signs and symptoms of one or several syndromes. He may even exhibit a combination of signs and symptoms from more than one syndrome.

## BROWN-SÉQUARD SYNDROME

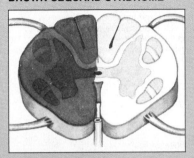

- Results from flexion-rotation injuries or from penetration injuries
- Causes complete motor loss on the ipsilateral side of the patient's injury
- Causes complete loss of pain and temperature sensation on the contralateral side of injury

## POSTERIOR CORD SYNDROME

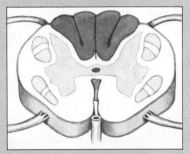

- Results from cervical hyperextension injuries
- Causes loss of light touch sensation and proprioception
- Motor function of extremities preserved

This means that even a minor fall can cause severe cord damage. In elderly women, osteoporosis can cause compression fractures even without a history of trauma.)

Ask your patient how his injury happened. Did he hyperextend, hyperflex, or compress his spine during the trauma? *Hyperextension* of the cervical spine, without fracture or dislocation, may cause central cord syndrome. *Hyperflexion* of the cervical spine, in contrast, may cause fracture and cord injury. *Spinal compression* may cause anterior cord syndrome.

Was your patient's spinal cord physiologically severed completely or only partially? Was his injury caused by herniation or by penetration? *Hemisection* of the cord (commonly caused by a traumatic lateral disk herniation or by a penetrating injury) may cause Brown-Séquard syndrome, whereas *complete transection* causes spinal shock and total loss of sensory and motor function below the level of injury. *Rotational* stress usually causes fracture, dislocation, or vascular injury and accompanying cord injury.

Assess your patient's gross motor and sensory function to help you determine the extent of injury. Ask him if he feels any weakness, numbness, or paralysis. Use his answers to guide your assessment of his motor and sensory function. Examine the patient's biceps, triceps, wrists, hands, hips, knees, and ankles. Ask him to flex both arms at the elbow, to open and close his fingers, to lift his legs from the bed, and to wiggle his toes. Press down against the patient's shoulder while he shrugs. Have him push against your hand with his hands, arms, legs, and feet so you can assess his motor strength (controlled by the pyramidal tracts). Grade his strength as normal, moderate, minimal, severe weakness, or paralysis. Be sure you re-

PATHOPHYSIOLOGY

# WHAT HAPPENS IN SPINAL CORD INJURY

Traumatic spinal lesions (such as contusions, lacerations, vertebral fractures, or hemorrhages) disrupt the intercommunication of the patient's spinal cord, brain, and the rest of his body. The injury may cause loss of both voluntary and autonomic motor activity. The lesion's location (cervical, thoracic, lumbar, or sacral) and the type of cord injury determine how much motor and sensory function the patient loses.

Types of spinal cord injuries include flexion, flexion-rotation, hyperextension, compression, and penetration injuries. Here's what you should know about how these types of spinal cord injuries occur.

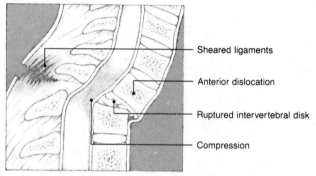

— Sheared ligaments

— Anterior dislocation

— Ruptured intervertebral disk

— Compression

*Flexion injury* frequently involves the cervical and lumbar spine. This type of injury generally results from impact to the posterior fossa that propels the patient's neck onto his chest, causing anterior dislocation, a ruptured intervertebral disc, or possibly, a fractured pedicle, vertebral body, or wedge fracture. With any vertebral fracture, if the ligamentous support to the vertebral column is also disrupted, the spinal cord's stability and integrity are jeopardized.

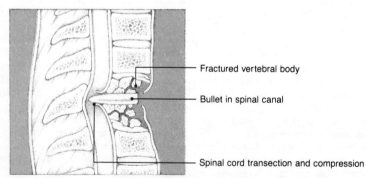

— Fractured vertebral body

— Bullet in spinal canal

— Spinal cord transection and compression

*Penetration injury* occurs when a penetrating object shatters a vertebral body or the ligamentous support on entry to the patient's spinal canal. Spinal cord tissue's damaged or transected, causing hemorrhage, compression, and infarction. In penetration injuries, as in all types of spinal cord injuries, edema may result from trauma, causing further compression above and below the level of injury.

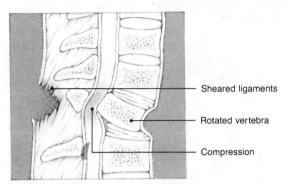

Sheared ligaments

Rotated vertebra

Compression

**Flexion-rotation injury** occurs when the patient's head and body are twisted in opposite directions, dislocating cervical vertebrae and shearing supporting ligaments. The resulting vertebral malalignment compresses the spinal column.

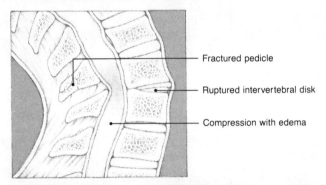

Fractured pedicle

Ruptured intervertebral disk

Compression with edema

**Hyperextension injury** occurs when the patient's head is thrown back sharply, disrupting various supporting ligaments, rupturing intervertebral disks, and fracturing one or more vertebral bodies or pedicles. This compresses the patient's spine and makes it unstable.

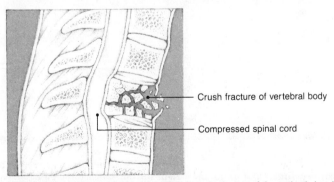

Crush fracture of vertebral body

Compressed spinal cord

**Compression injury** results from a vertical force to the top of the patient's head or from an upward force to his feet, often due to a fall from an extreme height. This causes a crush fracture of a vertebral body with impingement on the cord or nerve roots.

## NURSE'S GUIDE TO UNDERSTANDING MOTOR AND SENSORY IMPAIRMENT IN COMPLETE CORD INJURY

| | | SPINAL AREA AFFECTED |
|---|---|---|
| | Cervical nerve roots | C1 to C4 |
| | | C5 to C8 |
| | Thoracic nerve roots | T1 to T6 |
| | | T7 to T12 |
| | Lumbar nerve roots | L1 to L3 |
| | | L4 to L5 |
| | Sacral nerve roots | S1 to S5 |

cord all your findings.

Assess sensory function (spinothalamic tracts) with pinprick testing over the patient's hands, arms, chest, abdomen, groin, and thighs. Use a clean pin, and make sure you don't perforate the skin. Note any areas where the patient has *no* sensory response. Record these areas and those with some sensory loss by describing their distance from anatomical landmarks. Starting at the patient's toes, gently tap his skin

| TYPE OF MOTOR LOSS | AREA OF SENSORY LOSS (PAIN, TEMPERATURE, TOUCH, AND PRESSURE) |
|---|---|
| • Diaphragm paresis<br>• Intercostal paralysis<br>• Flaccid total paralysis in skeletal muscles below neck | • Neck and below |
| • Intercostal paralysis<br>• Paralysis below shoulders and upper arms | • Arms and hands, chest, abdomen, and lower extremities |
| • Paralysis below midchest | • Below midchest |
| • Paralysis below waist | • Below waist |
| • Paralysis in most leg muscles and in pelvis | • Lower abdomen and legs |
| • Paralysis in lower legs, ankles, feet | • Parts of lower legs and feet |
| • Ataxic paralysis of the bladder and rectum<br>• Paralysis of feet and ankles | • Posterior inner thigh, lateral foot, perineum |

over the same areas. Again, record your findings. You can test temperature sensation by applying test tubes filled with hot and cold water to the same areas, but this usually isn't necessary. Remember that if your patient has spinal shock, you'll see complete flaccid paralysis of all skeletal muscles and an absence of sensation and spinal reflexes.

Assess your patient's proprioception and vibration (posterior columns). Ask him to close his eyes and tell you if his finger or toe is being moved toward or away from his head. Hold a vibrating tuning fork to your patient's bony prominences and soft tissues, and ask if he feels the vibration. Remember that touch is controlled both by spinothalamic tracts and by posterior columns, so your patient may be able to feel the tuning fork itself but not its vibrations.

Check your patient's pupil size and response to light. If he has damaged cranial nerves due to cervical cord injury, watch for constriction of one or both pupils, for ptosis of the upper eyelid, and for a loss of sweating on the affected side of the face (Horner's syndrome).

Of course, record all your findings to establish a baseline and to detect any changes. Some of your patient's dysfunction may be the result of spinal shock, edema, or bleeding, so some function may eventually return. You may initially be unable to distinguish complete cord transection with spinal shock from a lesser injury with spinal shock; so *never* tell your patient, at this point, that his paralysis is permanent.

The doctor may want to complete the neurologic examination to explore the patient's spinal cord injury in greater detail.

Your patient may need further diagnostic tests to pinpoint his injury. The doctor may order:
• *spinal series*—to show dislocation or degeneration
• *CT scan*—to identify lesions difficult to see on X-rays
• *myelogram*—if he suspects occlusion of the spinal subarachnoid space or if the pathology's unclear.

Your patient may need surgery if the diagnostic test results show spinal cord compression—by bone, vertebral disk, or blood clot—or a spinal fracture that can't be reduced any other way. Surgery usually involves both fusion and wiring to prevent dislocation and to promote healing. Prepare your patient for surgery as necessary—make sure all ordered blood tests and X-rays are done

and recorded on his chart. Provide emotional support for your patient and his family.

## Therapeutic care

If your patient had surgery, he may return with a body cast. A special bed, such as a Stryker frame or Roto Rest bed, may be used to prevent long-term immobilization complications and to facilitate his care if the patient has a cast or traction. Provide wound, catheter, and skin care as necessary. Don't forget psychological support—these beds are frightening. If a special bed isn't used, you'll have to logroll your patient whenever you move him.

Monitor your patient's respiratory status closely. Of course, if his injury is in the C1 to C4 area, he'll stay on a ventilator. If his injury is in the C5 to C8 area, his diaphragmatic breathing will cause decreased tidal volume and vital capacity. Measure these parameters to detect progress or deterioration, and monitor his ABGs. Encourage your patient to deep breathe to maximally expand his lungs. The physical therapist will teach your patient diaphragmatic coughing to improve pulmonary function and to prevent infection and other pulmonary complications. You may provide humidified air (with or without additional oxygen) to help him clear secretions. Assess his breath sounds: if you detect rales, he may be receiving too much fluid. If your patient coughs up purulent sputum, send a specimen to the laboratory for culture and sensitivity testing so appropriate antibiotics can be ordered.

Monitor your patient's cardiovascular status, too. Watch his blood pressure—initial instability is usually self-limiting. When his blood pressure's stable, his arterial line will be removed. If he's intubated, remember to preoxygenate him and to suction for brief periods because, during suctioning, the vasovagal reflex can cause cardiac arrest. He may develop venous stasis and thrombosis in his legs and

# USING TRACTION TO IMMOBILIZE A SPINAL CORD-INJURED PATIENT

Your spinal cord–injured patient will have to be immobilized for as long as 1 to 3 months. For this, his doctor may use skull tongs, such as Gardner-Wells or Vinke, or halo-vest traction. Here's what you should know about these two types of skeletal traction units—and about caring for an immobilized patient.

## SKULL TONGS

Used to immobilize the patient's cervical spine after fracture or dislocation, invasion by tumor or infection, or surgery

**Nursing considerations**
• Reassure the patient and explain the procedure to him.

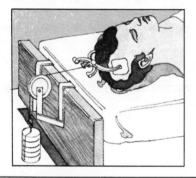

• Assess his neurologic signs, as ordered, with particular emphasis on motor function. Notify the doctor *immediately* if the patient experiences decreased sensation or increased loss of motor function: this may indicate *spinal cord trauma*.
• Be alert for signs and symptoms of loosening pins: redness, swelling, and complaints of persistent pain and tenderness. (Causes of loosening pins include infection, excessive traction force, and osteoporosis.)
• If the pins pull out, immobilize the patient's head and neck and call the doctor.
• Take action to prevent pressure sores. Remember, inadequate peripheral circulation can cause sores within 6 hours.
• Make sure the traction weights are hanging freely to maintain proper traction force. *Never add or subtract weights unless the doctor orders it.* (Inappropriate weight adjustment may cause neurologic impairment.)

## HALO-VEST TRACTION

Used to immobilize the patient's head and neck after cervical spine injury (allows

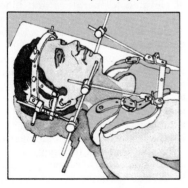

greater mobility than skull tongs; carries less risk of infection)

**Nursing considerations**
• Reassure the patient and explain the procedure to him.
• Assess his neurologic signs, as ordered, with particular emphasis on motor function. Notify the doctor *immediately* if the patient experiences decreased sensation or increased loss of motor function: this may indicate *spinal cord trauma*.
• Check the pin sites and use cleansing procedures, as ordered.
• Obtain an order for an analgesic if your patient complains of headache after the doctor retightens the pins.
• Never lift the patient using the device's bars.

pelvis from decreased blood flow due to paralysis. Expect to administer prophylactic anticoagulants, such as heparin, and apply antiembolic stockings (TEDS), if ordered.

Monitor the patient's electrolytes and check his ABGs again. He may develop *hypokalemia* or *alkalosis* from gastric suctioning, *extracellular volume excess* from overtransfusion, or *acidosis* from hypoperfusion. Expect to correct electrolyte imbalance and to change the I.V. fluid or rate of flow as the patient's volume status changes.

When the patient's bowel activity returns, so will his bowel sounds. This means you can remove his nasogastric tube, and he can start eating again. Provide a high-protein, high-calorie diet to help repair injured tissue and to prevent anemia, hypoproteinemia, and vitamin deficiencies. Initially, provide 2,000 to 2,500 calories per day, divided into numerous small meals. Monitor your patient's CBC and his hemoglobin and hematocrit levels. He may require transfusion to correct anemia and low blood volume from poor nutrition. Watch for melena, coffee-ground vomitus, or hematemesis—signs and symptoms of Cushing's ulcer, a type of stress ulcer common in patients with central nervous system injuries. Give stool softeners to prevent fecal impaction from decreased bowel activity or continued bed rest.

Force fluids (usually 3,000 to 4,000 ml/day) so your patient achieves a urine output of 1,500 to 2,000 ml/day. This will help to prevent urinary calculi, pyelonephritis, and urinary tract infection. Keep his calcium intake under 0.5 g/day; this will also help minimize the risk of urinary calculi.

If your patient's had complete cord transection, physiologic function will return to isolated sections of the cord in 3 to 6 weeks. Look for increases in his muscle tone and reflexes. You may also see spastic paralysis with increased deep tendon reflexes, clonus, plantar and extensor spasms of the limbs, and involuntary spasms in response to minor stimuli. Occurrence of these spasms doesn't indicate he's recovering from his paralysis. He may have them—and his paralysis—for the rest of his life.

If your patient is breathing diaphragmatically, keep encouraging him to cough, to deep breathe, and to turn frequently. These measures will improve his pulmonary function and prevent infections, such as pneumonia, which are always a risk for these patients.

Psychological support is very important for the patient with a spinal cord injury. He'll undergo a change in body image, and he'll have feelings of grief and dependence. If your patient is in spinal shock, let him know that his complete paralysis and flaccidity may *not* be permanent and that he may regain some function. Start a rehabilitation program for him as soon as possible, and let him know what benefits he can expect. Involve him in decisions about his care, to promote independence. Give him short-term, achievable goals to look forward to, such as the ability to dress himself or to use a wheelchair.

---

# Ischemic Cerebrovascular Accident

### Prediagnosis summary

Initial assessment findings in this patient may have included a sudden onset of elevated temperature and blood pressure, headache, stiff neck, photophobia, vomiting, and seizures. He also may have exhibited:

- aphasia, dysphasia, or slurred speech
- numbness around the lips or mouth
- dyslexia
- unilateral impaired vision, visual field cuts, or diplopia
- impaired coordination
- weakness, paralysis, or numbness on one or both sides of the body
- confusion, disorientation, personality changes, or amnesia
- incontinence
- dysphagia.

The doctor ordered diagnostic tests, such as an EKG, Holter monitoring, serology, CBC, coagulation studies, skull X-rays, brain scan, cerebral arteriogram, EEG, or CT scan.

## WHAT HAPPENS IN ISCHEMIC CEREBROVASCULAR ACCIDENT

Cerebrovascular accident (CVA) due to ischemia occurs when a thrombus blocks a blood vessel supplying an area of the brain. This causes ischemia, infarction, and edema in the affected brain tissue.

In *thrombotic ischemic CVA*, the most common type, a cerebral artery becomes obstructed, usually because of atherosclerosis. You may know that thrombotic CVA generally occurs in middle-aged and elderly patients, who have an increased incidence of atherosclerosis, hypertension, and diabetes. Usually an extracerebral vessel's obstructed, but sometimes an intracerebral vessel's involved. A transient ischemic attack (TIA) results in brief neurologic deficits followed by complete return to normal function. Causes of

TIAs include microemboli, released from the thrombus, and a temporary decrease in perfusion that results in a spasm.

*Embolic ischemic CVA*, the second most common type, can occur at any age. A clot or fat or air particle travels through the vascular system until it lodges in a small cerebral artery—most commonly the middle cerebral artery. Once it lodges, impaired circulation causes cerebral artery necrosis and edema. Embolic CVAs are prevalent among:

• patients with cardiac conditions—for example, atherosclerotic or rheumatic heart disease; valvular disease; or dysrhythmias, such as atrial fibrillation

• patients who've had recent myocardial infarctions or cardiac surgery.

---

The patient received supplemental oxygen through a nasal cannula or, if necessary, intubation and mechanical ventilation. An I.V. was started at a keep-vein-open rate. He may have been connected to a cardiac monitor.

### Priorities

Your first priority is to maintain your patient's respiratory status. Make sure he's adequately ventilated; he may need an artificial airway if the ischemic episode compromised his respirations.

The doctor may order medications, such as aspirin, to minimize your patient's risk of further embolic cerebrovascular accident (CVA). He may also have ordered anticoagulants, such as heparin sodium or warfarin sodium (Coumadin), to prevent further formation of emboli. (Be sure to test your patient's clotting profile *before* administering any anticoagulants.) Administer the patient's medications as ordered, and be alert for possible complications. For example, increased ICP often accompanies CVA (see the "Increased Intracranial Pressure" entry in this chapter).

### Continuing assessment and intervention

Perform a complete neurologic examination on your patient. The information you gather will provide important baseline data. Pay particular attention to his level of consciousness, motor and sensory functions, cranial nerve functions, and ability to speak. Remember to note the degree of your patient's signs and symptoms and whether they occur on one or both sides of his body.

Assess his level of consciousness first. He'll be in a coma only if the CVA is profound or if it involves the brain stem. If he's conscious, note any mental impairment, confusion, or disorientation, and repeat the assessment every 15 minutes to detect any changes.

Assess your patient's motor and sensory functions next. Deficits differ, depending on the artery affected, the severity of damage, and the extent of collateral circulation that develops. Remember that an infarct in the *left* hemisphere will produce local signs and symptoms on the *right* side, whereas an infarct in the *right* hemisphere will produce local signs and symptoms on the *left* side. (However, if the patient's cranial nerves are damaged, you'll see dysfunction on the *same* side as the ischemia.)

Check your patient's vital signs. He may have a fever or hypertension (which often accompanies CVAs that result from progressive atherosclerosis). A difference in blood pressure readings taken in both arms suggests carotid obstruction or subclavian steal syndrome (an occlusion of the subclavian artery, proximal to the origin of the vertebral artery, that causes diversion of blood from the vertebrobasilar system).

Obtain a detailed patient history. If he's conscious, ask him if he has a stiff neck, a headache, or photophobia. These symptoms suggest meningeal irritation, which may be caused by intracranial bleeding or infection (see the entries on "Hemorrhagic Cerebrovascular Accident", "Meningitis", and "Encephalitis" in this chapter).

Ask your patient (or his family, if he's unconscious) if he's noticed short episodes of motor impairment, vision loss, or aphasia. These episodes suggest TIAs, which are associated with atherosclerosis of the extracranial vessels and usually indicate an impending stroke. Also ask about a history of hypertension, diabetes, gout, cardiac dis-

ease, cigarette smoking, obesity, or use of oral contraceptives and about a family history of CVAs. All these are major risk factors.

You'll usually limit fluids to avoid increasing the patient's ICP. Make sure you maintain a low flow rate, and *never* give your patient a large amount of fluid in a short time. Offer him a bedpan every 2 hours and encourage him to urinate. Avoid urinary catheterization, if possible, because of the high risk of infection in these patients.

## Therapeutic care

Nursing care of a patient who's had a CVA is complex and requires keen observation and supportive care.

Repeat your neurologic assessment frequently (hourly for the first few days) to monitor any changes in your patient's condition. Report any changes to the doctor immediately.

Maintain your patient's respiratory function by changing his position frequently, suctioning secretions, and encouraging him to cough and deep-breathe. Remember that pneumonia is the most common cause of death in CVA patients. Your patient's decreased level of consciousness, inability to control secretions, or difficulty in swallowing may cause him to aspirate his secretions, so be sure to suction as necessary. Remember, too, that pulmonary embolism can result from the same process that sent an embolus to your patient's brain. Watch for the signs and symptoms of pulmonary embolism, which include dyspnea, tachypnea, and hemoptysis.

Monitor your patient's blood pressure frequently. Hypertension is common after a CVA; the doctor may prescribe antihypertensives if the patient's blood pressure doesn't return to normal after 24 hours. Report any sudden changes immediately. Monitor your patient's urinary output and his fluid and electrolyte balance.

Position him correctly to prevent complications of immobilization, such as pressure sores and contractures.

### BE PREPARED!

You know you must take seizure precautions for your patient with status epilepticus; but what about the patient with brain disorders (such as cerebrovascular accident, abscess, hematoma, or meningitis) or a history of head trauma? Remember, seizures often occur in these patients, too—so be sure you always have an oral airway at your patient's bedside. If a patient has a seizure, this device must be immediately available—so take a minute, at the beginning of your shift, to make sure it is.

Align his extremities and turn him frequently. Perform passive range-of-motion exercises on his affected extremities, and encourage active exercise of his unaffected extremities.

Make sure your patient is receiving adequate nutrition. If he isn't comatose or lethargic, he may be able to tolerate oral feedings and may even be able to assist in the feeding or to feed himself. Check your patient's gag reflex *before* you offer any food by mouth. If he has facial paralysis, he may have trouble even with soft or liquid foods. Don't rush him. Place the food where he can see it, and encourage him to try eating while lying on his unaffected side. This will also help prevent aspiration if he vomits. Check his stools for bleeding, which may indicate a stress ulcer. If your patient is constipated, give stool softeners, as ordered.

Your patient with ischemic CVA will probably be depressed, not just because of his brain injury, but because of the realization of his dependence on others. He may fear, quite reasonably, that the devastating loss of function he's experienced will be permanent. Reassure him, and try to help him overcome his fears and frustrations.

Communicate effectively with your patient. If he's aphasic, establish another form of communication (such as gestures, nods, or eye blinks) that utilizes his remaining functions. If he can write, give him a pencil and paper or an erasable slate. *Never* shout at your patient or talk to him as if he were a child—his inability to speak doesn't mean that his hearing or intelligence is impaired.

Start speech therapy and physical therapy as soon as your patient is able. Explain the goals of his rehabilitation program and what progress he can expect. Remember, your patient's family will also be frightened and concerned. Involve them in his care, and encourage them to be as supportive and responsive as possible, even if your patient expresses his frustration by lashing out at those closest to him.

# Hemorrhagic Cerebrovascular Accident

## Prediagnosis summary

The patient may initially have been unconscious if the amount of bleeding was severe enough to seriously increase his ICP. If awake, he complained of headache—sudden and excruciatingly severe if he suffered a *subarachnoid* hemorrhage; slow in onset and steadily developing if he suffered a *hypertensive* hemorrhage.

Additionally, he may have had:
- nausea
- vomiting
- seizures
- elevated temperature
- nuchal rigidity
- focal signs, such as hemiparesis, disturbances in vision, or aphasia.

The patient was given oxygen, and an I.V. was started for medication access. Blood was drawn for ABGs, CBC, electrolytes, blood glucose, BUN, and prothrombin time–partial thromboplastin time (PT-PTT). A bladder catheter was inserted, and cardiac monitoring was established. The doctor ordered a lumbar puncture to test the patient's CSF for blood and increased pressure (see *Nurse's Guide to Interpreting Cerebrospinal Fluid Test Results,* pages 288 and 289). The patient's CSF may have been bloody and his initial pressure elevated. The doctor also ordered a CT scan or cerebral angiography to determine the site and size of the hemorrhage.

The doctor diagnosed a hemorrhagic (as compared with embolic) CVA on the basis of the CT scan indicators.

## Priorities, assessment, and intervention

As soon as your patient's diagnosis is established, perform a thorough neurologic baseline assessment to deter-

## IDENTIFYING SITES OF HEMORRHAGIC C.V.A.

Your patient's had a hemorrhagic cerebrovascular accident. By observing his signs and symptoms, can you identify the site of his hemorrhage? Below you'll find a cross section of the brain, indicating possible sites of hemorrhage and associated signs and symptoms.

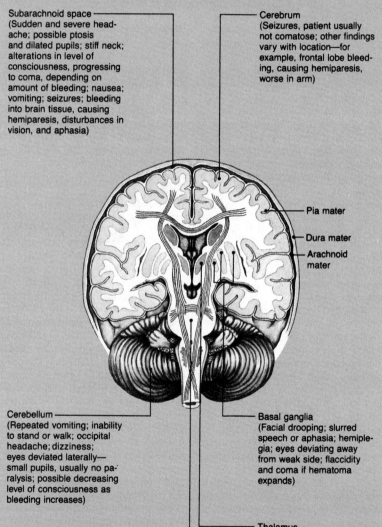

Subarachnoid space
(Sudden and severe head-
ache; possible ptosis
and dilated pupils; stiff neck;
alterations in level of
consciousness, progressing
to coma, depending on
amount of bleeding; nausea;
vomiting; seizures; bleeding
into brain tissue, causing
hemiparesis, disturbances in
vision, and aphasia)

Cerebrum
(Seizures, patient usually
not comatose; other findings
vary with location—for
example, frontal lobe bleeding, causing hemiparesis,
worse in arm)

Pia mater

Dura mater

Arachnoid
mater

Cerebellum
(Repeated vomiting; inability
to stand or walk; occipital
headache; dizziness;
eyes deviated laterally—
small pupils, usually no paralysis; possible decreasing
level of consciousness as
bleeding increases)

Basal ganglia
(Facial drooping; slurred
speech or aphasia; hemiplegia; eyes deviating away
from weak side; flaccidity
and coma if hematoma
expands)

Thalamus
(Hemiplegia or hemiparesis;
possible aphasia and
ocular disturbance, such as
eyes deviating downward
and unequal pupils that may
not react to light)

Pons
(Coma with total paralysis
or decerebrate posturing;
small pupils; bloody cerebrospinal fluid)

## WHAT HAPPENS IN HEMORRHAGIC CEREBROVASCULAR ACCIDENT

Either hypertensive or subarachnoid hemorrhage can cause hemorrhagic cerebrovascular accident. Hypertensive hemorrhage is often the result of chronic uncontrolled hypertension. A blood vessel, usually an artery, ruptures deep within the brain, causing intracerebral hemorrhage (hematoma). If the bleeding's significant, intracranial pressure increases and brain tissue's displaced and compressed. Coma and death may rapidly result.

The most common cause of subarachnoid hemorrhage is a ruptured saccular aneurysm located at one of the various arterial junction points on the circle of Willis at the base of the brain. Blood accumulates in the subarachnoid space surrounding the brain (bleeding within the brain may also occur). Unless the bleeding can be stopped, shock and death will follow.

mine the extent of damage and to alert you to subtle signs of deterioration. Elevate the head of the patient's bed to facilitate venous drainage. Then begin your emergency assessment.

Check your patient's blood pressure—if it's elevated, this may have caused his hypertensive hemorrhage. If it remains elevated, expect to give antihypertensive medications, which will lower his blood pressure and may help reduce the bleeding.

Assess your patient's level of consciousness. He may be restless or irritable or he may have personality or behavior changes, progressing to unconsciousness within minutes to hours after the initial event. He may even lapse into a coma. To keep the hemorrhage from expanding, the doctor may order aminocaproic acid (Amicar), which inhibits fibrinolysis and prevents clot breakdown. Monitor the patient's PT-PTT while he's on Amicar to assess his blood's clotting ability.

Watch for signs of increased ICP, which frequently accompanies hemorrhagic CVA. (See the "Increased Intracranial Pressure" entry in this chapter.) A deteriorating level of consciousness or deepening coma reflects this condition. In an awake patient, you may note vision disturbances or pupillary changes. Expect to administer corticosteroids and osmotic diuretics to reduce the patient's ICP.

Look for motor and sensory deficits that reflect the location of the bleeding (see *Identifying Sites of Hemorrhagic C.V.A.*). Remember that the majority of these hemorrhages occur deep within the *cerebral hemisphere.* You may see:
• hemiplegia
• deviation of the patient's eyes *toward* the site of the hemorrhage and *away* from the hemiplegia.

If the hemorrhage is in the *thalamus,* you may see:
• hemiplegia
• deviation of the patient's eyes inward, toward his nose; small, nonreactive pupils.

If the hemorrhage is in the *cerebellum* or *pons,* you may see:
• total paralysis or decerebrate posturing
• constricted pupils.

If the hemorrhage is in the *subarachnoid space,* you may note:
• visual disturbances
• ptosis
• dilated pupils.

Chart your assessment findings accurately. If later assessments yield different findings, this may indicate that the hemorrhage is expanding. History information you obtain may indicate that the patient's signs and symptoms developed abruptly and dramatically, while the patient was awake. However, your patient or his family may report a gradual onset of signs and symptoms over a few hours or even days. Ask about a past history of hypertension or cardiovascular disease.

### Therapeutic care

A patient who survives a hemorrhagic CVA will need strict bed rest for several weeks to prevent the recurrence of bleeding. Assess him frequently to identify developing complications, including signs and symptoms of further bleeding or increasing ICP. Reposition him frequently to prevent skin breakdown, contractures, and other complications of immobility. Perform *passive* range-of-motion exercises of the affected extremity, and encourage *active* range-of-motion exercise of his unaffected extremities.

Continue to give Amicar, if ordered, which will help stabilize clotting at the site of the hemorrhage. Remember, however, that Amicar may cause thrombus formation. Be alert for calf tenderness, possibly indicating a thrombus, or for sudden chest pain and dyspnea, possibly indicating pulmonary embolism from a thrombus that's broken loose. The patient may also develop hypotension or bradycardia.

Continue giving diuretics and corticosteroids, as ordered, to reduce the patient's ICP. Keep the head of the bed elevated, and give the patient stool softeners to prevent straining and Valsalva's maneuver. Restrict fluids (to prevent increasing ICP), keep an accurate intake and output record, and monitor your patient's electrolyte balance. If he's conscious, offer him a bedpan every 2 hours, and encourage him to urinate. You'll want to avoid catheterization, if possible, because a CVA increases the risk of infection. Expect to continue giving antihypertensive medications to reduce pressure on the bleeding site.

Begin rehabilitation for your patient as soon as he's stable, and arrange for physical and speech therapy, if needed.

You know that acute hemorrhagic CVA occurs without warning in young or middle-aged people who were previously healthy. So, your patient may experience great frustration as a result of his sudden transition to total dependence. He'll need all the emotional support you can provide, particularly before he's stable enough to begin a rehabilitation program.

---

# Generalized Tonic-Clonic Status Epilepticus

### Prediagnosis summary

Typically, the patient:
- was unconscious
- had continuous tonic-clonic seizure activity with incomplete recovery, or lack of recovery, between seizures.

However, he may have been in a coma with no evidence of seizures except sustained deviation of his eyes.

His other signs and symptoms probably included some combination of:
- incontinence
- diaphoresis
- labored breathing
- dyspnea
- apnea
- cyanosis
- mucus or saliva filling his mouth.

He was examined for signs of trauma, which may have precipitated the seizures.

An I.V. infusion and supplemental oxygen were started, and cardiac monitoring was established. Blood was drawn for electrolytes; blood glucose; ABGs; toxicologic studies; and anticonvulsant drug, BUN, creatinine, liver enzyme, and creatine phosphokinase (CPK) enzyme levels.

The patient's family or friends, if available, provided history information indicating whether the patient was a known epileptic or had a history of alcohol or drug abuse, diabetes, other chronic diseases, or an existing brain tumor. If no family or friends were available, the patient's belongings were searched for medications, cards, or Medic Alert symbols identifying him as an epileptic or diabetic. His body was examined for needle marks that might indicate drug abuse or insulin use.

The doctor diagnosed generalized tonic-clonic status epilepticus on the basis of the patient's continuous seizures.

## Priorities

Your first priority is to maintain adequate oxygenation while trying to stop the patient's prolonged seizure activity. Continuous seizures result in hypoxia and in metabolic and physical exhaustion; unchecked, this cycle leads to permanent brain damage and even death.

Make sure your patient's airway and oxygenation are adequate. Place the patient so that he's lying on his side, with his head in a semi-dependent position, to drain secretions and to prevent aspiration. Periodically, turn him onto his opposite side. Check your patient's ABG results for hypoxemia. Continue to administer supplemental oxygen by mask, and increase the flow rate if needed. If this doesn't ensure adequate oxygenation, expect to assist with intubation and mechanical ventilation. This will be difficult during seizure activity, especially if your patient's teeth are clenched. The doctor will try to wait until a time when severe seizure activity slows; then he may intubate the patient nasally.

The doctor will probably order diazepam (Valium) in a slow I.V. push, repeated two to three times at 10- to 20-minute intervals, to stop the patient's seizures. If the patient isn't a known epileptic, the doctor may order an I.V. bolus of dextrose 50% (50 ml) or of thiamine (100 mg). The dextrose may stop the patient's seizures if he's hypoglycemic; the thiamine may be effective if he's an alcoholic.

Expect to insert a nasogastric tube, once your patient's intubated, to prevent vomiting and aspiration. However, if the patient *hasn't* been intubated, the doctor may forego this procedure. Why? Because the nasogastric tube itself can trigger the gag reflex and cause vomiting.

## Continuing assessment and intervention

Assess the patient's neurologic status and vital signs frequently. If his temperature's elevated, a brain infection may be causing his seizures. If so, expect to give antibiotics after the sei-

**WHAT HAPPENS IN GENERALIZED TONIC-CLONIC STATUS EPILEPTICUS**

As a nurse, you know that status epilepticus is a life-threatening condition that can result from a wide variety of causes:
• cerebral trauma
• acute brain infection
• tumor
• cerebrovascular disease
• hypoglycemia
• alcoholism
• drug addiction
• chronic diseases, such as liver failure or uremia
• *failure of a patient with epilepsy to take his medication as prescribed*—the most

common cause.

When the patient goes into status epilepticus, he becomes unconscious, and his generalized tonic-clonic convulsions repeat so frequently that significant recovery of consciousness and function can't occur between them. Prolonged seizure activity leads to hypoxia, hypoglycemia, and hyperthermia. These, in turn, lead to continuing seizure activity, resulting in metabolic and physical exhaustion. Continuing oxygen and glucose deprivation may cause permanent brain damage or death.

DRUGS

## HIGHLIGHTING ANTICONVULSANT DRUGS USED IN STATUS EPILEPTICUS

| DRUG | ADVERSE EFFECTS | |
|---|---|---|
| **Diazepam (Valium)** | Respiratory depression, sedation, hypotension *(Side effects are much more common if phenobarbital's also given.)* | |
| **Phenytoin (Dilantin)** | Ataxia, slurred speech, nystagmus, diplopia, nausea, vomiting, bradycardia | |
| **Phenobarbital** | Sedation, drowsiness, hypotension, respiratory depression | |
| **Paraldehyde** | Pain with I.M. administration, sterile skin abscesses, skin sloughing, and muscular irritation; possible pulmonary edema or hemorrhage, circulatory collapse with I.V. administration | |

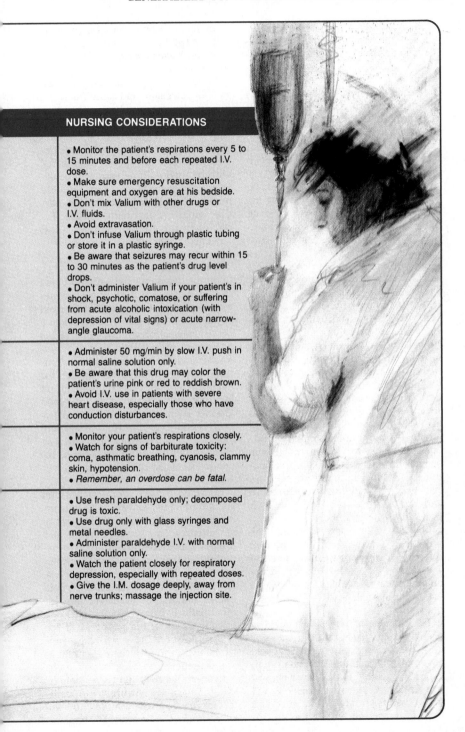

## NURSING CONSIDERATIONS

- Monitor the patient's respirations every 5 to 15 minutes and before each repeated I.V. dose.
- Make sure emergency resuscitation equipment and oxygen are at his bedside.
- Don't mix Valium with other drugs or I.V. fluids.
- Avoid extravasation.
- Don't infuse Valium through plastic tubing or store it in a plastic syringe.
- Be aware that seizures may recur within 15 to 30 minutes as the patient's drug level drops.
- Don't administer Valium if your patient's in shock, psychotic, comatose, or suffering from acute alcoholic intoxication (with depression of vital signs) or acute narrow-angle glaucoma.

- Administer 50 mg/min by slow I.V. push in normal saline solution only.
- Be aware that this drug may color the patient's urine pink or red to reddish brown.
- Avoid I.V. use in patients with severe heart disease, especially those who have conduction disturbances.

- Monitor your patient's respirations closely.
- Watch for signs of barbiturate toxicity: coma, asthmatic breathing, cyanosis, clammy skin, hypotension.
- *Remember, an overdose can be fatal.*

- Use fresh paraldehyde only; decomposed drug is toxic.
- Use drug only with glass syringes and metal needles.
- Administer paraldehyde I.V. with normal saline solution only.
- Watch the patient closely for respiratory depression, especially with repeated doses.
- Give the I.M. dosage deeply, away from nerve trunks; massage the injection site.

zures are under control.

Check the results of his blood studies to try to determine the cause of his seizures. Expect to correct any abnormalities, if possible. Of course, if the patient's a known epileptic and his blood test shows a low level of anticonvulsant drugs, expect to give these *immediately*. If the patient has an electrolyte imbalance, expect to correct it by replacing the appropriate electrolyte. If the patient's hypoglycemic, expect to give him more dextrose. If he has a drug overdose that's causing his seizures, expect to try to flush the drug out with fluids. Or you may give mannitol to promote diuresis that will eliminate the drug. Elevated liver enzymes point to liver failure as a cause of his seizures. Elevated BUN and creatinine levels may suggest uremia is the cause. If his ABGs show hypoxia, he'll need more oxygen—or intubation and mechanical ventilation.

Look for any injuries the seizures may have caused: shoulder dislocations are common. While your patient's having seizures, take steps to protect him from further injury. Avoid restraining him, and pad the side rails of his bed, if possible. Insert an oral airway—if your patient's mouth can be opened easily—to protect his tongue and his airway. *Don't* try to force anything into his mouth if his teeth are clenched; you may lacerate his mouth and lips or break off a tooth, which could lodge in his airway.

Continue your attempts to stop the patient's seizures or—if they've stopped—to prevent their recurrence. The doctor may order I.V. phenobarbital or phenytoin (Dilantin), repeated two to three times at 20- to 30-minute intervals.

The diazepam, phenobarbital, and phenytoin should stop the patient's seizures and prevent their recurrence; however, if his seizures still don't stop, expect to give I.V. paraldehyde slowly, repeated in an hour if necessary, or I.V. amobarbital slowly. Make sure you have appropriate ventilation equipment ready before you give amobarbital. Why? Because your patient may need respiratory assistance if he's given this drug I.V.

Remember this: Respiratory depression, hypotension, and coma can result if the patient receives *large amounts of these drugs,* so you need to assess his vital signs and neurologic status frequently. If his respirations become depressed, open his airway and assist with intubation, if necessary. If he develops hypotension, increase his fluid intake. Also check his heart rate, cardiac monitor, and temperature frequently for abnormalities—and document your findings carefully.

## Therapeutic care

Continue to monitor the patient's blood studies frequently. *New* abnormalities may result from the patient's prolonged seizures: for example, you may note a persistent electrolyte imbalance, or his ABGs may show respiratory and metabolic acidosis and hypoxemia. Continue to give supplemental oxygen for hypoxemia, and expect to give sodium bicarbonate for acidosis. If his blood glucose level continues to reveal hypoglycemia, expect to administer more dextrose to correct this problem. The patient's CPK level will probably be increased because of the continued seizures.

Continue to check your patient's vital signs frequently, as well. His temperature may be increased as a result of his seizures. So you may need to give a tepid sponge bath or to apply a hypothermia blanket to reduce the fever. Assess his BUN and creatinine levels, and keep an accurate record of his fluid intake and output to detect possible renal failure from myoglobinuria (a possible result of his seizures). If you notice increased BUN and creatinine levels, expect to give the patient fluids and diuretics.

Reassess your patient's neurologic status. You can expect him to be postictal (confused and drowsy) after his seizures, but he should gradually improve.

If, after all the treatment described, his seizures still haven't stopped, the doctor may use general anesthesia as a last resort. However, this is rarely necessary.

After the patient's baseline and subsequent blood levels of anticonvulsant drugs are evaluated, he'll be started on maintenance dosages of anticonvulsants—usually phenytoin (Dilantin) and phenobarbital.

After your patient's seizures have stopped, provide nutritional support and extra fluids, needed because the seizures have increased his body's metabolic demands. He'll also need a quiet environment with plenty of rest during his recovery period. Continue to assess him frequently and to record his vital signs and intake and output.

If your patient's a known epileptic who had seizures because of noncompliance with his anticonvulsant regimen, emphasize the importance of taking his medication properly. To help prevent further seizures while he's recovering in the hospital, keep his blinds closed at night and have defective lights fixed immediately. Why? Because flickering lights can precipitate seizures. Also keep an oral airway at the patient's bedside at all times.

If your patient's a child under age 4, he's at risk for permanent brain damage from uncontrolled status epilepticus. If he has febrile seizures, expect to try to control the fever by administering aspirin or acetaminophen in addition to medication for stopping the seizures. Sponging him with tepid water or using a hypothermia blanket may help, too.

---

# Myasthenia Gravis Crisis

## Prediagnosis summary
The patient's initial assessment findings probably included:

- a history of myasthenia gravis, with extreme exacerbation of the typical signs and symptoms—muscle weakness, fatigue, ptosis, diplopia, dysphagia, nasal vocalization, and lack of facial expression
- respiratory insufficiency that wasn't obviously apparent because of his weakened intercostal and diaphragm muscles.

He received supplemental oxygen, as needed, for respiratory distress. The doctor may have performed a Tensilon test to try to detect too little or too much cholinergic medication, which may have caused the patient's crisis. Blood was drawn for ABGs, and a chest X-ray was done.

(The Tensilon test is done by injecting edrophonium chloride [Tensilon] I.V. and measuring the patient's motor response. If the patient's signs and symptoms worsen after the injection, the crisis is *cholinergic;* if they improve, the crisis is *myasthenic.* After the injection, watch your patient closely to identify any changes, which should occur within a few minutes. Remember, however, that the test is often hard to interpret. This is because Tensilon may improve function in one muscle group while increasing weakness in another muscle group. If the results are questionable, anticholinesterase medications will be withdrawn for 24 to 72 hours, and the patient will be observed carefully. If his signs and symptoms worsen, the crisis is *myasthenic;* expect to give an anticholinesterase drug parenterally. If his signs and symptoms improve, the crisis is *cholinergic;* expect to give atropine, as ordered.)

## Priorities
Your first priority is to ensure that the patient's ventilation is adequate. His degree of respiratory insufficiency will be evaluated from his ABGs. Give supplemental oxygen by mask or nasal cannula if his respiratory difficulty is *mild to moderate.* If it's *severe,* expect to assist with intubation and mechanical ventilation.

PATHOPHYSIOLOGY

# WHAT HAPPENS IN MYASTHENIA GRAVIS

As you probably know, myasthenia gravis is a chronic disease that produces recurrent, progressive attacks of muscle weakness and abnormal fatigability. Exercise worsens these signs and symptoms.

A disturbance in nerve impulse transmission at the neuromuscular junction affects muscle contraction. Although the exact mechanism's unknown, researchers believe it involves insufficient acetylcholine synthesis, release, or binding at the neuromuscular junction. The causes of myasthenia gravis are also unknown, but an autoimmune disorder affecting postsynaptic receptor sites is suspected. Compare the following illustrations of a normal neuromuscular junction and one affected by myasthenia gravis.

## NORMAL NEUROMUSCULAR JUNCTION

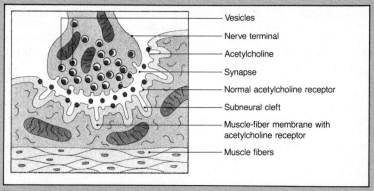

- Vesicles
- Nerve terminal
- Acetylcholine
- Synapse
- Normal acetylcholine receptor
- Subneural cleft
- Muscle-fiber membrane with acetylcholine receptor
- Muscle fibers

Nerve impulses reach the nerve terminal, causing the vesicles to release acetylcholine. The acetylcholine crosses the synapse and reacts with receptors in the muscle-fiber membrane, stimulating contraction.

## NEUROMUSCULAR JUNCTION AFFECTED BY MYASTHENIA GRAVIS

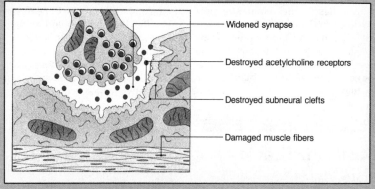

- Widened synapse
- Destroyed acetylcholine receptors
- Destroyed subneural clefts
- Damaged muscle fibers

In myasthenia gravis, antibodies destroy many acetylcholine receptors in muscle-fiber membranes. The synapse widens, and the number of clefts decreases. Affected muscles weaken because they're unable to contract normally.

## Continuing assessment and intervention

If the patient's been receiving inadequate anticholinesterase medication, he'll be treated for a *myasthenic* crisis.

If he's been overmedicated, this will cause persistent depolarization block and he'll be treated for a *cholinergic* crisis. (See *When Your Patient Goes Into Myasthenia Gravis Crisis.*)

---

### WHEN YOUR PATIENT GOES INTO MYASTHENIA GRAVIS CRISIS

Are you familiar with the nursing interventions for a patient in myasthenia gravis crisis? Can you differentiate the myasthenic type from the cholinergic? This chart shows you the causes and signs and symptoms of each type of myasthenia gravis crisis, along with appropriate nursing interventions.

| | MYASTHENIC CRISIS | CHOLINERGIC CRISIS |
|---|---|---|
| **Crisis Mechanisms** | • Respiratory muscles weaken, causing respiratory failure. | • Too much anticholinesterase medication causes respiratory failure. |
| **Causes** | • Exacerbation of disease, emotional stress, surgery, trauma, certain drugs, or infection; temporary resistance to anticholinesterase drugs or need for increased dosage | • Overmedication with cholinergic drugs |
| **Signs and symptoms** | • Acute respiratory distress with irritability, anxiety, extreme restlessness, decreased urine output, increased pulse, diminished cough and swallow reflexes, difficulty speaking, double vision, drooping eyelids, increased salivation<br>• Positive response to Tensilon test—muscle strength improves | • Extreme weakness with difficulty speaking; diminished cough and swallow reflexes with increased salivation; acute respiratory distress; micosis; nausea; vomiting; diarrhea; abdominal cramps; fine muscle tremors of eyelids, face, neck, or legs; bradycardia; pallor; sweating<br>• Negative response to Tensilon test—signs and symptoms worsen |
| **Nursing considerations** | • Be prepared to ventilate and suction your patient.<br>• Be prepared to assist with a tracheotomy or with insertion of an endotracheal tube.<br>• Monitor his vital signs.<br>• Be prepared to administer anticholinesterase agents, such as neostigmine or pyridostigmine, to improve neuromuscular transmission. | • Be prepared to ventilate and suction your patient.<br>• Be prepared to assist with a tracheotomy or with insertion of an endotracheal tube.<br>• Monitor his vital signs.<br>• Discontinue use of anticholinesterase drugs during the crisis until his condition improves.<br>• Be prepared to administer I.V. injection of 1 mg atropine to counteract the severe cholinergic reaction. |

Talking may worsen your patient's respiratory difficulty, so ask his family about the type and amount of anticholinesterase medication he's been taking. Also ask if he's had a recent cold, fever, or infection or if he's been under any increased emotional stress—all these can produce myasthenic crisis.

Find out if he's taking any other medications, too. The following drugs can exacerbate myasthenia gravis and produce myasthenic crisis:
- barbiturates
- narcotics
- antianxiety agents
- quinidine
- quinine
- procainamide
- aminoglycoside antibiotics (streptomycin, gentamicin, neomycin).

### Therapeutic care
If your patient's not on a ventilator, continue to monitor his respiratory status frequently. Give oxygen, as needed, because his coughing and swallowing reflexes are decreased. If he suffered respiratory failure and was intubated and put on a ventilator, check his respiratory status often by monitoring his serial ABGs and chest X-rays. Watch for signs and symptoms of respiratory infection—such as fever, yellow or green sputum, or productive cough—and expect to give prophylactic antibiotics. Remember, myasthenia gravis crisis can cause *acute respiratory failure.* (See this entry in Chapter 4.) Watch for signs and symptoms, such as dyspnea, tachypnea, and cyanosis, but remember that these may be difficult to detect because the patient's weakened respiratory muscles will prevent intercostal and suprasternal retraction.

The patient may be more susceptible to aspiration, too, because his oropharyngeal muscles are weakened. If he's not on a mechanical ventilator, give him soft foods, rather than liquids, to prevent choking. Aggressive pulmonary hygiene will be needed because the patient is highly susceptible to pulmonary infection. Encourage him to deep-breathe and to cough frequently, and provide chest physiotherapy—this will help loosen lung secretions.

Continue to administer your patient's medications, as ordered. In doing this, consistency is important. Unless you give the precise doses at the correct times, you may precipitate fluctuations of muscle weakness.

Once your patient's crisis has passed and his respirations become effective enough to ensure adequate oxygenation, he'll be placed on a medication regimen and be gradually weaned from oxygen therapy and from the ventilator. His readiness for this is determined by ventilator-weaning parameters, his ABG values, and his respiratory status prior to extubation.

When you gradually start to increase your patient's activity level, he may be acutely distressed about his muscular deterioration. Reassure him that his strength will probably return to its baseline level. Explain that while he's recovering in the hospital, you'll be monitoring him closely for any changes in his condition, and he won't be left alone.

# Meningitis

### Prediagnosis summary
On initial assessment, the patient had signs of meningeal irritation, such as:
- nuchal rigidity (patient resists when you try to flex his neck)
- positive Brudzinski's sign (patient's knees and hips flex when you bend his neck forward) (see *Two Quick Tests for Possible Meningitis,* page 290)
- positive Kernig's sign (patient resists leg extension after flexion at hip and knee) (see *Two Quick Tests for Possible Meningitis,* page 290)
- exaggerated, symmetrical deep-tendon reflexes
- opisthotonos (arched posture with the extremities and back bent backward).

He may also have had signs and symptoms of cranial nerve irritation:
- photophobia
- vertigo
- tinnitus
- diplopia
- ptosis
- unequal pupils.

He may also have been irritable, delirious, stuporous, or in a coma, and he may have had seizures.

Nonspecific assessment findings included some or all of the following:
- headache
- nausea
- vomiting
- fever
- chills
- malaise.

Blood was drawn for ABGs and a CBC, and the patient's blood, urine, mucus, and sputum were cultured to help determine the type and site of the infection. An I.V. infusion was started for later antibiotic therapy, and supplemental oxygen was given if he was stuporous or comatose. The doctor may also have ordered a chest X-ray, EKG, and CT scan. A lumbar puncture was probably necessary to confirm the diagnosis and to determine the organism causing infection.

Meningitis may be difficult to detect in children. You may see signs of infection, but sometimes an infant is simply fretful and anorexic. Watch for copious vomiting leading to dehydration—which can mask signs and symptoms of increasing ICP. Also keep alert for twitching, seizures, or coma.

Meningitis occurs most frequently in children ages 1 to 10 but may also occur up to age 16. Be alert for a rapid onset of signs such as petechiae, purpura, and hemorrhages into the mucous or serous membranes—these indicate meningococcemia. (See *Nurse's Guide to Pediatric Emergencies* in the Appendix.)

**Priorities**
Your first nursing priority is to administer the appropriate antibiotics and

fluids and to observe the patient closely for signs and symptoms of increasing ICP due to cerebral edema. (See the "Increased Intracranial Pressure" entry in this chapter.) If a *bacterial infection* caused the patient's meningitis, expect to give him I.V. antibiotics for at least 2 weeks, followed by oral antibiotics. If a *viral infection* caused the meningitis, antibiotics may still be given to prevent an overgrowth of bacteria—your patient's lowered resistance during viral infection predisposes him to further infection.

Keep in mind that cultures of the patient's blood, urine, mucus, and sputum usually take 24 hours for a preliminary report and up to a week for a final report. This means that the doctor may start the patient on a broad-spectrum antibiotic until the culture reports are back and antibiotics specific for the organism can be started. If the patient's ABGs show hypoxemia, give supplemental oxygen, as ordered.

Be alert for signs and symptoms of increasing ICP, such as altered level of consciousness, disturbances in vision, altered respirations, seizures, and increased temperature. Call the doctor *immediately* if you note any of these.

PATHOPHYSIOLOGY

## WHAT HAPPENS IN MENINGITIS

Meningitis is a bacterial or viral infection occurring most commonly when organisms—for example, meningococci—enter the meninges through the bloodstream, sinuses, or middle ear. They may also enter through a penetrating head wound, basilar skull fracture, lumbar puncture, or intracranial pressure (ICP) monitoring sensor, or during intracranial surgery.

The resulting infection may inflame all three meningeal membranes (dura mater, arachnoid, and pia mater). Inflammation leads to tissue and blood vessel congestion and to cortical irritation. If cerebral edema results, increased ICP may follow.

## NURSE'S GUIDE TO INTERPRETING CEREBROSPINAL FLUID TEST RESULTS

Have you ever received laboratory results from your patient's cerebrospinal fluid (CSF) specimens and wondered what they meant? Of course, the doctor interprets the test results. But what if you happen to see them first? Here's where your basic knowledge of CSF test abnormalities may benefit your patient. Study this chart so you'll know when CSF test abnormalities mean you should call the doctor.

| CSF CHARAC-TERISTICS | NORMAL RESULTS | ABNORMAL RESULTS |
|---|---|---|
| Pressure | 50 to 180 mm H$_2$O | • Increase<br>• Decrease |
| Appearance | Clear, colorless (*Note:* CSF can be clear if the patient has an intracranial lesion; however, if a lesion such as an abscess ruptures, the CSF may be colored.) | • Cloudy<br>• Xanthochromic or bloody<br>• Brown, orange, or yellow |
| Protein | 15 to 45 mg/100 ml | • Marked increase<br>• Marked decrease |
| Gamma globulin | 3% to 12% of total protein | • Increased |
| Glucose | 60% to 80% of true blood glucose; 40 to 80 mg/100 ml | • Increase<br>• Decrease |
| Cell count | 0 to 5 WBCs (lymphocytes)/µl<br><br>No RBCs | • Increase<br><br>• RBCs |
| Chloride | 118 to 130 mEq/liter | • Decrease |
| Gram stain | No organisms | • Gram-positive or gram-negative organisms |

Expect to give diazepam (Valium) for seizures.

### Continuing assessment and intervention

Assess your patient's vital signs and general condition often. You'll still need to watch him closely for signs and symptoms of increasing ICP and to notify the doctor if any appear. If your patient develops increased ICP, expect to give an osmotic diuretic, such as mannitol. Check his neurologic function frequently; persistent neurologic deficits, such as blindness, deafness, or hemiparesis, can result from meningitis.

Provide your patient with a quiet, darkened environment to relieve his photophobia, headache, and general discomfort. If his infection was *bacterial*, he'll be isolated for 24 hours following initiation of organism-specific I.V. antibiotics. If his infection was

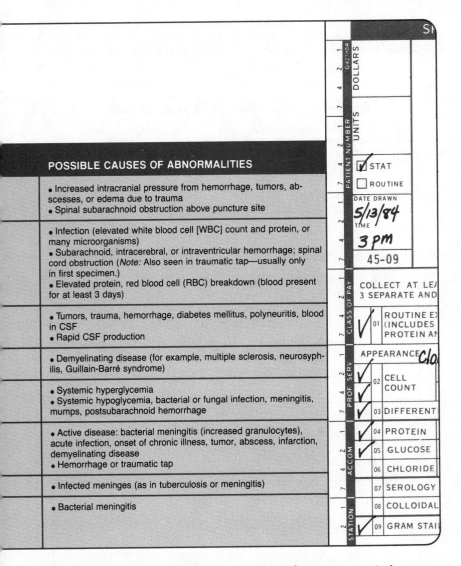

| POSSIBLE CAUSES OF ABNORMALITIES | | |
|---|---|---|
| • Increased intracranial pressure from hemorrhage, tumors, abscesses, or edema due to trauma<br>• Spinal subarachnoid obstruction above puncture site | | |
| • Infection (elevated white blood cell [WBC] count and protein, or many microorganisms)<br>• Subarachnoid, intracerebral, or intraventricular hemorrhage; spinal cord obstruction (*Note:* Also seen in traumatic tap—usually only in first specimen.)<br>• Elevated protein, red blood cell (RBC) breakdown (blood present for at least 3 days) | | |
| • Tumors, trauma, hemorrhage, diabetes mellitus, polyneuritis, blood in CSF<br>• Rapid CSF production | | |
| • Demyelinating disease (for example, multiple sclerosis, neurosyphilis, Guillain-Barré syndrome) | | |
| • Systemic hyperglycemia<br>• Systemic hypoglycemia, bacterial or fungal infection, meningitis, mumps, postsubarachnoid hemorrhage | | |
| • Active disease: bacterial meningitis (increased granulocytes), acute infection, onset of chronic illness, tumor, abscess, infarction, demyelinating disease<br>• Hemorrhage or traumatic tap | | |
| • Infected meninges (as in tuberculosis or meningitis) | | |
| • Bacterial meningitis | | |

*viral,* he may not require isolation. Administer mild sedatives such as diazepam (Valium), as ordered, to reduce his restlessness, but remember to watch for the respiratory depression these drugs may cause. Give aspirin or acetaminophen to relieve pain and fever. If his fever persists, expect to treat your patient with a hypothermia mattress or a tepid sponge bath. The doctor may order antiarrhythmics or anticonvulsants.

Remember to pay particular attention to your patient's skin, ears, and sinuses while performing your overall assessment. Observe his skin for petechial and hemorrhagic lesions and for purpura, all of which may indicate meningococcemia—a common complication of meningitis (especially in children). (*Note: Fulminating meningococcemia can be rapidly fatal* because of circulatory collapse and intravascular coagulation.)

After you complete your assessment, if you find no evidence of further complications, take a detailed *history*. Ask him (or his family) if he's had a recent infection, such as pneumonia, sinusitis, osteomyelitis, endocarditis, myelitis, or a middle ear infection. (Any of these can cause meningitis.) Also ask

## TWO QUICK TESTS FOR POSSIBLE MENINGITIS

When you suspect your patient may have meningitis, perform these two quick tests. Positive Brudzinski's and Kernig's signs—in the presence of such signs and symptoms as fever, chills, headache, stiff neck, and altered behavior and level of consciousness—indicate possible meningitis. Here's how to test your patient for Brudzinski's and Kernig's signs.

**BRUDZINSKI'S SIGN**

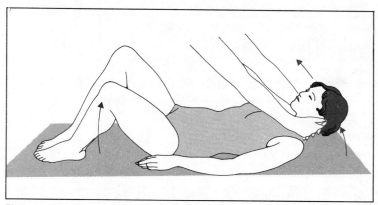

Place your patient in the dorsal recumbent position, putting your hands behind her neck and bending it forward. The sign's *positive* if pain and resistance are present and if the patient flexes her hips and knees in response to the maneuver.

**KERNIG'S SIGN**

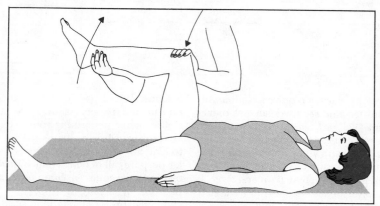

With your patient supine, flex her leg at the hip and knee, then try to straighten her knee. The sign's *positive* if pain and resistance are present.

if he's experienced a recent head trauma. If he's developed meningitis while hospitalized for another condition, find out from his chart whether he's had invasive procedures, such as lumbar puncture or ICP monitoring—these can cause meningitis.

## Therapeutic care

Keep your patient on complete bed rest. Position him carefully to keep him comfortable and to prevent his neck pain from worsening.

Monitor your patient's fluid level and electrolyte balance. Watch for signs and symptoms of dehydration—such as poor skin turgor or sunken eyes—and increase his fluids as needed. Expect to correct any electrolyte imbalance.

Because your patient will most likely be on a long-term I.V. antibiotic regimen, watch for signs and symptoms of the side effects common to these drugs. These include diarrhea and an overgrowth proliferation of *Candida,* causing vaginitis or thrush. Observe his I.V. site frequently for signs of phlebitis, such as redness, swelling, and warmth. Many broad-spectrum antibiotics are nephrotoxic, so monitor your patient's creatinine and BUN levels to detect any increases and his urine output for a possible decrease.

Your patient may need repeated—and painful—lumbar punctures to determine if the infection is improving. Provide emotional support as you assist in this procedure, and use relaxation techniques to help reduce his pain.

After your patient's received I.V. antibiotics for at least 2 weeks and his condition has improved, expect to remove the I.V. and to continue giving antibiotics orally. Continue to monitor his fluid intake and output, too, giving him plenty of fluids to prevent dehydration. (Don't restrict fluids—the patient should be in no danger of developing increased ICP at this time.) Encourage him to eat regular meals to build up his strength, and gradually increase his activity level as his energy begins to return.

Continue to watch your patient for any recurring signs or symptoms of infection. Take and record his temperature every 4 hours. Note any complaints of recurrent headache or other pain. When he's been afebrile for 3 days, antibiotics can be discontinued.

# Encephalitis

## Prediagnosis summary

The patient's initial assessment findings included a sudden onset of fever, headache, and vomiting. He may also have had:

● signs of meningeal irritation (stiff neck and back)

● signs of cerebral edema resulting in increased ICP, such as an altered level of consciousness (see the "Increased Intracranial Pressure" entry in this chapter)

● recent viral illness, such as mumps or infectious mononucleosis.

The doctor ordered a CT scan to detect brain lesions, and he cultured the patient's blood, stool, and throat to identify the infecting organism. He may have performed a lumbar puncture to obtain CSF for viral studies. Culture results were negative for bacteria, which helped the doctor determine that the patient's illness is not bacterial meningitis (the signs and symptoms are similar); the patient's history was also a determining factor, particularly if he lives in an area where encephalitis is known to be endemic. Viral studies of his CSF may have indicated the causative organism, confirming the diagnosis of encephalitis. However, many filterable viruses can't be identified this way, so the organism causing the patient's encephalitis may not have been identified.

## Priorities

A patient with encephalitis has a high risk of developing massive, asymmetrical cerebral edema, which, in turn, will

# WHAT HAPPENS IN ENCEPHALITIS

Encephalitis is a severe brain inflammation that can occur secondary to numerous other systemic viral infections. It may infect a single patient or spread (via mosquitoes) until it's epidemic.

Encephalitis causes lymphocytic infiltration of brain and meningeal tissues that results in cerebral edema, ganglion cell degeneration, and nerve cell destruction. In its most severe form, this process commonly ends in death.

cause increased ICP. Your first priority, then, is to take measures to prevent cerebral edema. If he already has cerebral edema, he may have pupil dilation on the affected side—a sign of pending temporal lobe herniation. (See the "ICP" entry in this chapter.)

The doctor may ask you to administer a rapidly acting osmotic diuretic, such as mannitol I.V., to lower the patient's ICP. However, you usually *won't* give high doses of corticosteroids because corticosteroids enhance the spread of the virus to unaffected areas of the brain. If the patient's cerebral edema is severe and osmotic diuretics can't control it, the doctor may order hypothermia treatments or barbiturate administration to the point of coma. Either of these treatments will reduce the metabolic rate, reducing his increased ICP. If these procedures fail, you may need to prepare him for immediate subtemporal surgical decompression.

## Continuing assessment and intervention

Assess your patient's neurologic status to provide a baseline. Be especially alert to signs of increasing ICP, such as decreasing level of consciousness, altered respiratory patterns, or a unilaterally dilated pupil. Infection and resulting edema may be more severe on one side

than the other, so look for asymmetrical reflexes and hemiparesis.

Your patient may have anosmia (an altered sense of smell) or olfactory hallucinations, indicating that his olfactory system is affected. You can test his sense of smell using familiar and nonirritating substances, such as coffee, tobacco, and cloves.

Watch for restlessness, vomiting, and seizure activity. Administer anticonvulsants, if ordered, and mild sedatives to help the patient rest. Provide a quiet, darkened environment to minimize his photophobia and headache. Restrict fluids to avoid increasing cerebral edema, as you would for any patient at risk for increased ICP. Monitor his intake and output and his electrolyte balance.

Obtain a history from your patient and his family, paying particular attention to recent viral illness, such as mumps, mononucleosis, chickenpox, or shingles. (As you know, the virus causing that illness may be the same one causing the encephalitis.) Determine if the patient lives in (or has recently visited) an area where eastern equine encephalitis is endemic.

## Therapeutic care

For your patient with encephalitis, care is mainly symptomatic and supportive. Administer sedatives, antipyretics, and analgesics, as ordered, to keep your patient comfortable and to reduce any fever. Provide adequate nutrition and fluid support, and watch for complications, such as increased ICP or neurologic deficits.

When cultures of the patient's CSF, blood, and stool return, the doctor may be able to identify the causative virus. If herpes simplex virus is identified (or if the doctor strongly suspects its presence, such as when the patient's encephalitis is an isolated case and he lives in an area where eastern equine encephalitis isn't endemic), he may ask you to administer the antiviral agent vidarabine monohydrate (adenine arabinoside; Vira-A), which inhibits multiplication of the herpes simplex virus. Give vidarabine I.V. infusion over 12 to 24 hours, and watch for side effects, such as nausea, vomiting, diarrhea, dizziness, or hallucinations.

As your patient's recovery continues, remember that *his ICP may increase at any time.* Assess him frequently for this. If his ICP increases, *call the doctor immediately,* or your patient may suffer permanent neurologic damage. Rehabilitative care should start as soon as the acute phase of his illness is over.

*Note:* Report any incidence of encephalitis to the board of health. Let them know if your patient has a history of recent viral illness, which may have precipitated the encephalitis, or if you suspect the virus was vector-borne.

# Brain Abscess

## Prediagnosis summary
Initial assessment findings were similar to those of a brain tumor and may have included:
- signs and symptoms of increasing ICP, such as severe headache, nausea, vomiting, seizures, disturbances in vision, pupillary changes, and altered levels of consciousness (progressing from drowsiness to coma)
- expressive aphasia
- hemiparesis
- ataxia
- central facial weakness.

The doctor confirmed the diagnosis of brain abscess by CT scan, brain scan, or angiography. An I.V. was started, and cardiac monitoring was established. Blood was drawn for CBC, electrolytes, and ABGs. Three blood cultures were drawn, ½ hour apart, and the patient was placed in isolation prophylactically, pending culture results.

## Priorities
Your first priority is to lower your patient's increased ICP (see the "In-creased Intracranial Pressure" entry in this chapter) and to start him on large doses of broad-spectrum I.V. antibiotics to combat infection.

## Continuing assessment and intervention
Perform a baseline assessment by taking your patient's vital signs and evaluating his neurologic status using the Glasgow Coma Scale (see *Assessing Your Patient's Level of Consciousness Using the Glasgow Coma Scale,* page 229). Then obtain a detailed history from your patient or a family member. Ask whether he recently suffered head trauma or had cranial surgery. Has he had a middle ear infection; sinusitis; mastoiditis; a dental abscess; congenital heart disease; bacterial endocarditis; pelvic, abdominal, or skin infections; or pulmonary or pleural infection? Closely monitor your patient's vital signs—check them at least hourly. Bradycardia, widening pulse pressure, or increasing blood pressure may be an indication of increased ICP. If you note any *significant* change, notify the doctor.

A patient with brain abscess has a high susceptibility to seizures, so take precautions to protect him from injury. Pad the bed's side rails, and keep an oral airway at the bedside.

## Therapeutic care
Treatment for a brain abscess is mainly surgical. However, surgery usually will be delayed until the abscess wall becomes sufficiently dense to withstand excision without rupturing. This may take up to 2 weeks; in the meantime, I.V. antibiotics will be continued, and follow-up CT scans will be done to determine when the abscess is sufficiently encapsulated. Sometimes, however, severe inflammation and cerebral edema may necessitate earlier surgical intervention to prevent cerebral herniation and death. Under these circumstances, excision may not be possible, so temporary aspiration and drainage will be performed.

PATHOPHYSIOLOGY

# WHAT HAPPENS IN BRAIN ABSCESS

A brain abscess is a collection of pus within the brain, most commonly in the cerebral hemispheres or the cerebellum. It may develop from direct, penetrating brain injury; brain surgery; infection elsewhere in the body that travels through the bloodstream; or neighboring infection in the mastoids, middle ear, or paranasal sinuses. (At least 50% of brain abscesses result from mastoid or ear infections.)

Brain abscess develops on the same side of the brain as the primary infection. Pus may be free at first, causing inflammatory necrosis and edema; but, over several weeks, the brain tissue surrounds the abscess with a thick capsule. The resulting mass produces clinical effects similar to those of a brain tumor.

Patients with brain abscess are most often between ages 10 and 35; the condition's uncommon in elderly patients and affects about 2% of children with congenital heart disease.

This four-part diagram shows you the pathophysiology of a brain abscess.

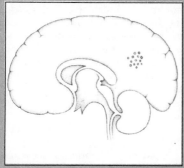

**1.** Infection (from the lungs, for example) spreads to an area of the brain; the site becomes edematous and infiltrated with white blood cells.

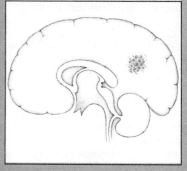

**2.** The center of the abscess becomes liquefied necrotic tissue.

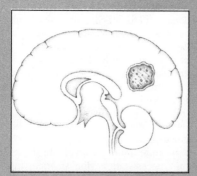

**3.** A thick, fibrinous wall encapsulates the abscess.

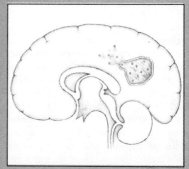

**4.** Without treatment, the capsule breaks, spreading satellite abscesses to white brain matter and ventricles and producing empyema and meningitis.

After your patient's surgery, monitor his neurologic function carefully. Watch for signs of meningitis—a common complication following brain surgery (see the "Meningitis" entry in this chapter). Continue to give antibiotics, as ordered. (Isolation precautions may be discontinued 24 hours after effective antibiotic therapy is initiated.) Position your patient on the side of the excision to prevent pus from reaccumulating and to promote drainage. Change his dressing frequently, noting the quantity and quality of the drainage. Continue to take precautions against seizures, including administering prophylactic anticonvulsants, as ordered.

## A FINAL WORD

As you're no doubt aware, the incidence of morbidity and mortality from neurologic emergencies is extremely high. Here are just two examples of the frustrating statistics associated with neurologic emergencies:

• Each year, EDs throughout the United States treat more than 400,000 people with *severe head injuries*. Of these, 33,000 die—more than half during the first 24 hours after surgery. Severe head injuries also cause death in many children and young adults who are trauma victims.

• Consider another common neurologic emergency—CVA, or stroke. Each year, 500,000 adults suffer CVAs, and more than 250,000 die. Many of those who survive must struggle to overcome CVA-induced disorders.

But this gloomy picture's getting brighter. Today, more patients with neurologic emergencies are recovering, with a reduced incidence of permanent damage. Why? Because of faster transport to hospitals, more sophisticated care on the way, new drugs and other new treatment methods, and advances in rehabilitation. *And* because more nurses are trained to respond to these patients' unique emergency-care needs in the ED and on the unit.

You know, if you've cared for very many patients with neurologic emergencies, that your nursing care extends far beyond initial treatment. When the medical emergency's passed and the patient's recovering, he's still at risk for a recurrence of his neurologic emergency. And for many of these patients, the quality of the emotional support they receive is a critical factor in their eventual recovery.

As a nurse, you can do a great deal to effectively combat the depression and frustration that so often accompany neurologic impairment. Your support may assist in restoring your patient's self-esteem. If you can help to instill the "I-can-do-it" attitude he'll need to get through the rehabilitation phase of his treatment, you can feel satisfied that you've met *all* his emergency-care needs.

## Selected References

Budassi, Susan A., and Barber, Janet M. *Emergency Nursing: Principles and Practice.* St. Louis: C.V. Mosby Co., 1980.

*Coping with Neurologic Disorders.* Nursing Photobook Series. Springhouse, Pa.: Springhouse Corp., 1982.

Davis, Joan, and Mason, Celestine. *Neurologic Critical Care.* New York: Van Nostrand Reinhold Co., 1979.

Kravis, Thomas C., and Warner, Carmen G., eds. *Emergency Medicine: A Comprehensive Review.* Rockville, Md.: Aspen Systems Corp., 1982.

Salcman, Michael. *Neurologic Emergencies: Recognition and Management.* New York: Raven Press Pubs., 1980.

Wilkins, Earle W., Jr. *MGH Textbook of Emergency Medicine,* 2nd ed. Baltimore: Williams & Wilkins, 1983.

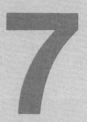

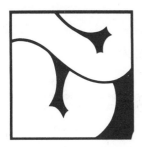

# Gastrointestinal Emergencies

## Introduction

You're working the night shift on the medical-surgical unit. One of your patients is Randy Stovers, age 55, an unkempt white male with a history of chronic alcohol abuse. Randy came into the hospital earlier in the day with complaints of weakness, fatigue, vague stomach pain, and loss of appetite. He has a history of cirrhosis, $B_{12}$ deficiency, malnutrition, and poor health habits, and he hasn't seen a doctor in 7 years. He was admitted for a thorough workup and for observation.

He seems fine during the early part of your shift, but later in the evening he becomes increasingly restless. His skin is cool and clammy. When you take his vital signs, his blood pressure is slightly decreased and his pulse rate is slightly increased. You continue to watch him closely; over the next hour, you note alterations in consciousness and a steady decrease in his blood pressure. You call the doctor to report this.

When you return to Randy's room, you find that he's vomiting and has diarrhea. His stools are black and tarry. You recognize the signs of possible GI bleeding. Suddenly, you have an emergency on your hands.

Would you know how to assess Randy's condition and intervene appropriately? What about other signs and symptoms of GI emergencies—are you confident that you can recognize them?

As you probably know, GI emergencies can occur as primary complaints, as consequences of non-GI disorders or injuries, or as complications of taking medications or undergoing diagnostic tests. Be particularly alert for a possible GI emergency in a patient:

• who has a history of chronic inflammatory bowel disease, which may flare up with acute signs and symptoms.

• who's had recent diagnostic tests such as endoscopy, which can cause perforation of the GI tract.

• who's had recent surgery that may result in bowel-obstructing adhesions or in peritonitis and sepsis from leaking anastomoses.

• who has a tumor or hernia, which can obstruct the bowel or other organs.

• who has atherosclerotic vascular disease, which may cause occlusion of mesenteric blood vessels.

• who has a history of taking large amounts of alcohol or drugs (such as aspirin, steroids, or antacids) that can irritate the GI tract or cause altered bowel function (or a history of low tolerance of these drugs).

This chapter will help you become familiar with the causes and the signs and symptoms of GI emergencies. You'll also learn assessment and intervention techniques that will build your confidence in managing patients with these types of emergency problems.

AT THE SCENE

# A G.I. BLEEDING EMERGENCY

What would you do if you were walking downtown and saw a man collapse in the street, vomiting blood? Assessing his condition and intervening appropriately at the scene would be difficult—but your help could save his life.

Here's what you could do:

First ask someone to call an ambulance; then quickly check the patient's airway, which may be filled with blood that's choking him. Use finger sweeps to clear blood and any vomitus from his airway, and listen for his respirations. If he isn't breathing, *start CPR immediately*, palpating for a pulse as you do so. Don't stop until he's breathing and has a pulse.

If you're able to stabilize his airway, breathing, and circulation, tilt his head to one side so he won't aspirate vomitus.

Next, check the patient's level of consciousness by shaking him and calling to him. If you can't arouse him, do a sternal rub to see if he'll respond to pain. (Recheck his vital signs periodically—if they deteriorate, you'll have to give CPR

again, possibly until the paramedics arrive.)

As you probably know, the patient's bloody vomitus may indicate GI hemorrhage, which can lead to hypovolemic shock. To help prevent shock, keep the patient warm by covering him with your coat. If you don't have one, borrow a jacket, a blanket, or even a newspaper and drape it over him. Next, elevate his legs with a rolled-up coat, a briefcase, or a few books—anything that will do the job. This will increase the blood volume return to his heart and other vital organs.

Now, what can you do about his bleeding? Obviously, pressure or dressings won't stop GI bleeding, but you may be able to slow it down with ice. Ask a passerby to get a bag of ice quickly from a nearby restaurant, soda fountain, or bar. Place the ice on the patient's upper abdomen: This will constrict his stomach wall and lower esophageal blood vessels so his GI bleeding should lessen.

Stay with him until the paramedics arrive, continuing CPR if necessary.

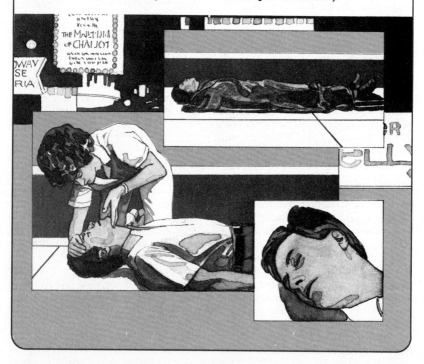

# INITIAL CARE

## Prehospital Care: What's Been Done

The rescue team's first priority, as always, is to stabilize the patient's airway, breathing, and circulation. But don't assume this has been done—particularly in a patient with a GI emergency, who may be choking on vomitus or blood or even suffering complete circulatory collapse. When the patient arrives in the ED, assess his airway, breathing, and circulation before you do anything else. If his airway's blocked, *clear it immediately.*

En route to the hospital, the rescue team will place the patient on his left side, or turn his head to one side, to keep him from aspirating vomitus or blood. If he's bleeding externally, they'll apply direct pressure at the bleeding site. They'll probably also start an I.V., with a large-gauge catheter, to replace lost fluids. If he has signs and symptoms of shock, the rescue team may put the patient in a modified Trendelenburg's position and apply medical antishock trousers (a MAST suit) to maintain sufficient blood circulation to the vital organs in his upper body. When you receive the patient, don't deflate all the compartments of the MAST suit at once. Why not? Because the external pressure the suit provides may be all that's keeping the patient from going more deeply into shock.

When the patient arrives in the ED, make sure he doesn't eat or drink anything, because:
• if he needs surgery, he won't be able to have certain anesthetics, and he may aspirate his stomach contents.
• having food and fluids in his stomach

will aggravate his condition.
• if he needs endoscopy, his stomach contents may obscure the view and prevent diagnosis.

## What to Do First

Unless you've already done so, assess your patient's airway, breathing, and circulation, and intervene as necessary. Then assess his general appearance and mental status to obtain further clues to his GI emergency problem.

### Airway
As you know, vomitus and blood com-

---

PRIORITIES

## INITIAL ASSESSMENT CHECKLIST

**Assess the ABCs first and intervene appropriately.**

**Check for:**
• vomiting and abdominal distention, possibly indicating bowel obstruction, peptic ulcer, or internal bleeding
• tachycardia, hypotension, diaphoresis, or pallor, possibly indicating occult bleeding and impending hypovolemia
• pain, guarding, or rigidity, indicating peritoneal irritation.

**Intervene by:**
• establishing an I.V. and infusing fluids
• inserting a nasogastric tube.

**Prepare for:**
• insertion of a Sengstaken-Blakemore tube
• peritoneal lavage
• emergency endoscopy
• insertion of a central venous pressure line.

# COMPARING GASTROINTESTINAL TUBES

## GASTRIC TUBES

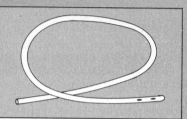

### Levin tube
This is a 50″ (127-cm), single-lumen, rubber or plastic tube with holes at the tip and along the side. It's used to remove stomach fluid and gas or to aspirate gastric contents. It may also be used for gastric lavage, drug administration, or feeding.

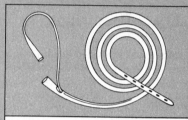

### Salem-Sump tube
This 48″ (122-cm), double-lumen tube has a small air-vent lumen (pigtail port) and a primary suction-drainage lumen. The air-vent lumen allows atmospheric air to enter the patient's stomach so the tube can float freely. This prevents the tube from adhering to the gastric mucosa and damaging it. The Salem-Sump tube is used for the same purposes as the Levin tube.

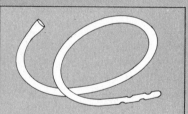

### Ewald tube
A wide-bore tube that passes a large volume of fluid quickly, it's used for stomach lavage in patients who've ingested poison or who have profuse GI bleeding.

### Nursing considerations:
• Attach the tube to low continuous or intermittent suction, or to straight gravity drainage, as ordered.
• Before instilling anything through the tube, always verify its placement by aspirating gastric contents or by auscultating the patient's stomach while injecting 50 cc of air into the tube. (If you hear a gurgling sound, the tube's in place.)
• To maintain patency, irrigate the tube with 30 cc of normal saline solution every 2 hours, or as ordered.

In an emergency, you may assist with the insertion of a GI tube to treat a patient's bowel obstruction, to aspirate his gastric or bowel contents, or to lavage his stomach. These are some of the tubes you may use. Be sure you're familiar with all of them.

## INTESTINAL TUBES

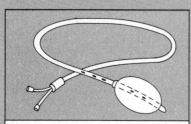

**Miller-Abbott tube**
This 10′ (3-m), double-lumen tube has one lumen for balloon inflation and one for drainage or suction. It's used in patients with bowel obstruction because it permits aspiration of bowel contents.

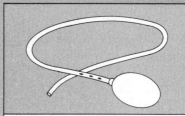

**Cantor tube**
This 10′ (3-m), single-lumen tube has a balloon at its distal tip, for mercury injection. It's also used in patients with bowel obstruction, because it permits aspiration of bowel contents.

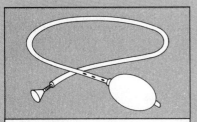

**Harris tube**
This 6′ (1.8-m), single-lumen tube has a metal tip and a balloon for mercury injection. Also used in patients with bowel obstruction, it permits intestinal tract lavage, usually with a Y-tube attached.

**Nursing considerations:**
• When using a *Miller-Abbott tube,* fill the balloon with mercury when the tube reaches the stomach, and clamp the balloon lumen to prevent accidental mercury withdrawal through suction. Label each lumen. With a *Cantor* or *Harris tube,* fill the balloon bag's upper portion with mercury before insertion, and aspirate all air from the bag.
• Place the patient on his right side for tube advancement.
• Drain the tube by gravity during insertion. If drainage stops, inject 10 cc of air.
• Confirm tube placement by X-ray.
• Attach the suction lumen to intermittent low suction when the tube reaches its mark (as ordered).

## USING THE TILT TEST TO EVALUATE HYPOVOLEMIA

A change in your patient's blood pressure or pulse rate when he changes his body position is an early warning sign of hypovolemia. To measure your patient's orthostatic vital signs, take his blood pressure and pulse rate when he's in three different postures: supine, sitting, and standing. (If you note significant changes when the patient sits up, *do not* have him stand up.) Record your findings in the following manner:

| Supine | BP 120/80 |
| --- | --- |
| | Pulse 86 |
| Sitting | BP 110/70 |
| | Pulse 96 |
| Standing | BP 80/48 |
| | Pulse 126 |

Consider a decrease of 10 mm Hg or more in systolic pressure, or an increase of 10 beats/minute or more in pulse rate, as a positive sign indicating volume depletion and possible impending hypovolemic shock. Keep in mind that dizziness, light-headedness, or disturbances in vision (such as blurred vision), occurring when your patient changes position, also may indicate a positive tilt test.

monly cause airway blockage in patients with GI emergencies. If the patient's chest isn't moving and you can't feel exhaled air over his nose and mouth, assume that his airway's completely obstructed and proceed *immediately* to clear it (see the "Life Support" section in Chapter 3). Use suction or a mouth sweep to remove food particles or blood. If you suspect that the patient's already aspirated vomitus or blood, notify the doctor immediately; he'll order a chest X-ray. If this confirms that the patient's aspirated foreign matter, the doctor will start him on antibiotics to prevent pneumonia.

To suction the patient's stomach contents and to reduce his risk of aspiration and airway obstruction, you may insert a nasogastric (NG) tube as ordered. (By indicating the presence or absence of blood, an NG tube can also help you determine if the patient has upper GI bleeding.)

Explain to your patient (if he's con-

scious) that insertion of the NG tube will feel uncomfortable at first, and assure him that he'll probably feel better once his stomach contents have been removed and his vomiting has stopped. (See *Comparing Gastrointestinal Tubes*, pages 300 and 301.) Begin meticulous mouth care.

### Breathing

Assess your patient's breathing for rate, depth, and pattern. If his respirations are inadequate, prepare to administer supplemental oxygen and to insert an artificial airway or to assist with intubation if mechanical ventilation is necessary.

You may note shallow tachypnea if your patient has:
• GI hemorrhage leading to hypovolemic shock or electrolyte imbalance
• severe abdominal pain, such as peritonitis can cause. (More men than women respond to severe abdominal pain by developing tachypnea. Why?

Because men use their abdominal muscles when they breathe.)

Your patient may breathe slowly and deeply to compensate for metabolic alkalosis resulting from loss of gastric acid and electrolytes, due to vomiting. Or he may have difficulty breathing because of abdominal distention or massive ascites—either can inhibit diaphragmatic excursion.

## Circulation

Because "GI emergency" so often means "GI bleeding," watch your patient closely for signs and symptoms of shock due to (possibly rapid) blood loss. Check his vital signs frequently and use the tilt test to assess him for hypovolemia. (See *Using the Tilt Test to Evaluate Hypovolemia.*)

As you may know, blood loss of 500 ml or less may cause no significant change in your patient's pulse rate, respiratory rate, or blood pressure. However, by the time the patient's lost 1,000 ml of blood, his pulse will be increased by approximately 20 beats/minute, his systolic blood pressure will be below 100 mm Hg (or will drop 10 mm Hg when he sits up), and he'll probably be thirsty, nauseated, or dizzy. With blood loss of about 2,000 ml, expect your patient to have frank signs and symptoms of hypovolemic shock (see the "Hypovolemic Shock" entry in Chapter 14):

• rapid, thready pulse
• cool, clammy skin
• restlessness
• confusion
• further decrease in systolic blood pressure.

Remember, hypovolemic shock may have other causes besides severe blood loss. For example, repeated bouts of vomiting or diarrhea can cause dehydration, leading to hypovolemic shock. So can a severe bowel obstruction.

If you think that your patient with a GI emergency is going into shock, place him in a modified Trendelenburg's position by elevating his feet on a pillow while keeping the head of his bed flat.

Start a large-bore I.V., in his right arm if possible. Why? Because your patient may require emergency endoscopy to determine the source of any GI tract bleeding, and if he does, he'll be positioned on his left side during the procedure. Use an 18G or larger needle to facilitate rapid fluid replacement and blood transfusion (if necessary). You may also assist with insertion of a central venous pressure (CVP) line to enhance fluid replacement and to allow you to monitor the patient's fluid status more accurately. Draw blood for typing and cross matching (in case transfusion is necessary) and for complete blood count (CBC), electrolytes, blood glucose, blood urea nitrogen (BUN), serum amylase, hemoglobin and hematocrit, platelet count, prothrombin time (PT), and partial thromboplastin time (PTT).

You may give crystalloids (except dextrose in water, which causes hypotonicity), colloids (such as plasma and albumin), blood, or Ringer's lactate. However, you *won't* use Ringer's lactate if the doctor suspects the patient has liver disease. This is because the patient's damaged liver won't be able to metabolize the lactate in this solution.

Start an intake and output record to keep track of the patient's fluid balance. Fluctuations are common in patients with severe blood loss, diarrhea, or vomiting. Include gastric aspirate, vomitus, or liquid fecal material in your output measurements.

If you suspect the patient's bleeding internally but you see no obvious signs (such as frank hematemesis or the passage of bloody stools), test his vomitus, gastric aspirate, and stool sample for occult blood, using a Hemoccult test. Remember, however, that if the patient's eaten red meat or other blood-containing foods recently, this may give you a false-positive result on the test.

## General appearance

A patient who's in distress because of a GI emergency will typically be weak and apprehensive, in pain, and, possibly, dehydrated or in shock. He may have a penetrating wound or signs (such as bruises) of internal bleeding or injury. Look for cool, pale, clammy skin—a sign that he's going into shock. If his skin feels dry, his skin turgor is poor, and his eyeballs are sunken, he's severely dehydrated, possibly from profuse vomiting or diarrhea.

Insert an indwelling (Foley) catheter to obtain accurate output measurements.

Look for bruises or wounds on the patient's body between the nipple line and midthigh. If he's suffered blunt trauma, keep in mind that he may have severe internal injuries even if you note few or no external signs. If he's been shot, remember that entry and exit wounds may not accurately demonstrate the bullet's path. Here's why: A bullet may ricochet off bones and organs, damaging them, before exiting the patient's body.

If your patient has a penetrating abdominal wound, find out when he had his last tetanus immunization. If he hasn't been immunized in the last 5 years, expect to give tetanus prophylaxis (see *Guidelines for Tetanus Prophylaxis,* pages 66 and 67).

Evaluate the patient's body position for clues to the location and severity of his pain. For example, if he's lying on his side with his knees flexed, he probably has severe abdominal pain.

### Mental status

Confusion, disorientation, anxiety—as you'd expect, a severely ill or injured patient can exhibit any of these signs. In a patient with a GI emergency, however, these signs may be due not only to stress but also to extreme fluid loss leading to shock. If you note these signs in a patient who *hasn't* lost excessive amounts of fluids, he may have liver disease.

Remember that the patient with a GI emergency may feel guilty if he suspects that his eating habits, excessive alcohol ingestion, or inability to handle stress

have caused his emergency problem. Provide emotional support, and do what you can to minimize stress on him at this time.

## What to Do Next

Once you've stabilized your patient's airway, breathing, and circulation, you're ready to gather baseline data that will help you evaluate his GI emergency. Remember, the success of his treatment may depend on the accuracy of this assessment. Why? Because although the signs and symptoms of different GI emergencies can be confusingly similar, a detailed and acccurate assessment will help clarify the patient's problem.

As you know, many GI emergencies cause hypovolemic shock, which can be rapidly fatal. You'll need to act quickly if your patient goes into shock (see Chapter 14). But this isn't your only consideration. You must do a thorough assessment that identifies his chief complaints. Don't forget to monitor his vital signs throughout your assessment. Be prepared to stop at once and *intervene* if his condition deteriorates.

Start your assessment by evaluating your patient's *abdominal pain.* Ask how long he's had the pain. Was its onset sudden or gradual? Have him show you where the pain's located— his response will indicate whether it's:

• *localized* (he can point to the painful area with one finger)

• *generalized* (he rubs, or holds, a specific area)

• *diffuse* (he complains that his entire stomach hurts; he may react to the pain by bringing his knees to his chest).

Diffuse pain typically indicates peritoneal irritation, whereas localized or generalized pain can indicate any of a host of GI disorders, depending on the pain's exact location. Localized pain in the lower right quadrant, for example, suggests appendicitis (see *Ap-*

## EVALUATING STOOL CHARACTERISTICS

As you probably know, the appearance of your patient's stool may help you identify the location of bleeding in his GI tract—and other GI problems as well. This chart characterizes abnormal stools and their possible causes.

| APPEARANCE | POSSIBLE CAUSES |
|---|---|
| **Black, tarry stool (melena)** | • Upper GI tract bleeding<br>• Slowly bleeding lesions in colon |
| **Black stool** | • Rapid elimination of bile<br>• Ingestion of iron |
| **Stool streaked with blood, or blood clots on stool surface** | • Bleeding in distal colon at site of fecal formation<br>• Hemorrhoids |
| **Red or maroon stool** | • Lower (sometimes upper) GI tract bleeding |
| **Mucoid stool** | • Colitis<br>• Mucus-producing tumor |
| **Large, bulky, foul-smelling stool that floats on water** | • Malabsorption of fat (steatorrhea) or large quantity of air or other gas in the stool |
| **Clay-colored stool** | • Liver disease (for example, hepatitis) or biliary obstruction<br>• Residue from barium studies |

pendicitis *Pain Pointer*, page 308). Generalized upper abdominal pain suggests gastric or biliary colic.

Ask your patient to describe the pain's character and severity:
• *Severe crampy, colicky pain* suggests gastroenteritis or bowel obstruction.
• *Severe steady pain* suggests peritonitis.
• *Dull steady pain* suggests cholecystitis or diverticulitis.

If the pain causes your patient to writhe about, it's probably colicky. If he's able to lie still in spite of the pain, it's probably generalized and steady.

While you're gathering data about your patient's pain, he'll probably ask you for pain medication. Explain that you don't want to mask his pain until its cause is pinpointed, and assure him that he'll receive pain medication soon.

Be sure to position him so he's as comfortable as possible in the meantime.

If your patient's a premenopausal woman, find out when her last menstrual period ended. If her period's due now or late, consider that an ectopic pregnancy may be causing her pain.

Other obstetric and gynecologic disorders can mimic the pain of GI problems. For example, pelvic inflammatory disease (PID) causes appendicitis-like signs and symptoms. (However, PID usually coincides with the woman's menstrual period, whereas appendicitis usually occurs between periods.)

If your patient's period is late or you suspect underlying obstetric or gynecologic problems, notify the doctor and prepare her for a pelvic examination, as described in Chapter 12.

During your initial assessment, you

### D.T. ALERT

Contrary to popular perception, delirium tremens (DTs) is no joke—in fact, mortality from DTs is about 15%. However, if the patient's treated early, his prognosis is good.

Watch for these signs and symptoms of impending DTs in *any* patient suspected of abusing alcohol:
- tremors
- agitation, confusion, and disorientation
- elevated vital signs
- signs of autonomic nervous system disorder (dilated pupils, fever, tachycardia).

If you see any of these signs and symptoms, intervene immediately. Notify the doctor, and prepare to administer tranquilizers as ordered. Try to calm your patient by creating a quiet, nonstressful atmosphere and by reassuring him in a soothing tone of voice.

identified any penetrating wounds your patient had and intervened appropriately. You also observed him for such signs of blunt trauma as bruises. Now, inspect his abdomen carefully for additional signs of blunt trauma, which may have caused his abdominal pain. Look for ecchymoses, Cullen's sign (a blue discoloration around the umbilicus), and Grey Turner's sign (a similar discoloration on his flanks). Ask him if he's been in an accident that caused a blow to his abdomen. If he has, have him describe the location of the blow and its force.

Measure the patient's abdominal girth at the level of his umbilicus. Check later measurements against this baseline: increased girth may indicate abdominal bleeding (or increased bleeding). Mark the place on the patient's abdomen where you took the measurement, so you'll always measure in the same place.

Closely watch a patient who's suffered blunt abdominal trauma. Remember that, even in a patient with few external signs, abdominal bleeding may be severe, and he may go into shock before you're aware of the extent of his bleeding.

When you're assessing abdominal pain, don't forget to ask your patient if he has pain anywhere else. If he does, it may be *referred* pain related to his GI emergency. For example, pain referred to the patient's shoulder may be due to cholecystitis, pancreatitis, or peritonitis.

But other disorders can also refer pain. Your awareness of this may help you uncover clues to additional emergency problems in your patient. Abdominal aortic aneurysm, for example, can refer pain to the patient's back. Or he may feel groin pain referred from the site of an arterial occlusion or a strangulated hernia.

Even though you're interested in whether he has rigidity and tenderness related to his chief complaint of pain, *don't* palpate his abdomen yet. Finish assessing his chief complaints. Then, auscultate his bowel sounds *before* you palpate his abdomen.

If your patient's *vomiting*, ask him when and how it started, and how often it occurs. Does he feel nauseous? Is the vomiting painful? If you can, collect his vomitus and measure its quantity. Then ask him about the color and quantity of his vomitus during earlier vomiting episodes. (He probably won't want to think or talk about this, but persist in asking. Explain that these details will help you evaluate his condition.) In particular, ask if he noticed blood, bile, or undigested food in his vomitus. Did it have a fecal smell? Undigested food in vomitus may indicate a gastric outlet obstruction; a fecal smell may indicate lower-bowel obstruction. Blood in the vomitus, of course, indicates upper GI bleeding.

If your patient's been vomiting for a prolonged period, he may develop a Mallory-Weiss syndrome—a tear in the esophageal wall that causes profuse bleeding—from the strain on his esophagus. If you see blood in his vomitus, call the doctor. Of course, you'll

# NURSE'S GUIDE TO
# SOME COMMON DRUGS THAT AFFECT
# THE GASTROINTESTINAL SYSTEM

| CLASSIFICATION | POSSIBLE SIDE EFFECTS |
|---|---|
| **ANALGESICS** | |
| **aspirin** | Nausea, vomiting, GI distress, occult bleeding |
| **indomethacin (Indocin)** | Nausea, vomiting, diarrhea, hemorrhage |
| **ibuprofen (Motrin\*)** | Nausea, vomiting, GI distress, occult bleeding |
| **phenylbutazone (Butazolidin\*)** | Nausea, vomiting, mucosal ulceration or hemorrhage |
| **ANTI-INFECTIVES** | |
| **gentian violet** | Nausea, vomiting, oral ulceration |
| **sulfonamides** | Nausea, vomiting, diarrhea, abdominal pain |
| **tetracycline (Achromycin\*)** | Nausea, vomiting, diarrhea, stomatitis, tooth discoloration |
| **penicillins** | Nausea, vomiting, diarrhea |
| **ANTACIDS** | |
| **aluminum hydroxide** | Anorexia, constipation, bowel obstruction |
| **magaldrate (Riopan\*)** | Mild constipation or diarrhea |
| **magnesia magma (Milk of Magnesia)** | Diarrhea, abdominal pain, nausea |
| **combination products (e.g., Gelusil\*, Mylanta\*, Maalox)** | Constipation, bowel obstruction, diarrhea, flatulence |
| **NARCOTICS** | |
| **codeine phosphate, codeine sulfate** | Nausea, vomiting, constipation |
| **meperidine hydrochloride (Demerol\*) methadone hydrochloride (Dolophine) morphine sulfate** | Nausea, vomiting, dry mouth, constipation, biliary tract spasm |

\*Available in U.S. and Canada. All other products (no symbol) available in U.S. only.

## APPENDICITIS PAIN POINTER

Your patient reports that his acute abdominal pain has suddenly ceased. A good sign? *Not necessarily*—it could be the first sign that his appendix has ruptured. Call the doctor if you observe *any* change in your patient's abdominal pain.

also continue to monitor his fluid balance and electrolyte levels closely, to forestall worsening dehydration and shock. Continue to check him for signs of dehydration and to assess him for the leg cramps and irregular pulse that can result from electrolyte imbalance. Be prepared to give I.V. supplemental fluids and electrolytes.

Ask your patient if he's had black and tarry or bright-red and bloody stools, which may indicate *GI bleeding*. Record a complete description of his stools' appearance, either by observation or by asking the patient what his last bowel movement looked like. Has he been taking regular doses of such medications as aspirin or steroids, which can irritate the GI tract and cause bleeding? (See *Nurse's Guide to Some Common Drugs That Affect the Gastrointestinal System*, page 307.)

Bloody vomitus, whether bright red or of a coffee-grounds consistency, indicates that your patient's bleeding is occurring above the ligament of Treitz in his duodenum. Bloody stools, however, don't always indicate the site of the bleeding. This is because blood may or may not darken as it passes through the GI tract. (See *Evaluating Stool Characteristics*, page 305, and the "Lower Gastrointestinal Tract Hemorrhage" entry in this chapter.)

If you note signs of bleeding, quickly check the patient's conjunctiva, oral mucosa, nail beds, and skin color for pallor—a sign that he has significant blood loss. If you haven't already drawn blood for hemoglobin and hematocrit levels and for typing and cross matching, do so now.

Your patient may report *changes in his bowel habits:* diarrhea or constipation. To avoid relying on the patient's subjective evaluation of these complaints, ask him for specific information. If he's "constipated," when was the last time he had a bowel movement, and the time before that? If he has "diarrhea," how many bowel movements did he have today? How many yesterday? Is he taking any drugs, such as laxatives or antacids, that can affect bowel function? (See *Nurse's Guide to Some Common Drugs That Affect the Gastrointestinal System*, page 307.) Ask if he has any food or drug allergies and whether he was recently exposed to a substance he's allergic to. Diarrhea, cramping, and even abdominal pain can indicate an allergic reaction.

Ask your patient if his *appetite* has increased or decreased lately. An increased appetite may mask a peptic ulcer that's soothed by food. Appendicitis causes a decrease in appetite.

After you've assessed your patient's chief complaints, auscultate his abdomen, noting the presence or absence of bowel sounds. Auscultate all four quadrants. If bowel sounds are present, note if they're *hypoactive* (occurring less than 5 times per minute) or *hyperactive* (more than 34 times per minute). The doctor will evaluate your patient's bowel sounds together with any changes in your patient's bowel or eating habits. Increased bowel sounds together with constipation may indicate acute bowel obstruction or hemorrhage; absent or decreased bowel sounds may indicate peritoneal inflammation or peritonitis.

Complete your abdominal examination by palpating and percussing your patient's abdomen. Begin by palpating *gently* for rigidity and for tender areas. If the patient's abdomen is rigid, he may have peritonitis. Stop palpating *immediately* and notify the doctor.

If the patient's abdomen yields to

your gentle palpation, continue to palpate all four quadrants. Save the quadrant where the patient's pain is located for last; otherwise, guarding in response to palpation in this quadrant could make palpation of the other quadrants difficult. Note any rebound tenderness, which may indicate peritoneal irritation. If your patient's suffered blunt trauma, ask him to contract his abdominal wall during palpation. This will help you distinguish muscle-wall tenderness from intraabdominal tenderness. (Muscle-wall contraction *increases* muscle-wall tenderness and *decreases* intraabdominal tenderness.)

Percuss your patient's abdomen for areas of tympany and dullness. Check for suprapubic dullness, indicating a distended bladder, and for increased areas of dullness over the liver, indicating liver enlargement, possibly due to trauma or liver disease. Identify the patient's spleen, and note if it's enlarged. Locate the tympany of the gastric air bubble in the area of the left lower anterior rib cage—an increase in bubble size, along with abdominal distention, suggests gastric dilatation. Percuss for shifting dullness, and note the line of demarcation between the dull and the tympanic areas. This allows you to detect free fluid and to roughly estimate volume. If you detect free fluid, assess for a fluid wave—an easily palpable fluid wave indicates ascites. Document your findings to provide a baseline for later comparison.

The doctor may do a peritoneal lavage if he suspects free blood, bile, or purulent material in the patient's abdomen. Assist him as necessary. (See *Assisting with Peritoneal Lavage,* pages 310 and 311.) If the lavage fluid's bloody, the doctor will ask you to prepare the patient for emergency surgery.

Finally, take a quick history. Ask your patient if he has any *chronic GI disorders* such as liver disease, ulcers, or inflammatory bowel disease. (As you know, chronic GI disorders can go into remission only to flare up later.) Find out if he's had surgery for any GI con-

dition; he may have developed adhesions that are causing bowel obstruction. Ask, too, if the patient has other chronic diseases, such as diabetes or cardiovascular disease—these may affect his care.

Ask your patient what *medications* he's taking. Note these on his chart, and find out if he's allergic to any medications—such as antibiotics.

Don't forget to ask your patient about his consumption of alcohol. As you probably know, alcohol abuse can lead to such GI emergency problems as acute pancreatitis and perforated ulcer. And its effects can complicate the patient's treatment.

When you question your patient about his drinking habits, be tactful. Don't display a judgmental attitude. If you do, he may refuse to discuss the matter or at least to give you accurate information about his drinking. Instead, emphasize that you need an accurate estimate of how much he drinks, and how often, to give him proper treatment. Ask specific questions:
• "What do you drink?"
• "How many drinks do you have each day?"
• "When do you drink?"

Be sure, too, that you find out when he had his last drink—if he develops delirium tremens (DTs), this will affect his medical care.

---

# Special Considerations

## Pediatric

Appendicitis in children may mimic other GI disorders, especially acute gastroenteritis. Be alert to the possibility of appendicitis in any child with abdominal pain. Remember, the child's condition may already have progressed to peritonitis by the time you see him. (See *Danger: Peritonitis,* page 332.)

Intussusception, most common in infants, may also occur in children. Signs include periods of crampy abdominal pain, alternating with pain-free periods, and currant-jelly-like or tarry stools.

### Geriatric
Sudden severe abdominal pain in an elderly patient is probably caused by ruptured diverticulum, acute bowel obstruction, tumor, or perforated ulcer.

As you may know, an elderly patient's pain threshold may be higher than normal. So pay particular attention to his complaints—even mild ones. They may indicate a severe emergency.

# CARE AFTER DIAGNOSIS

# Penetrating Abdominal Trauma

### Prediagnosis summary
The patient suffered recent invasive

---

PROCEDURES

## YOUR ROLE IN AN EMERGENCY

### ASSISTING WITH PERITONEAL LAVAGE

If the doctor suspects that your patient's suffered internal abdominal injuries, he may order a peritoneal lavage to detect bleeding in the patient's peritoneal cavity. Here's a review of this procedure and your role in it.

#### Equipment
• 3- to 5-ml syringe with 25G needle
• Peritoneal dialysis tray (with trocar, catheters, scalpel, hemostats, tubing, specimen containers and tubes, syringes, needles, gauze, tape)
• I.V. pole and macrodrip I.V. tubing (without a "non-backflow" filter)
• 1 liter of Ringer's lactate or normal saline solution
• Local anesthetic

#### Before the procedure
• Explain the procedure to your patient, and offer him emotional support.
• Take his baseline vital signs, and measure his abdominal girth.
• Insert a nasogastric tube to decompress his stomach, if ordered.
• If your patient's a woman, assess her for a gravid uterus.
• Shave, prepare, and drape the abdomen.
• Have the patient void, or insert a catheter if ordered.

#### During the procedure
• After the doctor's inserted the catheter into the patient's peritoneal cavity and

introduced the lavage solution through the I.V. tubing, clamp the tubing and tape the catheter to your patient's abdomen.
• Unless contraindicated (for example, if he has a spinal cord injury or fractured ribs), gently turn the patient from side to side or manually manipulate his abdomen, as ordered, to mix the lavage solution and the peritoneal fluids.
• Open the clamp to the bag, as ordered, so that peritoneal fluid drains by gravity.
• Drain 25 to 30 ml of peritoneal fluid.
• Place about 10 ml of the fluid in a sterile and labeled culture-and-sensitivity container (do this first, to prevent specimen contamination); then divide the rest of the fluid into labeled tubes. Send the specimens to the laboratory for red blood cell count, electrolytes, amylase, and bile, as the doctor ordered or according to protocol.

#### After the procedure
• After the doctor removes the catheter and sutures the incision, apply an antibiotic ointment and sterile dressing.
• Monitor the patient's urine output for hematuria, which suggests bladder perforation.
• Observe him for increased abdominal pain, which may indicate bowel perforation.
• Monitor his vital signs frequently, and periodically check his abdominal girth, comparing it to the baseline measurement.
• Remember to document all your findings.

trauma from a gunshot wound, a stab wound, or an embedded object from an explosion, and he had an open wound located between the nipple line and midthigh. In addition, he probably had:

• signs and symptoms of hypovolemic shock such as tachycardia, thready pulse, hypotension, pallor, weakness, diaphoresis, tachypnea, and altered mental status

• orthostatic hypotension—a fall in blood pressure and an increase in heart rate when the patient was raised from the supine to the seated position (see *Using the Tilt Test to Evaluate Hypovolemia,* page 302).

If an impaled object caused his wound, it was left in place and stabilized until the doctor could safely remove it.

Blood was drawn for a CBC and for typing and cross matching. Abdominal X-rays were taken, to help determine the site of the injury. A Foley catheter was inserted if the patient had no bleeding at the urinary meatus, and an NG tube was inserted to remove his stomach contents, to check for blood, and to prevent aspiration of vomitus.

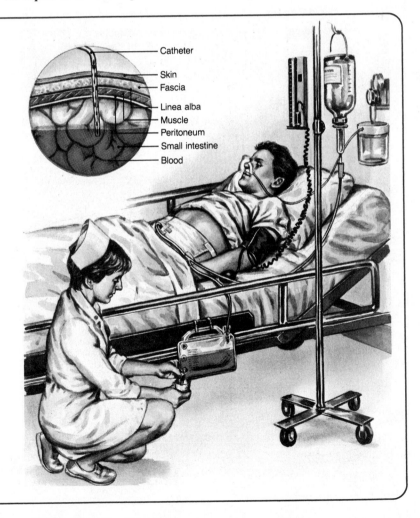

Catheter
Skin
Fascia
Linea alba
Muscle
Peritoneum
Small intestine
Blood

# EVALUATING PERITONEAL FLUID

While assisting with a peritoneal lavage, you can learn something about the patient's condition just by observing the appearance of his peritoneal fluid. Normal peritoneal fluid is clear to pale yellow. Here's what your patient's abnormal peritoneal fluid may indicate.

## BLOODY FLUID

**Possible causes:**
- Trauma
- Erosive tumor
- Acute hemorrhagic pancreatitis

## BILE-STAINED GREEN FLUID

**Possible causes:**
- Cholecystitis with bile duct obstruction
- Acute pancreatitis
- Perforated bowel or duodenal ulcer

## CLOUDY OR TURBID FLUID

**Possible causes:**
- Peritonitis from ruptured bowel
- Primary bacterial infection
- Pancreatitis
- Strangulated or infarcted bowel
- Appendicitis or ruptured appendix

## MILKY FLUID

**Possible causes:**
- Chyle (the cloudy liquid products of digestion taken up by the small intestine) escaping from a damaged thoracic duct
- Escaping barium following tests in the upper or lower GI tract

A large-bore I.V. (14G to 16G) was started for fluid replacement and medication access, and a CVP line was inserted. If the patient had signs and symptoms of shock, supplemental oxygen was given to decrease tissue hypoxia. Cardiac monitoring was initiated, and a MAST suit was applied.

## Priorities

Most patients with penetrating abdominal wounds require surgery. So your initial priority is to maintain the patient's hemodynamic status while the doctor determines the extent of his injury, and until the operating room is prepared. Expect to give crystalloids or colloids I.V. to help stabilize moderate hemorrhage. If the patient's hemorrhage exceeds 500 ml, expect to infuse whole blood and blood components as well.

The doctor will probably want to perform peritoneal lavage to determine if bloody fluid's present in the patient's peritoneal cavity. Expect to assist the doctor with the procedure and to collect the fluid drainage. (See *Assisting with Peritoneal Lavage,* pages 310 and 311.)

If the lavaged fluid's bloody, the patient will be rushed to the operating room for an exploratory laparotomy and further surgery as necessary. If the fluid isn't bloody, discontinue the lavage and thoroughly cleanse the wound site to prepare the patient for suturing. He'll probably be admitted for observation.

## Continuing assessment and intervention

*If your patient didn't require surgery,* continue to monitor his vital signs and to watch for signs and symptoms of peritonitis or wound infection (see *Danger: Peritonitis,* page 332). Perform a thorough baseline examination, and take your patient's history, including identifying the mechanism of injury. Take time, now that he's stabilized, to look for associated trauma that may have been overlooked initially. Remember to

### IMPROVISING A SPLINT PILLOW

Can't find an extra pillow or blanket for your patient who needs to splint his incision? You can make a good splint pillow out of linen savers (Chux). Simply fold four or five Chux in quarters and place them on one that's laid out flat. Then fold the whole package up and secure it with adhesive tape.

ask about associated blunt trauma to the patient's chest or abdomen that may have occurred along with the penetrating wound. (See the "Blunt Abdominal Trauma" entry in this chapter.) Remember, you may see no external signs of blunt trauma: signs and symptoms of underlying injury may not appear for several hours. Monitor your patient's vital signs closely during the observation period. Be sure to note any drug allergies, as your patient will require prophylactic antibiotics.

*If your patient's injury required surgical repair,* assess his vital signs frequently when he returns from surgery, including hourly CVP readings if he has a central line in place. Watch his abdomen for drainage, distention, tenderness, or rigidity. Thoroughly assess his bowel sounds in all four quadrants; a paralytic ileus may develop after surgery, causing decreased or absent intestinal motility. You may note vomiting and severe abdominal distention. If paralytic ileus persists more than 48 hours, you may need to insert an NG tube to aspirate the patient's gastric contents. You may be asked to administer cholinergic agents, such as neostigmine or bethanechol, to stimulate the patient's intestinal motility along with the nursing activity of increasing ambulation. Auscultate frequently for returning bowel sounds.

Watch for signs and symptoms of peritonitis—chiefly, a rigid abdomen with rebound tenderness, guarding, and severe abdominal pain. Early recognition and prompt treatment may minimize complications. Expect to give prophylactic antibiotics to reduce the risk of infection.

Start intake and output records, and monitor the patient's fluid and electrolyte balance closely after surgery.

Obtain a detailed history from the patient, his family, or his friends. This may not have been done if your patient needed emergency surgery, so be careful now to obtain any information that may have been missed earlier.

### Therapeutic care

After the patient's surgery, your care will center on preventing postoperative complications. Continue to monitor his vital signs and bowel sounds. He'll probably need aggressive pulmonary therapy with incentive spirometry, chest physical therapy, and mini-nebulizer treatments. Encourage the patient to cough and deep-breathe at least every hour, and teach him splinting techniques for minimizing stress on his surgical incision. (See *Improvising a Splint Pillow*, page 313.) Change his position at least every 2 hours, and medicate him for pain as necessary.

Continue to administer antibiotics, as ordered, and check the wound site frequently for drainage and signs of infection. If your patient's injury required a colostomy, start patient teaching to help him adjust to this alteration in body image.

# Blunt Abdominal Trauma

### Prediagnosis summary

The patient suffered a recent blow to the abdomen, with or without associated penetrating or multiple trauma. The organ(s) injured determined his signs and symptoms:

• *spleen*—left upper quadrant pain, accompanied by muscle spasm and rigidity; positive Kehr's sign (pain referred to the left shoulder)
• *liver*—right upper quadrant pain, accompanied by guarding, tenderness, and rigidity; positive Kehr's sign
• *duodenum*—transient pain and tenderness; positive Kehr's sign
• *large bowel*—subcutaneous emphysema; absent bowel sounds, blood noted upon rectal examination
• *pancreas*—increasing abdominal distention; positive Kehr's sign
• *stomach*—rapidly developing pain and tenderness.

The patient may have had signs and symptoms of hypovolemic shock: increased heart rate and pulse, decreased blood pressure, increased respirations, pallor, and diaphoresis. If he wasn't cared for immediately, he may also have had signs and symptoms of peritonitis (see *Danger: Peritonitis*, page 332).

A MAST suit may have been applied if the patient's hemorrhage appeared severe. A large-bore I.V. and a CVP line were inserted for fluid access and monitoring. The patient received supplemental oxygen to prevent tissue hypoxia and required an NG tube for aspiration of stomach contents and detection of blood. Blood was drawn for baseline CBC, electrolytes, blood glucose, BUN, serum amylase, SMA-12, PT-PTT, and typing and cross matching. Abdominal X-rays were taken to help determine the site of the patient's injury, and an intravenous pyelogram may have been done if associated kidney injury was suspected. Peritoneal lavage was performed to determine the presence of free fluid or blood in the patient's abdomen. Prior to this, a Foley catheter was inserted (if no obvious signs or symptoms of bladder injury were present), to minimize the risk of bladder perforation by the trocar. (See *Assisting with Peritoneal Lavage*, pages 310 and 311, and *Evaluating Peritoneal Fluid*, page 312.)

The doctor may not have been able to determine which of the patient's or-

# SEAT BELT SYNDROME:
## WATCH FOR HIDDEN ABDOMINAL INJURIES

You're working the Saturday night shift in the ED when an ambulance brings in Alex Harris, age 40, who's been in a head-on car crash. Miraculously, Alex says he feels fine, and your initial assessment reveals no obvious injuries except for a transverse band of bruising across his lower abdomen. He proudly announces that wearing a seat belt kept him from being seriously injured and may have saved his life.

Alex is probably right—wearing a seat belt may have prevented serious injury, particularly to his head. But you need to keep in mind that if he was using the belt improperly (wearing only the lap belt without the shoulder harness, or wearing the lap belt over his iliac crest), it may have *caused* injury—to his abdomen.

In a car crash, abrupt deceleration compresses a passenger's seat belt into his abdomen, greatly increasing intraabdominal pressure and the pressure within hollow organs—such as his stomach and bowel. This pressure may cause rupture, laceration, or herniation of abdominal organs. In addition, shearing stress from abrupt abdominal twisting and bending may cause tissue tearing, organ transection, or vertebral injury.

So you must *always* consider the possibility of hidden abdominal injuries in a car-crash victim who was wearing a seat belt. When assessing him, remember that not all his injuries (including the band of bruising across his abdomen) will be apparent immediately after the accident. Careful and continuous assessment is necessary to rule out injuries that are hidden—and perhaps life-threatening.

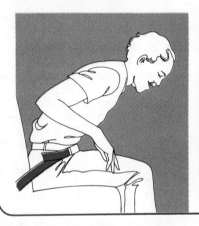 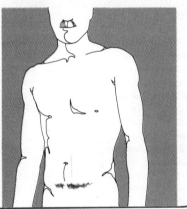

gans were injured without exploratory surgery; however, he was able to determine that the patient had an acute abdomen, based on positive peritoneal signs: guarding, rebound tenderness, decreased or absent bowel sounds, and severe abdominal pain.

## Priorities

Because any patient who's suffered blunt abdominal trauma may have severe internal hemorrhaging, your initial priorities are to perform a rapid assessment and to maintain the patient's hemodynamic status while his injury's evaluated. Continue to infuse fluids (and blood, if necessary) and to monitor his vital signs frequently. Administer oxygen to decrease tissue hypoxia.

If your patient's conscious prior to surgery, obtain a description of how the accident occurred and a brief history because identifying the mechanism of injury can help the doctor identify the injured organ(s). Find out, for example, if the patient was hit or fell or was thrown against a stationary object (such as a steering wheel) with great force. If he was in a motor vehicle accident, find out if he was wearing a seat belt—a hematoma across his lower abdomen or chest may indicate the area of underlying injuries. (See *Seat Belt Syndrome: Watch for Hidden Abdominal Injuries*, page 315.) However, *don't* waste time trying to determine which organ was injured. Determining if the patient has an acute abdomen is more important, because this will require immediate surgical intervention. Watch for these signs and symptoms:

- severe pain
- rigidity
- rebound tenderness
- decreased or absent bowel sounds.

If you note any of these, prepare the patient for surgery rapidly but thoroughly. Make sure the results of all his blood tests, X-rays, and diagnostic tests are available in his chart. Expect to administer prophylactic I.V. antibiotics if the doctor suspects that the patient's abdomen is contaminated.

Provide emotional support to the patient and his family, who'll be extremely anxious and upset at the prospect of this urgent, unexpected surgery. Ease their anxiety by explaining the procedures, several times if necessary, and by answering their questions.

Expect that your patient will be admitted for observation, even if he has very few or no signs and symptoms, because the risk that he has internal injury is high. Perform a thorough abdominal assessment for baseline data, and expect to repeat this examination frequently over the next 6 to 12 hours, watching for late-appearing signs and symptoms of GI tract disruption or peritonitis.

## Continuing assessment and intervention

Many patients will require immediate surgery to detect the injured organ(s) and to repair them as necessary. However, damage to some organs (such as the small or large bowel) may not be evident for several hours, until signs and symptoms of peritonitis appear.

Perform frequent abdominal examinations on the patient, including inspection, percussion, and palpation of all four quadrants. Auscultate for bowel sounds, and check for rebound tenderness. (Remember, increased tenderness accompanied by decreased bowel sounds may indicate developing peritonitis.) Report abnormal findings to the doctor immediately, and expect that the patient will require surgery. You may also note developing tenderness or rigidity, an enlarging abdominal mass, or a progressive drop in the patient's hematocrit and hemoglobin levels in the absence of hypotension. These findings may also indicate the need for surgery. Prior to surgery, take a complete history, including food and drug allergies, if you haven't had a chance to do this before.

## Therapeutic care

When your patient returns from surgery, continue to perform frequent assessments to detect complications. Administer analgesics for pain and antibiotics to prevent infection. Check your patient's wound dressings frequently; they may be left in place for several days if peritonitis is present. Reinforce or change them if they become wet or soiled. (As you know, wet dressings are an excellent medium for bacterial growth.)

Monitor the patient's vital signs, watching for an increase in temperature that may signal peritonitis or abscess. Assess his bowel sounds in all four quadrants. If they're absent, keep an NG tube in place until they return. Irrigate the tube every 4 hours or as needed, and remember to check it for position and patency *before* irrigation: It may have slipped into a lung. Maintain accurate intake and output records to monitor the patient's fluid balance; if necessary, the doctor may ask you to insert a Foley catheter to help measure output. You should see an output of 30 ml of urine per hour; if you don't, the patient may be hypovolemic. Notify the doctor, and expect that he'll ask you to increase the patient's I.V. fluid replacement.

Continue to monitor the patient's electrolytes. Imbalances may result from his injury or from NG tube drainage. Monitor his CBC results every 4 to 12 hours; it will alert you to internal bleeding (decreased hematocrit and hemoglobin levels) or to infection such as peritonitis (increased white blood cell [WBC] count).

When the patient's bowel sounds return, remove the NG tube and begin giving him oral fluids. If he tolerates the fluids well, the I.V. will be discontinued. Remove the Foley catheter, and help the patient ambulate as soon as possible. He'll probably receive aggressive pulmonary therapy (incentive spirometry, mini-nebulizer treatments, or chest physical therapy). Encourage him to cough, deep-breathe, and turn frequently, to prevent pulmonary complications.

*If your patient didn't require surgery,* he may be discharged if observation for 6 to 12 hours revealed no signs or symptoms indicating internal injury. Make sure you explain to the patient that abdominal injuries may still exist but that signs and symptoms may not appear for several days. Detail the warning signs and symptoms that the patient and his family should watch for:
- abdominal pain
- fever
- loss of appetite
- weakness
- fatigue.

Make sure you schedule him for a follow-up clinic appointment for 3 to 5 days later.

---

# Perforated Peptic Ulcer

## Prediagnosis summary

The patient's initial assessment findings included:
- sudden onset of intense, constant, generalized abdominal pain
- a history of previous cyclic pain that occurred when his stomach was empty
- melena (black, tarry stools)
- hematemesis
- signs of shock such as diaphoresis, pallor, palpitations, confusion, increased pulse and respirations, and decreased blood pressure
- a rigid and boardlike abdomen, with rebound tenderness
- absent bowel sounds.

A large-gauge I.V. was started for fluid administration, and Ringer's lactate was infused. An NG tube was inserted to aspirate the patient's stomach contents and to check for the presence of blood. Blood was drawn for clotting studies, CBC, electrolytes, hemoglobin and hematocrit, BUN, serum glutamic-oxaloacetic transaminase (SGOT), serum amylase, total bilirubin, and arterial blood gases (ABGs). Upper GI X-rays were taken, and emergency endoscopy was performed if the patient's condition permitted it.

## Priorities

Your patient may rapidly become hypovolemic as a result of both the hemorrhage and the fluid shift that occurs with developing peritonitis. (See *Danger: Peritonitis,* page 332.) Your first priority, then, is replacing lost fluids to maintain the patient's blood volume and to ensure his hemodynamic stability. Expect to infuse Ringer's lactate through a large-bore I.V., and assist in placing a CVP line, if possible. Make sure the patient's blood has been typed and cross-matched, and prepare him for transfusion. Monitor his vital signs and watch for developing hypovolemic shock. Insert a Foley catheter, to measure his output, and be prepared to apply a MAST suit if his condition deteriorates.

## Continuing assessment and intervention

Assess the level of your patient's bleeding, and control active bleeding with an iced normal-saline lavage. Instill

PATHOPHYSIOLOGY

# WHAT HAPPENS IN PEPTIC ULCER

A peptic ulcer is an ulcerative lesion of the upper GI mucosal membrane. Studies indicate that the two major forms of peptic ulcer, duodenal and gastric, occur when the GI tract's protective mucosa is unable to resist corrosion by acid-pepsin during digestion. Damaged duodenal or gastric mucosa permits further erosion of each layer of the abdominal wall, possibly causing bleeding and/or perforation. Although different factors may cause them, gastric and duodenal ulcers have essentially the same pathophysiology.

**Gastric**
Decreased mucosal resistance to normal or subnormal acid production, in the presence of conditions such as gastritis or irritants such as aspirin, steroids, alcohol, or caffeine, allows back-diffusion of gastric acids from the lumen to the mucosa. This leads to:

**Duodenal**
Acid hypersecretion may result from an overactive vagus nerve or from hyperparathyroidism, chronic pulmonary disease, chronic pancreatitis, or alcoholic cirrhosis. This leads to:

Erosion; histamines are released.

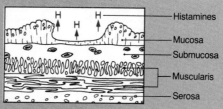

Further stimulation of acid secretion and increased capillary permeability to proteins cause mucosa to become edematous.

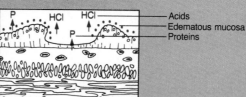

As erosion continues, mucosal capillaries and submucosal blood vessels are damaged, leading to hemorrhage and shock.

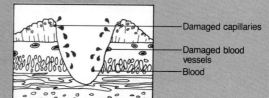

If erosion continues through the serosa, perforation and peritonitis will occur.

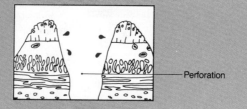

iced saline through the patient's NG tube or through a large Ewald tube, and lavage until the aspirate is clear. (See *Comparing Gastrointestinal Tubes*, pages 300 and 301.) Carefully record the amount of gastric drainage by subtracting the amount of saline you infused from the amount of drainage returned. If ordered, you may add norepinephrine to the iced saline; this induces vasoconstriction and helps reduce bleeding further. Note the color and character of the aspirate, which indicate the amount of the patient's bleeding and whether it's active:

• *Clear* aspirate indicates that prior bleeding, if any, has stopped.

• *Coffee-ground* aspirate indicates prior bleeding; if it clears after lavage, active bleeding has probably stopped.

• *Persistent pink* aspirate after repeated lavage indicates active bleeding.

Evaluate lavage results in the light of your other assessment findings. Decreasing blood pressure and increasing pulse are signs that the patient's hemorrhage may be continuing. Examine his abdomen for tenderness, boardlike rigidity, and absent or decreased bowel sounds, which may indicate continued bleeding or developing peritonitis.

If endoscopy wasn't performed initially, the doctor may do it now that the patient's stomach has been lavaged. Assist the doctor with this procedure by keeping the patient in the proper position, by providing emotional support, and by monitoring his vital signs frequently. Keep suction and emergency CPR equipment on hand. The doctor will examine the patient's esophageal and gastric mucosa and his upper duodenum in stages, as the flexible tube passes through the patient's upper GI tract (see *Assisting with Upper GI Endoscopy*, page 320).

If lavage or endoscopy indicates active bleeding, the doctor may instill a vasoconstricting agent, such as norepinephrine, through the patient's endoscope tube. An arteriogram may locate the bleeding site if the patient's blood loss rate is at least 0.5 ml/minute.

Or he may insert an intraarterial catheter under X-ray. The doctor may ask you to continuously infuse vasopressin (Pitressin) through the intraarterial catheter (see *Highlighting Vasopressin [Pitressin]*, page 326). Vasopressin induces vasoconstriction and helps control the active bleeding.

Your patient may require surgery if he's unresponsive to medical treatment and active bleeding continues. Take a complete history before the surgery. Your patient may report episodes of heartburn and indigestion after large meals; weight loss (if he has a gastric ulcer) or weight gain (if he has a duodenal ulcer); or midepigastric pain relieved by eating. Note any medications he's taking—if his ulcer was diagnosed previously he may be taking:

• antacids (to reduce gastric acidity)

• cimetidine (to reduce gastric secretions)

• anticholinergics (to reduce excessive gastric activity if his ulcer is in his duodenum)

• sedatives and tranquilizers (only if he has a gastric ulcer).

Ask if the patient's been taking aspirin regularly or frequently, drinking excessively, or smoking and if he's been under unusual stress. These factors, which can irritate the gastric mucosa, may have contributed to ulcer formation or perforation. Of course, you'll also note any food or drug allergies.

Your patient may require:

• *vagotomy and pyloroplasty*, which sever the vagus nerve, to reduce hydrochloric acid production, and enlarge the lumen of the pylorus, to facilitate gastric emptying

• *distal gastrectomy*, which resects the gastric ulcer and the surrounding margins.

Prepare the patient for surgery and explain the procedure to him and his family.

## Therapeutic care

*If the iced lavage or drug administration controlled your patient's bleeding,* your continued care will center on diet

## YOUR ROLE IN AN EMERGENCY

## ASSISTING WITH UPPER G.I. ENDOSCOPY

You may be asked to assist with emergency upper GI endoscopy if the doctor suspects an upper GI disorder. This procedure allows the doctor to visualize the patient's esophageal and gastric mucosa and his upper duodenum. It also allows him to instill blood-clotting agents through the tube if bleeding is a problem. Here's a review of this procedure and your role in it.

### Equipment
• Local anesthetic and lubricant
• Mouthpiece
• Flexible fiberoptic endoscope
• Suction machine
• Narcotic antagonists
• Syringes, needles, specimen bottles, gauze, alcohol

### Before the procedure
• Notify the doctor if your patient's eaten in the past 6 hours and document this.
• Explain the procedure to your patient.
• Obtain his baseline vital signs.
• Administer sedatives, as ordered.
• Remove dentures, if present.
• Insert an I.V. line, as ordered.
• Spray his throat with the local anesthetic, as ordered, to minimize gagging.
• *Keep suction and CPR equipment on hand.*

### During the procedure
• Place your patient in a sitting position for scope passage, then on his left side for the examination. (*Don't* have him sit up if he's in shock.)
• Tilt his chin toward his chest, keeping his head in midline.
• Tell him to let saliva drain from the side of his mouth and not to swallow it.
• Insert the mouthpiece; the doctor may ask you to hold it in place.
• Tell the patient to breathe deeply; this will help relax his abdominal muscles.
• Label any specimens and send them to the laboratory for analysis, as ordered.

### After the procedure
• Continue to monitor the patient's vital signs.
• Tell him to remain lying down until the sedative has worn off, and restrict his food and fluid intake until his gag reflex returns.
• Be alert for bleeding, dysphagia, fever, tachycardia, cyanosis, diaphoresis, hypotension, and neck, chest, or abdominal pain—these may indicate esophageal, gastric, or duodenal perforation. Notify the doctor if you note any of these signs or symptoms.
• Document specimens collected, assessment findings, and interventions.

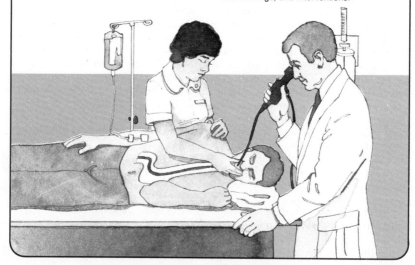

and rest while the perforation heals. Expect to administer medications such as:

• cimetidine (Tagamet) or ranitidine (Zantac)—histamine receptor antagonists that inhibit gastric acid secretion
• sucralfate (Carafate)—a barrier-forming drug that adheres to the ulcer and protects it against further attack by acids, enzymes, and bile salts.

When your patient's bowel sounds return, the doctor will order the NG tube removed. Start your patient on oral liquids. When he can tolerate sufficient oral fluids, remove the I.V. and the Foley catheter, as ordered. Before he begins eating solid foods, instruct him about dietary changes such as the need to restrict or avoid caffeine, alcohol, and certain foods. (You may want to set up an appointment with a dietitian to visit with your patient and explain the type of diet ordered and its accompanying restrictions.) Advise him to take antacids 1 hour before and after meals and to avoid bedtime snacks.

*If your patient needed surgery,* you'll provide postoperative care and watch for complications. Monitor his intake and ouput, including NG tube drainage. Replace fluids and electrolytes lost with NG tube drainage, and watch him for signs and symptoms of dehydration and electrolyte imbalance. Monitor his electrolyte levels, and check his CBC frequently—decreased hematocrit and hemoglobin levels may indicate new bleeding, and an increased WBC count may indicate peritonitis or wound infection. Assess his bowel sounds frequently until they return, when the doctor may order removal of the patient's NG tube. Then you'll probably start him on oral fluids, as ordered.

When your patient begins postoperative oral feedings, watch for *dumping syndrome*. As you probably know, a patient with this syndrome may experience early satiety—an intense feeling of fullness before finishing a meal—or nausea and vomiting shortly after eating. He may also experience abdominal cramps, flatulence, diarrhea, sweating, and palpitations. If your patient has this syndrome, teach him to lie down after eating and to drink fluids between meals rather than with meals. Provide frequent small meals that are high in protein and low in carbohydrates, rather than a few larger meals. Provide emotional support, too. Patients who experience dumping syndrome are likely to become very frustrated and depressed. Explain that this syndrome is common after gastric surgery and should resolve in time.

Prevent pulmonary complications by encouraging your patient to cough, deep-breathe, and turn frequently, and by encouraging early ambulation. Start patient teaching as soon as possible to help your patient adjust to changes in his life-style and diet.

---

# Ruptured Esophageal Varices

## Prediagnosis summary

The patient's signs and symptoms included some of the following:

• sudden, profuse hematemesis without pain or epigastric tenderness, with blood welling up in the back of his throat
• signs and symptoms of shock
• a history of heavy alcohol use, liver disease, such as cirrhosis or hepatitis, or schistosomiasis.

A large-bore I.V. was inserted, and rapid fluid replacement was started. Normal saline solution and colloids were started while the laboratory was preparing the proper type of blood. Blood was drawn for typing and cross matching and for CBC, electrolytes, hemoglobin and hematocrit, BUN, SGOT, serum amylase, total bilirubin, and ABGs. X-rays of the patient's upper GI tract were taken to help locate the source of his bleeding, and a gastroscopy was performed to visualize the

# WHAT HAPPENS IN
# RUPTURED ESOPHAGEAL VARICES

Ruptured esophageal varices result from portal hypertension—increased pressure in the portal vein due to an obstruction in portal circulation (for example, from cirrhosis).

Portal hypertension disrupts normal circulation so that blood bypasses the liver via collateral channels, instead of flowing through it via the portal vein. A common collateral channel is between the left and short gastric veins and the esophageal veins that open into the azygos vein. The excessive pressure causes these thin-walled esophageal veins to become varicosed. If the pressure continues, they may rupture. The resulting hemorrhage can lead to hypovolemic shock.

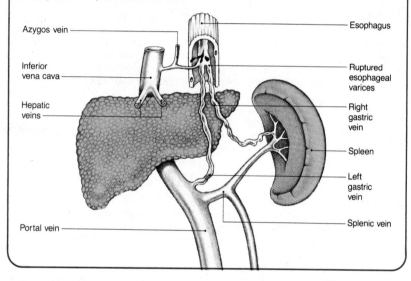

bleeding site and to confirm the diagnosis.

## Priorities

Ruptured esophageal varices cause profuse, severe bleeding that may be fatal without prompt intervention. Your first priorities in caring for the patient are to maintain a patent airway, to replace lost blood, and to control the bleeding.

Your patient will need multiple blood transfusions. Try to obtain fresh blood, if possible, because it contains less ammonium, which can't be readily metabolized by the patient's diseased liver. (You may know that ammonium can build up in the blood, causing hepatic encephalopathy and coma.) Insert a Foley catheter, and monitor the patient's intake and output carefully. The doctor may ask you to assist with insertion of a large-bore Ewald tube for lavaging the patient's stomach. If bleeding persists, you may assist the doctor with insertion of a Sengstaken-Blakemore tube, a triple-lumen tube used to tamponade the bleeding varices. (See *Using the Sengstaken-Blakemore Tube to Control Esophageal Bleeding,* pages 324 and 325.)

Start an infusion of vasopressin (Pitressin), if ordered; this will induce diffuse vasoconstriction. Expect to give this drug as an I.V. infusion or as an intraarterial infusion into the patient's superior mesenteric artery. Don't forget to support the patient's family during these procedures—the profuse bleeding is terrifying.

## Continuing assessment and intervention

Take a history from your patient or his family to determine the presence of underlying chronic liver disease or chronic alcohol abuse. Assess him for jaundice, dilated cutaneous veins, spider angiomata, palmar erythema, and ascites, and palpate for an enlarged liver—all signs of possible liver disease.

Monitor your patient closely for signs and symptoms of shock or of respiratory distress. Secure the tube carefully to prevent excessive traction or movement, and check the pressure within the gastric and esophageal balloons by attaching a manometer to the respective ports. Check the pressure frequently; excessive pressure will make your patient very uncomfortable and may cause esophageal and gastric mucosa ulcerations.

Keep a pair of scissors taped to the head of the patient's bed at all times— so you can cut and remove the tubing rapidly if the gastric balloon deflates or ruptures, causing airway obstruction from upward displacement of the esophageal balloon. Suction the patient's oral and nasal secretions frequently, because the tube will cause increased salivation and the inflated esophageal balloon will prevent him from swallowing his saliva. Unless a Minnesota tube is used, you may need to insert a small NG tube through the patient's opposite nostril, to drain secretions that collect above the esophageal balloon and to prevent aspiration.

Watch for signs of hepatic coma (altered mental status ranging from lethargy to coma, asterixis [flapping tremors of the outstretched hands], fetor hepaticus) related to your patient's underlying liver disease and the blood that's decomposing in his intestinal tract. As blood breaks down, it produces ammonium and raises blood ammonia levels; if your patient's liver is damaged, he won't be able to metabolize the ammonia, and its toxic levels will build up, affecting his brain function.

Draw blood for liver function studies and for electrolytes. You may administer magnesium sulfate, lactulose, or saline enemas as soon as your patient's condition permits. These will empty his intestinal tract of blood, thus preventing ammonia intoxication and hepatic coma. Also expect to give intestinal antimicrobial agents, such as neomycin, to decrease breakdown of the patient's blood by intestinal bacteria.

If your patient's receiving vasopressin, watch him closely for abdominal colic, facial pallor, and involuntary bowel evacuations—anticipated side effects. However, you should also be aware that vasopressin can cause systemic arterial hypertension, coronary artery vasoconstriction, and even myocardial infarction. Monitor your patient's vital signs closely. Call the doctor if you note decreased pedal pulses or increased blood pressure, and prepare to stop the infusion immediately (see *Highlighting Vasopressin [Pitressin],* page 326).

## Therapeutic care

Assess your patient for signs and symptoms of continued bleeding. Irrigate his stomach through the gastric aspirate port as ordered, and record the nature and color of the aspirate. If the Sengstaken-Blakemore tube and vasopressin administration can't control the bleeding, your patient may require emergency surgery—usually a portacaval shunt to decrease portal pressure and the pressure in the esophageal vessels.

If possible, the doctor will delay surgery until after bleeding has been controlled and the patient's condition has stabilized.

After surgery, watch the patient carefully for postoperative complica-

# YOUR ROLE IN AN EMERGENCY

## USING THE SENGSTAKEN-BLAKEMORE TUBE TO CONTROL ESOPHAGEAL BLEEDING

To help control bleeding when your patient has ruptured esophageal varices, the doctor may ask you to help him insert a Sengstaken-Blakemore (S-B) tube. Why? Because inflation of the tube's balloons will compress the varices and temporarily restrict bleeding.

As you can see in the illustration, the S-B tube has an esophageal balloon and a gastric balloon. Each of the three lumens attached to the tube has a specific function: One inflates the esophageal balloon, one inflates the gastric balloon, and one suctions gastric contents below the gastric balloon.

### Preparation

The doctor may ask you to prepare the S-B tube for insertion by chilling and lubricating it. He may also ask you to check for air leaks in the balloons by inflating them and holding them under water: if no bubbles appear, the balloons are intact.

Before the tube's inserted, elevate the head of the patient's bed to a semi-Fowler position (unless he's in shock). And, as always, explain the procedure to him and provide emotional support.

### Insertion and inflation

As the doctor inserts the S-B tube, encourage the patient to breathe through his mouth and to sip some water. Initial confirmation of tube placement involves injecting air into the gastric port, while auscultating the patient's abdomen, and aspirating gastric contents. Do this if the doctor orders it. The doctor will immediately order an X-ray to confirm the tube's position, but he won't wait for it. Instead, he'll proceed to inflate the gastric balloon with 250 to 500 cc of air.

When the gastric balloon's inflated, double-clamp its air intake port, and tape the nasal cuff in place on the S-B tube. This will minimize pressure on the patient's nostril. (To keep the patient comfortable with the tube in place, consider having him wear a football helmet—if one's available and the doctor okays its use. Then you can tape the tube to the helmet's face guard.)

Next, lavage the patient's stomach with normal or iced saline solution, as ordered, and attach the gastric suction port to an intermittent suction apparatus (Gomco). Doing this prevents nausea in the patient and allows evacuation of blood from his stomach as well as continuous observation of his gastric contents.

Now, the doctor will inflate the esophageal balloon. When he's finished, double-clamp the esophageal air intake port. To prevent accumulation and aspiration of esophageal secretions above the esophageal balloon, the doctor may ask you to insert a nasogastric tube through the patient's other nostril into his esophagus. Or he may insert it himself. (If you're using a Minnesota tube, be aware that it has a fourth lumen for this purpose.) Attach the port to suction, as ordered.

### Nursing considerations

• Check and record the patient's vital signs frequently. Be especially alert for signs and symptoms of esophageal rupture, shock, and increased bleeding and respiratory difficulty.

• *Keep a pair of scissors taped to the head of the patient's bed.* Then you'll be ready, if the patient develops acute respiratory distress, to grasp the tube at the nostril, to cut across it to deflate both balloons, and to remove it without delay.

• Maintain balloon pressures at the required levels—check the pressure every 4 to 6 hours. As ordered, deflate the balloons periodically, to prevent necrosis of the patient's stomach and esophagus. Be alert to recurrence of bleeding or aspiration of stomach contents—have suction available and be ready to reinflate if necessary.

• Maintain suction, as ordered, on the tube's gastric and esophageal aspiration ports.

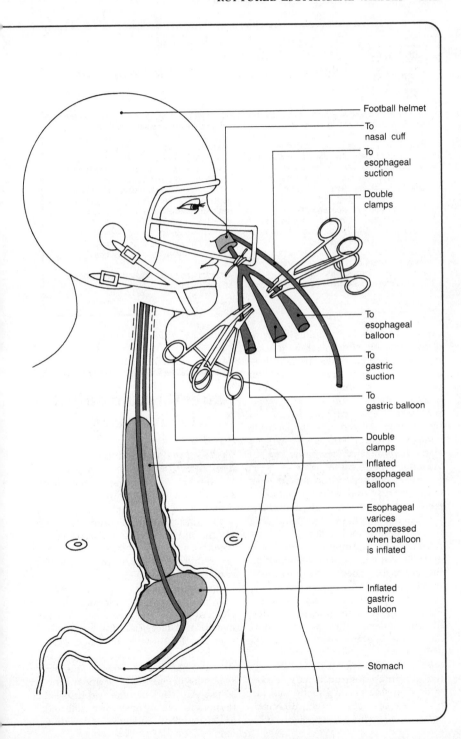

Football helmet

To
nasal cuff

To
esophageal
suction

Double
clamps

To
esophageal
balloon

To
gastric
suction

To
gastric balloon

Double
clamps

Inflated
esophageal
balloon

Esophageal
varices
compressed
when balloon
is inflated

Inflated
gastric
balloon

Stomach

DRUGS

## HIGHLIGHTING VASOPRESSIN (PITRESSIN)

You may be asked to administer vasopressin (Pitressin) as an adjunct to more conventional treatment for acute GI hemorrhage, such as use of the Sengstaken-Blakemore tube. Administered intravenously or intraarterially, vasopressin causes vasoconstriction that results in decreased blood flow, decreased portal pressure, and increased clotting and hemostasis. This action makes vasopressin particularly effective in the treatment of conditions precipitated by portal hypertension, such as ruptured esophageal varices.

Such treatment generally consists of an initial I.V. bolus of aqueous vasopressin for 5 to 30 minutes, with continuous I.V. infusion until 24 hours after the bleeding has stopped. While administering vasopressin, monitor your patient's heart rate, blood pressure, EKG, and renal function. Possible adverse effects include decreased heart rate and cardiac output, increased blood pressure, abdominal cramping, bowel infarction, and water intoxication.

*Warning:* When preparing vasopressin for administration, read the label carefully—different commercial products have confusingly similar names:
• Pitocin: oxytocin
• Pitressin: synthetic vasopressin
• Pitressin Tannate in Oil: vasopressin in oil diluent
• Pituitrin: posterior pituitary (vasopressin and oxytocin).

tions. Assess for signs and symptoms of hemorrhage from a leaking anastomosis—which may cause peritonitis—and for respiratory complications that may arise from your patient's reluctance to breathe deeply. Encourage your patient to deep-breathe, and turn him frequently. Watch for neurologic changes including lethargy, which may signal hepatic encephalopathy and developing hepatic coma.

Surgery will reduce the patient's risk of further ruptured varices, but it won't resolve the underlying liver disease. Explain the patient's new diet and drug regimen to him, and emphasize the importance of abstaining from alcohol.

If your patient is a poor surgical risk, the doctor may choose one of two new procedures that are currently being studied—electrocoagulation and sclerotherapy. *Electrocoagulation,* which directly cauterizes the varices, is similar to the treatment used in the operating room to cauterize bleeders. *Sclerotherapy,* performed after the initial bleeding's controlled, is injection of a sclerosing agent directly into the patient's esophageal varices. Both procedures offer hope to patients who

aren't able to tolerate surgery.

# Lower Gastrointestinal Tract Hemorrhage

### Prediagnosis summary
The patient initially had rectal bleeding and bloody diarrhea that may also have contained pus and mucus. In addition, he may have had:
• pain and abdominal cramping
• signs and symptoms of shock such as weakness, pallor, tachycardia, decreased blood pressure, and increased respirations.

He was given supplemental oxygen and had blood drawn for CBC, BUN, electrolytes, and typing and cross matching. A large-bore I.V. was established for fluid access, and Ringer's lactate or normal saline solution was started. If the patient showed signs and symptoms of shock, a CVP line was inserted. An NG tube was also inserted to check for bloody gastric aspirate and to determine if the source of bleeding was in the upper or lower GI tract. GI X-rays were also taken.

## Priorities

As with other forms of hemorrhage, your first priority is to maintain the patient's fluid balance while the site of hemorrhage is determined. Administer I.V. fluids and blood, as ordered. Monitor his vital signs closely while you prepare the patient for lower GI endoscopy. The doctor will use:

• an *anoscope*, if he suspects that the bleeding is from the patient's rectum or anus (for example, because of hemorrhoids or a foreign object)

• a *proctoscope* or *sigmoidoscope*, if he suspects that the bleeding is from the patient's rectosigmoid or rectum

• a flexible fiber-optic *colonoscope*, if he suspects that the bleeding is higher in the patient's GI tract (see *Comparing Types of Lower Gastrointestinal Endoscopy*, page 328).

Colonoscopy allows the doctor to visualize the patient's descending, transverse, and ascending colon and the cecum, as well as his rectosigmoid, rectum, and anus.

Prepare the patient for the procedure selected, and give enemas (as ordered) to clean the bowel. Monitor the patient's blood pressure closely during the procedure—a sudden drop may indicate perforation or, possibly, impending shock.

If the doctor's unable to locate the patient's bleeding site with endoscopy and the bleeding continues at a rapid rate, he may order angiography of the patient's superior and inferior mesenteric arteries—the most effective way to locate the source of active bleeding. Contrast material will be extravasated if the artery is bleeding at a rate of 0.5 ml/minute or more. Prepare the patient for angiography, and remember that the hypertonic contrast material may cause fluid balance problems, particularly in an older patient. Monitor his fluid and electrolyte status closely; be prepared to provide emotional support as necessary.

## Continuing assessment and intervention

Perform a thorough nursing assessment when your patient's bleeding is controlled and the bleeding site has been located. As you know, causes of lower GI hemorrhage include:

• ulcerative colitis
• diverticulosis
• fistulas
• cecal ulcers
• tumors
• angiodysplasia
• infarcted bowel.

Ask about any chronic GI diseases. Find out if the patient's experienced similar bleeding before and if he's noticed lower abdominal pain or cramping pain with bowel movements. Have his bowel habits changed? Inspect his abdomen, and auscultate all four quadrants for bowel sounds. Report any abnormal findings to the doctor.

Monitor the patient's vital signs regularly, and perform the tilt test for a quick gauge of fluid volume status (see *Using the Tilt Test to Evaluate Hypovolemia*, page 302). Monitor his fluid status and record his CVP readings and urine output hourly. Include all oral and I.V. fluids in your intake records; include urine, gastric aspirate, and an estimate of rectal blood loss in your output records.

Your patient may require surgery to remove the cause of his bleeding, such as a tumor or ruptured diverticuli. Prepare him for surgery by giving cleansing enemas as ordered. Expect to start him on antibacterial therapy as ordered 12 to 18 hours before surgery, to suppress the growth of bacteria in intestinal flora in his bowel and to decrease the risk of peritonitis. The doctor may ask you to insert a Foley catheter to make sure the patient's bladder remains empty during surgery; to monitor his fluid balance; and to keep his rectal dressings dry after surgery.

Your patient may have a temporary or permanent colostomy after surgical resection of the hemorrhagic area. Explain the procedure and start patient teaching *before* surgery, to help him come to terms with this change in body image. Ask an enterostomal therapist to come and speak to your patient before the surgery, if you know he'll def-initely have a colostomy.

## Therapeutic care

*If surgery isn't necessary,* direct your interventions toward allowing the pa-

---

### COMPARING TYPES OF LOWER GASTROINTESTINAL ENDOSCOPY

The doctor may perform an emergency lower GI endoscopy on your patient to locate and coagulate bleeding points and to diagnose such conditions as strictures, cancer and polyps. He'll do one of three procedures, depending on how far into the patient's lower GI tract he wishes to visualize.

Anoscopy is the examination of the anus and lower rectum with an *anoscope.* This quick procedure is used to check for obvious rectal or anal bleeding and to detect the presence of foreign objects.

Proctosigmoidoscopy is the examination of the lining of the distal sigmoid colon, the rectum, and the anal canal using a *sigmoidoscope* and a *proctoscope.* The procedure is done in three steps:
1. A digital examination, to detect any

obstruction that may hinder passage of the instruments
2. Sigmoidoscopy, to visualize the distal sigmoid colon and rectum
3. Proctoscopy, to examine the lower rectum and anal canal.

Colonoscopy is the examination of the descending, transverse, and ascending colon and the cecum with a *flexible fiber-optic colonoscope.* After insertion, the doctor advances the colonoscope through the large bowel (guided by the scope's optical system), palpating the patient's abdomen to aid passage of the scope through the intestinal bends. Because a colonoscope causes the patient less discomfort than a sigmoidoscope or a proctoscope, the doctor may also use it to perform a proctosigmoidoscopy.

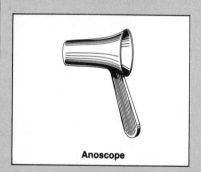

**Anoscope**

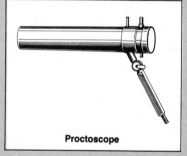

**Proctoscope**

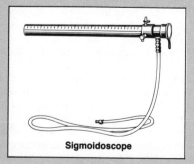

**Sigmoidoscope**

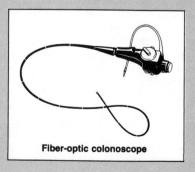

**Fiber-optic colonoscope**

tient's lower bowel to rest and heal. Give him nothing by mouth, and keep him on complete bed rest (decreased physical activity decreases intestinal motility). The doctor may order intraarterial administration of a vasoconstricting agent to reduce bleeding. If your patient receives this medication, assess his vital signs and bowel sounds frequently. Check his peripheral pulses, too; you may detect arterial occlusion.

*If the patient required surgery,* you'll provide postoperative care. Watch for such complications as peritonitis (see *Danger: Peritonitis,* page 332) and paralytic ileus. Monitor the patient's vital signs, and auscultate his bowel sounds frequently. Prevent pulmonary complications by encouraging him to cough and deep-breathe and to turn frequently.

When your patient's bleeding has stopped and his bowel sounds have returned to normal, the doctor may start him on oral fluids followed by a low-residue diet. Make sure the patient's meals are small, frequent, and high in calories, protein, and minerals.

# Bowel Obstruction

## Prediagnosis summary
Initial assessment findings depended on the location of the obstruction. If the patient had a *small-bowel obstruction,* his signs and symptoms may have included:
• crampy abdominal pain
• nausea
• profuse vomiting
• constipation
• abdominal distention.

If he had a *large-bowel obstruction,* his crampy pain may have developed slowly, accompanied by continuous hypogastric pain. Vomiting may have been absent, but abdominal distention probably appeared early. If distention did appear, it was very severe.

The patient was given supplemental oxygen. A large-gauge I.V. was inserted for fluid replacement (hypovolemic shock may develop as fluid shifts to the bowel). An NG or intestinal tube was inserted to relieve his abdominal distention. Blood was drawn for electrolytes, serum amylase, CBC, and blood glucose, and urine was obtained for urinalysis. Abdominal X-rays were ordered to detect distortion, distention, or localized air-fluid levels.

## Priorities
Monitor your patient closely. Watch for signs and symptoms of shock while you prepare for bowel decompression by GI tube or surgery. Pallor, rapid pulse, and a drop in the patient's blood pressure may indicate fluid loss from a strangulated hernia or from a drop in plasma volume as the bowel secretes fluid into the GI lumen (as much as 10 liters of fluid may collect). Administer I.V. fluids, and start careful intake and output records. Monitor the patient's electrolyte levels: An imbalance that's usually present because of the fluid shift into the bowel may become even more severe when decompression by NG tube is performed. Give the patient nothing by mouth, and help him find a comfortable position. The doctor will perform a rectal examination, digitally removing any fecal impaction he detects.

## Continuing assessment and intervention
Obtain a baseline assessment by asking your patient to describe where his pain is located, the type of pain, and how long he's had it.

If he has a mechanical small-bowel obstruction, he may have crampy, mid-abdominal pain. Pain may occur in paroxysms, with the patient relatively comfortable between episodes.

Large-bowel obstruction may cause either crampy, abdominal pain or continuous hypogastric pain. If strangulation's present in either the large or small bowel, the pain will be very severe and steady.

Vomiting may be present with either small-bowel or large-bowel obstruction. The higher the obstruction, the earlier and more severe the patient's vomiting will be; it may be a late finding in a patient with large-bowel obstruction. Note the color and character of the patient's vomitus: It will initially contain gastric juice, mucus, and bile, and it will remain that way if the obstruction's high in the bowel. If the obstruction's low in the ileum or in the large bowel, the patient may eventually vomit fecal contents. Auscultate his bowel sounds, which may be hyper-

---

PATHOPHYSIOLOGY

# WHAT HAPPENS IN BOWEL OBSTRUCTION

A partial or complete blockage of the small or large intestine results in bowel obstruction—a potentially life-threatening condition. Small-bowel obstruction is more common (because the ileum is the narrowest segment and most prone to obstruction) and is usually more serious (because of the accompanying fluid loss).

## COMMON CAUSES

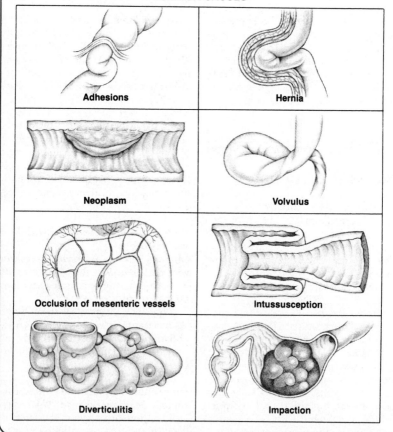

Adhesions

Hernia

Neoplasm

Volvulus

Occlusion of mesenteric vessels

Intussusception

Diverticulitis

Impaction

active and high pitched with a small-bowel obstruction, less frequent and lower pitched with a large-bowel obstruction.

Give your patient pain medication, as ordered. Expect to start prophylactic broad-spectrum antibiotics to reduce the risk of sepsis if the bowel perforates. Measure the patient's abdominal girth at the level of his umbilicus; this will provide a baseline for assessing the effectiveness of bowel decompression. Monitor the patient's intake and output—his urine output will steadily decrease unless his fluid volume is replaced.

## PATHOPHYSIOLOGY

Obstruction causes fluid, gas, and air to collect near the obstruction site. Peristalsis increases temporarily as the bowel tries to force its contents past the obstruction, injuring intestinal mucosa and causing further distention at and above the obstruction site.

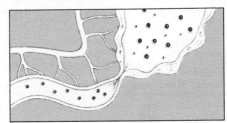

Distention impedes blood supply to the bowel wall and halts absorption. The bowel wall swells and—instead of absorbing—secretes water ($H_2O$), sodium (Na), and potassium (K) into pooled fluid in the bowel lumen, causing dehydration.

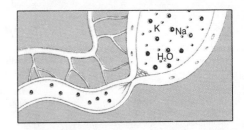

Gas-forming bacteria collect above the obstruction and further aggravate distention through fermentation.

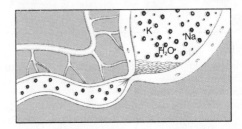

As more fluid pools, distention keeps extending proximal to the obstruction. If not treated early, this condition may lead to profound hypovolemia, shock, sepsis, and death.

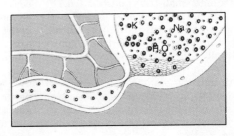

# DANGER: PERITONITIS

Peritonitis—a potentially life-threatening inflammation of the visceral and parietal peritoneum—results from bacterial infection or chemical irritation that occurs when a perforated abdominal organ leaks fluid and blood into the normally sterile abdominal cavity. Common causes of peritonitis are ruptured diverticuli, ruptured appendix, and penetrating abdominal trauma. But suspect it in *any* patient who has a GI disorder or a history of abdominal trauma, or who's had surgery of the abdominal cavity.

### Signs and symptoms
Be alert for these signs and symptoms:
• sudden abdominal *pain*, which may be localized or diffuse but is most intense in the area of the patient's primary GI disorder
• abdominal *distention* and rebound *tenderness*
• increased *temperature* (103° F., or 39.4° C.—or higher), with *chills*
• signs of *shock* (weakness, pallor, diaphoresis, tachycardia, decreased blood pressure)
• shallow, rapid *respirations* (due to diaphragmatic irritation).
    If you note any of these signs and symptoms, notify the doctor *immediately*. Remember, peritonitis can develop very rapidly.

### Diagnosis
The doctor will order a complete blood count to determine if the white blood cell count is elevated (20,000/mm³ or more). He'll also order abdominal X-rays, which may show a paralytic ileus, edema, distention of the small and large bowel, and upward displacement of the diaphragm. He may also perform a paracentesis to check for bacteria, exudate, pus, blood, or urine in the patient's abdominal cavity.

### Treatment
Treatment for peritonitis is in three steps:
• Identify the underlying cause and treat it.
• Treat the infection.
• Correct dehydration and paralytic ileus.
    Your patient may need surgery to remove or seal off the source of peritoneal contamination, or he may have an incision and drainage if the infection is localized.

### Nursing interventions
Expect to start antibiotics (such as gentamicin, tetracycline, or cephalosporin) promptly. Start an I.V. for fluid and electrolyte replacement, and insert a nasogastric tube, as ordered, to aspirate the patient's stomach contents. Give the patient nothing by mouth until his bowel sounds return and his gastric aspirate becomes scanty. Administer analgesics, usually morphine sulfate or meperidine, as ordered.

---

Your patient has an NG tube, initially inserted to remove his stomach contents and to prevent aspiration. Irrigate the tube with normal saline solution, and make sure it remains patent. (An NG tube may also relieve the distention of a high small-bowel obstruction.)

If your patient has a lower-bowel mechanical obstruction, the doctor may insert a single- or double-lumen GI tube—a long, weighted tube inserted nasogastrically and passed through the stomach to the bowel, where it may break up the obstruction. Assist with the insertion (see *Comparing Gastrointestinal Tubes,* pages 300 and 301).

Because GI tube insertion is uncomfortable and time-consuming, some doctors choose immediate surgery to decompress the patient's bowel. Also, a GI tube is only useful in breaking up an impaction. If the obstruction's caused by an adhesion, tumor, hernia, or volvulus, or by intussusception, the patient needs surgery after decompression with a short tube (such as a Levin tube). Prepare your patient for surgery as necessary, and explain the procedure to him and his family. Before the patient goes to the operating room, obtain a complete history, paying particular attention to current medications, past medical and surgical history, and food and drug allergies. Make sure all laboratory results and X-rays are included in the patient's chart.

## Therapeutic care

If your patient's had an intestinal tube inserted, your responsibility is to advance it once it's reached his stomach. Position your patient on his right side, with his knees flexed, to make him more comfortable and to facilitate the tube's passage. Every hour, slowly advance the tube 2″ to 3″ (5 to 7.6 cm), or as ordered. Encourage the patient to ambulate and to swallow frequently, so that gravity and peristalsis will help advance the tube. Lubricate the portion of the tube that's outside the patient's nose. Coil the extra tubing loosely and attach it to the patient's gown, so its weight doesn't interfere with its passage through his bowel. You may use Xylocaine jelly and a water-soluble lubricant to reduce the patient's nasal discomfort. If you're using a Miller-Abbott tube, make sure the port connected to the mercury balloon is taped shut and labeled, to prevent accidental suctioning of the mercury.

You can determine if the tube's reached the patient's duodenum by aspirating a small amount of fluid with a bulb syringe and testing it with red litmus paper. If the paper turns blue (indicating alkaline fluid), you know the tube's in the duodenum. The doctor will order an X-ray to confirm that the tube's in the proper place. Secure the tube, and connect it to suction as ordered by the doctor. The tube should relieve the patient's bowel distention.

If your patient's obstruction was managed surgically, he may have had a temporary colostomy if the bowel couldn't be anastomosed immediately. Prepare your patient for this possibility before surgery, and provide emotional support and reinforcement afterward. Arrange for an enterostomal therapist to visit the patient, and begin patient teaching. Provide stoma care, and irrigate the stoma as ordered. Help the patient become comfortable with the alteration in his body image by answering his questions openly and honestly and by making him familiar with ostomy equipment. Encourage the patient to ambulate and to resume activities of daily living as soon as possible.

# Appendicitis

## Prediagnosis summary

Initial assessment findings included some combination of:

• localized or generalized abdominal pain, possibly present for 12 to 48 hours, that may be epigastric or localized in his lower right abdomen and periumbilical region
• anorexia
• nausea
• vomiting
• positive McBurney's, Aaron's, and psoas signs (See *Eliciting Signs and Symptoms of Appendicitis*, page 335.)
• elevated temperature—99° to 102° F. (37.2° to 38.9° C.) if the appendix wasn't perforated, higher if it was.

If the patient's appendix was perforated, he may also have had:

• rebound tenderness
• absent bowel sounds
• abdominal rigidity.

An I.V. line was inserted, and the patient was given crystalloids for hydration. An NG tube was also inserted, and suction was started. Blood was drawn for CBC, electrolytes, and blood glucose. X-rays were taken and examined for free interperitoneal air, lesions, gas patterns suggesting obstruction, and an appendiceal fecalith.

## Priorities

Your patient will need surgery once the diagnosis of appendicitis has been confirmed. If his temperature's elevated, expect to administer antipyretics to reduce it. Place the patient in the Fowler position to reduce his pain and make

PATHOPHYSIOLOGY

# WHAT HAPPENS IN APPENDICITIS

Appendicitis—acute inflammation of the vermiform appendix—results from an obstruction of the bowel lumen such as stricture, viral infection, calculi, barium ingestion, or a fecal mass can cause.

Obstruction results in a collection of bowel secretions in the appendix, leading to its ulceration, distention, and inflammation. Distention and inflammation put pressure on the appendiceal artery; this results in decreased venous drainage of the appendix. Bacteria in the bowel lumen multiply and invade the appendix wall, worsening the inflammation.

If this process continues, ischemia, necrosis, and perforation may result, spreading infection into the patient's abdominal cavity. This may lead to *peritonitis*, the most common and serious complication of appendicitis.

him as comfortable as possible. Avoid giving him large doses of pain medications. Why? Because these may mask his symptoms of perforation. Continue I.V. fluids to keep your patient hydrated. Make sure you *don't* apply heat to his lower right quadrant, and *don't* give him enemas or cathartics. *These may cause the appendix to rupture.* Give him nothing by mouth. While you're preparing the patient for surgery, explain the procedure to him and to his family.

If the patient's appendix ruptured before surgery and he has signs and symptoms of peritonitis, you'll also need to monitor his fluid and electrolytes carefully and to give replacements I.V. Administer antibiotics as the doctor orders.

## Continuing assessment and intervention

After the appendectomy, monitor the patient's vital signs and maintain accurate intake and output records. Give analgesics as ordered, to keep your patient comfortable, and give prophylactic antibiotics I.V., to reduce his risk of infection. If the patient's appendicitis was complicated with peritonitis, an NG tube was inserted to decompress his stomach and to reduce his nausea and vomiting. Record drainage from the tube and watch for electrolyte imbalance, since electrolytes are lost with gastric aspiration.

Assess your patient's GI status frequently for return of bowel sounds, passing of flatus, and bowel movements, indications that bowel activity is returning. Document your findings, and expect that your patient may be ready to make the transition to oral fluids.

Watch him for signs and symptoms of infection. An increase in WBC count, temperature, and pain may signal peritonitis or formation of a surgical abscess. Notify the doctor if you note these signs and symptoms—surgical incision and drainage may be needed. Assess the patient's dressing frequently for wound drainage and for foul-smelling drainage, which may signal an infection.

## Therapeutic care

Prevent pulmonary complications by encouraging the patient to cough, to deep-breathe, and to turn frequently. Teach him splinting techniques; these will help to reduce stress on his surgical incision. Help the patient ambulate as soon as possible after surgery—usually within 12 to 24 hours. Start oral fluids as ordered; then introduce solid food gradually, when he can tolerate it. Continue to give antibiotics and analgesics. If no complications occur, the patient's wound will heal rapidly.

# ELICITING SIGNS AND SYMPTOMS OF APPENDICITIS

The signs and symptoms of appendicitis are often confusingly similar to those of other illnesses, such as gastritis, colitis, and diverticulitis. To help you differentiate appendicitis from other disorders, here are four characteristic signs to look for when examining your patient.

**McBurney's sign—** rebound tenderness and sharp pain occurring in the area of the patient's appendix when you palpate *McBurney's point,* located about 2″ (5.1 cm) below the right anterior superior spine of the ilium, on a line between the spine and the umbilicus

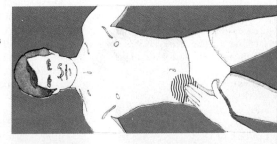

**Aaron's sign—**pain or distress occurring in the area of the patient's heart or stomach when you palpate McBurney's point

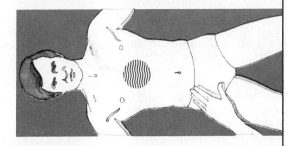

**Rovsing's sign—**pain in the patient's right lower quadrant when you apply pressure in the left lower quadrant

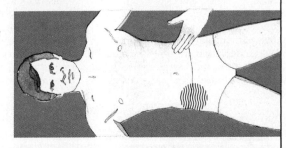

**Psoas sign—**increasing pain occurring in the patient's abdomen when he extends his right leg while lying on his left side, or when he flexes his legs while supine

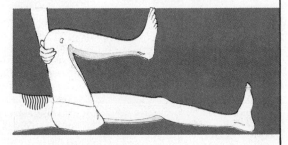

# Acute Pancreatitis

## Prediagnosis summary

Initial assessment of the patient may have revealed:

• an acute onset of severe epigastric pain, possibly radiating to his back and occurring within a few hours after a large meal or excessive alcohol intake

• nausea

• restlessness

• vomiting

• abdominal tenderness, rigidity, and distention

• Cullen's or Grey Turner's sign

• a history of alcoholism, biliary tract disease, or hyperlipidemia.

An I.V. was established for fluid and medication access, and blood was drawn for CBC, electrolytes, alkaline phosphatase, blood glucose, bilirubin, and serum amylase. Abdominal X-rays may have revealed no abnormalities, but ultrasonography or a computerized tomography scan may have revealed diffuse or local enlargement of the pancreas.

## Priorities

Your patient may suffer acute plasma volume depletion from hemorrhage or as a result of fluid sequestered in his abdomen, bowel, and other extracellular spaces. Your first priority, then, is to maintain his hemodynamic status. Infuse colloids and crystalloids I.V., as ordered, to replace lost fluid volume, and insert a Foley catheter as ordered to aid in accurate output measurements. Type and cross-match the patient's blood in case transfusion is necessary. Give the patient nothing by mouth—not even ice chips. You want to prevent *all* gastric stimulation, because gastric activity increases pancreatic secretions and makes pancreatic edema worse. Insert an NG tube, as ordered, and connect it to intermittent suction to remove the patient's stomach contents. Start a detailed intake and output record.

## Continuing assessment and intervention

Watch for signs of shock (increased pulse, decreased blood pressure, pallor, diaphoresis), which may indicate that your patient has *acute hemorrhagic pancreatitis*—which can progress to the most severe form: hemorrhage with necrosis. You may note mottled skin, tachycardia, and increased temperature (100° to 102° F., or 37.8° to 38.9° C.).

Vomiting may be persistent, and your patient's epigastric pain may be severe. Ask him when the pain and vomiting started and if it occurred after a large meal or a drinking bout. Auscultate his bowel sounds, which may be decreased or absent, and check for abdominal distention. Report these signs, which may indicate paralytic ileus, to the doctor. Monitor the results of your patient's blood glucose test and start doing urine fractionals every 6 hours—damage to the islets of Langerhans from severe hemorrhagic necrotizing pancreatitis may cause diabetes mellitus, which can progress to diabetic ketoacidosis if not treated (see Chapter 10).

Assess the patient's vital signs frequently, and continue colloid and blood replacement as needed. Be alert for signs of shock, which may develop as pancreatitis progresses. Watch for

PATHOPHYSIOLOGY

## WHAT HAPPENS IN ACUTE PANCREATITIS

The pathophysiology of acute pancreatitis (acute inflammation of the pancreas) isn't completely understood. But researchers do know that active proteolytic enzymes that the pancreas secretes somehow gain access to pancreatic tissue, instead of being excreted. This initiates autodigestion of the pancreas and leads to edema, abscess, vascular injury, and parenchymal and fat necrosis.

# CASE IN POINT: A MINOR'S CONSENT

You're working in the ED when an ambulance arrives with Frank McKenzie (who's unconscious) and his son Mike, age 17. You tell the paramedics to take Mike's father to the examining room; then you call the doctor and tell Mike to wait in the lounge.

You notice Mike's holding his stomach. He tells you it's been bothering him for a few days. Then, with no warning, he doubles over in pain.

After guiding him to an examining room, you find that Mike's temperature is 102° F. (38.9° C.), and you note rebound tenderness at McBurney's point. You call the doctor: he finds a positive psoas sign. Mike's white blood cell count is 12,500. The doctor, strongly suspecting acute appendicitis, recommends an immediate appendectomy.

But first, you and the doctor consider whether someone must sign a consent form. Neither of Mike's parents is available and the doctor feels that Mike's appendix could perforate at any time. So Mike's need for the surgery justifies operating immediately.

After discussing surgery with Mike, the doctor decides Mike seems mature and competent to make his own decision. Mike signs the form and subsequently undergoes successful surgery to remove his appendix.

When Mrs. McKenzie arrives at the hospital, she's upset about her husband but furious that her son's appendectomy was done without her permission. She threatens to sue you, the doctor, and the hospital. Does Mrs. McKenzie have a case?

In an actual case with a similar premise (*Younts v. St. Francis Hospital and School of Nursing,* 1970), Mrs. Younts was unconscious when her daughter's severed finger required emergency surgery. The defendants were found not liable. The court ruled that a minor who receives an explanation of the procedure and risks, and who's capable of making an intelligent decision, can give her own consent—especially in an emergency, when waiting for a parent's consent could endanger her life, limb, or function.

How can you avoid liability in a situation like this? The overriding legal rule here is: In a true emergency, treat first and obtain consent later. However, as in the *Younts* case, courts in some states have held that any mature minor, emancipated or not, may give a valid and binding consent to emergency treatment. So chances are you won't be liable if you're involved in emergency surgery on a minor—whether consent's been obtained for the surgery or not.

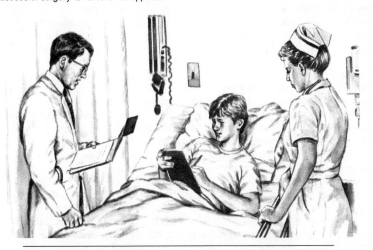

*Younts v. St. Francis Hospital and School of Nursing,* 205 Kan. 292, 469 P. 2d 330 (1970).

complications such as peritonitis, which may occur when pancreatic enzymes are released into the abdominal cavity (see *Danger: Peritonitis*, page 332).

Don't forget to assess respiratory status frequently in your patient with acute pancreatitis—20% to 50% of these patients develop pulmonary complications such as pleural effusions, alveolar infiltrates, and adult respiratory distress syndrome (ARDS). (See the "Adult Respiratory Distress Syndrome" entry in Chapter 4). Monitor his ABGs closely for evidence of hypoxemia, which often accompanies pancreatitis. Auscultate his lungs, and listen for rales or decreased breath sounds at the bases. Call the doctor if you note abnormal breath sounds—he'll want to determine the cause and start immediate medical intervention to prevent the patient from developing respiratory distress.

### Therapeutic care

When you've obtained a baseline assessment, your nursing intervention will focus on relieving the patient's pain and providing parenteral hyperalimentation to allow the pancreas to rest. Most patients will recover spontaneously with rest and supportive care. Expect to administer meperidine hydrochloride (Demerol) I.M., because the abdominal pain can be excruciating. You *won't* give morphine sulfate, because it can cause contraction of Oddi's sphincter. Position your patient on his side with his knees flexed to make him more comfortable. Monitor his fluid and electrolyte balance, and provide appropriate replacements as ordered. Continue to give the patient nothing by mouth until his signs and symptoms are resolved. And continue nasogastric suctioning during the acute phase of pancreatitis to allow the pancreas to rest (while the stomach is kept empty, the pancreas will not need to secrete enzymes for digestion). Nasogastric suction also appears to reduce abdominal pain and to keep paralytic

ileus from developing in most patients.

# A FINAL WORD

As a nurse, you probably know that GI emergencies are common, accounting for about 15% of all hospital admissions, 25% of all surgical operations (excluding tonsillectomies), and 20% to 30% of all trauma-related deaths. And GI emergencies have a wide variety of causes, so a patient's acute abdomen may be difficult to diagnose.

Fortunately, advances in GI diagnostic procedures and treatment are now available, and these make some aspects of patient care easier. But they're not a substitute for excellent nursing care. You need sound assessment skills, a knowledge of the pathophysiology of GI emergencies, and training in special treatment procedures to meet these patients' needs.

You'll be faced with constant challenges when caring for patients with GI emergencies:
• accurately assessing an uncomfortable, unstable patient
• successfully managing fluid balance in a patient with massive GI bleeding
• recognizing subtle signs of developing complications
• helping your patient cope with uncomfortable and embarrassing procedures.

These challenges, as you can see, include meeting the patient's emotional needs. Any GI emergency is painful; most are terrifying as well. A patient with massive upper GI bleeding, for example, may well fear for his life. In this frightening situation, your emotional support will reduce the inevitable stress and may actually help your patient recover.

Don't forget that the procedures you'll use to care for your patient are also uncomfortable and distressing. Take the time to explain to your patient what you're doing and why. Remember, too, that GI procedures—such as colonoscopy, proctosigmoidoscopy, or even routine rectal examinations—may embarrass your patient. By respecting his privacy and dignity, you'll help him tolerate the various procedures he needs.

## Selected References

Barry, Jean. *Emergency Nursing*. New York: McGraw-Hill Book Co., 1977.

Bates, Barbara. *A Guide to Physical Examination*, 3rd ed. Philadelphia: J.B. Lippincott Co., 1983.

Budassi, S.A., and Barber, J. *Emergency Nursing: Principles and Practice*. St. Louis: C.V. Mosby Co., 1980.

Burkhart, Carol. "Upper GI Hemorrhage: The Clinical Picture," *American Journal of Nursing* 81:1817-20, October 1981.

Cobert, B.L. "Diagnosis: Intestinal Obstruction," *Hospital Medicine* 19(7):57-65, July 1983.

Given, Barbara A., and Simmons, Sandra J. *Gastroenterology in Clinical Nursing*, 3rd ed. St. Louis: C.V. Mosby Co., 1979.

*Giving Emergency Care Competently*, 2nd ed. New Nursing Skillbook Series. Springhouse, Pa.: Springhouse Corp., 1983.

Kaye, Donald, and Rose, Louis F. *Fundamentals of Internal Medicine*. St. Louis: C.V. Mosby Co., 1983.

Kravis, Thomas C., and Warner, Carmen G. *Emergency Medicine: A Comprehensive Review*. Rockville, Md.: Aspen Systems Corp., 1982.

Lamphier, T.A., and Lamphier, R.A. "Upper GI Hemorrhage: Emergency Evaluation and Management," *American Journal of Nursing* 81:1814-17, October 1981.

Perdue, Patricia. "Abdominal Injuries and Dangerous Fractures," Part 4. *RN* 44:34-7, July 1981.

Smith, Carol E. "Abdominal Assessment: A Blending of Science and Art," *Nursing81* 11:42-9, February 1981.

Wyngaarden, James B., and Smith, Lloyd H., Jr., eds. *Cecil Textbook of Medicine*, 2 vols., 16th ed. Philadelphia: W.B. Saunders Co., 1982.

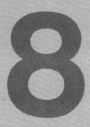

**8**

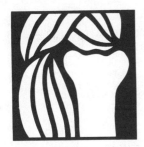

# Musculoskeletal Emergencies

## Introduction

Your small hospital's ED has been quiet all this rainy March day. Taking advantage of the lull, you're checking the emergency drug cabinet and making notes for restocking. Suddenly, a car pulls up outside. Three young men in wet suits get out and and splash through the rain to the entrance. The man in the middle has part of his wet suit cut away from his right arm and shoulder, and you notice he's wearing a makeshift sling. As they push through the ED door, Bob Kramer and Allen Jones begin explaining that they and their friend, Mike Murphy, have been kayaking on a nearby river, and that Mike injured his shoulder on a rock when his kayak overturned.

Mike's friends tell you they think he's dislocated his shoulder—a common kayaking injury. They also tell you they've tried to keep Mike warm and calm. Both men are experienced in first aid; when they pulled Mike out of the water, they checked him for obvious bleeding and didn't find any. However, they say, Mike complained of pain in his right shoulder, and he couldn't move his right arm at all. You note that Allen and Bob have immobilized Mike's shoulder and arm with a swathe and sling improvised from a couple of shirts. Mike says he's still in a lot of pain but that it lessened when his arm was immobilized. He seems relatively

calm, but his pale, tense face confirms his pain.

Although the circumstances will differ, you can expect to deal with patients who have injuries like Mike's hundreds of times in your career. This is because the complex interrelationship of the muscles, ligaments, tendons, cartilage, and bones that form the musculoskeletal system is easily disrupted by trauma—making fractures, dislocations, and other musculoskeletal injuries some of the most common problems you'll see, particularly in the ED.

Although fractures and dislocations are rarely life-threatening, they can result in severe disability and deformity if not attended to quickly, because underlying vital organs, blood vessels, and nerves may be injured. And when musculoskeletal injuries occur with other injuries (as in multiple trauma), the combination may threaten the patient's life. For example, hemorrhage and hypovolemic shock may develop in a patient with a traumatic fracture of the pelvis or the femoral shaft.

You'll have a great deal of responsibility for these patients—most often you'll be the first trained professional to see the patient who has a musculoskeletal emergency. Your care may determine how the patient's injury heals and whether disability results. To give him the best possible care, you

# PRIORITIES FOR MANAGING MUSCULOSKELETAL INJURIES IN MULTIPLE TRAUMA PATIENTS

A patient with multiple trauma presents a real challenge to your nursing skills. His injuries are so serious, he'll require several doctors and nurses to stabilize several body systems simultaneously. Here's what you need to know about prioritizing his *musculoskeletal injuries* once you've:
• assessed and stabilized his ABCs
• applied a cervical collar to immobilize his head and neck
• inserted an I.V. for fluid and medication administration
• performed a rapid head-to-toe physical examination, paying particular attention to deformities, mobility of extremities, and abnormal swelling. The data from this examination guide your setting of priorities for managing the patient's multiple injuries.

With injuries in *any* body system, the rule is to *care for the most life-threatening injuries first.* For musculoskeletal injuries, you'll generally prioritize your emergency assessment and intervention this way:
1. cervical spine
2. chest
3. pelvis
4. skull
5. abdomen
6. extremities.

Of course, you'll change this order if a lesser injury becomes life-threatening, such as a bone fracture that causes obvious cardiopulmonary compromise or neurovascular impairment. You'll also change priorities if the patient has a distended abdomen and decreased blood pressure, indicating life-threatening occult abdominal hemorrhage.

And remember: sometimes an obvious injury—an open fracture, for example—may *look* dangerous, but it may not be nearly as life-threatening as a closed fracture that's causing internal hemorrhage.

Use the following chart as a guideline for prioritizing your multiple trauma patient's musculoskeletal injuries.

| PRIORITY 1 | PRIORITY 2 | PRIORITY 3 | PRIORITY 4 |
|---|---|---|---|
| **Prepare the patient for X-rays of his:** | **Immobilize fractures or dislocations in this order:** | **Prepare the patient for X-rays of his:** | **Prepare the patient for further studies, as indicated:** |
| • lateral cervical spine <br> • chest (upright, if possible) <br> • pelvis, including a cystogram if he has hematuria. Watch for occult fractures not found by physical examination.) <br><br> If these X-rays show fractures, *intervene* as ordered. Expect to provide massive blood replacement and to assist with external skeletal fixation and laparotomy if life-threatening occult bleeding is also present. | • bones causing occult hemorrhage, such as the pelvis <br> • bones causing neurovascular impairment, such as posterior dislocation of the hip <br> • large bones with obvious fractures, such as the femur or humerus <br> • smaller bones with obvious fractures, such as the ulna | • skull <br> • abdomen <br> • extremities <br> *Intervene* as ordered if injuries are found in these X-rays. Close lacerations and dress wounds. | • CAT scan <br> • IVP <br> • additional X-rays <br> • surgery <br> • ICU monitoring |

need to understand the musculoskeletal system and its relationship to other organ systems. For example, your ability to carefully but quickly assess the patient's circulatory and neurologic status distal to his injury can help prevent neurovascular complications. In addition, your familiarity with and skilled handling of various methods of immobilization will minimize the patient's pain and prevent further damage to the injured area.

In this chapter, you'll learn about musculoskeletal emergencies such as fractures, dislocations, amputations, crush injuries, and serious lacerations. Consult Chapter 6, NEUROLOGIC EMERGENCIES, for skull and cervical spine fractures; Chapter 4, RESPIRATORY EMERGENCIES, for rib fractures; and Chapter 9, EYE, EAR, NOSE, AND THROAT EMERGENCIES, for facial fractures.

PRIORITIES

## INITIAL ASSESSMENT CHECKLIST

**Assess the ABCs first and intervene appropriately.**

**Check for:**
• deformity, local swelling, decreased range of motion, immobility or bruises, indicating fracture or dislocation
• poor capillary refill, absent or diminished pulses, pallor or cool skin, possibly indicating vascular compromise
• paralysis, numbness, or decreased sensation, indicating nerve injury.

**Intervene by:**
• immobilizing the injured part
• preserving an amputated part.

**Prepare for:**
• compartment pressure measurement
• traction
• surgical interventions
• transfer to a replantation center.

# INITIAL CARE

# Prehospital Care: What's Been Done

Unlike emergencies involving other body systems, musculoskeletal emergencies are usually the result of trauma. Although the diagnosis for this type of emergency may seem self-evident—for example, if the patient fell and one of his legs is crooked and very painful, it's probably fractured—rescue personnel will assume the patient has a serious (possibly underlying) injury and give the patient care based on this assumption.

Rescue personnel first assessed the patient's airway, breathing, and circulation—especially if he suffered multiple trauma. Then they assessed him for spinal injuries and immobilized him appropriately. During their assessment (and throughout transport) they paid particular attention to the possibility of shock if the patient had a partial or complete traumatic amputation or if they suspected an open fracture or a closed femoral or pelvic fracture. Rescue personnel also assessed the patient's peripheral pulses, warmth, and color in the area distal to the injury, to detect internal bleeding.

If the patient had a thigh injury, they may have measured for increased circumference of the affected thigh as compared to the unaffected thigh's circumference—an increase may indicate hemorrhage from a closed femoral fracture. Similarly, they assessed the patient for signs of internal abdominal bleeding if they suspected hemorrhage from a pelvic fracture. Of course, they assessed his pulse and blood pressure frequently.

If rescue personnel were qualified, and if they suspected blood loss, they probably started an I.V. of Ringer's lactate; they may have also applied medical antishock trousers (a MAST suit).

If your patient suffered *traumatic amputation* of a limb, digit, or part, the rescue personnel first tried to stanch the bleeding. They applied large absorbent dressings with direct pressure and elevated the remaining part. If direct pressure and elevation—and pressure applied to pressure points—failed, rescue personnel may have applied a tourniquet despite the tissue damage it would inevitably cause. If your patient arrives in the ED with a tourniquet in place, *don't remove it.* This is the doctor's responsibility. Instead, find out from the rescue personnel when the tourniquet was applied, and tell the doctor.

Rescue personnel may also have attempted to salvage the amputated part and to preserve it for possible replantation. If they did this, they wrapped the amputated part in a dressing saturated with normal saline solution, placed it in a plastic bag, and put it on ice. Make sure you keep the part wrapped in the wet gauze and away from direct contact with ice. (See *Caring for an Amputated Part.*)

Additional prehospital care of a patient with a suspected fracture or dislocation consisted primarily of immobilization. Rescue personnel assessed the patient's affected area for swelling, deformity, and obvious fractures or open wounds. They dressed a major laceration or open fracture with a sterile saline dressing. They may have applied cold packs to reduce swelling, and may have elevated the limb. Then they splinted the area as necessary, using standard cardboard or plastic splints, air splints, or splints improvised from pillows or other available material. They may have used a sling, as well, to further immobilize an upper extremity fracture. If rescue personnel suspected a pelvic or hip fracture, they placed a backboard under him to prevent further movement; they may also have applied a MAST suit. If the rescue personnel had the necessary training and specialized equipment, they may have applied a traction splint (such as a Hare traction splint) to a patient with an obvious femur fracture. Traction splinting of this type of serious fracture reduces pain and also reduces the chance that the patient will go into shock during transport. If the patient arrives in the ED with a traction splint in place, promptly assess the neurovascular status of the limb in traction. If it's compromised, ask the doctor to examine the patient immediately so the traction can be removed.

# What to Do First

Although your patient's musculoskeletal injury may be as simple as an uncomplicated dislocation or a small-bone fracture, *don't* make assumptions about his condition. Your first priority—even if he's been brought in by rescue personnel—is to assess his airway, breathing, and circulation and to intervene if necessary. Then you'll assess his general appearance—possibly taking longer than usual in order to pay particular attention to open fractures and to areas of deformity, swelling, and angulation. Your prompt assessment and intervention by elevating and immobilizing the injured area and by applying a cold pack will help minimize your patient's pain and avoid serious complications.

### Airway
Airway assessment is especially important in a patient with obvious multiple injuries. Why? Because upper chest injuries or facial fractures, for example (see Chapters 4 and 9), may directly occlude his airway. (Of course, if your patient's airway is compromised, you'll clear it first, even if his other injuries appear serious.)

## YOUR ROLE IN AN EMERGENCY

### CARING FOR AN AMPUTATED PART

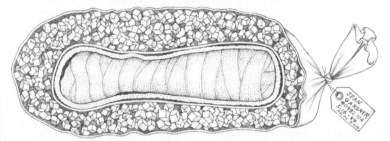

If a patient arrives in the ED with a traumatic amputation, you may be asked to preserve the amputated part for possible replantation. Here's a four-step procedure to follow:
1. Put on sterile gloves; then flush the part with normal saline or Ringer's lactate solution. *Never use any other solution,* and don't try to scrub or debride the part.
2. Gently pat the part dry with sterile gauze. Then wrap it in saline-soaked sterile gauze. Wrap the gauze with a sterile towel. Then put the whole thing in a watertight container or bag and seal it.

3. Fill another plastic bag with ice water and place the part, still in its watertight container, inside. Seal the bag. (Always protect the part from direct contact with ice—and *never* use dry ice—to prevent irreversible tissue damage, which would make the part unsuitable for replantation.) Keep this bag ice-cold until the doctor's ready to do the replantation surgery.
4. Label the bag with your patient's name, identification of the amputated part, the hospital identification number, and the date and time when cooling of the part began.

## Breathing

Although patients with musculoskeletal injuries are most often stable, watch your patient carefully for tachypnea. This may be a result of occult blood loss from severe fractures. If you suspect blood loss, tell the doctor and expect to give supplemental oxygen by mask or cannula.

## Circulation

Your next important consideration about your patient is the threat of hypovolemic shock. Remember, injury to the musculoskeletal system can cause hypovolemic shock in various ways:
• from occult blood loss due to fractured bones (particularly the pelvis or the femur)
• from injury to organs and blood vessels underlying injured bones
• from major lacerations
• from traumatic amputation.
Blood may be drawn for hemoglobin and hematocrit levels (to assess blood loss) and for other laboratory studies.

When you check your patient's vital signs, watch particularly for signs of volume depletion. For example, hypotension may signal blood loss that can lead to shock.

If your patient has signs and symptoms of shock, insert at least one large-bore I.V. line to facilitate fluid replacement and blood transfusion, and administer fluid and blood as ordered. You may also put him in a MAST suit to increase circulation to his vital organs, if rescue personnel haven't already done this.

Of course, if your patient has an obvious hemorrhage, you'll try to control the bleeding with direct pressure, pressure on a pressure point, or a pressure dressing. Elevate the part, if possible. *Don't* use a tourniquet except when it's absolutely necessary—when the choice is between saving your patient's limb or saving his life. This is particularly important with traumatic amputations, because a tourniquet may destroy tissue distal to the injury, making replantation impossible. If you must apply a tourniquet, use a wide bandage or a blood pressure cuff (*not* a narrow tubing or band), and apply it as close to the injured end as possible. Remember, if your patient arrives with a tourniquet in place, be sure to ask rescue personnel when it was applied. Why? Because injured nerves and blood vessels cause increasing damage over time. And *don't* take the tourniquet off—the doctor will do this.

Traumatic amputations are a double challenge: you'll have to act quickly to stabilize the patient and to prepare the amputated part for possible replantation. (Ideally, replantation should be done within 6 hours.) You *must* keep the amputated part hypothermic, or ischemia will cause irreversible tissue and blood vessel damage and muscle necrosis within 6 hours. (See *Caring for an Amputated Part,* page 345.)

The doctor will decide if replantation is possible, depending on the extent of the patient's injury and the viability of the amputated part. (Replantation usually won't be attempted if the patient has other major injuries.) If the doctor decides the conditions are right, he'll make arrangements for a replantation center to accept the patient. Stabilize the patient prior to transfer by:

• replacing lost fluids
• keeping the stump elevated and in anatomic alignment, to maintain bone stability
• keeping the stump cool, possibly covering it with a sterile dressing that has been soaked in normal saline solution or Ringer's lactate solution.

Expect to give pain medication and tetanus prophylaxis (see *Guidelines for Tetanus Prophylaxis,* pages 66 and 67) prior to your patient's transfer. The doctor may also order aspirin, to decrease platelet activity, and a broad-spectrum antibiotic I.V., such as cephalothin sodium (Keflin) or cefazolin sodium (Ancef).

If your patient has a partial amputation, he may actually bleed *more* than if he has a complete amputation because when an artery's completely severed, it goes into spasm and retracts into the remaining muscle, and both actions reduce hemorrhage. These mechanisms don't occur in partial laceration of an artery, so you'll have to use direct pressure to control your patient's bleeding. If he has an arterial bleeder, you may have to continue pressure until the doctor can suture the artery. If you can control the bleeding with pressure, place the part as close as possible to its correct anatomic position. Wrap the area in sterile saline gauze and place a watertight plastic bag over it, covering the area above the injury, as well. Place a second plastic bag over the first one and fill it with crushed ice; seal the bag with tape. Elevate the patient's limb, maintaining correct anatomic alignment. (You may need to use sandbags or pillows to keep an arm or leg aligned correctly.)

If your patient isn't visibly hemorrhaging (or the hemorrhage is under control), check for occult blood loss. When you're assessing his circulation, remember to evaluate accompanying cutaneous signs, including pallor, patchy cyanosis, discoloration, ecchymoses, and petechiae. These signs usually indicate neurovascular compromise due to disrupted blood supply. Pallor or patchy cyanosis *above* the injury site indicates venous impairment; *below* the injury site, it indicates arterial impairment. Check for weak or absent pulses distal to the affected area. (Notify the doctor *immediately* if an extremity is pulseless.) Test capillary refill time by compressing a nail bed on

the patient's affected side. Report a refill time of longer than 3 seconds, because this indicates significant
circulation impairment.

Discoloration and ecchymoses usually indicate that blood is seeping into
the subcutaneous tissues surrounding
a patient's fracture. An advancing or
extending ecchymosis may indicate internal hemorrhage. Keep in mind that
pelvic fractures may have ruptured vital internal organs, causing additional
blood loss. If you suspect internal hemorrhage, notify the doctor and:
• recheck your patient's vital signs
• administer oxygen
• immobilize the affected area
• measure the circumference of the affected area (an increase indicates blood
accumulation)
• start a large-bore I.V.

### General appearance
Because most musculoskeletal emergencies are traumatic injuries, even a
quick assessment of your patient's general appearance is likely to provide
substantial clues to his condition. Look
for cervical spine or head trauma (see
Chapter 6), open wounds, deformity,
and swelling. If you suspect your patient's spine is injured, don't move him
until X-rays have ruled out this possibility.

Look for major lacerations and for
open wounds associated with fractures; these may appear on the skin
surface near the fracture site. Cut away
the patient's clothing surrounding the
wound, to prevent contamination. Apply a sterile saline dressing to an open
wound. Don't attempt to cleanse and
debride the wound, because you'll risk
increasing contamination deep within
it. Administer analgesics as ordered to
relieve pain, and anticipate the need
for prophylactic broad-spectrum antibiotics and tetanus prophylaxis (see
*Guidelines for Tetanus Prophylaxis*,
pages 66 and 67).

You may see such obvious deformities as bone protruding through an
open wound, a crush injury, obvious

shortening of a limb, or malposition of
a part. Always compare the affected
side with the unaffected one. Cover
open fractures and crushed areas with
sterile saline gauze to prevent further
bacterial contamination. (Contamination may result in osteomyelitis, a serious bone infection.) Joint deformity,
coupled with the patient's inability to
move the extremity, may indicate dislocation. Keep in mind that edema surrounding the joint may obscure the
degree of deformity. Deformity may be
associated with fractures and may be
produced or altered by muscle spasms
surrounding the fracture site. Document the deformity as you first see it—
it may change in appearance as appropriate treatment progresses and edema
and muscle swelling decrease. Check
the patient's pulses and his sensation
distal to the deformity to assess for neurovascular compromise. *Don't* attempt
to straighten an angulated joint—this
is the doctor's responsibility.

If the patient was brought in by rescue personnel, they probably splinted
obvious fractures or dislocations to increase the patient's comfort and to reduce suspected internal hemorrhage
from broken bone ends. If this wasn't
done, immobilize each affected part
now by splinting it.

Edema will occur in the soft tissue
surrounding the area of your patient's
injury. This reaction to trauma may
indicate the severity of the underlying
damage. In addition, keep in mind that
edema may cause further damage by
compressing nerves and blood vessels
and causing ischemia. After splinting,
elevate the injured area and apply a
cold pack to reduce congestion.

### Mental status
When you assess your patient's mental
status and level of consciousness, remember that most patients with musculoskeletal emergencies are awake
and alert. Although he's probably in
pain and anxious, your patient should
be coherent and able to describe the
circumstances of the injury. If he isn't,

# TESTING FOR PERIPHERAL NERVE DAMAGE

When you're assessing a patient's fracture or dislocation, always check for peripheral nerve damage. Shown here are the most commonly used tests of sensory and motor function. Decreased sensation or inability to perform the range-of-motion tests indicates possible nerve damage.

## UPPER EXTREMITIES

### Median nerve

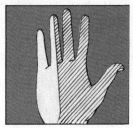 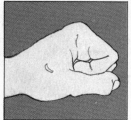 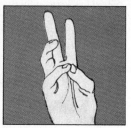

*Sensory:* Test sensation over the palmar side of the patient's thumb, index and long fingers, and half of ring finger.

*Motor:* Ask the patient to rotate his thumb to a grasp position.

*Motor:* Ask the patient to oppose his thumb to his little finger.

### Radial nerve

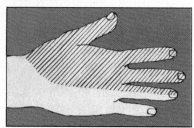 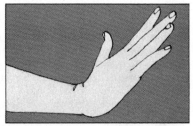

*Sensory:* Test sensation over the dorsum of the patient's thumb, index and long fingers, and one half of the ring finger.

*Motor:* Ask the patient to extend his wrist and fingers at the metacarpophalangeal joint and his thumb at all joints.

### Ulnar nerve

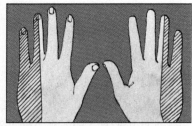 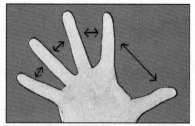

*Sensory:* Test sensation of the patient's dorsal and palmar side over his little finger and the ulnar half of his ring finger.

*Motor:* Ask the patient to spread and close his fingers or to flex his metacarpophalangeal joints without interphalangeal flexion.

## UPPER EXTREMITIES (*continued*)

**Axillary nerve**

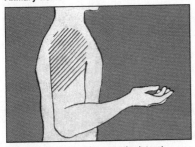

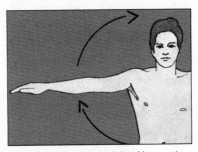

*Sensory:* Test sensation over the lateral aspect of the patient's upper arm and shoulder (military patch area).

*Motor:* Ask the patient to abduct his arm at the shoulder joint.

## LOWER EXTREMITIES

**Peroneal nerve**

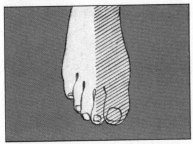

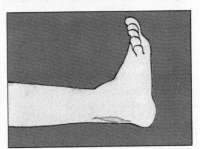

*Sensory:* Test sensation over the dorsum of the patient's foot in the area adjacent to his great and second toes.

*Motor:* Ask the patient to dorsiflex his foot or to extend his toes.

**Tibial nerve**

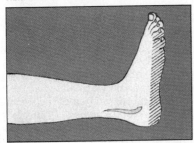

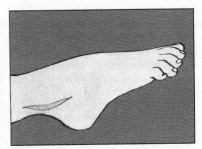

*Sensory:* Test sensation over the lateral part of the patient's foot.

*Motor:* Ask the patient to plantar flex his ankle and toes.

or if his mental status deteriorates and he becomes confused, agitated, or obtunded, suspect shock and assess him for other signs such as hypotension, tachycardia, decreased pulse pressure, tachypnea, and cool, clammy skin. If the patient's unconscious when you first see him, suspect shock or neurologic injury. Notify the doctor *immediately* if you see any of these signs.

# What to Do Next

Once you've assessed your patient's airway, breathing, and circulation and intervened as necessary, you're ready to perform a rapid and detailed emergency assessment.

Even if a patient's musculoskeletal injuries are visually evident, hidden damage to underlying organs, tissue, vessels, and nerves may require more immediate intervention. To help you estimate the location and extent of any internal injuries your patient may have, try to build a mental image of how they may have occurred. Do this by:

• getting a detailed description of the traumatic event

• determining the mechanism of injury and the type of force involved

• visualizing the probable internal damage sequence.

To save time, get the patient's history while performing the physical examination. Your patient may describe an event that caused a blunt or penetrating injury. With *blunt trauma,* the patient may have serious internal injuries even though he has no skin perforation or other obvious external signs. Ask him to point to the area of impact and to describe the object's size and shape and the direction of impact. Try to visualize the event and its probable internal effects; then you can quickly determine and assess the most likely areas of underlying injury.

*Penetrating trauma* perforates the skin but usually causes less secondary damage than blunt trauma does. If the patient has penetrating trauma, use his description of the object, what you can determine about its direction at impact, and the location and depth of the entrance wound to help you estimate and assess the damage.

When you're assessing a patient with *crush injuries,* remember the possibility of crush syndrome (see *What Happens in Crush Syndrome,* page 382).

Of course, most musculoskeletal injuries result from traumatic events. But remember, for the patient who's elderly or has bone disease, even a minor insult—such as stepping off a curb the wrong way—can cause a major musculoskeletal injury.

Be sure to ask your patient what he heard and felt at the time of the injury:

• Did he hear a snapping, cracking, grating, or popping sound?

• Can he describe any other sensations he noticed?

• Could he move the affected area right after the injury?

• When and where did the injury occur?

• What steps were taken to manage the injury before he arrived at the hospital?

Organize your assessment of his primary musculoskeletal injury by the *five Ps*—pain, paresthesias, paralysis, pallor, and pulses.

If your patient complains of *pain,* ask questions that will help you narrow down and define that complaint. Ask about the character, severity, and location of the pain. Find out if his pain's relieved by immobilization, elevation, or cold-pack application. Most important, find out whether his pain is increasing. If he says yes, he may be developing neurovascular impairment or compartment syndrome. These complications require *immediate* intervention, usually surgical. (See *Understanding Compartment Syndrome,* pages 370 and 371.)

In a patient with compartment syndrome, muscle swelling in the compartment causes increased pain due to muscle ischemia, especially on passive movement. For example, if your patient has a lower extremity injury and is developing compartment syndrome, he'll experience intense pain when you flex his toes and foot.

If your patient's developing neurovascular impairment, he may complain of a constant *burning* distal to the injury, due to nerve and muscle ischemia. As the area becomes progressively ischemic, the pain will become deep, throbbing, and constant. It may be accompanied by motor or sensory impairment such as paresthesias or paralysis.

If you think your patient may be developing either compartment syndrome or neurovascular impairment, send someone to notify the doctor *immediately*. While you wait for the doctor, elevate the immobilized extremity, make sure the splint isn't too tight, and remove any constrictive dressings to try to decrease the edema-ischemia cycle.

If your patient has a fracture or dislocation, he'll usually describe the pain as deep, throbbing, and constant. Gently palpate the area for point tenderness. Ask if moving the injured part intensifies the pain. Remember that pain associated with fractures and dislocations may be very intense due to edema, muscle spasm, and soft tissue injury compressing blood vessels and nerves. Another possible cause of pain is bone fragments impinging on muscle, blood vessels, and nerves. Ask your patient to rate his pain on a scale of 1 to 10, with 10 as the worst he's ever experienced. Then you and your patient will have a common reference point for subsequent assessments of his pain. For example, later, when you ask him to describe his pain, which was an 8, he may say, "Now it's a 5."

Now assess your patient for *paresthesias*. Pinch the involved area lightly, or touch it with the point of a paper clip or another blunt object. Check sensation both distal and proximal to the injury site; note any increase or decrease in sensation, lack of sensation,

numbness, or tingling. Check the same areas on his unaffected side and compare your findings. Paresthesias indicate neurovascular impairment, which may result from edema, muscle spasms, or bone fragments impinging on nerves, or from actual severing of the nerve fibers by sharp bone fragments or a penetrating injury.

Your patient will usually tell you if he has any *function loss* or *paralysis* of the affected area. Always confirm these reports yourself. Have him flex, abduct, and adduct the injured part. The patient with a fracture will complain of inability to move the affected part or of increased pain and muscle spasm with movement. You may notice excessive motion of the bone at the fracture site, especially if the site isn't near a joint or isn't splinted by surrounding soft-tissue structures. Ask the patient to move his fingers or toes distal to the injury—if he can't, suspect nerve or tendon damage. Don't attempt passive range of motion on the injured part if you suspect nerve damage; you may aggravate it.

Assess the patient's skin on his injured side for *pallor* and *coolness*, which may indicate reduced blood supply. Do the same for his unaffected side and compare your findings.

Increased capillary refill time may also indicate reduced blood supply. Check this by pressing on one of your patient's nail beds distal to the injury. Does it blanch and then rapidly return to normal? If not, suspect his blood supply's reduced.

Check all *pulses* distal to your patient's injury. If he has an upper extremity injury, check his axillary, brachial, radial, and ulnar pulses. If he has a pelvic, hip, or lower extremity injury, check his femoral, popliteal, posterior tibial, and dorsal pedal pulses. As you know, a decreased or absent pulse indicates reduced blood supply.

While you're assessing the five Ps, listen for a characteristic sign of fracture—crepitation. This sound is from

## USING IMMOBILIZERS

Some musculoskeletal injuries, such as dislocations and sprains, don't require a cast for immobilization. For injuries like these, and for postreduction immobilization of some fractures, the doctor may use an immobilizer. Here's what you should know about the uses and fitting of some types of immobilizers.

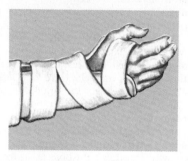

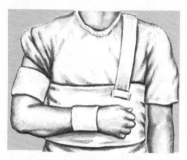

**Wrist immobilizer**
*Uses:* immobilizes the wrist after a severe sprain or surgery
*Tip:* Check the patient's neurologic and circulatory status frequently.

**Belt-type shoulder immobilizer**
*Uses:* immobilizes shoulder dislocations and clavicle fractures
*Tip:* Assess the patient's respiratory status frequently to make sure that tight straps don't restrict his breathing.

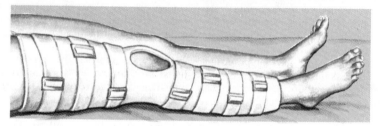

**Knee immobilizer**
*Uses:* immobilizes the knee after a severe sprain or strain, or after surgery
*Tips:*
• Measure the patient's thigh and calf circumference and consult the manufacturer's chart to select the correct size.
• The doctor will specify the length and contour of the immobilizer he wants to use for a particular patient.

broken bone ends rubbing together. You may hear it when the patient moves the injured part or when you gently palpate his skin over the injured area. Remember: *Don't* try to elicit this sound by moving the patient's injured limb—in addition to causing pain, you may convert a closed fracture into an open one, by penetrating his skin, or you may cause further soft tissue, nerve, and vessel injury.

To complete your initial assessment, ask about your patient's medical history. Find out if he's ever had a similar injury. If so, was any disability associated with it? What treatment was given? Has he had any pulmonary problems, such as chronic obstructive pulmonary disease? If he has, prolonged immobilization resulting from his musculoskeletal injury may predispose him to pulmonary complica-

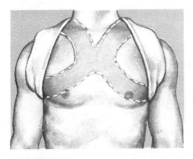

**Clavicle strap**
*Use:* immobilizes clavicular fractures
*Tip:* Make sure the strap doesn't apply excessive pressure under the patient's arms—this could cause nerve damage.

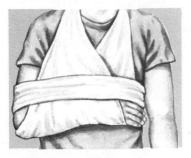

**Sling and swathe bandage**
*Uses:* immobilizes shoulder dislocations and some fractures of the humerus and elbow
*Tips:*
• Remove any rings or bracelets the patient's wearing; swelling may impair circulation.
• Make sure the sling supports your patient's fingers to the first interphalangeal joints. This will help prevent nerve damage, which can lead to wrist drop.

tions. Of course, a past medical history of hemophilia or blood dyscrasias signals potential bleeding problems, particularly bleeding into the joints. Ask if your patient has diabetes—if so, his musculoskeletal injury may alter his insulin needs, healing may be more difficult and prolonged, and infection is more likely to occur.

An accurate medication history will help prevent complications. Determine

if your patient's taking an anticoagulant, such as warfarin (Coumadin), or any medication that prevents platelet aggregation, such as sulfinpyrazone (Anturane) or aspirin. Remember, if your patient has arthritis, he may take large quantities of aspirin so routinely that he won't think to mention it. So ask him about aspirin specifically. Ask, too, if your patient is taking corticosteroids. Corticosteroid therapy increases your patient's risk of developing vascular necrosis following femoral or humoral fracture; it may also predispose him to pathologic fractures.

Find out if your patient has allergies to any medications, particularly antibiotics, analgesics, and anesthetics. This information is especially pertinent, because these drugs are likely to be used in his treatment.

# Special Considerations

## Pediatric
Greenstick fractures occur more commonly in children than in adults. The bone may partially break or buckle rather than breaking completely. Be alert to the possibility of a greenstick fracture if your pediatric patient has pain and a history of trauma, particularly in the lower arm—these fractures often go unrecognized.

Fracture may also occur in an epiphyseal plate, which can be highly vulnerable to traumatic force. (See the discussion of epiphyseal fractures in *Nurse's Guide to Pediatric Emergencies* in the Appendix.) An epiphyseal fracture is most common in the distal radius. Early closure of the fractured epiphyseal plate may prevent further growth in the affected bone and require extensive follow-up care by an orthopedic surgeon.

If your patient or his parents can't explain how his fracture occurred, or the mechanism of injury seems unusual, consider the possibility of child abuse. (See the "When to Make a Report" entry in Chapter 2 and *Nurse's Guide to Pediatric Emergencies* in the Appendix.)

### Geriatric
The elderly are especially prone to fractures, because their bones grow brittle during the aging process. When an elderly patient falls on an outstretched arm or hand or suffers a direct blow to his arm or shoulder, he's very likely to fracture his shoulder or humerus.

Osteoporosis affects women more than men and occurs most often in postmenopausal women over age 60. Be partic ularly alert to the possibility of serious hip and pelvic fractures if your elderly female patient has suffered even a minor fall.

# CARE AFTER DIAGNOSIS

# Upper Extremity Dislocations

### Prediagnosis summary
On initial assessment, the patient had:
• a history of trauma
• severe pain and point tenderness
• inability to move the affected joint
• swelling.
He may have had:
• deformity and displacement of the joint
• hematoma over the injury site
• tingling or numbness distal to the injury
• nausea elicited by flexion or pressure on the injured area.

The patient's joint was immobilized, probably with a sling and swathe, in whatever position it was found. (See *Using Immobilizers*, pages 352 and 353.) A cold pack was also applied to

reduce swelling and pain. If the patient's condition was stable, a multiview X-ray was taken to determine the site and extent of the injury.

### Priorities, assessment, and intervention
Your first priority is to perform a thorough neurovascular assessment of the function of the patient's axillary nerve and brachial plexus (median, radial, and ulnar nerves) and of his axillary, brachial, radial, and ulnar arteries. Remember that edema from the dislocation can cause nerve and vessel compression. So be alert for signs of developing compartment syndrome (see *Understanding Compartment Syndrome,* pages 370 and 371).

Check to make sure your patient's limb is sufficiently immobilized and comfortable. Administer analgesics, if ordered. Continue cold-pack application to his injured area to help reduce swelling and pain.

When assessing your patient for nerve impairment, watch for abnormal or altered sensation, for weakness, or for burning—distal to the injury—which may become dull and throbbing. Report these signs to the doctor *immediately.*

Fully assess the function (motor and sensory) of the patient's axillary, ulnar, median, and radial nerves. (See *Testing for Peripheral Nerve Damage,* pages 348 and 349.) For example, *axillary* nerve compression may cause impaired ability to abduct his shoulder and a sensory loss over the deltoid of the patient's arm or the lateral aspect of his forearm. Compromised *ulnar* nerve function may affect his ability to abduct all his fingers: If you place his hand flat, can he move his middle finger from side to side? Check for sensory loss in the distal fat pad of his little finger, too. If his *median* nerve function's compromised, he'll have difficulty opposing his thumb and little finger and sensory loss on the distal palmar surface of his index finger. Suspect *radial* nerve damage if he has trouble hyperextending

## YOUR ROLE IN AN EMERGENCY

### PERFORMING PIN CARE

Once your patient has a pin in place—for skeletal traction or an external fixation device—the doctor will order pin care. Here are some general guidelines to follow when giving pin care—specific procedures vary according to hospital protocols.
• Examine the patient's skin around the pin for tautness, pain, tenderness, and redness from inflammation and infection.
• Note any crusted serous drainage around the pin site. *Gently* remove the crust to prevent it from obstructing wound drainage.
• Give skin care every 4 hours.
• Note any signs and symptoms of pin looseness—such as increased or purulent drainage or free turning of the pin in the patient's skin.
• Don't prod the patient's skin around the pin—you may cause additional pain or skin abrasions that can lead to infection.
• Clean the pins once or twice a day, using povidone-iodine or hydrogen peroxide, as ordered. For an external fixation device, work proximally to distally on one side, then on the other. Afterwards, wipe the device's frame with a sterile cloth moistened with sterile water. Cover the pin ends with pin caps, corks, or rubber plugs from blood-sampling vials.

---

his thumb or wrist against resistance or if he has sensory loss in the web between his thumb and index finger, on the dorsal surface.

To assess your patient's circulatory status, check all his distal pulses and his capillary refill time. Look for cool, pale, cyanotic, or mottled skin. Report *any* signs or symptoms of neurovascular compromise right away, because the patient's injured joint will need immediate relocation.

### Therapeutic care

At this point in your patient's care, be prepared to assist in the relocation procedure. You'll probably administer a muscle relaxant, such as diazepam (Valium), and an analgesic, as ordered, to make the patient as comfortable as possible and to make performing the procedure easier for the doctor. Local anesthesia may also be needed. You may have to maintain traction during the relocation. Your patient may require surgical fixation—using wires, nails, pins, or plates and screws—particularly if he has an elbow dislocation. If the patient is elderly and has osteoporosis, general anesthe-

sia will probably be used to obtain full muscle relaxation and satisfactory relocation.

Following relocation, repeat the neurovascular assessment described earlier, and compare your findings with the patient's baseline data. The doctor will order a follow-up X-ray to confirm relocation. You'll use a splint, sling and swathe, or another immobilizing device to stabilize the joint after relocation. For example, for *acromioclavicular* separation, expect to apply a shoulder sling or acromioclavicular support. The support provides downward pressure on the clavicle by the shoulder strap; the sling supports the forearm and keeps the acromion in place; and the halter pulls both the shoulder strap and the sling downward.

For a *posterior or anterior shoulder* dislocation, a shoulder immobilizer or a sling and swathe may be applied. An *elbow* dislocation should be splinted in the position most comfortable for the patient (if he didn't have open reduction with pin or wire insertion, under general anesthesia). For an *elbow* or *wrist* dislocation, the doctor may cast the limb (see *Your Role in Cast Care,*

# UNDERSTANDING DISLOCATIONS

A sports injury, a motor vehicle accident, or other trauma may exert a forceful impact on a person's extended limb, causing a joint to exceed its range of motion. The result? A dislocation.

A dislocation may cause soft tissue damage, neurovascular damage, and even a fracture at the injury site. Signs and symptoms include severe pain, deformity, immobility, swelling, and point tenderness.

Here are some illustrations to help you understand how dislocations occur and how they disrupt bones and joints.

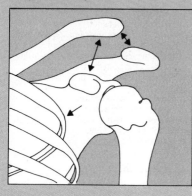

### Acromioclavicular separation
*Mechanism*—A fall or application of a force causes upward displacement of the acromial process of the scapula while the clavicle remains fixed, separating the acromion and the clavicle.

### Glenohumeral dislocation
*Mechanism*—A fall on the patient's extended arm abducts and externally rotates it; the force pushes the head of the humerus anterior to the shoulder joint.

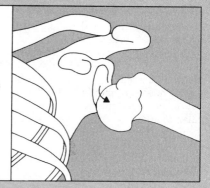

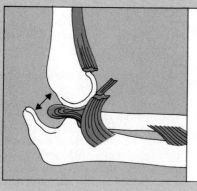

### Elbow dislocation
*Mechanism*—A fall on the patient's outstretched hand, with his elbow extended and his forearm either supine or prone, forces his forearm upward and backward and causes posterior dislocation.

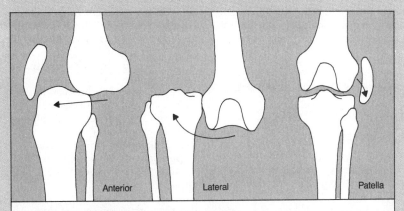

Anterior          Lateral          Patella

## Patella and knee dislocation

*Mechanism*—This type of dislocation can occur in either of two ways:
• Severe direct trauma produces abnormal abduction, adduction, internal and external rotation, extension, or forward or backward displacement of the knee joint, causing anterior, posterior, lateral, or rotational dislocation.
• A sports injury directs force to the inner aspect of the knee, driving the patella laterally and slightly downward.

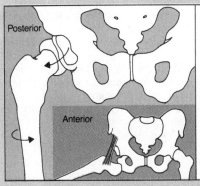

Posterior

Anterior

## Hip dislocation

*Mechanism*—A fall or motor vehicle accident violently impacts the patient's hip, causing:
• *posterior dislocation.* The hip flexes, adducts, and internally rotates so that the head of the femur is thrust backward.
• *anterior dislocation.* The hip flexes, abducts, and externally rotates so that the head of the femur is driven out of the acetabulum.

## Ankle dislocation

*Mechanism*—A sports injury causes exaggerated plantar flexion and strong forward thrust of the patient's leg, producing a posterior dislocation.

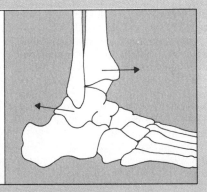

page 360). A splint may be used for a *finger* dislocation. To avoid joint stiffness, the doctor will probably have the patient begin graduated exercise of the limb while the support's still in place.

# Lower Extremity Dislocations

## Prediagnosis summary
The patient had a history of trauma and may have had:
- extreme pain with localized tenderness, swelling, and deformity
- the feeling that his joint was "locked"
- severe muscle spasms in the extremity.

If the injury was a dislocated *hip*, the femoral head may have been felt on gentle palpation of the inguinal area, and hip flexion, abduction, or adduction or external rotation may have been found.

If the *knee* was dislocated, it may have had a bowed or knock-kneed appearance. A dislocated *ankle* probably showed deformity with abnormal protrusion medially or laterally.

The patient's injured joint was immobilized, in its "frozen" position, with a splint or pillows and sandbags. Cold packs were applied to reduce swelling. If he also had an open fracture, a sterile dressing was applied to the wound to prevent contamination, an I.V. line was inserted, and antibiotics were given (see the "Lower Leg Fractures" and "Hip and Femur Fractures" entries in this chapter). Blood may have been drawn for typing and cross matching and for a complete blood count (CBC). An X-ray was taken to locate the site of the injury and to determine its extent.

## Priorities
Your first priorities are to keep the patient's dislocated joint immobilized, to administer analgesics as ordered, and to continue cold-pack treatment. Make sure his splint is tight enough to keep the joint immobilized but loose enough to ensure adequate circulation to the limb. You'll have to assess your patient's neurovascular status carefully, because extreme swelling can lead to nerve and vessel compression that can cause ischemia and further neurovascular injury. This degree of impingement on major arteries can result in compartment syndrome and possibly in amputation of the limb (see *Understanding Compartment Syndrome,* pages 370 and 371).

## Continuing assessment and intervention
Perform a thorough baseline assessment of your patient's neurovascular status. Check his *tibial* nerve function by testing plantar flexion of his ankle; also test sensation over his medial and lateral foot surfaces. Check his *peroneal* nerve function by testing his ankle dorsiflexion and toe extension; test sensation over the dorsum of his foot, too, especially in the area near the great and second toes. If he has *sciatic* nerve damage (common in patients with posterior hip dislocation), he'll have a combination of motor and sensory loss (tibial and peroneal nerves) and pain on knee extension when his hip is flexed.

An inability to perform these actions—or loss of sensation in these areas—indicates nerve damage. Notify the doctor *immediately* if you see these signs; he'll want to do an immediate reduction of the dislocation.

Next, check your patient's circulatory status distal to the dislocation. Check all his distal pulses, the color and temperature of the extremity, and his capillary refill time. Swelling can cause compression, resulting in vessel damage unless it's treated promptly. In a patient with a knee dislocation, for example, gross swelling can compromise the popliteal artery.

When you're assessing a patient with a dislocated knee, remember that a pedal pulse doesn't necessarily mean no arterial damage is present. If the popliteal artery is damaged, the collateral circulation around the knee will initially produce an effective pedal pulse. However, it won't be sufficient to prevent eventual circulatory compromise in response to swelling. Expect to prepare your patient for an arteriogram if the doctor suspects popliteal artery damage. (Some doctors will order an arteriogram for *every* patient with a knee dislocation.)

### Therapeutic care

Be prepared to assist in the closed reduction of your patient's dislocation, usually within a few hours of the injury. Why is the time element important? Because waiting longer than 4 hours to reduce a patient's dislocated *hip* can result in necrosis of the femoral head. A delay of more than 8 hours to reduce a *knee* dislocation—especially if the patient has arterial damage—can ultimately result in loss of the limb.

Before the reduction, expect to give your patient a muscle relaxant, such as diazepam (Valium), and an analgesic to aid in the relocation procedure. The doctor may also use a local anesthetic. Usually you'll assist by maintaining traction while the doctor does the reduction. Or, your patient may need surgery for:
• reduction of his dislocation
• repair of an artery, vein, or ligament
• insertion of a pin, nail, or wire.
Local or general anesthesia may be used.

After the procedure, reassess the patient's neurovascular status. The doctor will order a follow-up X-ray to confirm successful reduction. Once the joint has been reduced successfully, a patient with a *hip* dislocation may require bed rest with skeletal traction for 6 to 12 weeks, to allow the ligaments to heal. A patient with a *knee* dislocation will require postreduction bed rest, with knee elevation and cold-pack treatment, for 7 to 10 days. Then, a long-leg cast will be applied. A patient with

an *ankle* dislocation may have a cast applied immediately after the reduction procedure.

The doctor will probably prescribe a regimen of graduated activity to prevent joint stiffness.

# Upper Extremity Fractures

### Prediagnosis summary

On initial assessment, the patient had a history of trauma to the affected part, and he may also have had:
• pain with point tenderness
• swelling
• ecchymoses
• crepitation
• paresis or paralysis
• an open wound.

The patient's injured extremity was temporarily immobilized (with a splint, a sling and swathe, or pillows and sandbags) and elevated, and cold packs were applied. If he had an open wound, it was covered with a sterile saline dressing. If an open fracture was suspected, an I.V. line was started for fluid and blood replacement and for drug administration.

Blood was drawn for typing and cross matching and for a CBC. An X-ray was taken to assess the site and extent of the injury. (A portable X-ray machine may have been used if the patient's condition was unstable.)

### Priorities, assessment, and intervention

Your first priority is to make sure your patient's fractured extremity is properly immobilized. (As you know, immobilization helps reduce pain and swelling resulting from the fracture.) If he has excessive bleeding and his fluid volume is depleted, expect to administer crystalloids, such as normal saline solution or Ringer's lactate, and, possibly, blood transfusion. If he has

## YOUR ROLE IN CAST CARE

After the doctor applies your patient's cast, you must:
- make sure it dries properly
- check it for drainage stains
- assess your patient's condition frequently.

Use this checklist to ensure proper care of your patient *and* his cast.

☑ Make sure your patient's casted extremity is elevated above his heart level.

☑ Place bed-saver pads between the moist cast and any pillows or sheets, to absorb moisture. To ensure proper drying, *never* put a wet cast directly on plastic.

☑ Periodically check the cast for flat spots or dents. These may cause pressure areas, resulting in skin breakdown.

☑ Reposition the patient every 2 hours, as ordered, to ensure even cast drying. (Use the palm of your hand, not your fingertips, to avoid denting the cast.) Make sure bony prominences, such as heels, ankles, and elbows, are pressure free.

☑ Routinely assess your patient for signs and symptoms of neurovascular impairment—swelling, pallor, numbness, tingling, and cool skin in areas around the cast. Notify the doctor *immediately* if the patient develops any of these signs or symptoms.

☑ Monitor the cast for drainage stains. Notify the doctor if:
- drainage from a wound increases significantly during the first 48 hours after casting.
- drainage stains the cast bright red.
- drainage occurs even though no wound was originally present.
- drainage odor changes (this may indicate infection).

☑ Protect the cast from getting wet.

☑ Place waterproof material, such as plastic wrap, around the perineal edge of a hip spica or body cast to prevent soilage from urine or stool.

☑ Provide skin care.

an open wound, make sure it's been covered with a sterile saline dressing. Continue cold-pack treatment and elevation of your patient's fractured extremity to further reduce or control swelling and pain.

Frequent assessments of the patient's neurovascular status are important to help you detect nerve and vessel damage and intervene promptly. Keep in mind that nerve and vessel compression and occlusion from swelling can

ultimately lead to serious complications, such as compartment syndrome (see *Understanding Compartment Syndrome*, pages 370 and 371). If the patient suffers neurovascular compromise, delaying immediate intervention can result in loss of the limb. You'll need to assess the motor function and sensation of his ulnar, median, and radial nerves (see *Testing for Peripheral Nerve Damage*, pages 348 and 349).

Remember, *don't* try to check motor nerve function in a patient with an open fracture; you could cause further damage. With any fracture, your patient will have some degree of pain on active motion. Tell him not to force any movement if the pain is excessive. If your patient can't abduct all his fingers or move his middle finger from side to side when his hand lies flat, he may have *ulnar* nerve damage. Check sensation loss in the distal fat pad of his little finger; any loss there may also mean ulnar nerve damage. Your patient should be able to oppose his thumb and little finger; if he can't, he may have *median* nerve damage. Check for sensation loss, which may indicate median nerve damage in the distal palmar surface of his index finger. If your patient can't hyperextend his thumb or wrist against resistance, suspect *radial* nerve damage. Test this possibility by checking for sensation loss in the dorsal surface of the web between the thumb and index finger. *Axillary* nerve damage will compromise shoulder motion and cause a sensory loss over the deltoid of the arm or the lateral aspect of the forearm.

To assess his vascular status, first check his distal pulses. If these are weak or absent, be sure you tell the doctor *immediately*. Also note capillary refill time and the color and temperature of the skin distal to the injury; pallor, coolness, or slow capillary refill can also indicate reduced blood supply.

Watch for signs and symptoms of increasing compartment pressure—increased swelling, pain on passive movement, taut skin, and increasing

## CASE IN POINT: A PATIENT FALL

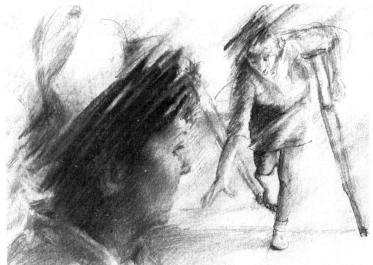

Angie Mariana, age 12, fell during cheerleading practice; X-rays confirmed a fractured right tibia/fibula. Now, in the ED, the doctor applies a cast, then asks you to fit Angie's crutches and teach her crutch walking. Because the ED's getting very busy, you quickly guide Angie into the hallway and briefly show her how she should balance on the crutches. She's doing pretty well, so you let her try to walk without your help. She's taken only a few steps when a commotion down the hall distracts you. When you turn back to watch Angie, she's falling to the floor. You rush to her and are relieved to find that her leg seems no worse than before. But then you discover that her right wrist is broken.

Angie's parents are furious. Now their little girl has a broken leg *and* a fractured wrist. They intend to file suit against you and the hospital.

If you were really involved in this situation, could you be liable for Angie's fall?

In *Butler v. Lutheran Medical Center* (1971), an elderly patient sustained a fracture after falling from her crutches. After hearing evidence that the attending nurse failed to give the patient adequate in-

struction in crutch walking, the court ruled she'd breached the applicable standard of care. The nurse was found negligent.

Patient falls are probably the most common cause of negligence suits filed against nurses and hospitals. Why? Because patients can fall for so many reasons. For example, they can fall from crutches, from their beds, or while they wait in the ED to see the doctor. Here are some guidelines for preventing patient falls:

● Make a thorough assessment of every patient's ability to take care of himself if left alone. If you have doubts, have a coworker or family member stay with him.

● Periodically assess your patient's condition; deterioration may precipitate a fall.

● If a doctor asks you to teach crutch walking, you're responsible for giving adequate instructions. Make sure you support your patient until he gains confidence on the crutches, and stay close while he tries using them without your support. If you're called away, make sure that another staff member stays with the patient.

● Be sure bed side rails are in place when indicated, especially if the patient's very young or elderly.

*Butler v. Lutheran Medical Center*, 36 A.D. 2d 640, 319 N.Y.S. 291 (2d Dept. 1971).

pain despite analgesia. These can indicate developing compartment syndrome, a devastating complication that can lead to Volkmann's contracture or loss of the limb. Tell the doctor *immediately* if you see these signs, and expect to assist in measuring compartment pressure. If this syndrome is developing, your patient may need an emergency fasciotomy (see *Understanding Compartment Syndrome,* pages 370 and 371, and *Measuring Compartment Pressure,* page 368).

Carefully document *all* your findings during this assessment so you'll have a baseline to measure future changes against. If your assessment has detected any signs of nerve or vessel damage,

---

## UNDERSTANDING TYPES OF FRACTURES

Suppose you've been floated to the orthopedic unit and assigned to care for a patient in skeletal traction. You know that he has a lower leg fracture, so you scan his chart to find out what type. When you read, "comminuted, oblique fracture of the fibula-tibia," you understand the terms—but a few seconds pass before a complete picture of the patient's injury forms in your mind. You wish that the various fracture types were easier to remember.

The information given here will help. A fracture may be classified as:

- *compound (open)*—a fracture in which the bone fragments penetrate the skin
- *simple (closed)*—the fracture site does not communicate with the exterior of the body
- *complete*—an interruption in the continuity of bone
- *incomplete (partial)*—an incomplete interruption in the continuity of bone.

Once a fracture's classified, the next step is to describe it in terms of *direction of fracture line* and *position of bony fragments.* (Of course, a fracture may combine several fracture types.)

### DIRECTION OF FRACTURE LINE

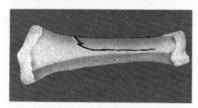

**Longitudinal**
Fracture line that runs parallel to the bone axis

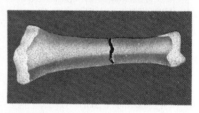

**Transverse**
Fracture line that crosses the bone at a right angle to its axis

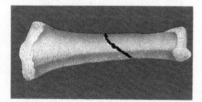

**Oblique**
Fracture line that breaks the bone at a slanted angle to the bone's axis

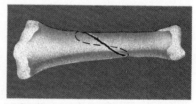

**Spiral**
A fracture line that runs through the bone in a coil-like manner

report these to the doctor *immediately*. Your patient may require prompt surgical intervention for repair of nerves or vessels.

Expect to give an analgesic for pain. Assess the degree of pain your patient's experiencing, both *before* and *after* the analgesic should have taken effect: Has the medication relieved his pain partially, completely, or not at all? This will give you baseline information for measuring any increases or decreases in his pain level.

## Therapeutic care

If your patient shows no evidence of neurovascular compromise or compartment syndrome, and if he doesn't

---

## POSITION OF BONY FRAGMENTS

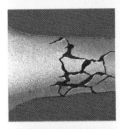

**Comminuted**
Three or more fragments

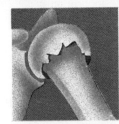

**Impacted**
One fragment forced into or onto another bone fragment

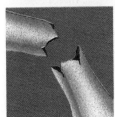

**Angulated**
Fragments deviating from their normal linear alignment so that they're at angles to each other

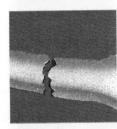

**Nondisplaced**
Fragments maintain essentially normal alignment

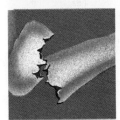

**Displaced**
Disrupted anatomic bone relationships with deformity

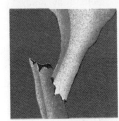

**Overriding**
Fragments overlapping and shortening total bone length

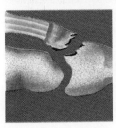

**Avulsed**
Fragments pulled from their normal position by forceful muscle contractions or ligamentous resistance

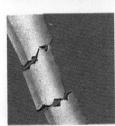

**Segmental**
Fractures in two adjacent areas with an isolated central segment

need surgery, prepare him for reduction of his fracture and for application of stabilizing devices. Reduction may be either open or closed, with application of a cast or another immobilizing device. *Open* reduction (with pins, rods, an external fixation device, or skeletal traction) may be needed for a severe fracture (see *The Hows and Whys of External Fixation Devices*). The patient may also need surgery for bone fragment removal and/or wound debridement.

If your patient requires *closed* reduction followed by application of a cast or other immobilizer, you may assist with these procedures. Before the reduction, expect to give an analgesic and a muscle relaxant, as ordered.

One of several types of immobilizers may be applied. (See *Using Immobilizers,* pages 352 and 353.) For example, expect to apply a figure-eight support for a *clavicular* or *shoulder* fracture. Have the patient sit with his shoulders squared and chest out as you apply this support. Sprinkle talcum powder or cornstarch under each axilla (or pad them), to prevent skin irritation.

Another example is the commercial immobilizer, or sling and swathe, used to support an *uncomplicated humeral* fracture. If the patient has a fracture of the *humerus,* the doctor may wish to apply a long cast from just below the shoulder to the elbow, instead of an immobilizer. Support the patient's arm in a triangular sling. If he has a *finger* fracture, a plastic or aluminum splint may be applied.

Cast application generally extends from the joint above the fracture to the joint below it. For example, if your patient has an *elbow* fracture, he may need a cast extending from the axilla to the base of the fingers, with the elbow acutely flexed and the forearm fully supinated.

If your patient needs *open* reduction, you'll have to prepare him for surgery. Ask him if he has any known allergies, is taking any medications, or has any preexisting diseases. Make sure you re-

## THE HOWS AND WHYS OF EXTERNAL FIXATION DEVICES

You may encounter a patient with a fracture so severe that the doctor can't use a cast, traction, or internal rods, wires, or plates to immobilize it. Such a patient may require an external fixation device.

External fixation involves inserting metal pins above and below the fracture, to hold bones and bone fragments together, then securely attaching them to the device's frame. The pins transfix individual bone fragments—but not necessarily the limb.

The doctor may use an external fixation device for a patient with:
• a massive open fracture with extensive soft tissue damage
• a comminuted fracture
• infected nonunion of a fracture
• multiple fractures
• a bone graft.

Once it's in place, an external fixation device immediately stabilizes bone and soft tissue, minimizes trauma to other injured parts, and relieves pain. When it's used to immobilize an open fracture, the device permits irrigation, debridement, dressing changes, and more accurate assessment. It also allows the doctor to adjust bone alignment during healing.

To help you care for a patient fitted with an external fixation device, here are some general tips. The illustrations will help you understand how some common devices work so you'll be able to answer patients' questions. Remember, the doctor's selection of a device will depend on the severity of the patient's fracture and the type of bone alignment needed.

**Nursing considerations**
• Prepare your patient. Tell him that an external fixation device, once in place, doesn't hurt. Explain that it will decrease possible swelling, muscle atrophy, and stiffness and thereby hasten mobility.
• Elevate the immobilized limb to reduce swelling.
• If the patient has a tibial fracture, make sure a sling or foot board is in place, to prevent ankle joint deformity.
• Monitor the patient's neurovascular status frequently.
• Watch for inflammation and drainage at the pin insertion sites, as well as for loosening of the pins.
• Give pin care, as ordered.
• Encourage the patient to do isometric and active exercises, as ordered.

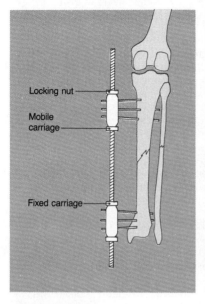

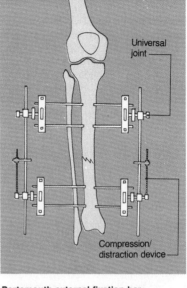

**Universal day frame**
*Use:* manages tibial fractures
*Characteristics:*
• The universal joint allows readjustment of the position of bony fragments by angulation and rotation.
• The compression/distraction device allows compression and distraction of bony fragments.

**Portsmouth external fixation bar**
*Use:* manages complicated tibial fractures
*Characteristics:*
• The locking nut adjustment on the mobile carriage *only* allows bone compression, so the doctor must accurately reduce bony fragments before applying the device.

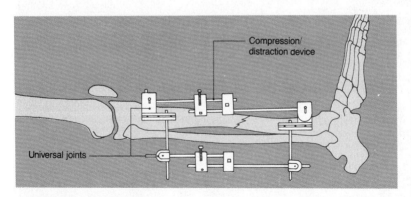

**Hoffman external fixation system**
*Use:* manages complex tibial fractures and fractures of the femur, upper limbs, and pelvis
*Characteristics:*
• The doctor may assemble the frame before he reduces the fracture, then adjust it later.
• Each component of the system can be readjusted to correct angulation and rotation and to apply distraction and compression.

cord all pertinent history information on his chart. The doctor may order an I.V. broad-spectrum antibiotic, especially if the patient has an open wound, to achieve therapeutic blood levels preoperatively and to help prevent infection.

If your patient had *closed* reduction and he now has a cast or immobilizer, a follow-up X-ray will be done to check for proper bone alignment and for successful reduction. He may be discharged at this time. Make sure the patient's cast is neither too loose (which may prevent proper bone alignment) nor too tight (which may impair his circulation). Before discharge, teach him how to care for his cast at home. He should:

• report any swelling (or cast tightness), pain, numbness, tingling, coldness, burning, skin color changes, or foul odors

• keep the cast elevated (above his heart level, when possible, to prevent excess swelling) until it's dry (48 to 72 hours later)

• avoid inserting objects into the cast

• keep the cast dry

• exercise the fingers of his casted extremity four times daily.

If your patient's had *open* reduction, he'll have an X-ray done to check it. You'll need to perform frequent assessments of his vital signs and neurovascular status, as described earlier, and to check your findings against his baseline. Check his motor and sensory nerve function, too, and assess his distal temperature, skin color, pulses, and capillary refill time. Watch for signs and symptoms of developing compartment syndrome (increased pain despite analgesics, pain on passive movement of the distal part, and edema).

If debridement was necessary and the bone ends weren't clean, the wound will be left open, and you'll apply fresh dressings often. After several days, reirrigate the wound. A cast may be applied at that time.

Continue I.V. fluid replacement for the patient after surgery, as ordered. Expect to continue I.V. antibiotics if they were started preoperatively. If they weren't, the doctor may order them af-

---

## HOW FORCES CAUSE FRACTURES

Bones have a degree of elasticity that lets them absorb forceful pressures, up to a point, without breaking. When a bone does break because excessive force is applied to it, the result is a *fracture*—a partial or complete disruption in the bone's continuity. Forces that cause fractures are classified as direct or indirect and of high or low energy.

**Direct force**—a high-energy, violent force powerful enough to cause serious fractures. Direct forces include:

• *wedging force*, which fractures the bone and propels a fragment into another fragment or into a joint

• *compression force*, which propels bones together, causing an incomplete fracture so that the cortex breaks on one side, bends on the opposite side

• *crushing force*, which splinters bones into fragments.

**Indirect force**—a less violent, lower-energy force that can fracture bones at a distance from the site where the force is applied.

Indirect forces include:

• *torsion force*, a twisting force strong enough to fracture bones

• *shearing force*, a force exerted when part of the bone is fixed, fracturing the part above or below

• *angulatory force*, a force exerted on an angle so that the bone fractures at that angle.

Sometimes a fracture will occur when only *minimal force* is applied. For example, minimal force exerted on a bone that's lost elasticity because of disease or tumor can cause a pathologic fracture. Or a stress fracture may occur when fatigue and exercise have caused a small crack in a bone. Then only minimal force may be needed to extend the crack to a complete fracture.

After a fracture, the force that caused it (or bone fragments) may also damage surrounding soft tissue, blood vessels, nerves, ligaments, muscles, and tendons. This may cause edema, bleeding, hematoma formation, and nerve or vessel damage.

ter surgery to prevent infection. Expect to give analgesics as needed.

Make sure your patient's injured extremity is in proper anatomic alignment. This will enhance circulation to the fracture and to distal areas. Encourage him to move his hand and fingers—unless he has an elbow fracture—to prevent contractures and to help his distal circulation.

If your patient's had an open wound, watch for signs and symptoms of infection, even if he's been given prophylactic antibiotics. (Drainage, indicating infection, may not be visible if his extremity's in a cast, so be alerted by any foul smell and check for drainage seeping through the cast or around its edges.)

Cleanse any exposed skin areas and, if your patient's had pins inserted, be sure to provide scrupulous pin care (see *Performing Pin Care,* page 355).

Also watch for signs and symptoms of fat emboli syndrome—a common *and serious* complication of long-bone fractures—so you can notify the doctor *immediately* if you suspect this syndrome's developing. (See *Assessing for Fat Emboli Syndrome,* page 376.)

If this syndrome develops, the doctor will order supplemental oxygen and, possibly, intubation and mechanical ventilation.

Expect that your patient will begin an early program of graduated exercise to prevent postreduction joint stiffness in the noncasted or nonpinned joints of the injured extremity. This activity is *contraindicated,* however, for a patient with an elbow fracture. Why? Because exercise may cause calcification leading to fibrosis.

# Lower Leg Fractures

## Prediagnosis summary
Initial assessment revealed that the patient had a history of direct, indirect, torsion, or stress trauma to his lower

leg. He may also have had:
- pain with point tenderness
- deformity
- angulation
- crepitation
- swelling
- ecchymoses
- weakness or partial paralysis of his foot or toes on the affected side
- an open wound over the injured area, with possible bone protrusion.

Gentle palpation may have revealed a disruption of the regular anterior edge of the tibia. The patient's leg was elevated and temporarily immobilized by either a rigid-board or an air-inflated splint extending well above and below the fracture. If he had an open wound, a culture specimen was taken, and a sterile saline dressing was applied. Application of pressure was used if he had excessive external bleeding. Cold packs were applied to reduce swelling and pain.

An X-ray was taken of the patient's lower leg—including the joints above and below the injury—to determine the fracture's exact site and extent. (A portable X-ray machine was used if the patient's condition wasn't stable.) Blood may have been drawn to test for hemoglobin and hematocrit levels, for typing and cross matching, and for a CBC. An I.V. line may have been started to expedite drug and fluid administration.

## Priorities, assessment, and intervention
Your first priorities in caring for a patient with a lower leg fracture are ensuring that the leg is properly immobilized and replacing blood and fluids if necessary. If the patient's blood loss was significant, expect to give crystalloids, such as normal saline solution or Ringer's lactate, and, possibly, blood transfusions.

Continue cold-pack treatment and elevation of the fractured leg to help reduce pain and swelling.

Next, perform a thorough neurovascular assessment because of the like-

PROCEDURES

# YOUR ROLE IN AN EMERGENCY

## MEASURING COMPARTMENT PRESSURE

Here's what you need to know about measuring compartment pressure.

### Equipment
- Mercury manometer
- Two anesthesia extension-tubing sets
- Three-way stopcock
- 20-ml syringe with plunger pulled back to 15-ml mark
- 20-ml bottle of normal saline solution
- Several 18G or 19G needles

### Procedure
- Explain the procedure to the patient.
- Assemble the equipment as shown.
- Ask a co-worker to stand by to help you.
- Attach a needle to the extension tubing and draw sterile saline into the tubing, forming a meniscus.
- Prepare, with povidone-iodine, all the patient's skin over the compartments to be measured.
- Assist the doctor as he inserts the needle through the patient's skin, subcutaneous tissues, and fascia and into the muscle.
- Push the syringe plunger in very slowly.
- Ask your co-worker to watch the manometer and record its pressure as soon as the meniscus moves toward the patient's skin. At this point, manometer pressure equals compartment pressure.
- To measure the pressure in each affected compartment, change the needle and repeat this procedure.

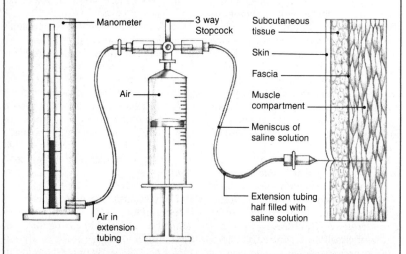

| What compartment pressures mean | |
| --- | --- |
| 20 mm Hg or less | Normal |
| 21 to 40 mm Hg | Decreased nerve conduction and tissue perfusion |
| 41 mm Hg and above | Impaired perfusion with ischemia (emergency fasciotomy needed) |

lihood of injury to your patient's nerves and vessels. (You also want to establish a baseline for comparison with your later findings.) Nerves and vessels may be compressed if excessive swelling occurs around the fracture site. Delays in intervention, if damage isn't found quickly, can allow neurovascular compromise to cause ischemia and compartment syndrome, which may lead to Volkmann's contracture and limb loss (see *Understanding Compartment Syndrome*, pages 370 and 371). So assess your patient's vascular status by checking for any increasing swelling, taut skin, pallor, or cyanosis and for increased pain (despite analgesics) or pain on passive movement of his ankle or toes. Check your patient for reduced capillary refill time and for pulse weakness or absence in his lower extremity. (Report any of these signs to the doctor *immediately*.) You may have to measure and record your patient's compartment pressures, too. (See *Measuring Compartment Pressure*.)

Next, check your patient's neurologic status by assessing the sensory functions of his tibial and peroneal nerves. Check for any decrease or loss of sensation over the medial and lateral surfaces of the foot on the fractured leg; if you detect any, suspect *tibial* nerve damage. Also check for lack of sensation in the lateral surface of the patient's great toe and the medial surface of his second toe; if you note this, suspect *peroneal* nerve damage. If you find a decrease or lack of sensation in *all* of these areas, suspect *sciatic* nerve damage. (See *Testing for Peripheral Nerve Damage*, pages 348 and 349.)

Check motor response of the tibial and peroneal nerves *only* if your patient's fracture was closed. (As you know, any fracture will cause some pain on active movement, but tell your patient not to force any movement if it causes excessive pain.) Look for any paresis or paralysis when the patient attempts to plantarflex or dorsiflex the affected ankle (indicating tibial and peroneal nerve impairment, respec-

tively). Call the doctor *immediately* if you see any of these signs of neurovascular compromise. The patient will need *immediate* surgical intervention to repair damaged nerves or vessels or fasciotomy to relieve increasing compartment pressure.

If the doctor ordered analgesics to relieve the patient's pain, administer them as needed. Remember to assess his degree of pain (on a scale of 1 to 10) *before* and *after* the analgesic should have taken effect. This will give you a baseline for measuring any changes in his pain level.

## Therapeutic care

If your patient has no neurovascular deficit requiring surgery, prepare him for permanent stabilization and fracture reduction at this time. Reduction may be either open or closed, with application of a cast or other type of immobilizer.

If your patient needs *closed* reduction, you'll assist in cast or immobilizer application. Expect to give analgesics to decrease the patient's pain and, possibly, a muscle relaxant prior to reduction, to aid in the procedure. Casts and immobilizers typically extend from the joint above the fracture to the joint below it.

If your patient's fracture needs *open* reduction, however, expect to prepare him for surgery. A severe fracture may require pin or rod insertion or application of external fixation devices or skeletal traction. (See *The Hows and Whys of External Fixation Devices*, pages 364 and 365.) Surgery may also be required to remove bone fragments or to debride the open wound. Before the surgery, take a brief history, asking the patient what medications he's taking and what (if any) allergies or preexisting diseases he has. Record all pertinent information on his chart. You may need to shave and cleanse the affected area before surgery, according to your hospital's protocol. You may also be asked to give I.V. antibiotics preoperatively—especially if your pa-

WARNING

## UNDERSTANDING COMPARTMENT SYNDROME

**Cross section of mid-lower leg**

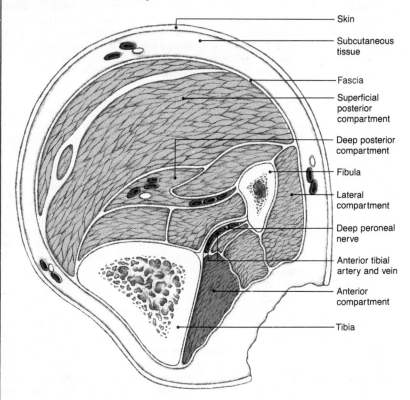

- Skin
- Subcutaneous tissue
- Fascia
- Superficial posterior compartment
- Deep posterior compartment
- Fibula
- Lateral compartment
- Deep peroneal nerve
- Anterior tibial artery and vein
- Anterior compartment
- Tibia

If your patient develops compartment syndrome, you have a serious emergency on your hands. Failure to detect it early and to intervene quickly—within 6 hours—may allow irreversible muscle and nerve damage to develop. Your patient could end up permanently deformed and handicapped.

Compartment syndrome may arise suddenly, right after a patient's injury, or gradually, over several days. Primary causes include elbow, forearm, and lower leg fractures; crush injuries; and soft tissue injuries with hemorrhage and edema. But other traumatic injuries—such as

animal bites, burns with edema, and missile injuries—as well as tight bandages and casts may also bring it on.

**What causes it**

As you may know, muscle groups are arranged in compartments surrounded by connective tissue called fascia. Each compartment has only enough room for major arteries and nerves to pass through.

After an injury, tissue swelling compresses arteries and nerves, causing muscle ischemia and releasing histamines. These make the swelling worse. As the swelling increases, it further compresses the veins and arteries within the muscle compartment, and reflex muscle spasms compromise large arteries entering the compartment.

The compression decreases blood flow, causing ischemia that permanently damages the sensory and motor functions of the patient's peripheral nerves. After 24 to 48 hours, the limb becomes contracted, paralyzed, numb, functionless, and possibly gangrenous. Volkmann's contracture is a common result.

### Signs and symptoms
• Progressive intense pain in the injured limb, unaffected by immobilization, elevation, or analgesic administration (traction may *increase* the pain)
• Increased pain on passive motion
• (With leg muscle compartment swelling) numbness, tingling, or loss of sensation in the web space between the first and second toes
• (With forearm superficial flexor compartment swelling) paresthesias on the hand's medial and ulnar surfaces

When you assess a patient who may have compartment syndrome, remember that peripheral pulses may be present, even with severe compartment ischemia, and the limb may *not* become pale or cool or exhibit decreased capillary refill. Keep your index of suspicion high.

### Nursing interventions
If your patient may be developing compartment syndrome, intervene as follows:
• Quickly decrease the edema-ischemia cycle by elevating the patient's affected limb, applying cold packs, and removing anything constricting the limb—such as an elastic bandage or a tight dressing.
• Immediately notify the doctor.
• Expect to assist with measuring the compartment pressure.
• Administer an analgesic for pain, as ordered.
• Anticipate that the doctor will perform emergency fasciotomy if initial interventions don't provide relief within 30 minutes. Fasciotomy is a surgical procedure to incise the fascia enclosing the muscle, allowing it to swell beyond its compartment. The incision may be left open, to heal by granulation. Later, split-thickness skin grafts will be applied.

tient has an open wound—to achieve therapeutic levels preoperatively and to help prevent infection.

### Postreduction care
If your patient's had closed reduction, and if a cast or immobilizer was applied, the doctor will check for proper bone alignment and reduction by ordering a follow-up X-ray. The patient may be discharged at this time. Make sure the cast isn't too loose or too tight. (Proper alignment won't occur if it's too loose; circulation may be compromised if it's too tight.) Before he's discharged, teach him how to care for his cast at home. He should:
• note any swelling (or cast tightness), pain, tingling, numbness, coldness, burning, skin color changes, foul odors
• keep the cast elevated above heart level, to prevent excessive swelling, until it's dry (48 to 72 hours later)
• avoid inserting objects into the cast
• keep the cast dry
• exercise his toes four times daily.

If your patient had open reduction, he'll also have a follow-up X-ray to check for proper bone alignment and successful reduction. Assess his vital signs and neurovascular status frequently. Check his motor and sensory nerve functions; assess distal skin temperature and color, his pulses, and his capillary refill time, just as you did earlier; and compare your findings with his baseline. Also watch for increased pain despite analgesic administration, pain on passive movement, and edema—which may indicate developing compartment syndrome. (After cast application, check the cast periodically for increasing tightness, a sign of increasing edema.)

If your patient's injury required debridement, and if the bone ends weren't clean, the wound will be left open and you'll have to apply fresh sterile dressings often. Reirrigate the wound after several days. A cast may or may not be applied at that time.

Expect to continue I.V. antibiotics after surgery if they were started pre-

# CARING FOR A PATIENT IN TRACTION

The doctor may order traction for a patient to treat a fracture or dislocation, to decrease muscle spasms, or to immobilize an injury before surgery.

*Skin traction* is used to treat fractures in small children or to reduce pain in adults by temporarily immobilizing their injuries.

*Skeletal traction* is used to treat long-bone fractures and cervical spine fractures.

Both types of traction work by exerting a pulling force on a body part. For skin traction, the doctor connects the weight system to a bandage made of moleskin and elastic; for skeletal traction, he connects it to a pin or wire. (You may be asked to apply some forms of skin traction.)

The following traction-care tips and illustrations will help you care for patients with skin or skeletal traction.

**Nursing tips**
• Check for wrinkles in the moleskin; they may cause skin blisters.
• Monitor a patient with skin traction for itching, burning, or pain, possibly indicating an allergic reaction.
• Relieve pressure against bony prominences by placing sheepskin under them.
• Check for circulatory and neurologic impairment from an elastic bandage that's too tight or from splint pressure on the popliteal area.
• Maintain ropes and pulleys in straight alignment, with weights hanging free.
• For a patient in a pelvic sling, watch for signs and symptoms of abdominal organ injury. These include inadequate output, hematuria, rectal bleeding, abdominal pain, spasm, rigidity, distention, and shock from internal bleeding.

**Buck's extension:** immobilizes dislocated hips after reduction, hip fractures before surgery, total hip replacements, locked knees, femur fractures before surgical reduction, or irritated hip or knee joints

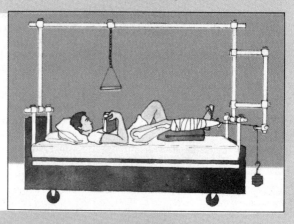

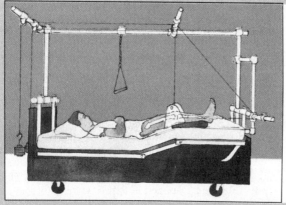

**Skeletal split Russell's:** immobilizes tibia and fibula fractures and femoral shaft fractures (in adolescents)

**Balanced suspension using Thomas' splint with Pearson attachment:** immobilizes fractures of femoral shaft, hip, and lower leg (allows the patient to move freely in bed; Pearson attachment supports his lower leg off the bed, allowing knee flexion)

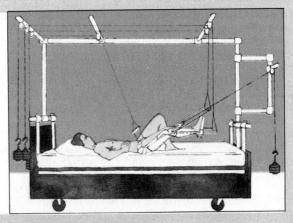

**Overhead skeletal traction (90°-90°):** immobilizes fractures of humerus, elbow, or femur; may also immobilize shoulder fractures or injuries

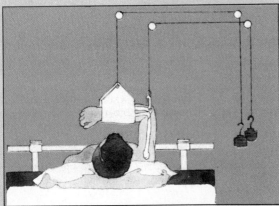

**Pelvic sling:** immobilizes pelvic injuries or treats low back pain

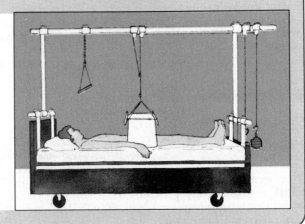

operatively. If they weren't, the doctor may start antibiotics now, to prevent infection. Fluid replacement may be continued as well. Expect to give analgesics as needed.

Make sure your patient's fractured leg is in proper anatomic alignment, which will enhance circulation to the fracture and to distal areas. Encourage toe, foot, and ankle movements, if possible, in order to prevent contractures. (This will also aid distal circulation.)

Even though he's received prophylactic antibiotics, watch a patient who's had an open wound for signs and symptoms of infection.

(Note: The drainage may not be directly visible if your patient has a cast, so be alerted by any foul smell and by drainage seeping through the cast.)

Cleanse any exposed skin areas and, if your patient's had pins inserted, provide scrupulous pin care (see *Performing Pin Care*, page 355).

Also watch for signs and symptoms of fat emboli syndrome (see *Assessing for Fat Emboli Syndrome*, page 376)— a common complication with long-bone fractures—so you can notify the doctor *immediately*.

If the patient develops fat emboli syndrome, the doctor will order supplemental oxygen therapy and may order intubation and mechanical ventilation. You may perform *passive* range-of-motion exercises on his affected extremity. Encourage him to move in bed and to do *active* range-of-motion exercises of his uninjured extremities. The doctor will set up a program of graduated activity for your patient.

---

# Hip and Femur Fractures

## Prediagnosis summary
Initial assessment of the patient revealed a history of trauma, with intense localized pain. He may also have had:

• swelling and discoloration in the hip or thigh area
• reluctance or inability to move the affected leg or to put weight on it
• deformity (such as a shortening of the leg and outward foot rotation)
• crepitation on gentle palpation.

If the patient had a suspected femur fracture, the circumferences of both thighs were measured to assess the amount of edema in the affected leg. His pant leg was cut away so a traction splint (either Hare or Thomas) could be applied for immobilization.

His vital signs were monitored to determine his general status and the severity of his blood loss. If his blood loss was so great that hypovolemic shock was imminent, an I.V. infusion of Ringer's lactate or normal saline solution was started. He was also given supplemental oxygen.

Blood was drawn for a CBC, typing and cross matching, electrolytes, and prothrombin time and partial thromboplastin time. An X-ray was taken to determine the precise site and extent of the injury. (A portable X-ray machine was used if the patient's condition was unstable.)

The diagnostic X-ray confirmed whether the fracture was of the femoral head or neck (hip) or of the femoral shaft.

## Priorities
Your first priorities in caring for a patient with a hip or femur fracture include immobilization of the fracture, fluid replacement (if he's had significant blood loss), and pain relief.

For a patient with a hip fracture, be sure the area's immobilized with a splint and with pillows between the patient's legs. Place a trochanter roll at the hip joint for further support. Immobilization will help relieve painful muscle spasms and prevent further damage to soft tissue, vessels, and nerves around the fracture. Make sure the leg is anatomically aligned—this will also help reduce the patient's pain. Provide additional pain relief by applying cold packs around the hip and administering analgesics as ordered. Assess the patient's vital signs; if signs and symptoms of significant blood loss develop, expect to administer replacement I.V. fluids and blood.

To immobilize a femoral shaft fracture and to reduce associated muscle spasm, make sure a long leg splint (Hare or Thomas) has been used. In this type of fracture, spasm of the patient's hamstrings, quadriceps, and adductor muscles can produce *severe* pain and also overriding and angulation of the bony fragments. Apply cold packs to the area to help reduce swelling, pain, and blood loss.

Because this patient may lose significant amounts of blood, assess him for signs and symptoms of hypovolemic shock, checking his vital signs and his hematocrit level. If an I.V. hasn't been inserted, expect to do so now to replace lost blood and fluids. A MAST suit may be applied if the blood loss appears to be severe. If the fracture's open, use pressure to control the bleeding, and cover the wound with a sterile saline dressing or pack it with sterile saline gauze. *Don't* try to clean the wound; this may facilitate infection by pathogens. The doctor will clean the wound during surgery—but you should remove any grossly contaminating objects, such as pieces of glass, wood, or metal. Remember, don't try to force protruding bone ends back into the wound.

Once the patient's been stabilized, you'll probably give him an analgesic to relieve his pain. (Intramuscular pain medication probably won't be given if the patient's hypovolemic. This is because the medicine won't take effect until the patient's fluids are adequately replaced; then it will take effect all at once and may cause respiratory depression.)

## Continuing assessment and intervention

Once your patient's condition is hemodynamically stable, perform a thorough assessment. Remember to continue checking his vital signs every 5 to 10 minutes during your assessment. Because a patient with a femur fracture probably suffered a high-impact trauma, assess him for associated nerve or vessel injuries. Broad-spectrum antibiotics may be infused to prevent infection from an open femur fracture.

Your next step is to perform an assessment of your patient's neurovascular status. Check the five Ps as described in the "What to Do Next" section in this chapter. Watch for suddenly increasing pain, excessive puffiness, and decreased or absent leg pulses. In a patient with a *femur* fracture, check peroneal nerve function by testing for decreased sensitivity across the top of the foot, which may be most apparent adjacent to the great and second toes. If the patient's fracture is closed, also check for foot drop and an inability to extend the toes. To assess him for tibial nerve damage, look for any decrease in sensitivity over the lateral aspect and the sole of the foot, and check for loss of plantarflexion of the ankle and toes. *Never* assess motor response if your patient has an open fracture; you may cause bone fragments to move so they cause further damage.

A patient with a *hip* fracture may have sciatic nerve impairment. To assess for this, look for a combination of signs of both tibial and peroneal nerve damage. Another sign of sciatic nerve injury in a patient with a hip fracture is severe pain when he extends his knee while his hip is flexed. Assess his distal circulation by checking all his pulses, his capillary refill time, and the color and temperature of the affected leg.

Expect to prepare your patient for surgery; he'll probably require open fracture reduction, insertion of an internal fixation device, application of skeletal traction, and, possibly, debridement. A patient with a femur fracture may require skeletal traction by means of a Kirshner wire or a Steinmann's pin. Or the patient may require an internal fixation device that extends into the neck of the femur. (This is commonly used to repair a hip fracture.)

The type of internal fixation device used depends on the precise fracture site. For example, the surgeon will usually correct an intracapsular fracture by inserting an Austin-Moore prosthesis, because vascular necrosis of the femoral head is a common complication of this type of fracture. To correct an extracapsular fracture, the usual procedure is internal fixation with hip nails or screws.

Expect to give I.V. broad-spectrum antibiotics before surgery to achieve therapeutic levels preoperatively. Make sure that all information needed before surgery, such as allergies, current medications, and last meal eaten, is on your patient's chart. If time permits, complete your history by focusing on preexisting medical conditions. In particular, ask if your patient has diabetes; if he does, his insulin dosage will be adjusted for surgery. Ask about prior pulmonary disease, too. If the patient's had any, inform the anesthesiologist of

this so he can determine the best approach for general anesthesia. Note any preexisting heart disease, as well, so the surgeon can anticipate possible complications.

Before surgery for a patient with a hip fracture, the doctor may apply Buck's extension traction with the straps below the knee, using about 5 to 8 pounds of weight. (Surgery may be delayed if your patient is elderly, to allow improvement in his fluid and nutrition status.)

## Therapeutic care

After your patient returns from surgery, gather baseline neurovascular information for use in assessing any subsequent changes. Watch for increasing swelling, which may compress and injure nerves and vessels. Check all the patient's pulses, and assess his nerve function for paresis or paralysis. Circle any areas of bleeding on the patient's wound dressing, and use the circle to assess any further increase in bleeding.

Initially, check your patient's vital

---

⎡ WARNING ⎤

## ASSESSING FOR FAT EMBOLI SYNDROME

One of the most serious complications of long-bone fractures is fat emboli syndrome (FES), which may occur 24 to 72 hours after the patient's injury. If FES isn't treated quickly, it can cause acute respiratory distress and death. So notify the doctor *immediately* if you detect the development of FES.

Watch your patient for the following signs and symptoms, and be prepared to intervene appropriately.

**Signs and symptoms**
• Altered mental status (in early FES stages)
• Complaint of chest pain on inspiration
• Changes in EKG waveforms (due to chemical irritation)—prominent S waves, T-wave inversions, multiple dysrhythmias, right bundle-branch block
• Cardiovascular collapse
• Gradually increasing tachypnea and

tachycardia, rales, wheezing
• Arterial blood gas measurements showing respiratory alkalosis, hypoxemia, pulmonary shunt
• Petechiae (lasting 4 to 6 hours) over the patient's torso, in his axillary folds, in his conjunctival sacs and retina, and on the mucosa of his soft palate
• Fever due to brain-center irritation
• Localized muscle weakness, spasticity, and rigidity from muscle irritation.

**Nursing interventions**
• Administer fluids to prevent shock and to dilute free fatty acids.
• Administer corticosteroids, as ordered, to counteract the inflammatory response to free fatty acids.
• Administer digoxin, as ordered, to increase the patient's cardiac output.
• Reassure the patient. He may be frightened or anxious from the hypoxemia.

# WHAT HAPPENS IN
# FAT EMBOLI SYNDROME

Although the pathophysiology of fat emboli syndrome (FES) isn't well understood, its effects are. A fracture initiates the pathophysiologic process that leads to pneumonitis from lipase release; this may eventually cause death.

Two theories have been formulated to explain the pathophysiology of FES. This flowchart will help you compare and understand them.

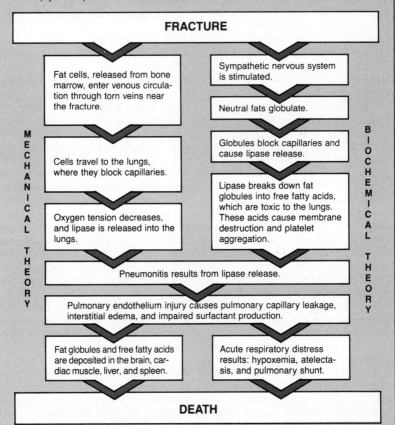

**FRACTURE**

**MECHANICAL THEORY**

**BIOCHEMICAL THEORY**

Fat cells, released from bone marrow, enter venous circulation through torn veins near the fracture.

Sympathetic nervous system is stimulated.

Neutral fats globulate.

Cells travel to the lungs, where they block capillaries.

Globules block capillaries and cause lipase release.

Oxygen tension decreases, and lipase is released into the lungs.

Lipase breaks down fat globules into free fatty acids, which are toxic to the lungs. These acids cause membrane destruction and platelet aggregation.

Pneumonitis results from lipase release.

Pulmonary endothelium injury causes pulmonary capillary leakage, interstitial edema, and impaired surfactant production.

Fat globules and free fatty acids are deposited in the brain, cardiac muscle, liver, and spleen.

Acute respiratory distress results: hypoxemia, atelectasis, and pulmonary shunt.

**DEATH**

signs every 15 minutes for 1 hour; then reduce the frequency to every ½ hour for 1 hour; and then to every hour until his condition is stable.

Your patient may still require blood replacement, especially if he has a femoral shaft fracture. You'll need to monitor his hemoglobin and hematocrit studies frequently. Either the doctor will give new orders for blood replacement each time you report the results, or he'll write a general order on the patient's chart. If your patient's elderly and has a hip fracture, be sure to assess him for signs and symptoms of dehydration and to provide adequate I.V.

fluid replacement. Why? Because an elderly patient who's broken a hip may have been unable to get up to seek help. By the time a neighbor or relative found him, he may have become dehydrated and developed electrolyte imbalances. So check his electrolytes often and expect to correct any imbalance.

Continue to administer analgesics to relieve the patient's pain or discomfort. Check his wound or pin insertion site often for signs of infection. (See *Performing Pin Care,* page 355.) Keep in mind that your patient with a femur fracture may be in traction with a pin inserted for 6 weeks or more. While his fracture heals, he'll need your emotional support to reassure him that he's getting better.

You'll probably give your patient a stool softener because this will help him avoid straining with bowel movements. (Remember, his peristaltic reflexes will be reduced after his injury, surgery, and prolonged bed rest.)

Have your patient cough and deep-breathe frequently to prevent the pulmonary complications that can occur during a prolonged period of bed rest. The respiratory therapist may initiate incentive spirometry, and you'll supervise subsequent repetitions. You'll also need to watch for any signs and symptoms of fat emboli syndrome so you can call the doctor if you note any (see *Assessing for Fat Emboli Syndrome,* page 376).

Help your patient change position often so he's as comfortable as possible. Be sure to perform passive range-of-motion exercises of your patient's foot on the affected side, and encourage active range-of-motion exercise of all his other extremities.

---

# Pelvic Fractures

## Prediagnosis summary
The patient had a history of direct or indirect trauma to the pelvic region.

He may also have had:
- pelvic pain or tenderness increasing with compression of the iliac crests
- muscle spasm in the pelvic region
- sacroiliac joint tenderness
- bruising over the pelvis
- inability to walk, to bear his weight without pain, or to raise his legs when lying supine
- backache
- hematuria
- external foot rotation on the affected side
- signs of blood loss or shock
- deformity (shortening of one leg, for example)
- hematoma or ecchymoses in the perineum, groin, suprapubic area, or flank (Grey Turner's sign).

A large-bore I.V. line was inserted; Ringer's lactate was given if the patient was hypovolemic. A MAST suit may have been applied if the patient's hypovolemia was so severe that he had signs and symptoms of shock. Blood was drawn for typing and cross matching, CBC, electrolytes, arterial blood gases (ABGs), prothrombin time, and partial thromboplastin time. If the patient was able to void, a urinalysis was done. He may have been given supplemental oxygen and placed on a cardiac monitor.

An X-ray of the patient's pelvis was done. If his condition was too unstable to permit transport, a portable X-ray machine was used.

## Priorities
Your first priorities are to stabilize your patient's hemodynamic status and to keep him immobilized. Continue giving him fluids and Ringer's lactate, as needed, and keep him in the MAST suit, if one was applied, to promote circulation to his vital organs and to enhance immobilization. Take his vital signs frequently (watch particularly for changes in his systolic blood pressure), and observe his cardiac monitor for any dysrhythmias.

If the doctor suspects the patient has intraabdominal bleeding, he may per-

# WHAT HAPPENS IN PELVIC FRACTURES

As you probably know, crush injuries and the application of severe direct or indirect force cause most pelvic fractures.

Because the pelvis is a bony ring, fractures usually occur in at least two separate places, often with separation of one or both sacroiliac joints. The illustrations below show you two common sites of pelvic fractures.

Complications of pelvic fractures may also be serious. These include injuries to:
• the peripheral and central nervous systems
• the great vessels
• the bladder, urethra, vagina, or uterus
• the liver, kidneys, spleen, or lower intestines
• other bones.

Because many major blood vessels lie in the pelvic region, a pelvic fracture can also result in a significant loss of blood (2 to 8 pints) from arterial bleeding into the extraperitoneal space. Hemorrhage, with or without subsequent sepsis, is another life-threatening complication.

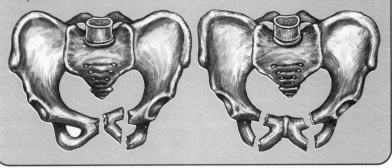

form peritoneal lavage (see *Assisting with Peritoneal Lavage,* pages 310 and 311). Check the lavage fluid when it returns. If it's clear, assume this rules out peritoneal bleeding—but remember, this *doesn't* rule out *retro*peritoneal bleeding. Abdominal X-rays may be taken to assess your patient for free air in his abdomen or for any signs of internal injury.

If your patient's still hypovolemic, expect to give him a total of 2 liters of a crystalloid, such as Ringer's lactate. If he's not stable within 30 minutes, you'll probably start a blood transfusion (don't remove the MAST suit). The doctor may order an arteriogram, either immediately or within 2 hours, to detect and locate arterial bleeding. If the results are positive, expect to prepare your patient for surgery to repair

or occlude the damaged artery, using embolization with an autologous clot or absorbable gelatin sponge.

If the arteriogram results are *inconclusive* and your patient's still hemodynamically unstable, a venogram may reveal the cause. Surgical repair may be necessary. If the venogram fails to reveal venous damage and your patient's still hypovolemic, expect to prepare him for a laparotomy. This procedure should locate the source of his bleeding and allow for the necessary surgical repair.

The doctor may order a spleen-liver scan to rule out rupture of either organ. If your patient's been kept in a MAST suit during these procedures, monitor his ABGs frequently—the constant pressure on his diaphragm can impair respiratory exchange. If he also has a lower leg fracture, deflate that leg of his MAST suit to minimize the possibility of compartment syndrome (see *Understanding Compartment Syndrome,* pages 370 and 371).

Immobilizing your patient is extremely important, because any movement can shift unstable bone fragments and cause further injury to underlying vessels, nerves, and organs. Use pillows and sandbags for support. If you must shift your patient from one surface to another, use a draw sheet. If you have to turn him onto his side (for example, to prevent aspiration of vomitus), first place pillows between his knees to avoid further pelvic stress. Then turn his body as a unit, in a logrolling fashion.

## Continuing assessment and intervention

Once your patient's immobilized and you've started measures to stabilize his hypovolemia, assess him thoroughly for secondary injuries related to his pelvic fracture. Expect to administer analgesics for pain, as ordered, if his blood pressure's stable.

Pay special attention to possible urinary tract injuries, common with pelvic fractures. Look for supraumbilical swelling, which may indicate bladder distention or a hematoma around the bladder. Ask him when he voided last and if he can void now; if he can, take another urine specimen for analysis to detect changes in his status.

If he can't void but has bladder distention and a sense of urgency, expect to insert an indwelling (Foley) catheter to relieve bladder pressure and to drain any urine. *However,* if you see any blood on the urinary meatus (indicating probable urethral injury), check with the doctor. He may decide *against* Foley catheter insertion and may have a urologist perform one or more of the following procedures:

• suprapubic cystotomy, to avoid possible further damage to the urethra
• retrograde urethrography, to determine if the urethra's ruptured

• cystography, if the urethra's intact, to reveal subtle tears or rupture of the bladder, extravasation of urine, or a hematoma
• intravenous pyelography, to reveal retroperitoneal hematoma, rupture of the urinary tract, or kidney damage.

Indicators of a ruptured *posterior* urethra include inability to void, blood at the meatus, bladder distention, and hematoma (or discoloration) in the perianal area, possibly diffusing onto the patient's thigh.

A localized hematoma in or around the patient's perineum, penis, or scrotum may indicate a ruptured *anterior* urethra.

When you assess your patient for signs or symptoms of urethral laceration or rupture, keep in mind that urethral damage is more common in men because of the greater length of the urethra. Monitor his electrolytes for any imbalances, which may point to urinary tract rupture. An increased potassium level is a common indicator. (See Chapter 13, GENITOURINARY EMERGENCIES.)

Observe the patient's perineum and rectum or vagina for signs of an open pelvic fracture (ecchymoses, swelling, or lacerations), which isn't always obvious during the initial external examination.

If the patient's male, the doctor will palpate his prostate to check for urethral injury; if she's female, he'll examine the vagina for signs of pregnancy or a cul-de-sac hematoma.

To test for spinal cord integrity, the doctor will check the patient's rectal sphincter tone.

Fracture of the patient's sacroiliac joint or of the sacrum can injure the spinal nerve root, lumbosacral plexus, and peripheral (especially sciatic) nerves. Excessive swelling can compress nerves and damage them further. Sharp bone fragments may lacerate nerves, so perform a thorough neurologic assessment. Check the patient's ability to plantarflex and dorsiflex both his ankles without experiencing weakness or pain. Observe his distal skin color for any pallor or cyanosis, and ask if he feels tingling, numbness, or weakness in any distal areas.

Continue checking your patient's vital signs often, recording all your findings and comparing them with earlier baseline data. Be constantly alert for any signs or symptoms of developing hypovolemic shock. Gently palpate your patient's abdomen for signs of liver, spleen, or bowel injuries:
• organ enlargement
• swelling
• distention
• rigidity
• guarding.

### Therapeutic care
If your patient has an open pelvic fracture, expect to infuse broad-spectrum antibiotics to prevent infection. As soon as a culture of the wound site has been assessed, the antibiotic can be adjusted accordingly. If the patient has an open wound, watch for signs and symptoms of infection that may occur in spite of prophylactic antibiotic therapy.

Your next step will probably be to prepare your patient for surgical stabilization of his pelvic fracture. Plates, pins, or screws will be inserted to fix the bones in place. The doctor may also use skeletal traction or an external fixation device. If the fracture isn't severe, the doctor may decide to apply a pelvic sling or simply to keep the patient on bed rest.

After the patient's surgery, continue to administer pain medication as ordered. Expect to start him on a soft diet, too. You'll also need to check his traction or external fixation device frequently. Continue to watch for signs of infection, and change the sterile dressing around his pins as ordered.

Be particularly alert for signs and symptoms of fat emboli syndrome: this common and serious complication of pelvic fractures can develop within the first 3 days after the injury. (See *Assessing for Fat Emboli Syndrome,* page 376.)

Encourage your patient to cough and deep-breathe frequently to help prevent pulmonary complications. Change his position often to keep him as comfortable as possible and to prevent pressure sores. Help your patient do passive range-of-motion exercises with his legs. Record any deterioration or improvement you note during these exercise sessions. Encourage your patient to move his feet, to bend his knees, and to wiggle his toes, as the doctor allows.

# Crush Injuries

### Prediagnosis summary
Initial assessment of the patient disclosed a history of traumatic compression of an extremity by a heavy object (such as the rollers in an industrial machine). He may have had:
• considerable edema
• an obvious wound
• hematomas
• sizable ecchymotic or avulsed areas with bleeding, abrasions, and cyanotic or reddened areas on the skin.

Or he may have had no obvious damage. In either case, he was unable to move the affected extremity, and he had severe pain.

The patient was given supplemental oxygen and placed on a cardiac monitor. A large-bore I.V. was inserted for fluid replacement and drug administration. Blood was drawn for a CBC, electrolytes, blood sugar, blood urea nitrogen, creatinine, ABGs, prothrombin time and partial thromboplastin time, and typing and cross matching. The doctor may have ordered an X-ray to detect bone fractures accompanying the injury.

The diagnosis of a crush injury was made on the basis of the patient's history information and the data the doctor gathered from inspecting the injured extremity.

### Priorities
Crush injuries are very serious because

PATHOPHYSIOLOGY

# WHAT HAPPENS
# IN CRUSH SYNDROME

Severe crush injuries may lead to crush syndrome—hemorrhage, destruction of muscle and bone tissue, and fluid loss resulting in hypovolemic shock, renal failure, coma, and possibly death. Here's a flowchart that explains how crush injuries can lead to crush syndrome.

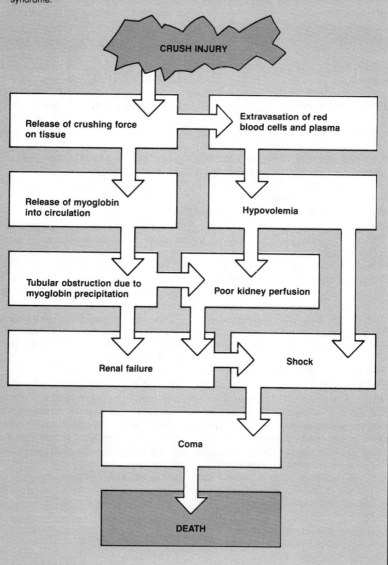

extensive muscle and tissue damage can alter the patient's hemodynamic status and metabolic processes and can also lead to eventual loss of the limb. Your priorities for a patient with a crush injury are restoring his circulating blood volume and maintaining an adequate urinary output of 75 to 100 ml/hour to prevent myoglobinuric renal failure—which can result from severe muscle damage and release of myoglobin. You'll do this by administering blood, plasma, and an electrolyte solution, such as Ringer's lactate. Expect to insert an indwelling (Foley) catheter to measure the patient's urinary output.

A central venous pressure (CVP) line may be inserted to assess the patient's circulating blood volume in relation to his heart function. An arterial line may be inserted or an external blood pressure device may be used for constant monitoring of his blood pressure.

### Continuing assessment and intervention

You'll need a baseline from which to gauge any changes, so perform a thorough assessment now.

First, if your patient has avulsed areas, estimate the amount of skin he's lost. (Remember, large areas of denuded skin have the same effect as burns; see Chapter 15). Assess your patient's motor function in the area distal to the injury. When checking the patient's flexion and extension against resistance, expect to find paresis and decreased or absent distal sensory perception. Assess your patient's circulation distal to the injury by checking his pulses and observing the skin color and capillary refill time of the affected extremity. Also measure the circumferences of both the affected and the unaffected extremity and compare them. Take the time to document *all* your assessment findings so you can compare later findings easily.

If your patient has an open wound, cleanse it with a mild antiseptic soap and irrigate it with warm sterile water. You may apply a bulky sterile saline dressing to the patient's open wound. Keep the extremity elevated, and administer analgesics, as ordered.

Because of the potential of crush syndrome, expect to increase your patient's I.V. fluid intake and to alkalize his serum and urine by adding sodium bicarbonate to the I.V. infusion. Alkalization prevents (or treats) acidosis that can occur with extensive muscle damage. When combined with alkalization, increased fluid intake prevents renal insufficiency due to myoglobin precipitation in the renal tubules; thus, it prevents subsequent renal failure and shock. Your patient's urine output should be 75 to 100 ml/hour. If it isn't, notify the doctor. He'll probably order more fluid or mannitol to increase your patient's urine output. His urine will probably be a port-wine color due to heme pigment from myoglobin and hemoglobin breakdown as a result of tissue and muscle damage. Expect to monitor your patient's serial ABGs frequently to check his *serum* alkalization, and test his urinary pH to check his *urine* alkalization.

Assess your patient's fluid status frequently by checking his vital signs and CVP every 15 minutes. Watch him carefully for signs and symptoms of developing compartment syndrome, which occurs commonly with crush injury: increasing edema, pain on passive motion, and increasing pain despite analgesics.

Compare your latest assessment findings with your baseline findings. Notify the doctor if your comparison indicates your patient's condition is worsening. You may be asked to measure compartment pressures (see *Understanding Compartment Syndrome*, pages 370 and 371, and *Measuring Compartment Pressure*, page 368). The doctor may do an emergency fasciotomy if pressure in a tissue compartment is increasing.

Your patient may require surgical debridement of any nonviable tissue to prevent further necrosis and infection. You'll probably infuse broad-spectrum antibiotics if he has an open wound.

Expect to start these preoperatively to achieve therapeutic blood levels.

When you take your patient's history, pay careful attention to these factors, which affect the severity of the injury:
• the length of time the extremity was compressed
• the extremity's size
• (if the injury was caused by rollers) whether the rollers were reversed, subjecting the extremity to a second compression
• the weight or force of the object that compressed the limb.

Also pay particular attention to any preexisting medical condition the patient has that may affect healing and his ability to recover from this type of injury. Examples include diabetes, peripheral vascular disease, and blood disorders.

### Therapeutic care
Continue to assess your patient's vital signs every 15 minutes until his condition's stable, and at frequent intervals thereafter—whether he had surgery or not. Check his neurovascular status frequently in the area distal to the injury. Watch for any signs of increasing edema. Remember that measuring the circumference of the affected limb at regular intervals and comparing your findings can be a helpful tool. Keep the injured limb elevated and immobilized to help control edema.

Administer analgesics to your patient as ordered, and expect to continue I.V. antibiotic and fluid therapy. Check his CVP to monitor his hydration level, and measure and record his urinary output accurately. Continue to monitor his serum and urinary alkalization by checking his ABGs and urine pH frequently.

You'll need to keep on the alert for signs and symptoms of fat emboli syndrome, which commonly occurs between 1 and 3 days after a crush injury (see *Assessing for Fat Emboli Syndrome*, page 376).

Continue to observe your patient for signs and symptoms of infection. Remember, a patient with a crush injury is vulnerable to sepsis because of the overwhelming stress on his body and resultant lowered resistance.

Because crush injuries are very serious, all attempts to save the limb may fail. If this happens, your patient and his family will need your support and reassurance throughout his care. Make sure you allow time for the family to visit the patient alone, too, so they can talk about their feelings. And don't forget to be available to the family to explain your patient's care and to answer questions.

# Major Soft Tissue Injuries

### Prediagnosis summary
On initial assessment, the patient may have had:
• a history of severe blunt or penetrating trauma with avulsion or shearing
• a large open laceration with regular or irregular edges
• small or large areas of skin and subcutaneous tissue separated from the underlying fascia
• a large ecchymosis with swelling, a hematoma, and taut skin over the affected area.

An I.V. infusion may have been started for fluid and drug administration. Tetanus prophylaxis was given (see *Guidelines for Tetanus Prophylaxis*, pages 66 and 67).

### Priorities
Your first priorities are to control frank bleeding and to replace fluids if necessary. For a patient with an open wound, direct pressure with a pressure dressing and elevation will usually control the bleeding. If the patient has a severed artery, the doctor may need to clamp it with a hemostat before he can suture it. (You'll have to replace lost fluids if the bleeding is extensive.)

## WHAT HAPPENS IN MAJOR SOFT TISSUE INJURIES

Traumatic injuries can have devastating effects on underlying soft tissue. Here are descriptions that will help you understand how major soft tissue injuries occur.

**Severe contusions**
Blunt trauma often causes severe contusions, which damage large blood vessels without disrupting the skin. This type of injury produces significant internal blood accumulation (hematoma) between the muscle fascia and subcutaneous fat and within the subcutaneous tissue.

**Complicated lacerations**
A sharp object penetrating the skin may cause complicated lacerations (irregular or stellate) with partially avulsed tissue

flaps. These wounds cause bleeding and are often deep enough to injure muscles and tendons in the underlying area.

**Degloving injuries**
Shearing forces usually cause degloving injuries, which separate the skin from the underlying fascia. The result is disruption of circulation and tissue necrosis. Patients with this type of injury require debridement and skin grafting.

**Severe avulsions**
Severe avulsions occur when a large amount of soft tissue is forcefully torn away from the body. Bleeding occurs, and a significant amount of overlying tissue is destroyed.

Use normal saline solution, dextrose 5% in water, or Ringer's lactate; a blood transfusion usually isn't necessary to stabilize a patient with this type of injury.

Keep a sterile saline dressing on the patient's open wound to prevent further bacterial contamination.

If your patient's wound isn't open, but he has a large ecchymotic area with a hematoma, expect to immobilize the area, to elevate it if possible, and to apply a cold pack to aid in controlling edema. Give analgesics as ordered.

### Continuing assessment and intervention

You'll have to thoroughly assess his neurovascular status distal to the injury, because edema can cause compression of vessels and nerves as well as ischemia and necrosis of surrounding tissue.

First, look for digital cyanosis and assess the capillary refill of his extremity. Then assess him for peripheral nerve damage. (See *Testing for Peripheral Nerve Damage*, pages 348 and 349.) If your patient's hand was injured, you may do a complete hand examination. Test tendon function by

holding the digits in extension while asking him to flex each finger joint separately. Remember, extensor tendons—lying immediately beneath the skin on the dorsal side of the fingers and hand—are very susceptible to injury.

This examination should reveal most functional tendon deficits. But be sure to use adequate resistant force when testing these motor responses, especially for the extensor tendons, because otherwise you may see apparent finger motion despite tendon laceration. So test strength by asking your patient to push against your finger, using flexion and extension. The doctor will thoroughly examine the patient's laceration for tendon damage. He'll evaluate the wound in the position it was in when injured and try to find the end of the damaged tendon if it retracted. This procedure will cause the patient some pain, so explain why it must be done.

If your patient's injury was to a lower extremity, you'll have to assess him for nerve and tendon damage distal to the injury. A pretibial laceration or contusion requires special attention and treatment because of the nearness of the tibia to the skin and the minimal amount of subcutaneous tissue and fat

## TESTING FOR TENDON DAMAGE

When your patient's had a major laceration of his hand or arm, *be sure to check for hidden tendon damage.* Why? Because untreated tendon damage can lead to permanent deformity.

You should always test a lacerated hand for deep and superficial tendon damage. Begin by asking your patient to spread his fingers apart; then ask him to make a fist. This test assesses *general tendon function.*

Next test for *deep tendon damage* by immobilizing the proximal interphalangeal joint of your patient's lacerated finger, as shown. Then ask him to flex the finger. If he can't, he may have deep tendon damage.

Now, test for *superficial tendon damage* by immobilizing the two fingers on either side of the patient's middle finger, as shown. Then ask him to wiggle the middle finger. If he can't, he may have damage.

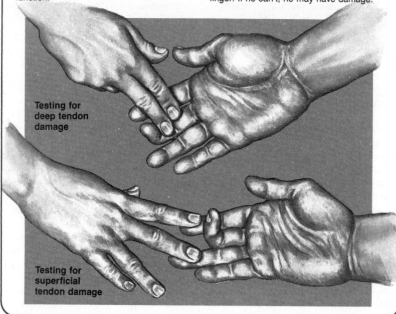

Testing for
deep tendon
damage

Testing for
superficial
tendon damage

in this area. Check for motor nerve damage by asking the patient to plantarflex and dorsiflex his ankle. If he shows signs and symptoms of weakness or paralysis, notify the doctor *immediately.* Measure the patient's strength by using a resistant force when you test his motor responses. Also check pulses and capillary refill time; swelling from the contusion or laceration can compress vessels as well as nerves.

Following your neurovascular and tendon assessment distal to your patient's injury, expect to assist in cleansing and examining his wound. He may need analgesics or anesthesia (or both)

30 to 45 minutes before the procedure to eliminate pain and to reduce his anxiety. If the wound's open, remove any large foreign bodies; then cleanse it with a broad-spectrum antimicrobial such as povidone-iodine. You may need to scrub it to get it thoroughly clean. Expect to irrigate the wound with normal saline solution. *Rinse,* instead of *irrigating,* for a patient with a degloving or an avulsion injury.

If the wound is closed (severe contusion), cleanse the area *gently,* also with a broad-spectrum antimicrobial such as povidone-iodine.

Your patient may need *surgery* to repair his injury, or the doctor may debride and repair the injury with your assistance. (He may insert a drain in a large laceration.) Any of several surgical techniques may be used. For a patient with an avulsion injury, the doctor may do a local flap or free skin graft; repair of a degloving injury may require debridement and a skin graft. A patient with an enlarging hematoma, such as one in a pretibial contusion, will need excision of any necrotic tissue, evacuation of any hematoma, and a skin graft. If your patient does need surgery, expect to start I.V. antibiotics now.

### Therapeutic care

After your patient's wound has been repaired, expect to cover it with an occlusive dressing that provides some degree of pressure and immobilization. If he had surgery, he'll return with this type of dressing. (The pressure is necessary to prevent hematomas and excessive edema; these can delay primary wound healing.)

Sometimes, especially if the patient's injured area was the hand or a finger, you may assist in splint application following tendon repair.

Once the dressing, splint, or cast has been applied, the patient will require bed rest with the injured part elevated and immobilized. Immobilization is important because activity produces unnecessary blood oozing and increases inflammation and the possibility of infection. Check his vital signs and distal circulation frequently. Assess the surgical site or wound often for signs of bleeding and for the degree of edema. Notify the doctor *immediately* if edema's extreme at the surgical site; he may want to release a stitch to prevent tissue necrosis. Watch closely for signs or symptoms of developing compartment syndrome (see *Understanding Compartment Syndrome,* pages 370 and 371).

Expect to administer pain medication, to continue I.V. antibiotics, and to observe your patient for signs and

symptoms of infection—which can occur despite antibiotics.

The doctor will gradually increase the patient's activity over a period of time, depending on the healing process and his evaluation. You may have to do passive range-of-motion exercises of the injured part.

---

# Traumatic Amputations

## Prediagnosis summary

Initial assessment of the patient revealed a partial or total severing of a body part, with some degree of hemorrhage and soft tissue damage. He may have had an accident at work, with heavy machinery, or a motor vehicle accident. If his bleeding was excessive, he probably had signs and symptoms of hypovolemic shock. The doctor's first decision was whether replantation was possible. If he decided it was, the part was preserved, and the patient was prepared for transfer to a replantation center.

If *replantation wasn't possible,* the patient's hemorrhage was brought under control by use of pressure rather than a tourniquet, if possible. He was given supplemental high-flow oxygen by nasal cannula. Two large-bore I.V. infusions were started, and broad-spectrum antibiotics, such as cephalothin (Keflin), were administered. Blood was drawn for typing and cross matching, and transfusions were given (if needed). The patient may have been given analgesics to help relieve his pain, but he was permitted nothing by mouth.

## Priorities

Your first priorities are continued care of the patient's stump and pain control while the patient is being prepared for surgery. Continue the I.V. fluid and blood replacement during this period, as needed. Pain medication may also be given. Be sure all stump hemor-

## PHANTOM PAIN IS REAL PAIN

When your patient experiences phantom pain—pain he feels in the missing limb, as though the amputation hadn't taken place— remember that it's *real pain*. Although his limb has been severed, nerve tracks that register pain in that area are still sending this message to his brain. Continue to treat him with analgesics (or other medications as ordered), and explain that his pain may not subside for a long time. Explain this phenomenon to family members, too, so they will know that it's a normal reaction to the patient's amputation.

rhaging has been controlled; continue applying pressure if the bleeding continues. After it stops, keep a large tourniquet at the patient's bedside at all times for use in case the stump begins to hemorrhage again.

You'll need to take a brief history before the patient goes to surgery. Ask about any allergies he has; what (if any) medications he's currently taking; when he last ate anything; and whether he has any preexisting diseases or other medical conditions. Make sure all the pertinent information is transferred to his hospital chart.

Your patient's just had a major debilitating trauma, so you should understand its effect on his psychological status. He'll be very fearful about being able to continue with his previous lifestyle and about the need to change his body image and to start doing basic things differently. Encourage him to ventilate his feelings about this to you, and provide emotional support. Assure him that, with proper rehabilitation and with practice, he'll eventually find alternate ways to enjoy many of the things he did before his injury.

### Continuing assessment and intervention

After your patient returns from sur-

gery, perform a thorough baseline assessment, taking his vital signs every 15 minutes until his condition is stable. Continue I.V. fluid replacement throughout your assessment, too, and expect to give analgesics as needed.

Evaluate your patient's vascular status hourly by checking his proximal pulses, skin color and temperature, capillary refill time, and tissue turgor. Look for dusky or cyanotic skin color or pallor. With the backs of your fingertips, note the temperature of your patient's skin—it should feel warm. Turgor should be full rather than taut or shriveled.

After *leg* amputation, your patient may return from surgery with a prosthesis; some doctors feel this lessens the psychological impact of amputation and allows rehabilitation to begin immediately. Most often, however, you'll see a rigid dressing (a light dressing with plaster molded over it), which some doctors believe enhances healing. A rigid dressing controls edema and hematoma formation and immobilizes the injury, so your patient will be more comfortable and will usually require less analgesia. (The doctor may also have inserted a drain during surgery, to allow fluids to flow from the wound and to prevent excessive edema.)

If the patient's stump was allowed to remain open, and no flap closure was done because the wound was grossly contaminated, expect to change the sterile saline dressings frequently.

### Therapeutic care

Your patient will require continued I.V. antibiotic therapy to prevent infection. And don't neglect to watch him for signs and symptoms of infection, which may occur in spite of the antibiotics.

Keep the stump elevated for no longer than 48 hours. (Elevation for a longer period can lead to joint contractures.) Avoid external rotation and abduction of the stump (if it's his leg); this can also cause contractures.

Encourage your patient to exercise his stump, as the doctor permits. Continue administering analgesics for pain, as ordered.

Expect to assist in drain removal the day after the patient's surgery. Then you'll probably assist with application of a cast, to be worn for 7 to 10 days, unless signs of infection are present. If necessary, teach your patient how to walk on crutches with his cast. Explain that once he's fitted with a prosthesis, he'll learn to walk on his own.

Following cast removal, assess how well the patient's stump is healing. If no signs of infection are present and healing is complete, the patient will be fitted for a prosthesis.

# A FINAL WORD

Your nursing responsibilities for patients with musculoskeletal emergencies have expanded in recent years. Advances in medical and surgical treatment mean your patient has a better chance than ever of recovering from his injury without crippling disability.

Surgical replantation of digits and limbs is perhaps the most dramatic advance. Where traumatic amputation might once have left your patient disabled, new techniques make significant return of function possible in many cases. When you know how to care for the patient's amputated part before surgery, replantation has an increased likelihood of success.

For a patient with a hip fracture, new prosthetic hip devices and surgical techniques have significantly increased the chances of improved function. And the incidence of complications, such as pulmonary embolism and pneumonia, has been reduced, now that prolonged bed rest and traction are no longer used. Here again, *your* role in patient care is critical. You have a major role in helping your patient achieve early mobility through your encouragement, support, and coordination of services.

Always keep in mind that, while musculoskeletal injuries are rarely life-threatening, they *can* result in permanent disability and deformity. You can help prevent this by providing early assessment and intervention and thorough follow-up care.

## Selected References

Connolly, John F., ed. *DePalma's the Management of Fractures and Dislocations: An Atlas*, 2 vols., 3rd ed. Philadelphia: W.B. Saunders Co., 1981.

Farrell, Jane. *Illustrated Guide to Orthopedic Nursing*, 2nd ed. Philadelphia: J.B. Lippincott Co., 1982.

Glancy, G.L. "Compartment Syndromes," *Orthopedic Nurses' Association Journal* 2(6):148-50, June 1975.

Hogan, K.M., and Sawyer, J.R. "Fracture Dislocation of the Elbow," *American Journal of Nursing* 76:1266-68, August 1976.

Kuska, B.M. "Acute Onset of Compartment Syndrome," *Journal of Emergency Nursing* 8(2):75-79, March/April 1982.

Lupien, A.E. "Head Off Compartment Syndrome Before It's Too Late," *RN* 43:38-41, December 1980.

Martin, Sandi. "Fat Embolism Syndrome," *Dimensions of Critical Care Nursing* 2(3):158-61, May/June 1983.

Rosse, Cornelius, and Clawson, Kay. *The Musculoskeletal System in Health and Disease*. Philadelphia: J.B. Lippincott Co., 1980.

Whitehead, D.J. "Emergency Care in Orthopedic Injuries," *Nursing Clinics of North America* 8(3):435-40, September 1973.

*Working with Orthopedic Patients.* Nursing Photobook Series. Springhouse, Pa.: Springhouse Corp., 1982.

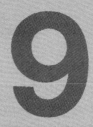

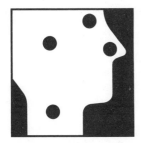

# Eye, Ear, Nose, and Throat Emergencies

## Introduction

Just before the end of a quiet shift in the ED, Officer McKenna brings in Marian Whitmore, age 63. She's complaining of a severe headache—so severe that she can't lie down to take a nap. Practically in tears, she covers her right eye—it, too, hurts badly. "Maybe it's just a migraine," Mrs. Whitmore tells you. "I get 'em sometimes, and I've been feeling nauseous all day...even spit up a little, too."

Suddenly, Mrs. Whitmore says she can't see. Extremely frightened, she grasps for your arm, saying, "What's wrong with me.... why can't I see? This never happened to me before!" You realize this is *not* a migraine, but you can't be certain of what's causing Mrs. Whitmore's signs and symptoms. They could be due to acute closed-angle glaucoma, hyphema, or retinal detachment, among numerous other possibilities. You quickly complete your initial assessment and call the doctor to examine Mrs. Whitmore.

Now the triage nurse calls you to help three young men, dressed in muddied baseball uniforms, who are carrying a fourth man. He's Ricky Macer, age 23, a shortstop for their company's baseball team. "He was hit in the face with a baseball," one teammate informs you. "Yeah!" another continues, "He was hit by a line drive... smack in the face. Blood all over the place." Placing Ricky on a stretcher, you immediately note that his right eye's displaced downward. His nose is displaced, too, and his face is swollen. Asking if he has pain, you discover that when he tries to speak, his teeth get in the way. He can't speak clearly, but he's able to tell you he's in pain and seeing double. Ricky obviously has facial fractures, and his eye requires emergency treatment. With all these problems, you're naturally concerned about setting priorities so that Ricky gets the timely care he needs.

As in all other emergencies, your first priority is *still* quickly assessing your patient's airway, breathing, and circulation. Even though eye, ear, nose, and throat (EENT) emergencies can result in loss of sight or hearing, you can't afford to forget that they can also compromise your patient's life-support systems. For example, epistaxis can block his nasal passages at the same time edema is obstructing his airway.

Even when your priorities are clear, EENT emergencies can offer a special challenge. Here's why: Your patient's signs and symptoms may not be as directly indicative of EENT problems as Ricky's were. For example, a seriously ill patient may only report nausea or a headache at first—like Mrs. Whitmore. So you need especially sharp emergency assessment skills to set priorities

# A CHEMICAL BURN TO THE EYE

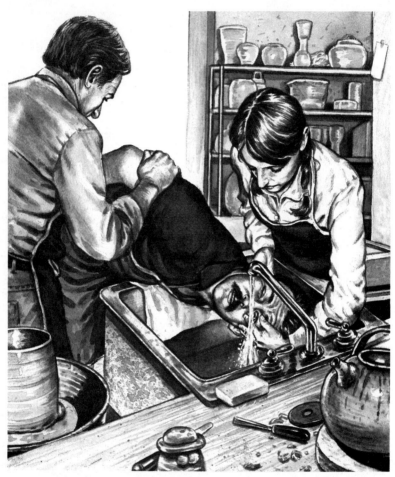

As a nurse, you've probably assessed many eye injuries and intervened as necessary. But how often have you been called on to do this at the scene of an emergency, with the patient's vision in serious jeopardy? Probably not often enough that you feel fully confident about your role in such emergencies. For example, if you were in a pottery painting class and one of the students accidentally splashed some brush-cleaning solution into his eye, would

you know just what to do? Here are the emergency assessment and intervention steps to follow:

First, find out what's in the patient's eye. If it's a caustic solution, his eye will need *immediate* attention to prevent a severe chemical burn and blindness. If the patient's panicky, your next priority will be to calm him down. Prevent him from thrashing around and hurting himself or others by talking to him firmly, but calmly, and telling

and to intervene appropriately when a patient has an EENT emergency. Reading this chapter will ensure that you have these skills.

him that you're going to help. Have someone restrain him, if necessary.

Ask someone to call an ambulance or to get a car so you can take the patient to the hospital. Then check quickly to see if he's wearing contact lenses. If he is, no matter how urgent the emergency, you must remove them first. Then, lead the patient to the nearest sink to flush his eyes with water.

First, adjust the tap water to a tepid temperature and moderate pressure. Then place his head sideways under the faucet, with the affected eye downward. (This keeps the caustic solution from splashing into his other eye.) Tell the patient to keep his eyes open and to roll them so the water can wash out as much of the solution as possible. Make sure he doesn't rub his eyes with his hands. Keep him restrained, if this was necessary in the first place. Remember, he may become panicky again at any time.

While you flush his eyes, ask someone to fill a large container with fresh water and to find a cup. You'll need the extra water and cup to flush the patient's eyes on the way to the hospital. Also have someone carefully pour a little of the caustic solution into a bottle. The ED will use this solution sample to identify what's burning the patient's eye.

Suppose you're in some other situation, not your painting class, when this type of emergency happens. If you aren't close to a sink, you can flush the victim's eyes using a water fountain, garden hose, shower, or even a watering can that has water in it. You can even use contact lens rinsing solution. *(Make sure it's not cleaning solution!)* If you can't move the victim because of other injuries, have other people bring water to you in any *clean* vessels available, such as bottles, jugs, pans, or coffee mugs. Then, when the patient can be moved and taken to the hospital, take a large bottle or basin of water and a cup, turkey baster, or some other clean vessel to flush his eyes on the way. Flush his eyes continuously until you reach the hospital.

At the ED, give the nurse the sample of the caustic solution, describe the accident, and tell her exactly how you intervened up to this point.

# INITIAL CARE

## Prehospital Care: What's Been Done

Prehospital care of your patient with an EENT emergency depended on the cause and severity of his injury or illness. As you probably know, EENT emergencies cause a wide spectrum of problems. Some are life-threatening (for example, airway obstruction); others directly threaten the patient's functioning (for example, by causing blindness). So EENT emergencies, although they're confined to a small area of the patient's body, nevertheless can cause big problems.

Rescue personnel took steps to stabilize the patient's airway, breathing, and circulation. If his airway was obstructed (for example, with broken teeth or bone fragments), they attempted to clear it. If he was unconscious, the rescue team may have inserted an artificial airway to keep his tongue from falling backward and occluding his oropharynx. Suppose blood was clogging his airway: they tried to clear it using a large-bore or tonsil-tip suction catheter.

If swelling from a facial fracture impaired the patient's breathing, rescue personnel elevated his head and gave him oxygen by face mask, nasal cannula, or Ambu bag.

If the patient was bleeding heavily from the nose, rescue personnel applied external pressure by gently pinching his nostrils temporarily to-control blood flow and to avoid compromising his circulation. The patient may have shown signs of hypovolemia (such as hypotension or increased pulse) from excessive blood loss. In this situation, rescue personnel (if qualified) inserted a large-bore I.V. and began rapid infusion of normal saline solution or Ringer's lactate for fluid replacement.

If the patient suffered head or neck trauma, rescue personnel assumed that his cervical spine was damaged. So they attempted to stabilize his neck by using a Philadelphia (hard) cervical collar or sandbags.

---

PRIORITIES

### INITIAL ASSESSMENT CHECKLIST

**Assess the ABCs first and intervene appropriately.**

**Check for:**
• decreased sensation, facial asymmetry, limited extraocular movements, and hearing or vision loss, indicating possible neuromuscular damage
• local swelling, redness, drainage, fever, tenderness, and lesions, indicating possible infection
• nasal or neck swelling and stridor, dyspnea, or tachypnea, indicating respiratory compromise.

**Intervene by:**
• administering supplemental oxygen by nasal cannula or mask
• applying ice packs
• irrigating your patient's eyes
• administering eye medication.

**Prepare for:**
• eye protection
• intraocular pressure testing
• visual acuity and hearing testing
• fluorescein staining
• nasal packing
• carbogen therapy
• ear irrigation.

---

# What to Do First

As in any emergency, your immediate priority is to make sure that your patient's airway, breathing, and circulation are stabilized. A patient with head or neck trauma will need close, continuing assessment, because edema can progress to partial or even total airway obstruction, compromising his breathing.

### Airway

If your patient's airway is obstructed, quickly assess whether the obstruction's partial or complete and intervene appropriately. (See the "Life Support" section in Chapter 3.) You may have to assist in artificial airway insertion. But *first* make sure your patient doesn't have cerebrospinal fluid (CSF) leakage. (The quickest way to check for this is to test any watery fluid draining from his nose or ears for the presence of glucose.) If he has CSF leakage, *don't* use a nasal airway—use an oral airway instead. Why? Because CSF leakage indicates that he has a tear in his dura mater, and nasal airway introduction can cause further damage or introduce infection. Remember, the cause of his airway obstruction could be edema from anaphylactic shock (see Chapter 14, SHOCK), from tracheobronchial injuries (see Chapter 4, RESPIRATORY EMERGENCIES), or—if your patient's a child—from epiglottitis (see *Nurse's Guide to Pediatric Emergencies* in the Appendix).

As a nurse, you know you should always suspect cervical spine injury if your patient has head or neck trauma. To clear such a patient's airway, don't hyperextend his neck or you may damage his cervical spine further. (For example, don't use the head-tilt maneuver—instead, try a modified jaw-thrust or chin-lift.) Keep his neck stabilized with a cervical collar, and logroll him onto his side to prevent aspiration. Expect that your patient will be intubated, and be prepared to assist. Keep suction equipment, a suction catheter, and an Ambu bag ready for an emergency tracheotomy or cricothyrotomy. You may also need normal saline solution (in unit doses of 3 to 5 ml, if available) to loosen and clear blood, food, or thick secretions from your patient's airway.

## Breathing
Traumatic injuries to a patient's head or throat are likely to cause nasal or oral breathing difficulties. So assess your patient with an EENT emergency for signs of ventilatory compromise— pallor, cyanosis, abnormal or absent chest movements, rapid pulse, or absent or irregular respirations. Hold your hand over the patient's nose and mouth; if you don't feel any flow of air, act quickly to restore his breathing (see the "Life Support" section in Chapter 3). Once he's breathing normally, you may need to administer supplemental oxygen. Your patient's arterial blood gases (ABGs) will be tested to assess his ventilatory status. If it's inadequate, expect to assist with intubation and mechanical ventilation. Monitor your patient's ABGs frequently.

A patient who's suffered nose trauma may develop edema that can block his nasal passages and compromise his breathing. To slow the development of edema, apply ice packs and keep your patient's head elevated and turned to the side.

## Circulation
Frank bleeding from your patient's nose may cause him to panic and start swallowing blood, which will cause him to vomit later. If this happens, notify the doctor *immediately*. Then reassure your patient, lean his head forward over a basin to catch the blood, and tell him to breathe through his mouth. You may be asked to assist with nasal packing or cauterization. (See *Understanding Nasal Packing*, pages 422 and 423.)

If your patient's nose isn't broken, apply direct gentle pressure by squeezing his nostrils to stanch the flow of blood.

For a patient who has open external wounds, apply ice packs to the bleeding sites to help reduce blood flow and edema. Monitor his blood pressure and pulse, and watch for signs and symptoms of shock from excessive blood loss. You may need to initiate I.V. therapy, as ordered, or to assist with insertion of a central venous pressure line to monitor his blood volume status. Blood will be drawn for typing and cross matching, complete blood count (CBC), prothrombin time (PT), and partial thromboplastin time (PTT).

## General appearance
Observe your patient for signs of trauma—lacerations, bruises, and swelling—not only to his head and neck, but also to his chest, abdomen, and extremities.

If you see bruises or swelling around his eyes, ask your patient if he's seeing double. If he is, he may have sustained ocular nerve or muscle damage.

If you haven't already checked for CSF leakage, do so now by looking for any discharge from the patient's nose and ears. Do a glucose test on any watery leaking fluid to determine if it's CSF; if it is, notify the doctor *immediately*. Don't try to clean dried discharge with cotton-tipped applicators or probes until CSF leakage has been ruled out. Why? Because if your patient's dura mater is torn, this procedure might introduce infection directly into his CSF and thus into his brain.

The doctor will suture most facial lacerations as soon as possible. This will ensure minimal scar formation and reduce the risk of infection.

## Mental status
A patient with an EENT emergency may lose consciousness because of an upper airway obstruction, extreme blood loss, or associated head trauma. Assess your patient's airway frequently, and intervene as needed. ABGs will be taken to determine if any respiratory

insufficiency is present.

Check a conscious patient frequently for signs and symptoms of mental status deterioration—for example, confusion, restlessness, or anxiety. These may be early warning signals of shock or hypoxia. (As you know, confusion can also result from cranial trauma.) If your patient's hypoxic, give supplemental oxygen as needed.

A patient who complains of dizziness or losing his balance may have an inner ear disorder. Protect him from injury until the doctor can intervene.

# What to Do Next

Now that your patient's airway, breathing, and circulation are stabilized, you're ready to perform a quick emergency assessment that will help you identify his chief complaint.

## Eye complaints

If the patient arrived in the ED with a *laceration* or a *penetrating object* in his eye, *don't* attempt to manipulate his eye. Send someone for the doctor *immediately* while you cover the area with a metal shield to prevent further movement—or, if the object is protruding, use a protective device, such as a cup. Tell the patient not to squeeze his eye shut.

If your patient has had *sudden, painless, unilateral vision loss*, contact the doctor *immediately*. This is a sign of central retinal artery occlusion—one of the most serious eye emergencies. Intervene quickly by performing light external eye massage (over his closed eyelid) and increasing his carbon dioxide level, as ordered—this will dilate the artery and, possibly, restore blood flow to the retina. Expect to administer either a set flow of oxygen and carbon dioxide through a Venturi mask or the "brown bag treatment"—your patient rebreathes in a paper bag to retain exhaled carbon dioxide.

Notify the doctor if your patient claims to suddenly see *floaters*—moving spots, "lightning flashes," or "sparks." The doctor will want to do a detailed eye examination right away, with the patient's pupils dilated. Why? Because sudden onset of these symptoms may indicate retinal detachment, which requires immediate intervention. Expect to keep your patient's head immobilized in a specified position to allow the detached retina to settle back in place. (See *Pillow Talk*, page 414.) Explain to your patient the importance of maintaining this position.

Whether a patient's had a chemical substance splashed in his eyes and is complaining that he has a *burning sensation*, or he has a small foreign body in his eye and is complaining that he has *painful tearing* and can *"feel something in there,"* your initial interventions will be the same:

• Check for and remove contact lenses (see *Removing Contact Lenses*, page 399).

• Begin irrigating the eye with normal saline solution (see *Irrigating the Eye*, page 402).

If your patient's eyes are *sensitive to light* and he complains of severe pain, he may have a corneal abrasion, corneal ulcer, infection, or inflammation from a foreign object in his eye. Notify the doctor *immediately*, and be prepared to perform or assist with eyelid eversion. (See *Performing Eyelid Eversion.*)

If the patient says he removed something from his eye earlier but came to the ED because his eye *still feels irritated*, he may have a corneal abrasion or laceration. He'll need a thorough eye examination. You may assist the doctor with eyelid eversion to expose the entire conjunctival surface of the eye for a thorough examination.

If your patient suffered *minor eye trauma* or complains of *blurred* or *diminished vision*, assess his visual acuity. Do this by performing a Snellen test. Position the patient 20 feet away from the Snellen chart. Have him cover one eye with an opaque card or shield, and

# YOUR ROLE IN AN EMERGENCY

## PERFORMING EYELID EVERSION

You may perform eyelid eversion to assess an eye injury, to remove a contact lens, or to irrigate the eye. (If your patient has a foreign body in his eye, the doctor will evert the eyelid.)

Here's what you need to know about everting a patient's upper and lower eyelids and performing double eversion of the upper lid.

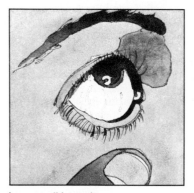

**Lower eyelid eversion**
Gently pull the lower lid downward; then ask your patient to look down, left, and right. This exposes the sclera beneath the transparent conjunctiva and lets you assess the entire inner lid.

**Upper eyelid eversion**
Ask your patient to look downward while you grasp his upper eyelashes and gently pull the lid down. Next, place a sterile cotton-tipped applicator across the outer lid and fold the lid back over the applicator, exposing its inner side. Now remove the applicator and keep the lid everted with your fingers.

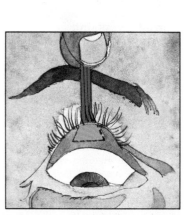

**Double eversion of the upper eyelid**
Grasp the lid's eyelashes and pull them downward. Then place the eyelid retractor so that its curved end is facing the eyelid's outer surface. Point its handle toward the patient's cheek, then gently push the retractor down. As his eyelid folds over the retractor, raise the handle above his forehead. Pull the eyelid upward with the retractor to expose the conjunctival fornix.

**Nursing considerations**
• Wash your hands before and between everting eyelids to prevent cross-contamination.
• Return the lid to its normal position by pulling the lashes forward and telling the patient to look up and then blink.

ask him to read each line as you point to it. Then repeat the same procedure while he covers the other eye. Be sure you assess his vision both with and without corrective lenses, if he wears them. The fractions at the sides of the lines tell you his visual acuity; they also provide a baseline that will help the doctor make the diagnosis and determine the appropriate treatment.

If your patient complains of *decreased light perception,* this suggests cataracts, retinal damage, or hemorrhage. Assess his visual acuity, using the Snellen test, to help the doctor make the diagnosis.

*Severe, constant eye pain* is difficult to diagnose in the ED. If it's accompanied by *blurred vision, severe sudden headache, nausea,* or *vomiting,* increased intraocular pressure (IOP)—for example, from acute closed-angle glaucoma—could be the cause. Pain occurring with no other signs or symptoms may originate in the patient's sinuses or orbit. An ophthalmologist will be consulted to perform a more detailed eye examination.

## Ear complaints
If your patient complains of *hearing loss,* ask whether he's had recent head or neck trauma or surgery or if he's been exposed to loud noise. If none of these applies, then check his ears for impacted cerumen. Each of these may cause transient or (except for cerumen) permanent hearing loss.

Ask your patient what drugs or medications he's taking, too, and what prior medical problems he's had. As you probably know, hearing loss can be an adverse effect of some antibiotics, such as streptomycin, gentamicin, or quinine. And certain organic or physical disorders, such as otosclerosis or perforated eardrum, as well as several common childhood diseases, such as mumps, also cause some degree of hearing loss.

Assess the patient's hearing loss using a watch tick, whisper, or tuning fork. Remember, this assessment is an emergency screening measure. The doctor may order audiometry tests later for more definitive information.

## Facial complaints
If your patient has facial trauma, check for evidence of fracture and nerve damage. Look for *dental malocclusion, midface elongation, periorbital swelling,* and *bruises*—all signs of facial fracture. Assess the patient's face for point tenderness and pain. Apply an ice pack to reduce the swelling of simple soft tissue injuries. If your patient has wounds that require extensive debridement or closure of multiple tissue layers, the ED doctor will probably consult an EENT specialist or plastic surgeon for specialized emergency treatment.

To assess for facial nerve damage, have your patient raise his eyebrows, squeeze his eyes tightly shut, and wrinkle his nose. Do you note *facial asymmetry*? Again, an EENT specialist will be consulted if nerve damage is present.

A patient who complains of *nasal or facial pain* or *inflammation* and who has no signs of trauma may have an underlying disorder. Ask your patient whether he has a history of headaches or sinusitis, and apply ice packs to reduce pain and swelling.

## Throat complaints
Assess a patient with throat or neck trauma for *bruises, lacerations,* and *swelling,* and keep his neck immobilized to protect his cervical spine.

*Severe pain on swallowing* is characteristic of a number of throat disorders, of course; but the most serious emergency is a patient who's swallowed a caustic substance. Try to find out what he ingested, and administer the proper antidote. (See Chapter 17, POISONING AND SUBSTANCE ABUSE.)

If your patient's recently had throat or neck surgery, he may be experiencing complications. Look for signs and symptoms of *infection*—foul-smelling breath, redness in the throat, fever, and

## YOUR ROLE IN AN EMERGENCY

### REMOVING CONTACT LENSES

Suppose a patient who wears contact lenses comes to the ED with facial injuries. Or a patient has chemical irritants or foreign bodies trapped under his contact lenses. In these and similar situations, you'll need to remove the lenses before you can care for him.

Here are the methods to use.

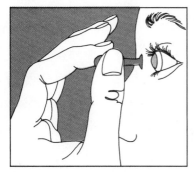

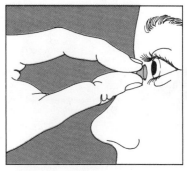

**Suction bulb removal (hard and soft lenses)**
Gently place the cup end against the contact lens, then pull the bulb away from the eye in a straight line. (Make sure you don't touch the cornea with the suction bulb. If you do, you may cause permanent damage.)

**Manual removal (soft lens)**
Make sure your hands are clean and dry. Place your index finger directly on the lens; then slide it gently down and away from the cornea. Pinch the lens between your thumb and index finger, and lift it out.

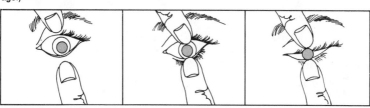

**Manual removal (hard lens)**
Pull the eyelids apart so you completely expose the contact lens. Press down with your right thumb, tipping the lens forward. Then gently pinch the patient's eyelids together to expel the lens.

**Nursing considerations**
• Never use force to remove a lens. If you have difficulty, slide the lens onto the sclera, then call the doctor.
• Look for "lost" lenses in the upper cul-de-sac of the eye—their most common hiding place.
• Preserve each lens in a separate sterile container (marked *left* or *right*) filled with sterile saline solution.
• Don't replace a lens until an ophthalmologist examines the patient. Then, before you replace it, cleanse it—and the patient's eye, as well.

PATHOPHYSIOLOGY

# WHAT HAPPENS IN CHEMICAL BURNS OF THE EYE

Chemicals splashed into the eye can cause varying degrees of burn injuries, depending on whether the chemical is an acid or an alkali. Alkalis (which have a high pH) cause more damage than acids because they burn longer and often penetrate Bowman's membrane, causing permanent scarring.

The full extent of the damage may not be known for 3 to 4 days because the alkali will probably continue to destroy tissue unless the destructive process is stopped through copious irrigation.

Use these flowcharts to compare the pathophysiologic processes of acid and alkali burns in the eye.

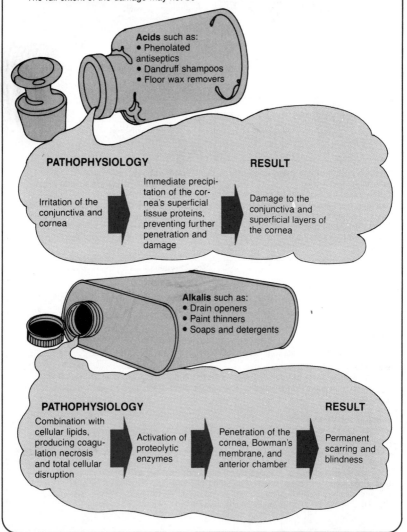

**Acids** such as:
- Phenolated antiseptics
- Dandruff shampoos
- Floor wax removers

**PATHOPHYSIOLOGY**

Irritation of the conjunctiva and cornea → Immediate precipitation of the cornea's superficial tissue proteins, preventing further penetration and damage →

**RESULT**

Damage to the conjunctiva and superficial layers of the cornea

**Alkalis** such as:
- Drain openers
- Paint thinners
- Soaps and detergents

**PATHOPHYSIOLOGY**

Combination with cellular lipids, producing coagulation necrosis and total cellular disruption → Activation of proteolytic enzymes → Penetration of the cornea, Bowman's membrane, and anterior chamber →

**RESULT**

Permanent scarring and blindness

swollen tonsils or neck lymph nodes. Remember, *drooling is a red-alert sign* that indicates your patient's unable to swallow because of extreme pain or swelling. Notify the doctor *immediately*, and be prepared to assist with emergency intubation—continued swelling may occlude your patient's airway.

---

## Special Considerations

### Pediatric
Thanks to the preventive measures required by law (silver nitrate or antibiotic drops instilled in the eyes of newborns), gonococcal conjunctivitis occurs today in less than 0.03% of all infants born in the United States. When it does occur, however, treatment involves a race against time to save the infant's sight. If you assess a newborn infant with such signs and symptoms as *bilateral lid edema, itching, lacrimation*, or *copious discharge*, notify the doctor *immediately*. Treatment involves isolation and administration of penicillin, erythromycin, or tetracycline ointment for several days.

### Geriatric
Preexisting cardiovascular disease can cause spasm or blood clots to occlude the central retinal artery. If an elderly patient comes to the ED with sudden, painless unilateral vision loss—without an abnormal external eye appearance or a history of trauma or inflammation—atherosclerosis may have caused his condition. Shine a penlight in his eye. If the pupil doesn't constrict, he probably has central retinal artery occlusion. Notify the doctor *right away*, and expect to perform external eye massage and to administer carbogen therapy, as ordered. To dilate the occluded artery, have your patient rebreathe his exhaled carbon dioxide by using a mask or paper bag. This may save your patient's sight.

If your patient is over age 50 and complains of *deep aching* in his eyes, of *"smoky"* or *"misty"* *vision*, or of *seeing red and blue halos around points of light*, he may have acute closed-angle glaucoma. (The diagnosis may be missed because of the nausea and vomiting that often accompany these ocular symptoms.) The doctor will perform a tonometry test to detect IOP. This will be elevated in a patient with acute closed-angle glaucoma. An ophthalmologist will be consulted for further examination and treatment.

---

# CARE AFTER DIAGNOSIS

---

## Chemical Burns of the Eye

### Prediagnosis summary
Initial assessment findings for the patient who came to the ED with a chemically burned eye included some or all of the following:
• eye pain (notable if absent, indicating severe damage)
• inability to keep the eye open
• impaired vision in the eye
• a white, opaque cornea
• a pale conjunctiva.

### Priorities
You must act quickly if you're to prevent permanent damage. Your first priority is to check for and remove contact lenses (see *Removing Contact Lenses*, page 399). Then begin continuous irrigation of your patient's burned eye(s) and surrounding tissue. (See *Irrigating the Eye*, page 402.) This will flush out the caustic substance and may prevent permanent damage. Irrigation will also help soothe his pain.

## YOUR ROLE IN AN EMERGENCY

### IRRIGATING THE EYE

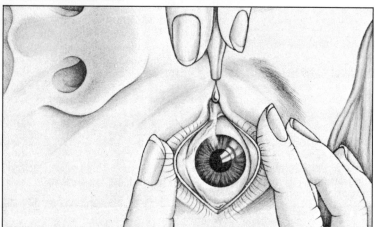

To care for a chemical burn or a foreign body in your patient's eye, perform eye irrigation immediately and continue it as long as necessary. Here's how to perform eye irrigation using I.V. tubing and normal saline solution. (An alternative—and less common—method involves inserting a special contact lens, attached to I.V. tubing, into the patient's eye. This allows continuous irrigation.)

#### Equipment
• Towels
• Eyelid retractor
• Cotton balls or dry tissues
• Topical anesthetic (such as proparacaine hydrochloride)
• Normal saline solution at room temperature (1,000 ml)
• I.V. infusion set without needle
• Plastic trash bag
• Trash can

#### Procedure
• Explain the procedure to your patient to ease his anxiety.
• Wash your hands.
• Place your patient supine, with his head turned so the solution won't flow into the nonirrigated eye.
• Place towels so they'll soak up the irrigating solution. Or place a plastic trash bag under the patient's head, then drape it

off the bed and into a trash can that will catch the solution.
• Evert the patient's eyelid and instill a topical anesthetic, as ordered, to ease his discomfort during irrigation.
• Holding the patient's eyelids open with your fingers, ask him to rotate his eyes clockwise during irrigation. Then hold the tubing at a 45° angle and irrigate the lower cul-de-sac and the superior fornix. (A lid retractor may help you irrigate the superior fornix.) Make sure the solution flows across the cornea to the outer canthus.

*To irrigate both eyes,* alternate between them, moving the flow of solution from the inner to the outer canthus of each eye. To prevent cross-contamination, don't touch the tubing to either eye.
• When you're irrigating a chemically burned eye, use litmus paper—after irrigating for 10 minutes—to test the pH of the palpebral conjunctiva. If the pH isn't neutral, continue irrigating until it is. If you don't have litmus paper, irrigate for at least 10 minutes with 1,000 ml of normal saline solution.
• When you've finished irrigating, dry the patient's eyelids with cotton balls (so he won't feel the urge to rub his eyes). Wipe from the inner to the outer canthus, using a *new* cotton ball for each wipe.

## Continuing assessment and intervention

Continue to irrigate your patient's eye for 10 minutes. During this procedure, ask your patient if he knows the name or type of the chemical agent. If he doesn't know but brought a sample with him, have someone test it quickly for acidity or alkalinity while you continue irrigation. This information will help you anticipate the extent of the damage to his eye. (See *What Happens in Chemical Burns of the Eye,* page 400.)

Remember, acid chemicals, such as floor wax removers or dandruff shampoos, usually damage only the superficial layers of the cornea; but alkaline chemicals, such as those in strong detergents and drain openers, cause extensive damage to the cornea's deeper layers and can cause blindness.

After 10 minutes of continuous irrigation, check the pH level of your patient's conjunctiva. If his pH level *hasn't* reached the normal range (approximately 7), continue irrigation until it does.

Once your patient's conjunctival pH *has* returned to the normal range, you can stop irrigation. Then test his visual acuity using a Snellen chart (even if the burn seems severe) to help evaluate the extent of damage.

Next, apply corticosteroid ointments (as ordered) to reduce inflammation, and apply an eye patch. (See *Patching Pointers,* page 404.)

As always, take and record the patient's vital signs as a baseline.

### Therapeutic care

The doctor will prescribe antibiotics to prevent infection. But if your patient's cornea is severely damaged, the doctor may treat the eye with collagenase inhibitors. Why? To stop collagenase, secreted by injured epithelial cells, from eroding the corneal layer. If scarring has occurred, the patient may require a corneal transplant.

A patient with only minor eye damage probably won't be admitted to the hospital. Instruct him to call the doctor

---

### UNDERSTANDING FLUORESCEIN STAINING

Fluorescein staining of a patient's eye helps the doctor detect foreign bodies, corneal abrasions, or other corneal injuries.

Fluorescein dye applied to the patient's palpebral conjunctiva temporarily turns the sclera orange. Then, when the doctor shines a cobalt blue light on the eye, damaged epithelium shows up as bright green, indicating a corneal injury.

The illustration shows how to apply fluorescein dye to a patient's eye. If you perform this procedure, always use fluorescein strips instead of drops, which can easily become contaminated with *Pseudomonas.* Have your patient gently roll his eyes, with his lids closed, so the dye spreads over his cornea. After the examination, irrigate his eye with normal saline solution to remove the excess dye.

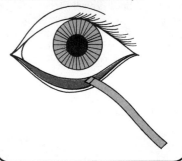

---

if he has pain, fever, or a discharge from the eye—these may indicate infection.

---

# Corneal Foreign Bodies, Abrasions, and Lacerations

### Prediagnosis summary

The patient came to the ED complaining that something was in his eye. Initial assessment revealed some combination of the following signs and symptoms:
• sharp or stabbing eye pain
• eyelid spasm

- squinting, blinking
- profuse lacrimation
- diminished pupil size
- sensitivity to light (photophobia).

The patient's visual acuity was quickly tested using a Snellen chart. (If the patient was sensitive to light, the room may have been darkened.) His visual acuity was found to be normal or only slightly decreased. An emergency eye examination may have revealed one or more foreign bodies, a corneal abrasion, or a corneal laceration.

## Priorities

Whether you or the doctor does it, prompt removal of a corneal foreign body is the first priority. First check for and remove contact lenses. Then, if the foreign body is easily accessible, try to remove it with a moist cotton-tipped applicator. Remember, the corneal epithelium tears easily, so be careful not to push the object across the epithelium.

If the foreign body's not easily accessible, start irrigating the patient's eye with normal saline solution and try to gently flush it out (see *Irrigating the Eye,* page 402). If this doesn't work, the doctor will try to remove the foreign body with a foreign body spad (a very fine sterile spatula) or a 25G hypodermic needle. You may assist by instilling anesthetic eye drops before he begins the procedure. A metallic foreign body may leave rust rings, which should be removed if possible.

In most patients, this procedure will remove the foreign body. If it doesn't, the doctor will try to flush the object out of your patient's eye with normal saline solution, but he'll use a syringe to focus the stream more directly.

## Continuing assessment and intervention

After removal of the foreign body, expect to give your patient cycloplegic and antibiotic eye drops. After any foreign body is removed, assist the doctor in everting your patient's eyelid to detect whether any additional foreign bodies are present. (See *Performing Eyelid Eversion,* page 397.)

## Therapeutic care

The foreign body's been removed, so your patient should be more comfortable now. Your next step is to assess his eye for corneal lacerations or abrasions. To do this, you may use fluorescein strips to stain the cornea. (See *Understanding Fluorescein Staining,* page 403.) Small lacerations heal by themselves, but an ophthalmologist must suture a large one. After this surgery, you'll probably apply an eye patch or eye shield to decrease eye movement, allowing undisturbed healing. (See *Patching Pointers.*) Expect to give your patient antibiotic eye drops and appropriate tetanus toxoid therapy, if needed. (See *Guidelines for Tetanus Prophylaxis,* pages 66 and 67.)

If your patient has a *corneal abrasion,* expect to instill antibiotic eye drops to guard against infection. Apply a pressure patch to ease the pain and irritation that can occur when the lid, opening and closing, rubs the abrasion.

---

### PATCHING POINTERS

Your patient may need an eye patch to prevent contamination, to discourage eye movement, and to promote healing. The next time you're asked to apply an eye patch, keep the following pointers in mind:

- Use as many gauze pads as you need to fill the orbital depth so the patch is level with the patient's frontal edge.
- Tape the patch diagonally from the medial orbital rim to the lateral cheek bone. (Remember to use paper tape so you won't irritate your patient's skin when you remove the patch later.)
- After you've applied the patch, ask your patient to try to open his eye. He shouldn't be able to do this if the patch is of the right depth and correctly placed.

## CASE IN POINT: TRANSMITTING INFECTION

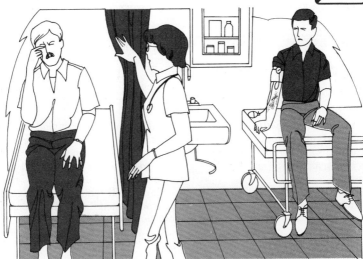

You've just begun your shift in the ED. Your first patient is Daniel Jamison, age 28. His problem? Fever and malaise. Pulling up his sleeve to take his blood pressure, you notice a rash on his lower forearm— Daniel tells you he first noticed it yesterday. The doctor arrives to examine Daniel just as you finish documenting your findings on his chart. You then go directly to the examining room where your next patient is waiting. He's Arthur Manula, age 43. He's "lost" his right contact lens in his eye, which is very irritated. You quickly examine the eye, locate the lens, and retrieve it from under Arthur's upper eyelid. The doctor finds no abrasions on Arthur's cornea, so Arthur is discharged from the ED.

Later in the day, you learn that Daniel— your patient with the rash—was admitted to the hospital with a diagnosis of recurrent gonococcal bacteremia. Two days pass; then Arthur Manula returns to the ED, complaining of pain and discharge in his right eye. Cultures reveal *Neisseria gonorrhoeae*. In considering how this organism may have gotten into Arthur's eye, the doctor checks the ED records and makes an incriminating connection. You treated Arthur Manula after you assessed Daniel Jamison. The doctor did this,

too, but he washed his hands before examining Arthur, and you didn't. You probably transmitted Daniel's infection to Arthur.

What if this were a real event? Could you be held liable for the patient's infection? In a court case involving a similar situation (*Helman v. Sacred Heart Hospital*, 1963), the nurse was found liable for transmitting a staphylococcal infection from one patient to another. The court reasoned that by failing to follow sterile techniques according to her hospital's policy, she failed to take reasonable precautions to avoid spreading infection.

To reduce your risk of liability for causing infection in patients, especially during hectic shifts in the ED, follow these tips:
- Every time you care for any patient, take the time to wash your hands afterward.
- Always wash your hands before examining a patient's eyes or administering treatment. You may even want to wash your hands again before touching the patient's second eye, to prevent cross-contamination.
- Whenever you suspect a patient has an infectious disease, isolate him according to hospital policy, double-bag and label his clothes and linens, and caution his family members to avoid direct contact with him.

---

*Helman v. Sacred Heart Hospital*, 62 Wash. 2d 136; 381 P. 2d 605 (1963).

Corneal abrasions usually heal within 24 to 72 hours because epithelial tissue regenerates rapidly. Remember, topical anesthetics are contraindicated during healing because they retard healing and may obscure signs of infection.

# Penetrating Injury to the Eye

## Prediagnosis summary
The patient had a history of penetrating trauma and some combination of these signs and symptoms:
• pain
• bleeding
• profuse lacrimation
• decreased visual acuity
• a visible corneal or scleral wound, possibly together with laceration of the lid.

An ophthalmologist was called to perform a complete eye examination, which may have revealed any of the following:
• a soft eye due to reduced or absent IOP
• hemorrhage into the anterior chamber
• vitreous hemorrhage
• laceration of the iris
• dislocated lens
• increased intraocular swelling
• orbital floor fracture
• retinal hemorrhage or detachment.

## Priorities
With this patient, your first priority is to remember what *not* to do. If an object's impaled in your patient's eye, *don't* remove it. And *don't* manipulate the patient's eyeball—you may expel the contents and cause permanent blindness. Instead, place a metal shield over your patient's eye to prevent further damage while you're waiting for the ophthalmologist to arrive. (If your patient's a child, you may also need to apply hand restraints.) Insert an I.V.,

and begin antibiotic therapy, as ordered. Administer prophylactic tetanus toxoid, too, as ordered, if the patient hasn't received a tetanus booster in the last 5 years. (See *Guidelines for Tetanus Prophylaxis,* pages 66 and 67.)

## Continuing assessment and intervention
Prepare your patient for X-rays or for ultrasonography to locate the penetrating object. The doctor may also order a computerized tomography (CT) scan, if necessary.

Take a quick history and perform a brief physical examination before you prepare your patient for surgery. Make sure you note any allergies and current medications on his chart. The ophthalmologist will remove the foreign body that penetrated the eye and repair your patient's corneal or scleral laceration or his retinal detachment and any associated injuries.

## Therapeutic care
When your patient returns from surgery, your care will focus on protecting the injured eye. He'll be wearing an eye shield for maximum protection. Expect to continue antibiotic treatment to prevent infection and to start him on corticosteroids to reduce inflammation and edema. Give analgesics as necessary to relieve mild pain. However, if your patient's pain is severe, notify the doctor, because this may indicate hemorrhage or infection.

# Acute Vitreous Hemorrhage and Hyphema

## Prediagnosis summary
Initial assessment findings for the patient included some or all of the following signs and symptoms:
• some degree of pain
• blood partially or completely filling

# WHAT HAPPENS IN ACUTE VITREOUS HEMORRHAGE AND HYPHEMA

**Acute vitreous hemorrhage**

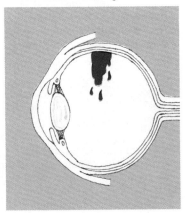

**Hyphema**

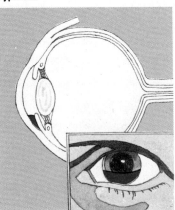

Acute vitreous hemorrhage and hyphema are two serious eye disorders that can cause temporary or permanent blindness.

Acute vitreous hemorrhage occurs when trauma, an ocular tumor, or a disease process (such as diabetes mellitus or hypertension) causes hemorrhage in retinal vessels, the choroid, or the ciliary body. Blood leaks into the vitreous, which becomes opaque and blocks passage of light rays to the retina. The patient becomes blind in the affected eye.

In a patient with a hyphema, blunt trauma to the eye tears the ciliary body and iris, causing bleeding into the anterior chamber. The blood may be reabsorbed spontaneously within 72 hours; if it isn't, it may cause secondary glaucoma and blood staining of the cornea. Loss of vision in the eye may occur if the glaucoma becomes severe.

Another variation of hyphema, so-called eight-ball hyphema, occurs when dark, clotted blood fills the eye's anterior chamber. Intraocular pressure becomes extremely high and can be lowered only by removing the blood. The hyphema may recur 3 to 5 days after the initial hemorrhage because of reflex congestion of the iris and ciliary body.

---

the anterior chamber
• a report of seeing a reddish tint
• a report of moving spots that seem to drift in front of the patient's eye (floaters)
• a history of recent blunt trauma to the eye (more likely in a patient with a hyphema).

The patient was placed on bed rest, and an ophthalmologist was called.

## Priorities

Your first priority is to check your patient's visual acuity, using the Snellen test, to provide baseline data. Report your results to the doctor—together with his complete ophthalmologic examination, your results will provide a baseline for evaluating changes in your patient's condition.

## Continuing assessment and intervention

Take a detailed history to help determine the cause of your patient's hemorrhage. If he's suffered blunt trauma, find out when and how the accident happened. If he didn't experience trauma, ask if he has diabetes mellitus or hypertension, because these may precipitate acute vitreous hemorrhage. And ask if he's ever experienced a sudden decrease of vision in one eye—he may have had a prior venous occlusion that caused vascularization leading to vitreous hemorrhage.

The ophthalmologist will do a complete examination to identify the bleeding site—into the anterior chamber (*hyphema*) or behind the lens (*vitreous hemorrhage*). When he's finished examining the patient, he may ask you to apply bilateral eye shields to restrict eye movement. (See *Patching Pointers*, page 404.)

Keep the patient on bed rest and administer medications as ordered. You may give:
• cycloplegics, to paralyze iris movement and to reduce the risk of new bleeding from weakened iris blood vessels
• carbonic anhydrase inhibitors, such as acetazolamide (Diamox) or mannitol (Osmitrol), to reduce IOP.

If your patient has a *hyphema*, regularly check the blood level line in the eye's anterior chamber. Why? Because a second, larger hemorrhage may occur after the initial hemorrhage. If the bleeding becomes so extensive that it fills the anterior chamber, your patient may need surgery.

If your patient has a *vitreous hemorrhage*, he may need surgery to remove the hemorrhagic fluid and to simultaneously replace it with clear, normal saline solution. Eventually, the aqueous fluid that the eye continually produces will replace this solution.

### Therapeutic care
If your patient's had surgery, he may return with bilateral eye patches or shields. Monitor his vital signs every 15 minutes until he's stable, then at least once every shift.

He'll need continued bed rest, with bathroom privileges only, whether he's had surgery or not. Orient your patient to his environment (remember, he can't see), and encourage him to perform active range-of-motion exercises. Ask him to deep-breathe 15 times every hour, to prevent postsurgical respiratory complications.

Expect to administer prophylactic antibiotics and to give analgesics as needed for pain. Try to visit with your patient for at least 5 minutes every hour to reduce his anxiety and disorientation.

# Blow-out Fracture

### Prediagnosis summary
The patient had blunt facial trauma with accompanying periorbital swelling and ecchymoses. On initial assessment, he had some combination of the following signs and symptoms:
• facial swelling at the injury site
• double vision (diplopia)
• a sunken eyeball
• decreased sensation on the inside or outside of the cheek on the affected side
• blood in the nostril on the affected side of his face
• pain on the affected side of his face when he looked up
• globe displacement (downward and inward)
• inability to elevate the eye
• subconjunctival hemorrhage
• restricted extraocular movements in the affected eye.

To confirm the diagnosis of orbital fracture, an ophthalmologist applied traction to the patient's inferior rectus muscle (forced duction test) to detect the eye's inability to move upward due to extraocular muscle entrapment.

### Priorities
Your first priority is to obtain baseline data concerning your patient's visual acuity. To do this, use the Snellen test. If his eye isn't ruptured and he doesn't have a hyphema, apply an ice pack to

## WHAT HAPPENS IN BLOW-OUT FRACTURE

A blunt blow to the eye that compresses orbital tissues causes pressure within the orbit to increase. The result? The orbital floor, the weakest portion of the orbit, gives way—"blows out." This causes prolapse of the orbital fat and the globe, entrapping the inferior rectus and inferior oblique muscles and, possibly, the infraorbital nerve as well.

The eye thus loses its full range of upward and downward motion. The patient may also have decreased sensation in his lower eyelid from infraorbital nerve entrapment.

This diagram shows you how a blow-out fracture affects the eye.

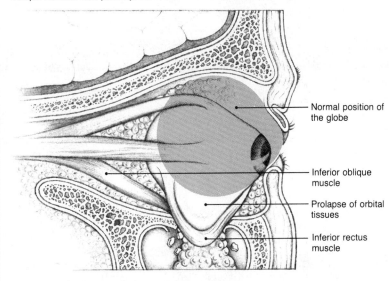

Normal position of the globe

Inferior oblique muscle

Prolapse of orbital tissues

Inferior rectus muscle

---

reduce pain and swelling. The ophthalmologist will perform a complete eye examination.

### Continuing assessment and intervention

Expect to accompany your patient to the radiology department for facial X-rays or a CT scan to identify the extent of the fracture and to determine if other fractures are present. Your patient will be on bed rest. Explain to him that he shouldn't lift objects or bend over, because these movements may cause strain that increases IOP.

After his facial swelling has been reduced (usually 7 to 10 days after admission to the hospital), your patient will have surgery to release the entrapped orbital muscles. During the period leading up to your patient's surgery, be alert for signs of associated intraocular injuries or disorders, such as hemorrhage or infection. (See the "Acute Vitreous Hemorrhage and Hyphema" entry in this chapter and *Comparing Eye Infections*, pages 410 and 411.)

### Therapeutic care

Following his surgery, assess your patient's vital signs every 15 minutes until they're stabilized. Check for signs and symptoms of postsurgical infection:

## COMPARING EYE INFECTIONS

All eye infections have similar signs and symptoms, so telling them apart can be difficult. Here's a chart to help you differentiate common eye infections.

| INFECTION | Pain | Photophobia | Lacrimation | Eyelid spasm | Visual disturbances | Discharge/drainage | Decreased visual acuity | Fever | Itching | EYE EXAMINATION RESULTS |
|---|---|---|---|---|---|---|---|---|---|---|
| **Keratitis** (inflammation of cornea) | 👁 | 👁 | 👁 | 👁 | 👁 | 👁 | 👁 | | | • Pinpoint corneal lesions that stain with fluorescein • Gray-white flecks on anterior epithelial surface • Conjunctival injection (redness) |
| **Iritis** (inflammation of iris) | 👁 | 👁 | | | 👁 | | 👁 | | | • Circumcorneal injection • Dull and swollen iris • Small and irregular pupils • Turbid aqueous humor • Poor light reflex in affected pupil • Upper eyelid edema • Possible corneal precipitates |
| **Corneal ulcer** (local necrosis of corneal tissue from microorganisms) | 👁 | 👁 | 👁 | 👁 | 👁 | 👁 | 👁 | | | • Blepharospasm (eye twitching) • Dull gray film over the ulcer • Green stain with fluorescein • Pus in anterior chamber • Possible constricted pupil |
| **Conjunctivitis** (inflammation of conjunctiva) | 👁 | | 👁 | | 👁 | | | | 👁 | • Peripheral injection of conjunctiva (brick-red) • Clear cornea • Equal size pupils with normal light reaction • Lid edema |
| **Endophthalmitis** (inflammation of entire eye) | 👁 | 👁 | 👁 | 👁 | 👁 | | 👁 | 👁 | | • Lid edema • Mild proptosis (forward displacement or bulging of the eye) • Conjunctival and ciliary injection |

| TREATMENT: Antivirals | Topical antibiotics | Systemic antibiotics | Corticosteroids | Mydriatic or cycloplegic drops | SPECIAL CONSIDERATIONS |
|---|---|---|---|---|---|
| ◉ | ◉ | | ◉ | ◉ | • Infection may be acute or chronic.<br>• Residual vision impairment is rare. |
| | | | ◉ | ◉ | • Infection may signal systemic disease, such as sarcoidosis or inflammatory bowel disease. |
| ◉ | ◉ | | | ◉ | • Infection may spread over the width of the cornea or penetrate deeply.<br>• Permanent scarring may result from deep penetration.<br>• Mild iritis may occur. |
| | ◉ | | ◉ | | • Gonococcal conjunctivitis may result in corneal perforation.<br>• Gonococci may cause infection even if the epithelium's unbroken.<br>• Viral conjunctivitis is generally self-limiting, lasting 1 to 2 weeks. |
| | ◉ | ◉ | ◉ | ◉ | • If his infection's bacterial, the patient's placed on wound and skin isolation.<br>• The prognosis for improved visual acuity is poor.<br>• Fever and infection may accompany systemic blood-borne infection or a penetrating injury. |

pain, fever, foul-smelling drainage. *Important:* Infection may be confined to the eye or may spread to other areas of the body. (See the "Eye Infections" entry in this chapter.) Be especially alert for signs of meningeal irritation—as you know, these include neck pain, irritability, and changes in level of consciousness (see the "Meningitis" entry in Chapter 6).

# Eye Infections

## Prediagnosis summary
Initial assessment of the patient revealed some or all of the following signs and symptoms:
• purulent discharge
• pain
• sensitivity to light (photophobia)
• lacrimation
• decreased visual acuity
• intense itching
• fever.

An ophthalmologist was called. His examination of the patient's eye(s) identified some or all of the following signs and symptoms:
• pinpoint corneal lesions
• ciliary injection
• a small, irregular pupil
• turbid aqueous humor
• pus in the anterior chamber.

## Priorities
Treating the patient's infection and keeping it from spreading are your first priorities for this patient. Expect to begin antimicrobial therapy (topical or systemic).

## Continuing assessment and intervention
Take a complete history including other medical problems your patient has (or had) and information on medications he's taking, if any. You may be asked to apply warm compresses to his eye; this will increase drainage and soothe irritation. Expect to culture the af-

fected eye for culture-and-sensitivity testing. This will identify the organism causing the infection (and the antibiotics it is sensitive to). Remember, any patient with an eye infection requires strict wound and skin isolation. Explain to your patient the importance of not rubbing his eyes, because cross-contamination can easily occur. (See *Comparing Eye Infections,* pages 410 and 411.)

## Therapeutic care
Check the patient's culture-and-sensitivity results—is he receiving the correct antibiotic to kill the organism that's causing his infection? (If he isn't, notify the doctor.) Expect to administer topical corticosteroids to decrease inflammation *only* if the causative agent isn't viral. Why? Because in viral infections, corticosteroids decrease immunity and allow the virus to proliferate. Emotional support is particularly important for a patient whose eye infection has caused permanent vision loss. Visit with this patient frequently (for at least 5 minutes every hour) so he can ask questions and talk about his concerns.

# Retinal Detachment

## Prediagnosis summary
The patient's chief complaint was altered vision. On initial assessment, he had some combination of the following signs and symptoms:
• seeing light flashes or floaters
• a partially obscured visual field
• absence of pain
• cloudy vision
• decreased visual acuity.

An ophthalmologist was called. His funduscopic examination determined the location and extent of the patient's suspected retinal detachment. The retina was gray and opaque, with an indefinite margin. A visual acuity test was performed; the degree of the patient's vision loss depended on how much retina was detached, and where.

The patient was placed on bed rest, with bilateral eye patches to restrict eye movement.

## Priorities

Your first priority is to assist in restricting your patient's eye and body movement. This is important, because once his detached retina's settled back

# WHAT HAPPENS IN RETINAL DETACHMENT

Trauma or degenerative changes cause retinal detachment by separating the nervous tissue layers of the retina from the retinal pigmented epithelium. This permits fluid, such as the vitreous, to seep into the subretinal space (between the pigmented epithelium and the rod and cone layer) and to balloon the retina into the

vitreous cavity away from choroidal circulation. A retina detached from its blood supply can no longer function: without prompt surgery, the patient may become permanently blind in the affected eye.

Here's an illustration to help you understand the process of retinal detachment.

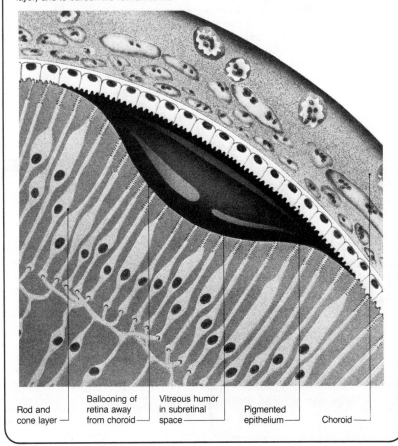

Rod and cone layer — Ballooning of retina away from choroid — Vitreous humor in subretinal space — Pigmented epithelium — Choroid —

into its proper position, the ophthalmologist can perform reattachment surgery.

Place eye patches over both the patient's eyes to restrict their movement. (See *Patching Pointers,* page 404.) Then check the doctor's orders regarding the head position he wants your patient to maintain. Place pillows or folded towels behind your patient's head (see *Pillow Talk*). Take the time now to explain to your patient why positioning is so important; this will help to ensure his cooperation. Warn him not to touch or rub his eyes and to avoid straining or sudden body motions.

## Continuing assessment and intervention

Your patient will probably be disoriented (remember, he can't see), anxious, and afraid. So try to visit him for 5 minutes every hour to provide emotional support and reassurance. Try to keep his environment calm and relaxing, too. Expect to administer sedatives or tranquilizers to keep him comfortable and to minimize eye strain. Keep his side rails up, and place the call bell within his easy reach.

Ask your patient whether he's had any other medical problems—especially hypertension, myopia, or diabetes mellitus (these conditions can

cause retinopathy, which may lead to retinal detachment). Also ask whether he has a history of facial trauma or eye surgery, which can predispose your patient to retinal detachment.

Myopia and previous eye trauma are also predisposing factors in retinal detachment. Most incidences of retinal detachment in children, however, are hereditary; so, if your patient's a child, be sure to ask whether his family has a history of retinal detachment.

### Therapeutic care

Prepare your patient for surgery. First, wash his face with warmed liquid surgical soap. Then administer antibiotics, as ordered. Expect to instill two types of eye drops (one drop of each, in each eye), 5 minutes apart:

• mydriatic eye drops, such as phenylephrine (Neo-Synephrine), to dilate the pupil

• cycloplegic eye drops, such as cyclopentolate hydrochloride (Cyclogyl), to paralyze the intraocular muscles. (This decreases the patient's tendency toward eye movement and allows the doctor to visualize the retina easily.)

After surgery, your patient will be placed on bed rest for 1 or 2 days. Make sure he maintains proper body position and restricts his eye movement. If your patient isn't required to wear eye patches, caution him not to use rapid eye movements, such as for reading. He may look straight ahead, however, which means that he can watch television.

Notify the doctor *immediately* if your patient begins vomiting. This can signal increased IOP—or, of course, can cause it.

Your patient's eyes may appear swollen and discolored after surgery. Explain that this is normal.

Apply an antibiotic ointment to your patient's eyes, as ordered, and expect to give analgesics if he has pain. Remove crusts that form on his eyelashes; apply warm, moist compresses to the area for a few minutes to soften the crusts for easier removal.

## PILLOW TALK

As you're probably aware, a patient with a retinal detachment needs to maintain the proper head position without moving. A pillow or two can help while the patient's awaiting surgery.

For example, if the patient's retina is detached at its right periphery, the doctor may ask you to elevate the patient's head 30° and to have him lie on his right side. To maintain the patient in this position, place pillows behind his head. (The presence of the pillows will also remind him not to roll over.)

Continue regular assessments of your patient's eyes. Notify the doctor if your patient complains of sharp eye pain, which could indicate intraocular hemorrhage or an infection.

If your patient shows no evidence of developing an infection or hemorrhage, expect to discharge him within 3 to 5 days. Before he leaves the hospital, prepare him for making the trip home. How? By instructing him to lie down on the car's backseat in the same position he maintained in bed in the hospital. Taking this precaution will reduce stress on the newly repaired retina during the ride. Also remind the patient to avoid reading or rapidly moving his eyes for several weeks. Be sure he realizes that his affected eye will be swollen and discolored for 1 or 2 weeks after his surgery.

# Central Retinal Artery Occlusion

## Prediagnosis summary
The patient, with no history of trauma, had sudden, painless loss of vision in one eye. Initial assessment revealed sluggish pupil constriction in response to direct light.

An ophthalmologist was consulted, and his funduscopic examination revealed:
- retinal edema
- a cherry-red spot on the macula
- narrowed arterioles (and, possibly, optic atrophy)
- splinterlike (rather than round) hemorrhages
- fluffy, white exudates.

The patient was placed on bed rest; external eye massage and carbogen therapy were started.

## Priorities
As you probably know, the central retinal artery is the retina's major blood supply. When it's occluded, the retina

PATHOPHYSIOLOGY

**WHAT HAPPENS IN CENTRAL RETINAL ARTERY OCCLUSION**

Causes of central retinal artery occlusion (CRAO) include:
- atherosclerosis of the carotid artery
- rheumatic heart disease
- mitral valve prolapse
- prolonged and abnormal pressure on the globe
- intraorbital swelling
- improperly applied eye dressings
- lying prone, with feet elevated.

Patients over age 50 are most susceptible, probably as a consequence of atherosclerosis.

In a patient with CRAO secondary to atherosclerosis or heart disease, emboli dislodge from the carotid artery or heart valves and travel into the retinal artery, occluding it. For a short time thereafter, the retina still receives blood from the choriocapillaries, which are attached to Bruch's membrane. So it survives—for a short time. But the retina needs the full flow of the central retinal artery; it's the retina's major blood supply. If the artery's flow isn't fully restored within 2 hours, the retina becomes edematous and necrotic.

becomes edematous and necrotic within 2 hours unless treatment to open the occlusion is instituted. This means that your immediate priority is to assist in decreasing the patient's IOP rapidly. Start an I.V., and be prepared to administer medications and to assist with IOP-reducing procedures. Continue eye massage and carbogen therapy, as ordered. Keep the head of the patient's bed elevated, and tell the patient to try to avoid coughing, sneezing, or bending over—these actions *increase* IOP.

Medications to reduce IOP include:
- *acetazolamide (Diamox)* I.V. A diuretic, acetazolamide may cause vomiting, nausea, and confusion, so watch your patient carefully during infusion.
- *mannitol (Osmitrol)* as a rapid infusion over 30 to 60 minutes. An osmotic diuretic, mannitol may cause dehydration and fluid and electrolyte

imbalances. Start intake and output records for your patient, and check his electrolyte levels frequently. Remember to use an in-line filter when giving mannitol, to avoid infusing microcrystals.

• *timolol (Timoptic),* one drop in the affected eye. An ophthalmic beta-blocking agent, timolol reduces aqueous formation.

• *nitroglycerin* sublingually. This decreases arterial spasm and aids in opening the affected artery. Check your patient's vital signs after you give nitroglycerin, because it can cause hypotension.

• *anticoagulant.* The doctor may order this given I.V. or subcutaneously to inhibit clot formation.

### Continuing assessment and intervention

Perform a quick assessment to see how your patient is tolerating his medication. Ask him if he has a history of cardiovascular disease (this is particularly important if he's elderly—atherosclerosis of the carotid artery is by far the most common cause of central retinal artery occlusion). Explain the medication you're giving, and ask the patient to tell you *immediately* if he regains any vision in his affected eye—even if he can only see a dark haze or a flicker of light.

The doctor may ask you to assist with paracentesis of the anterior chamber of the patient's eye or with a lateral canthotomy.

During paracentesis, he'll withdraw fluid through a fine needle, causing a rapid decrease in IOP (it will be close to zero after he removes 0.2 to 0.3 ml of fluid). As the IOP drops, arterial pressure may push the occlusion into the peripheral retinal circulation, restoring retinal blood flow and the patient's vision.

Lateral canthotomy (surgically dividing the outer canthus) is indicated if severe intraorbital edema or an orbital mass caused the occlusion. Canthotomy allows the orbital contents to push forward, decreasing pressure on the artery. This sometimes reopens the central retinal artery.

Remember, you'll be expected to give these medications and to assist with these procedures quickly—if the patient's occlusion lasts more than 2 hours, his retinal damage and loss of vision will probably be permanent.

### Therapeutic care

Once treatment begins, check your patient's visual fields and visual acuity frequently for signs of improvement. However, you should be aware that most patients *don't* recover vision in the affected eye. So the prognosis is generally poor—in spite of expert and aggressive medical, surgical, and nursing intervention.

Your patient will also need medical treatment for the underlying cause of his occlusion (usually atherosclerosis). After that, your continuing care will probably focus on helping your patient adjust to loss of vision in the affected eye. You'll provide emotional support, of course—sudden loss of vision is devastating for anyone. But beyond that, be prepared to provide teaching that helps your patient adjust to his disability.

# Acute Closed-Angle Glaucoma

### Prediagnosis summary

Initial assessment of the patient revealed some or all of the following signs and symptoms:

• decreased visual acuity
• nausea and vomiting
• sudden, severe pain starting in one eye and then radiating to his head
• a fixed semi-dilated pupil
• blurred vision
• a report of seeing rainbow-colored halos around lights (such as streetlights or automobile headlights).

# WHAT HAPPENS IN ACUTE CLOSED-ANGLE GLAUCOMA

In a normally functioning eye, the ciliary body produces aqueous humor, which flows from the posterior to the anterior chamber, then through the trabecular meshwork to the canal of Schlemm (outflow channel). From there it travels into the venous circulation.

When the iris comes in contact with the trabecular meshwork, this flow is blocked, causing a sudden increase in intraocular pressure—acute closed-angle glaucoma. The resulting compromise in the optic nerve's blood supply can lead to blindness.

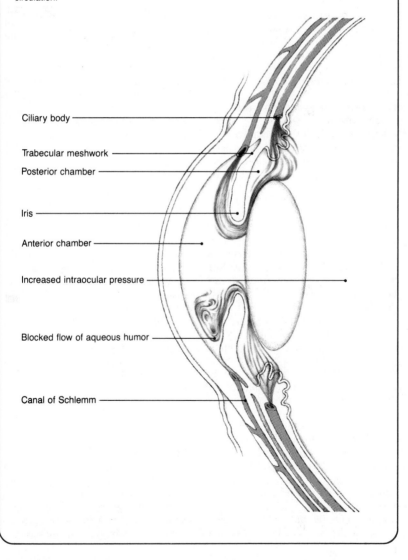

Ciliary body

Trabecular meshwork

Posterior chamber

Iris

Anterior chamber

Increased intraocular pressure

Blocked flow of aqueous humor

Canal of Schlemm

An ophthalmologist was called and the patient's eyes were tested for increased IOP using applanation tonometry. The patient was questioned about past visual disturbances and eye pain.

## Priorities

Once acute closed-angle glaucoma has been diagnosed, the first medical priority is to reduce the patient's IOP. The doctor will order topical therapy first: timolol (Timoptic) and miotic eye drops. Once you've administered these medications, expect to start an I.V. line to administer either a carbonic anhydrase inhibitor or a hyperosmotic agent. This medication will decrease formation of aqueous and so decrease the patient's IOP.

## Continuing assessment and intervention

Assess the patient's vital signs; then, to relieve his pain, expect to administer analgesics, such as Demerol (meperidine) or morphine sulfate I.M. If the patient's pain persists, continue to administer analgesics as ordered. To control the patient's nausea and vomiting, the doctor may ask you to administer an antiemetic, such as prochlorperazine maleate or trimethobenzamide hydrochloride, by suppository or I.M. Remember to provide continuous emotional support because your patient's impaired vision and pain will make him anxious and frightened.

As the patient's IOP falls, his peripheral vision and visual acuity should progressively improve. Assess him for this. The doctor will also monitor the patient's IOP, adjusting the amount and frequency of his medication accordingly.

Although some of the drugs the patient receives will increase his thirst, give the patient nothing by mouth. Why? Because he may need surgery. To provide some relief, periodically give him a water-moistened gauze sponge to suck on.

Remember, the patient's depth perception is distorted, so he's vulnerable to injury. Keep his bed side rails up at all times and explain that this precaution is for his safety.

## Therapeutic care

Usually the IOP of a patient with acute closed-angle glaucoma drops to normal 30 minutes to 2 hours after drug therapy begins. If this doesn't happen, the patient may need peripheral iridectomy or laser surgery.

# Facial Fractures

## Prediagnosis summary

The patient came to the ED with facial trauma and the following signs and symptoms:
• facial swelling and asymmetry
• ecchymoses
• palpable fracture or fractures
• pain.

Palpation was performed and X-rays were taken to locate the fracture site.

If the patient had a *nasal fracture,* he may also have had these signs:
• deviated septum
• epistaxis.

A patient with *mandibular* or *maxillary fractures* may have had some combination of these signs and symptoms:
• malocclusion of teeth
• inability to open his mouth due to muscle spasm
• midface elongation.

If the patient had more than one facial fracture, the doctor may have assigned a Le Fort classification to define the extent and severity of the injury. (See *Understanding Le Fort's Classifications.*)

## Priorities

Your first priority is to watch the patient for signs and symptoms of respiratory distress (including airway obstruction) from increasing edema. Apply an ice pack to the fracture site to reduce swelling, pain, and bleeding.

## UNDERSTANDING LE FORT'S CLASSIFICATIONS

The doctor may diagnose your patient's facial fracture as *Le Fort I, II,* or *III.* Do you know what this means? It's a quick way to describe the location and extent of facial fractures. Here are illustrations and descriptions of the three Le Fort classifications.

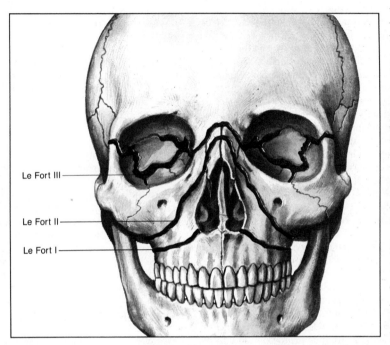

Le Fort III —
Le Fort II —
Le Fort I —

**Le Fort I:** Fracture of the transverse alveolar process involving the front teeth in a bilateral fracture extending up to the nose. This patient's airway may become occluded if he's aspirated a loose tooth.

**Le Fort II:** Fracture of the pyramidal area including the central part of the maxilla, the nasal area, and the medial aspects of the orbits. This patient will bleed profusely (from the nose and pharynx) and his airway may be compromised.

**Le Fort III:** Total craniofacial separation including a tripod fracture and craniofacial detachment. This patient may have airway occlusion and cerebral spinal fluid (CSF) leaking through his nose (CSF rhinorrhea).

Remember, keep a patient who's bleeding from his nose upright, and tilt his head forward to prevent him from swallowing the blood. If he has a facial fracture, don't squeeze his nostrils to stop the blood flow. Instead, catch the blood with a gauze sponge or place a bowl under the patient's nose. If your patient has an open fracture, expect to insert an I.V. and to begin prophylactic antibiotic treatment immediately.

## Continuing assessment and intervention

Find out when, where, and how the injury occurred, and expect to give analgesics to relieve pain. A patient with a mandibular or maxillary fracture should be given nothing by mouth, so you'll need to administer his medications I.M.

Check your patient's vital signs. If he has a fever, the doctor may ask you to administer antibiotics to prevent infection. Ask the patient when he had his last tetanus shot. If he can't remember, assume it was more than five years ago, and begin tetanus prophylaxis as ordered (see *Guidelines for Tetanus Prophylaxis*, pages 66 and 67).

Continue checking your patient frequently for possible upper airway obstruction due to massive swelling from soft tissue injury. Perform a neurologic assessment to establish a baseline, and repeat it every hour to detect any changes. Why? Because any force strong enough to fracture bones is also likely to cause neurologic damage, which may not be apparent until several hours after the injury. So even if your patient sustained only a mild nasal fracture and is being discharged, be sure you teach his family members how to perform a neurologic assessment at home.

### Therapeutic care

The goal of mandibular or maxillary surgery is to stabilize the fracture by wiring the patient's jaws closed. Explain that he won't be able to talk or open his mouth for the first 24 hours after surgery. Help him to communicate by writing or simple sign language during that time.

Tape wire cutters by your patient's bed where you can reach them easily, and have suction equipment at the bedside. Then, if your patient develops respiratory distress or starts to vomit, you can prevent aspiration by cutting the jaw wiring, suctioning the vomitus, and allowing your patient to spit out the blood or vomitus. Expect to give analgesics I.M., such as Demerol (meperidine) or morphine, to relieve your patient's pain. (He'll return from surgery with an I.V., which you can discontinue when he's able to tolerate a normal liquid diet.)

Explain to your patient and his family that he'll need to eat and drink through a straw until his fracture heals and the wires are removed. Of course, your patient won't be able to brush his teeth during this time, so his oral hygiene should include frequent rinsing with mouthwash.

---

# External Ear Trauma

## Prediagnosis summary

The patient came to the ED with obvious ear trauma. On initial assessment, he had some combination of the following signs and symptoms:
- pain
- edema
- ecchymoses
- localized bleeding
- diminished hearing
- hematoma
- fluctuant swelling
- partial or total loss of ear tissue.

The patient was kept in an upright position and an ice pack was applied to reduce local swelling and bleeding, if present. If the patient's ear was avulsed, the wound was cleansed and a sterile 4″ x 4″ gauze pad was applied. A plastic surgeon was notified for possible replantation.

## Priorities

If your patient's ear was avulsed and he has the detached portion of the ear with him, your first priority is to preserve it for future replantation. Saturate a gauze sponge with normal saline solution; then wrap the avulsed fragment in it. Place the sponge in a plastic bag and store it over ice.

Be prepared to assist the doctor while he examines your patient's internal ear. You may need to immobilize your patient's head during the examination.

Completely examine any patient who has a hematoma on his ear. Why? Because the blunt trauma that caused the hematoma may also have caused other injuries.

## Continuing assessment and intervention

Test your patient's hearing with the

Rinne and Weber tests. Administer analgesics to relieve his pain, and provide emotional support.

When you take your patient's history, be sure to ask when he last had a tetanus booster. (See *Guidelines for Tetanus Prophylaxis,* pages 66 and 67.) Administer tetanus prophylaxis, as ordered. For a patient with a hematoma, cleanse the affected area and shave 1″ around his ear to prepare him for drainage of the hematoma.

### Therapeutic care
If your patient's ear is avulsed, saturate a gauze pad with povidone-iodine and use it to cover the area the detached portion was torn from. If the *entire ear* is avulsed and the detached portion was salvaged, the doctor may surgically bury the ear cartilage in soft tissue, to provide a secondary blood supply and to preserve the ear cartilage for later reconstruction. If only *part of the ear* is avulsed, the doctor will suture it immediately. Prepare the equipment you'll need to assist the doctor with suturing your patient.

If your patient has a hematoma, the doctor will drain it by aspirating it with a large-gauge needle (15G). If a blood clot impedes aspiration, he'll make an incision, remove the blood clot, and insert a plastic drain. When this process is complete, apply a sterile fluff dressing using cotton or gauze moistened with sterile saline solution.

Expect to begin administering antibiotics, and check your patient regularly for signs and symptoms of ear infection, particularly pain (aggravated when he opens his mouth) or diminished hearing.

---

# Epistaxis

## Prediagnosis summary
Initial assessment of the patient revealed one of the following signs:
- active bleeding from his nose
- dried blood in his nostrils
- no obvious signs of bleeding, but a sensation of blood trickling down the back of his throat.

### Priorities
Your first priority is to try to control the bleeding. Apply external pressure by pinching your patient's nostrils firmly—*except* if the epistaxis accompanies a nasal fracture (see the "Facial Fractures" entry in this chapter). Ask your patient to tilt his head forward to minimize the amount of blood draining down the back of his throat. Give him an emesis basin and tell him to spit out the blood instead of swallowing it.

### Continuing assessment and intervention
As you know, extreme blood loss can cause your patient to go into shock. Monitor such a patient's vital signs closely, and perform a tilt test (see *Using the Tilt Test to Evaluate Hypovolemia,* page 302). If you detect positive orthostatic signs in the patient, start an I.V. and administer replacement fluids.

Question the patient about the following:
- a history of recent nasal trauma
- the frequency and usual duration of any prior episodes of epistaxis, and the amount of blood usually lost
- a history of previous nasal packing or surgery in the sinus area
- a history of recent upper respiratory tract infection, such as sinusitis or allergies
- a past history of anemia; hypertension; cardiovascular, respiratory, or liver disease; or alcoholism
- past or present use of anticoagulants, aspirin, or antihypertensives.

A patient with nasal trauma may have associated neurologic injuries (such as cerebral contusion or concussion), eye injuries, or facial fractures. Assess him for these, and intervene as necessary.

The doctor will order blood drawn for a CBC, which will help him estimate the amount of blood the patient's

## UNDERSTANDING NASAL PACKING

Uncontrolled nasal bleeding can affect your patient's vital signs in a hurry. But the doctor can avert potentially severe hemorrhage by inserting nasal packing in a patient with *severe* epistaxis. Depending on the location and severity of the bleeding, the doctor will insert an anterior or a posterior nasal pack—or both. This chart will show you the differences between the two.

|  | ANTERIOR PACKING | POSTERIOR PACKING |
|---|---|---|
| **Uses** | bleeding in anterior nose | • bleeding in posterior nose or if anterior bleeding flows posteriorly after anterior packing is in place |
| **Materials** | petrolatum gauze strips | • a gauze pack tied to rubber catheters by three heavy sutures |
| **Procedure** | The doctor layers gauze in a stair-step fashion. | 1. The doctor pulls the catheters back through the patient's nostrils, leaving the pack behind the soft palate. 2. He ties the free ends of the sutures to a dental gauze roll, which rests under the patient's nose and keeps the posterior roll in place. 3. He tapes the third suture to the patient's cheek for later use in removing the pack. 4. He inserts anterior packing to help maintain traction and to prevent excess pressure on the patient's nostrils. |
| **Care required** | hospitalization possibly required for sedation and observation, for bilateral anterior packing, or after drainage and packing of a septal hematoma | • hospitalization possibly required for *all* posterior packing |

lost and detect anemia. The doctor will also order a PT and PTT to test your patient's coagulation time (it may be prolonged if your patient's taking anticoagulants or aspirin).

When the doctor examines the patient's nose, he may ask you to administer a sedative, such as diazepam (Valium). This will help to relax the patient for the examination. Gather the EENT and suction equipment the doctor will need, and be prepared to assist him.

Once the doctor identifies the source of the patient's epistaxis, he'll probably apply a vasoconstrictive agent or silver nitrate (a cauterization agent) directly on the site. If this doesn't stop the bleeding, he'll insert an anterior nasal pack made from petrolatum gauze. If the patient complains of feeling blood trickling down his throat, the doctor will insert posterior nasal packing with either a balloon catheter or gauze. (See *Understanding Nasal Packing.*) For a patient who receives either type of

**Nasal gauze packing**

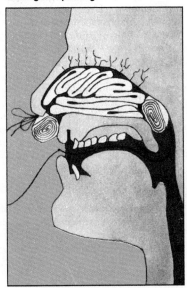

**Double-cuffed nasal balloon catheter**

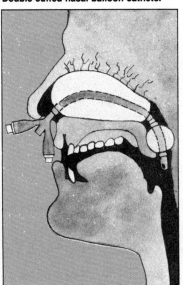

If your patient has nasal packing, keep these points in mind while you're caring for him:
• Your patient can't breathe through his nose once the nasal pack's in place. If he panics, remind him to breathe through his mouth; then calm him and elevate the head of his bed.
• The nasal pack can slip out of place and fall down the patient's throat, occluding his airway. If this happens, quickly cut the dental roll sutures, untape the suture on his cheek, and pull the pack from his mouth.
• Watch your patient for signs and symptoms of hypoxia. This can happen when the

posterior pack depresses his soft palate, causing airway resistance.
• Look for signs and symptoms of hypertension or hypotension. Sedatives or tranquilizers may cause either disorder; severe bleeding and hypovolemia may cause hypotension.

In some EDs, doctors use a disposable single- or double-cuffed nasal balloon catheter instead of gauze packing for posterior bleeding. When inflated, the balloon cuffs compress blood vessels, controlling bleeding. (Anterior packing is also inserted to prevent pressure necrosis of the nostrils from the catheter.)

packing, the doctor will ask you to insert an I.V. and to begin administering broad-spectrum antibiotics. Expect to administer a decongestant, too, to prevent sinusitis.

### Therapeutic care

If your patient's bleeding couldn't be stopped and he required posterior nasal packing to control his epistaxis, he'll be admitted for close observation. Assess him frequently, watching for signs and symptoms of respiratory dis-

tress. Nasal packing restricts a patient's breathing, so expect to give supplemental oxygen by mask to prevent hypoxia.

If the balloon catheter slips back and occludes your patient's airway, quickly cut the catheter and pull it out. Be prepared for this emergency: keep scissors taped near your patient's bed.

Because your patient has an open blood vessel that allows bacteria to freely enter his circulation, he's vulnerable to infection. Assess his vital signs frequently. (Remember that chills or pain over his sinus area, eyebrow, or forehead may indicate sinusitis.) Start him on a full-liquid or semisolid diet, as ordered. If your patient's appetite is poor, explain that this is probably because he can't smell the food. Remember, nasal packing is not only uncomfortable for your patient but frightening, as well. Give him your emotional support.

# Peritonsillar Abscess

## Prediagnosis summary

Initial assessment of the patient revealed some or all of these signs and symptoms:
• a history of sore throat lasting 5 to 10 days
• increasing unilateral throat pain
• swollen cervical lymph nodes
• trismus
• drooling
• foul breath
• muffled speech
• fever and chills.

The doctor examined the patient's throat and found that the tonsillar pillars and soft palate were edematous and that the uvula was displaced away from the abscess.

## Priorities

Watch your patient closely for signs and symptoms of respiratory distress, particularly airway obstruction due to increasing edema or to pus from the ruptured abscess sac. If necessary, administer oxygen by nasal cannula, and call the doctor *immediately*. Expect to assist him with emergency intubation.

Administer analgesics, as ordered, to relieve the patient's pain. If he has trismus, the medication will also help to relieve his muscle spasms.

## Continuing assessment and intervention

The doctor will ask you to obtain a throat culture specimen for culture-and-sensitivity testing and then to start an I.V. for antibiotic therapy and fluid replacement. Ask your patient if he has any drug allergies—particularly to the drug of choice, penicillin. When the culture results return, check to see if the organism causing the infection is sensitive to the antibiotic you've administered. If it isn't, the doctor will change the medication.

One way or another, the abscess must drain. Either it will rupture spontaneously or the doctor will incise it. Provide an emesis basin so your patient can spit out the drainage.

## Therapeutic care

Continue to administer analgesics for pain, as needed, and watch your patient for signs and symptoms of respiratory distress. His condition should improve within 24 to 48 hours after the start of antibiotic therapy.

# A FINAL WORD

As a nurse, you're probably aware that mortality among patients with EENT emergencies is low—about 20%. The primary *threat to life,* of course, occurs when a patient's upper airway is obstructed. But many EENT emergencies can affect the *quality of life* without necessarily threatening it. For example, ear trauma can diminish the patient's hearing, and many common eye emergencies—such as chemical burns or penetrating injuries—can reduce or destroy a patient's vision.

Fortunately, this threat is becoming less common every day. One reason for this is the development of sophisticated surgical techniques, such as laser technology and cryosurgery. These techniques, which are less invasive than traditional surgery, allow the patient to recover more quickly with less risk of postsurgical complications.

Here are some more examples: Implanting permanent artificial lenses in the eyes—a technique that was unheard-of 10 years ago—now restores sight to cataract patients. And breakthroughs in replantation surgery—such as surgically burying the amputated portion of an ear to allow revascularization before replantation—have greatly increased the chances that the surgery will be successful. Of course, this means that such a patient's related hearing disability will be minimal—or may never occur.

What about *your* role, as a nurse, in successfully managing patients with EENT emergencies? Here's where your ability to respond quickly and to anticipate needed interventions can help ensure minimal loss of function for your patient—and a return to the quality of life he enjoyed before his emergency occurred.

## Selected References

Bates, Barbara. *A Guide to Physical Examination*, 3rd ed. Philadelphia: J.B. Lippincott Co., 1983.

Brown, Melissa M. "Symposium on Opthalmic Nursing. Retinal Vascular Disorders: Nursing and Medical Implications," *Nursing Clinics of North America* 16(3):415-32, September 1981.

Cavalier, J.P. "When Moments Count... The Two Eye Emergencies that Demand Instant Intervention," *RN* 44:41-3, November 1981.

Henkind, Paul, and Chambers, Jerre. "Arterial Occlusive Disease of the Retina," in *Clinical Ophthalmology*, 5 vols. and index. (Loose Leaf Reference Service.) Edited by Thomas Duane.

Kilroy, J.L. "Symposium on Opthalmic Nursing. Care and Teaching of Patients With Glaucoma," *Nursing Clinics of North America* 16(3):393-404, September 1981.

Kinney, Marguerite, et al. *AACN's Clinical Reference for Critical Care Nursing.* New York: McGraw-Hill Book Co., 1981.

Lanros, Nedell E. *Assessment and Intervention in Emergency Nursing*, 2nd ed. Bowie, Md.: Robert J. Brady Co., 1982.

Luckmann, Joan, and Sorenson, Karen C. *Medical-Surgical Nursing: A Psychophysiologic Approach*, 2nd ed. Philadelphia: W.B. Saunders Co., 1980.

Paton, David, and Goldberg, Morton F. *Management of Ocular Injuries.* Philadelphia: W.B. Saunders Co., 1976.

Saunders, William, et al. *Nursing Care in Eye, Ear, Nose, and Throat Disorders, Nineteen Seventy-Nine*, 4th ed. St. Louis: C.V. Mosby Co., 1978.

Smith, Joan F., and Nachazel, Delbert P. *Ophthalmologic Nursing.* Boston: Little, Brown & Co., 1980.

Snow, James B. *An Introduction to Otorhinolaryngology.* Chicago: Year Book Medical Pubs., 1979.

# 10

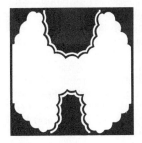

# Endocrine and Metabolic Emergencies

## Introduction

You're on ED duty early one afternoon when you notice a police car pulling up to the entrance. Two policemen get out and lift an unkempt woman, about age 65, out of the backseat. She's obviously extremely weak—she's barely able to walk. The policemen seem to be half carrying and half dragging her.

You rush out with a wheelchair to meet them; the two men unceremoniously drop the woman into it. "She's just drunk," one of them says contemptuously. "Name's Edith Olenik. She collapsed in a bar down on South Street and the owner called us. We thought you'd better check her out before we take her in."

Of course, as a nurse, you know better than to assume that Edith's "just drunk." True, she collapsed in a bar and her breath smells faintly of wine. But you know that many other conditions could be responsible for her lethargy, confusion, and weakness.

In the ED, you begin your assessment by noting that Edith's flushed and that her skin's warm, dry, and loose. When you quickly take her vital signs, you find a rapid, weak pulse, low blood pressure, and a slight fever. And Edith seems to be getting weaker and more lethargic by the minute.

"Did she have a purse?" you ask. One of the policemen runs out to the car for it. Quickly, you sort through Edith's wallet, looking for clues. With many patients, this effort proves futile. Today, however, you're lucky—you find a small card identifying Edith as a diabetic.

Edith's card doesn't say whether she's a Type I (insulin-dependent) or a Type II (non-insulin-dependent) diabetic. Without that knowledge, you can't be sure what's happening. But her condition leads you to suspect that she's suffering from either diabetic ketoacidosis (DKA) or the early stages of hyperglycemic hyperosmolar nonketotic coma (HHNC). You'll need to perform a thorough physical assessment, to obtain a history, and to get the results of blood and urine tests before you can be sure. But at least now you know where to start.

Do you *always* know where to start when you see a patient who may have an endocrine emergency? As your own experience has probably demonstrated, these emergencies can be difficult to recognize. Some of them (for example, myxedema crisis or acute hypoparathyroidism) are relatively rare—so health-care professionals don't get practice in recognizing them. Others, particularly those related to diabetes (DKA and HHNC, for example), are fairly common—but resemble each other so closely that telling one from the other during an emergency is extremely difficult. These problems, however, don't change your responsibility for recognizing endocrine and metabolic emergencies. Remember, an endocrine emergency is *always* a crisis because hormones affect all the body's functions. A patient with *any* of these emergency conditions needs your immediate intervention.

As you can see, endocrine emergencies provide a unique set of nursing challenges: first, to recognize them; second, to differentiate among them; third, to respond to them quickly and correctly. Be sure you're prepared to meet these challenges. You just may prevent a misdiagnosis—and save a patient's life.

# INITIAL CARE

## Prehospital Care: What's Been Done

If rescue personnel brought the patient to the ED, chances are they were called because the patient was *confused, lethargic,* or in a *coma.* They took steps to stabilize his condition during transport, but they probably had few or no clues to the cause of his signs and symptoms.

Initially, rescue personnel cleared the patient's airway. If the patient was vomiting, they turned him on his side to prevent him from aspirating his vomitus. They assessed the patient's breathing and provided supplemental oxygen by nasal cannula or mask, if necessary.

If his respirations were severely depressed (as may occur in a patient with hypoglycemia or myxedema coma) and the rescue personnel were qualified and equipped, they intubated him or

they may have inserted an esophageal obturator airway. They also assisted his ventilation with an Ambu bag.

Next, rescue personnel assessed the patient's pulse rate, blood pressure, and temperature. They may have found signs of dehydration—common in these emergencies. If the patient had signs of dehydration, and if the rescuers were qualified, they started an I.V. and infused dextrose 5% in water ($D_5W$), normal saline solution, or dextrose 5% in 0.45% sodium chloride, for fluid replacement.

Rescue personnel may have tested a drop of the patient's blood with glucose-testing tape, such as Dextrostix, to check his blood glucose level. If the level was low or borderline—or if the patient was unconscious—rescue personnel probably gave 50 ml of 50% dextrose as an I.V. push, to reverse the effects of possible hypoglycemia.

If the patient's temperature was very high, rescue personnel removed his clothing and applied ice packs—or cool, wet cloths—to his axillae and groin.

Rescue personnel also initiated cardiac monitoring (if the transport vehicle was equipped for this), and they may have noted dysrhythmias.

When you receive the patient, obtain a thorough report of what's been done for him. Be especially careful to note and document his vital signs, any dysrhythmias, the results of his blood glucose test, and his response to I.V. dextrose (if given).

## What to Do First

As you know, an endocrine emergency affects *all* of a patient's body systems. Your patient won't have an obvious traumatic injury, and he's unlikely to have clear-cut signs and symptoms of respiratory, cardiovascular, neurologic, GI, or other body system disorders. Instead, he may have vague and

## UNDERSTANDING HORMONAL CONTROL SYSTEMS

"Together, the endocrine and neurologic systems control body metabolism and maintain homeostasis." This simple sentence sums up a highly complex group of processes that defy quick comprehension. But if you take the time now to review how hormonal control systems work, you'll have a clearer idea of what's happening when one of your patients has an endocrine emergency.

One type of control, a *negative feedback system,* consists of an endocrine gland and a target tissue (illustration A). This system's activated by the imbalance that results from too much or too little hormone secretion. A hormone deficiency triggers the responsible endocrine gland, which releases its hormone to a specific target tissue. Once the target tissue's hormone level is adequate, it signals the endocrine gland to reduce secretion. For example, in response to an insufficient blood calcium level, the parathyroid glands release additional amounts of parathyroid hormone (PTH), which stimulates calcium reabsorption from bones (the target tissue) into the bloodstream. This raises the circulating calcium level; once it's sufficient, the parathyroid glands decrease PTH secretion.

This negative feedback system maintains hormone concentrations at relatively stable levels. Any disruption of this feedback system—for example, if the parathyroid gland is injured or removed during thyroid surgery—will mean the target tissue's demand for increased PTH can't be met, and the patient may develop hypocalcemia secondary to acute hypoparathyroidism.

In a second type of hormonal control system, nerve impulses stimulate an endocrine gland to release its hormone (illustration B). For example, a rapidly falling blood glucose level (hypoglycemia) will be brought back to normal when it triggers compensatory mechanisms, via the sympathetic nervous system (SNS), that stimulate glycogenolysis and gluconeogenesis. One such mechanism stimulates the adrenal medulla to secrete catecholamines (primarily epinephrine), which in turn help stimulate glycogenolysis and gluconeogenesis. If the SNS is unable to compensate for a falling blood glucose level, as it may for a diabetic with autonomic neuropathy, serious problems can develop. If the neuropathy is very severe, it may prevent the SNS from sending impulses to the adrenal medulla to secrete catecholamines. And without the catecholamine response that stimulates glycogenolysis and gluconeogenesis, severe hypoglycemia may develop.

A third hormonal control system combines elements of the negative feedback system with neurologic system controls, as an endocrine gland interacts with the hypothalamus and the pituitary gland (illustration C). Thyroid hormone regulation is an example of this control system. The hypothalamus secretes a thyrotropin-releasing factor (TRF), which stimulates the anterior pituitary gland to release thyroid-stimulating hormone (TSH). Then, TSH stimulates the thyroid gland to secrete its hormone. When the thyroid hormone level is sufficient, the hypothalamus reduces TRF secretion.

Any disruption of this control system will also have serious consequences; examples include myxedema crisis—a life-threatening complication of deficient thyroid hormone production—and thyroid storm, which results from thyroid hormone overproduction.

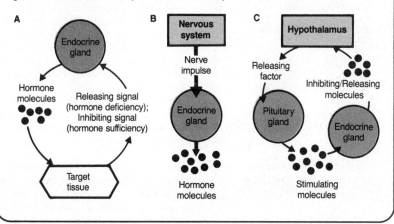

**A**  
Endocrine gland  
Hormone molecules  
Releasing signal (hormone deficiency); Inhibiting signal (hormone sufficiency)  
Target tissue

**B**  
Nervous system  
Nerve impulse  
Endocrine gland  
Hormone molecules

**C**  
Hypothalamus  
Releasing factor  
Inhibiting/Releasing molecules  
Pituitary gland  
Endocrine gland  
Stimulating molecules

confusing signs and symptoms that appear to reflect systemic illness.

Remember to *suspect* an endocrine emergency whenever you see an obviously sick, distressed patient with an altered level of consciousness and signs of increased or decreased metabolism. As in any emergency, your first steps with such a patient are to rapidly assess

PRIORITIES

## INITIAL ASSESSMENT CHECKLIST

**Assess the ABCs first and intervene appropriately.**

**Check for:**
• wheezing or stridor, indicating airway obstruction from laryngeal spasm related to hypocalcemia from hypoparathyroidism
• tachypnea, indicating hypermetabolism, such as in thyrotoxic crisis; bradypnea, indicating hypometabolism, such as in myxedema coma; or Kussmaul's respirations, indicating diabetic ketoacidosis (DKA)
• alterations in level of consciousness, indicating DKA, hyperglycemic hyperosmolar nonketotic coma (HHNC), or hypoglycemia
• dry mucous membranes, dry skin, and decreased skin turgor, indicating severe dehydration from DKA, HHNC, or adrenal crisis
• decreased blood pressure, increased pulse rate, and cool, clammy skin, indicating hypovolemia such as in DKA, HHNC, or adrenal crisis.

**Intervene by:**
• inserting a large-bore I.V. line and administering fluids, as ordered

**Prepare for:**
• an EKG tracing to check for dysrhythmias and electrolyte imbalances
• administration of glucose, potassium, sodium bicarbonate, or other electrolytes, and hormones.

his airway, breathing, circulation, general appearance, and mental status (including life-threatening signs of central nervous system alterations) and to intervene as appropriate. Your assessment of his general appearance and mental status is particularly important because you'll find clues to the severity of his endocrine emergency. Remember, *endocrine emergencies share many common characteristics*.

### Airway

Start by assessing the patency of your patient's airway. (If he's unconscious, his tongue may fall back, occluding his airway.) Insert an oral airway or assist in endotracheal intubation, as necessary.

Listen for wheezing or stridor. Wheezing results from small-airway obstruction, such as may occur if your patient aspirates vomitus. (Vomiting—from gastric dilatation and decreased peristalsis—is a sign common to many endocrine emergencies, so be particularly alert to this possibility.) If your patient has aspirated food particles, remove them immediately, using a finger sweep or suction, as necessary. Turn your patient on his side to decrease the risk of further aspiration. If his level of consciousness is decreased, he may be unable to clear his own secretions or vomitus. Insert a nasogastric (NG) tube, if necessary, to prevent aspiration and to decompress his stomach.

You may hear stridor if the patient has laryngeal spasm from tetany due to hypocalcemia. (Severe hypoparathyroidism decreases blood calcium levels and can result in tetany.) If your patient has respiratory distress or stridor, and you suspect laryngeal spasm, call the doctor *immediately*. Without immediate intervention your patient may die within minutes.

Get ready to administer I.V. calcium gluconate to relieve the spasm, and prepare for an emergency tracheotomy. (The doctor may have to do a tracheotomy to provide an airway until the calcium can relieve the spasm.) Remember that you must give calcium gluconate *slowly,* despite the urgency of your patient's condition, because calcium given too quickly can cause severe hypotension and cardiac arrest. Administer the calcium over 5 minutes, even if this means that the doctor must perform an emergency tracheotomy.

## Breathing

Assess the quality of your patient's respirations, noting their rate, rhythm, and depth. Remember, acute endocrine disorders cause alterations in metabolism that can influence the mechanics of ventilation.

Watch for tachypnea—a common manifestation of the hypermetabolism that occurs with thyrotoxic crisis, diabetic ketoacidosis, hyperglycemic hyperosmolar nonketotic coma, and adrenal crisis (see these entries in this chapter). Tachypnea may also be due to fluid and electrolyte imbalance or to infection—common precipitating factors of endocrine emergencies. Watch a patient with tachypnea closely; if his breathing suddenly slows and becomes bradypneic, his condition is deteriorating. Be sure to call the doctor *immediately.*

Watch your patient also for Kussmaul's respirations—slow, deep respirations indicative of metabolic acidosis (see *Understanding Metabolic Acidosis,* page 465). Kussmaul's respirations occur as your patient's respiratory system attempts to compensate for his metabolic acidosis by blowing off $CO_2$. As he reduces his blood levels of $CO_2$, his pH will start to shift back to normal.

If you note this breathing pattern, report it to the doctor *immediately,* and expect him to draw blood for arterial blood gases to determine the extent of the patient's acidosis.

Your patient's respirations may also be severely depressed, reflecting the hypometabolism that occurs with myxedema coma or hypoglycemia. As you know, respiratory depression may lead to respiratory arrest. Provide supple-

mental oxygen by nasal cannula or mask, and anticipate the need for intubation and mechanical ventilation.

## Circulation

With your patient's breathing stabilized, quickly assess his circulatory status. Your most important considerations are impending circulatory collapse and possible dysrhythmias—emergencies common to many endocrine crises. Check his vital signs and note any indications of hypovolemia, such as hypotension and tachycardia. You may see signs and symptoms of hypovolemia if your patient has:

• *thyrotoxic crisis (thyroid storm)* — Profuse diaphoresis causes dehydration leading to hypotension and circulatory collapse.

• *myxedema coma*—Fluid shifts may cause diminished plasma volume leading to hypovolemia and circulatory collapse.

• *DKA or HHNC*—Hyperglycemia causes massive osmotic diuresis leading to hypovolemia and circulatory collapse.

• *adrenal crisis*—Fluid depletion from the crisis and cortisol inadequacy from stress cause severe hypotension leading to circulatory collapse.

If you note hypotension, place the patient supine with his feet elevated 20° to 30° unless his other signs and symptoms—for instance, possible congestive heart failure (CHF) occurring with thyrotoxic crisis—contraindicate this. Insert at least one large-bore I.V. line and administer volume expanders, such as normal saline solution, as ordered. Draw blood for laboratory tests, as ordered—the results will help you understand why the patient's dehydrated. If possible, obtain a urine sample for routine analysis and for culture-and-sensitivity and osmolarity tests.

Obtain a 12-lead EKG tracing and start cardiac monitoring to check for dysrhythmias. These may result from:

• the effects of hypometabolism or hypermetabolism on cardiac muscle

• electrolyte disturbances from exces-

## AN ADDED RISK

Your diabetic pregnant patient is more likely than most diabetics to develop hypoglycemia, especially during the first trimester. Why? One reason is that to ensure healthy fetal growth, her doctor will try to tightly control her blood glucose through a balance of insulin dosage, diet, and a specified amount of daily exercise. Any disruption of this delicate balance can cause a drop in her blood glucose. Another reason is that glucose passes through the placenta to nourish the growing fetus, possibly decreasing your patient's insulin requirements. Still another reason is that patients with morning sickness tend to skip breakfast and are likely to develop hypoglycemia.

Suspect hypoglycemia in any diabetic pregnant patient who's confused, diaphoretic, and weak, and who complains of tingling sensations, tremors, and palpitations. Give her oral or I.V. glucose promptly. When the episode's under control, make sure she talks with her doctor—he may want to adjust her insulin dosage.

sive diuresis or from alterations in aldosterone levels
• changes in myocardial contractility due to hypocalcemia, as seen in patients with acute hypoparathyroidism.

Of course, call the doctor *immediately* if you note any dysrhythmias (see the "Cardiac Dysrhythmias" entry in Chapter 5). Cardiac arrest may occur at any moment—be sure you're prepared to intervene.

### General appearance

Check your patient's skin color, temperature, moisture, and turgor. He may be very pale if he's hypovolemic, or flushed and hot with the fever of thyrotoxic crisis. If the patient's skin is very cool and dry, he may have myxedema coma. Profuse diaphoresis may accompany hypoglycemia or thyrotoxic crisis. Check your patient's skin turgor by pinching a fold of skin and noting its elasticity. If he's extremely dehydrated (as with DKA or HHNC), his skin may be very loose even over his forehead, and his eyeball may feel soft when you *gently* palpate it (through his closed lid, of course). Report your findings to the doctor, and start an intake and output record. The doctor may ask you to increase the patient's I.V. infusion rate.

Assess your patient for tremors, restlessness, or nervousness—possible signs of increased sympathetic nervous stimulation or of altered electrolyte balance.

Check your patient's breath for a sweet, fruity smell, which may indicate DKA.

### Mental status

Assess your patient's mental status and neurologic function—sensitive indicators of hypo- or hypermetabolism. Alterations in level of consciousness may range from hyperactivity and restlessness to lethargy, deep stupor, or coma. If your patient's level of consciousness is decreasing, he may have seizures prior to coma. Possible causes of these seizures include:
• metabolic acidosis
• high serum osmolarity
• carbon dioxide intoxication
• low blood glucose level
• decreased calcium level.

Keep an oral airway near the patient in anticipation of seizure activity. If he does have a seizure, protect him from injury during his convulsions, and observe the type of seizure activity: note tonic and clonic stages, the body parts involved, and the order of their involvement. Immediately after the seizure, check the patient for a patent airway and for any apparent injury. Notify the doctor *at once*—seizures indicate that the patient's underlying endocrine crisis is worsening and requires immediate medical treatment. Without treatment, the patient will continue to have seizures (see the "Generalized Tonic-Clonic Status Epilepticus" entry in Chapter 6) and may progress to coma.

Always suspect hypoglycemia if your patient has an altered level of consciousness. Blood tests will confirm this, but you can't wait until they return from the laboratory. Instead, test a drop of your patient's blood with a blood glucose reagent strip such as Visidex, Chemstrip bG, or Dextrostix. (Remember, however, that these strips are susceptible to deterioration from light, heat, and moisture. Make sure you get accurate results by using *fresh* glucose-testing strips.) If you note a low blood glucose level (below 60 mg/dl), notify the doctor and give some readily available form of glucose *immediately*—orange juice, candy, nondiet soda, or corn syrup if the patient's conscious and able to take food by mouth; I.V. dextrose (50%) if he's unconscious or unable to swallow. (As soon as the patient regains consciousness, give him glucose by mouth.)

You may note high blood glucose levels during your test—400 or more mg/dl. If you find this result, test a drop of your patient's urine with a ketone reagent strip such as Ketostix or Keto-Diastix. Notify the doctor of your results—*positive* ketones combined with a high blood glucose level indicate that your patient has DKA, whereas *negative* ketones combined with a high blood glucose level indicate HHNC. Your quick test can help the doctor differentiate between these confusingly similar conditions.

# What to Do Next

After you've completed your primary assessment and intervened as necessary, take a few minutes to determine your patient's chief complaints and to perform a quick physical assessment. Remember that endocrine emergencies affect *all* body systems, so your patient's signs and symptoms may mimic illnesses found in other body systems and may appear in seemingly paradoxical combinations. Don't overlook complaints that seem vague or generalized—in combination with your patient's history, they may help the doctor make his diagnosis.

When you're identifying your patient's chief complaints, ask him if he's ever been diagnosed as having a *chronic endocrine disorder,* such as diabetes, thyroid disease, Addison's disease, or hypoparathyroidism. As you probably know, almost all endocrine emergencies occur in patients with chronic endocrine disorders that have been aggravated by stress or illness. If your patient has a history of endocrine disease, determine if he's experienced illness or emotional stress recently. Find out how long he's had his endocrine disorder, what medical treatment he's had, if he takes his medications as ordered, and what difficulties he's experienced in the past. Don't forget to ask if he's ever had an episode similar to the one he's having now and, if so, what happened. This information will provide an important clue to his condition.

If he's never been diagnosed as having an endocrine disorder, remember that some patients may have an *undiscovered* endocrine disease for years. Ask if his weight has fluctuated—changes may indicate long-standing endocrine disease predisposing him to particular endocrine crises. Take a quick look at his skin and hair. Fine, soft hair and a history of weight loss, for instance, may indicate long-standing *hyper*thyroidism, predisposing him to thyrotoxic crisis. Or, coarse, dry hair; cool, dry skin; and a history of weight gain may indicate long-standing *hypo*thyroidism, predisposing him to myxedema crisis. Hyperpigmentation (abnormally tanned skin) may indicate Addison's disease, meaning he's at risk for adrenal crisis.

Ask your patient if he's experienced *increased thirst* (polydipsia) or *increased urination* (polyuria). These alterations of internal fluid balance may occur in a patient whose diabetes has

## EKG CHANGES IN ELECTROLYTE IMBALANCES

Do you know that your patient's EKG strips can provide valuable information on his electrolyte status? A potassium, calcium, or magnesium imbalance—either an excess or a deficiency—will have a marked effect on your patient's cardiac conduction system, as

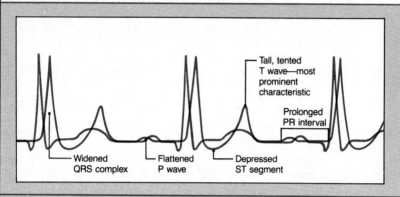

Tall, tented T wave—most prominent characteristic

Prolonged PR interval

Widened QRS complex

Flattened P wave

Depressed ST segment

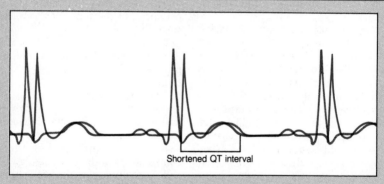

Shortened QT interval

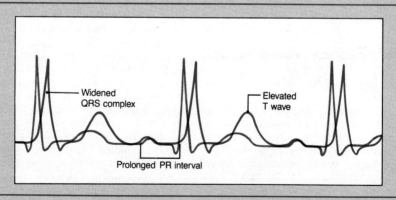

Widened QRS complex

Elevated T wave

Prolonged PR interval

**KEY:**    ▮ Abnormal    ▮ Normal

shown on his EKG strip. Learn to recognize these EKG abnormalities—they may help you prevent serious and possibly life-threatening problems.

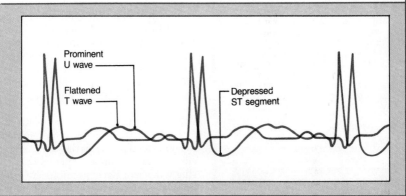

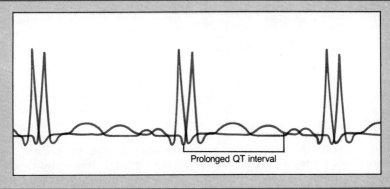

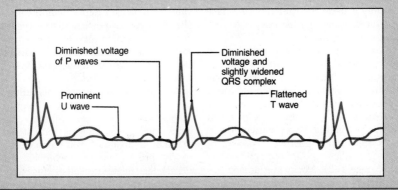

## STORM WARNING

Your patient in thyrotoxic crisis (thyroid storm) will be treated with a number of drugs to control his signs and symptoms and to reduce his thyroid hormone levels. But, before administering drugs, find out what he's *already* taking. Watch for two drugs, in particular, that can cause complications in this patient:

• **aspirin,** which your patient may be taking for a condition such as arthritis. Large doses of aspirin *may* increase free thyroxine levels and exacerbate thyrotoxic crisis.

• **propranolol** (Inderal), which your patient may be taking for a cardiovascular condition, such as angina or hypertension. Thyrotoxic crisis may precipitate congestive heart failure; if so, propranolol *may* be contraindicated.

If your patient's taking either of these medications, notify the doctor at once—he may want to adjust his patient's medical therapy appropriately.

progressed to DKA or HHNC and may cause severe dehydration. Continue fluid replacement as ordered by the doctor, and insert an indwelling (Foley) catheter as ordered to monitor fluid output accurately. Remember—if your patient's had polyuria and polydipsia for several days, he may have severe *electrolyte imbalances* accompanying his fluid imbalance. So watch his cardiac monitor closely for dysrhythmias (see *EKG Changes in Electrolyte Imbalances,* pages 434 and 435).

Ask your patient if he's experienced *paresthesias, muscle cramps,* or *muscle spasms,* which may be caused by the hypocalcemia that accompanies acute hypoparathyroidism. If he's experienced any of these, check for latent tetany by looking for a positive *Chvostek's sign* and a positive *Trousseau's sign* (see *Eliciting Signs of Latent Tetany,* page 468). Notify the doctor immediately if these are positive, because they're a warning that laryngeal spasm may occlude the patient's airway. Administer calcium gluconate, if ordered, to correct his hypocalcemia.

Your patient may complain of *abdominal pain, nausea,* or *vomiting.* Auscultate his bowel sounds—they may be hypoactive if your patient has myxedema crisis. Continue NG suctioning, as ordered, to decompress his stomach. Palpate his abdomen gently; you may detect localized tenderness suggestive of infection—an important finding because infection may have precipitated your patient's endocrine crisis. Or you may detect an enlarged liver, which often accompanies DKA or thyrotoxic crisis.

Your patient may also complain of *fatigue* and *weakness*—symptoms of hypometabolism, occurring with myxedema crisis; neuroglycopenia, occurring with hypoglycemia; or electrolyte imbalance, occurring with any of many endocrine crises. Ask him if these are constant or intermittent, how long he's felt this way, and when they occur.

Continue your assessment by determining other important history findings. Your patient may have *chronic diseases* that may further compromise his condition. Ask particularly about cardiovascular disease—such as atherosclerosis, angina, or past myocardial infarction—because cardiovascular complications are very real possibilities in your patient with an altered metabolism. His weakened heart may not tolerate the increase in heart rate that results from hypermetabolism or the decrease in perfusion that results from hypometabolism. If your patient has a history of cardiovascular disease, be alert for signs of developing CHF or myocardial infarction.

Also ask about chronic respiratory or renal disease, which may require alterations in treatment of the endocrine emergency. If your patient has asthma, for instance, you won't expect to give propranolol hydrochloride (Inderal) for the treatment of thyrotoxic crisis, because Inderal may cause acute respiratory distress in this patient. If your patient has renal failure, the dosage of insulin he receives for the treatment of DKA or HHNC will usually need to be decreased.

Ask your patient what other *medications* he's taking, because medications often alter hormonal levels. For example, aspirin increases free thyroxine ($T_4$) levels, increasing hypermetabolism due to thyrotoxic crisis. And steroid therapy makes your patient particularly vulnerable to adrenal crisis, because steroids suppress the adrenal glands' production of hormones. Of course, if your patient is taking insulin for Type I diabetes, you'll determine the type, the dosage, and when he took his last dose. This information will help the doctor calculate the patient's insulin infusion rate.

Determine if your patient has any food, drug, or environmental *allergies*. If he does, an allergic reaction may have precipitated his endocrine crisis. Ask specifically about allergies to antibiotics, because your patient will probably receive these drugs if he has an infection.

Document all your findings carefully. They'll provide a baseline that you and other health-care personnel can use to measure your patient's progress.

# Special Considerations

### Pediatric

Don't forget to consider that sudden acute illness in a child may signal the onset of an endocrine disorder. You may, for example, see a child with severe dehydration and altered mental status—with no previous history of an endocrine disorder—who now has DKA. Ask the parents if the child's had a recent illness. If he has, did the parents note weight loss, lethargy, polyuria, and polydipsia? They may have assumed that these were aftereffects of the illness when, in fact, they were early signs of Type I (insulin-dependent) diabetes. Always check blood glucose levels in a child with these signs and

symptoms—the results of a glucose reagent strip test can provide a quick clue to your patient's condition.

### Geriatric

Consider the possibility of acute myxedema in an elderly patient who's lethargic or comatose. The onset of myxedema may be insidious and may simulate such expected signs of aging as dry skin and hair loss. Myxedema is also especially common in older women who have significant atherosclerosis, and it occurs *after* hospital admission in up to 50% of these patients. If you're caring for a hospitalized geriatric patient with a history of hypothyroidism, be alert for this possibility.

# CARE AFTER DIAGNOSIS

# Diabetic Ketoacidosis

### Prediagnosis summary

On initial assessment, the patient had some combination of these signs and symptoms:
- decreased level of consciousness (which may have been as mild as drowsiness or inattentiveness or as severe as coma)
- fatigue and weakness
- abdominal pain and tenderness
- nausea and vomiting
- warm, dry, loose skin with decreased skin turgor (indications of dehydration)
- hypotension
- tachycardia and thready pulse
- oliguria
- acetone breath (fruity breath odor)
- Kussmaul's respirations
- polyuria and polydipsia
- fever
- a history of diabetes (usually Type I).

PATHOPHYSIOLOGY

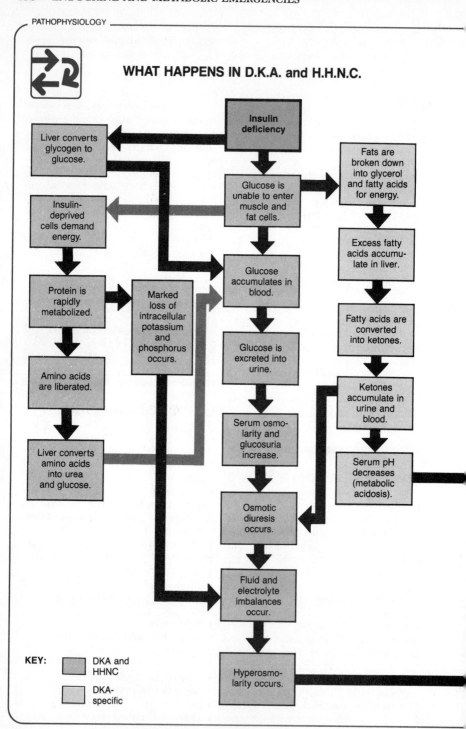

## WHAT HAPPENS IN D.K.A. and H.H.N.C.

Insulin deficiency

Liver converts glycogen to glucose.

Glucose is unable to enter muscle and fat cells.

Fats are broken down into glycerol and fatty acids for energy.

Insulin-deprived cells demand energy.

Glucose accumulates in blood.

Excess fatty acids accumulate in liver.

Protein is rapidly metabolized.

Marked loss of intracellular potassium and phosphorus occurs.

Fatty acids are converted into ketones.

Amino acids are liberated.

Glucose is excreted into urine.

Ketones accumulate in urine and blood.

Liver converts amino acids into urea and glucose.

Serum osmolarity and glucosuria increase.

Serum pH decreases (metabolic acidosis).

Osmotic diuresis occurs.

Fluid and electrolyte imbalances occur.

Hyperosmolarity occurs.

KEY:
DKA and HHNC

DKA-specific

Diabetic ketoacidosis (DKA) and hyperglycemic hyperosmolar nonketotic coma (HHNC) are acute complications of hyperglycemic crisis that may occur in your diabetic patient. If not treated properly, either may result in coma and death.

DKA occurs most often in patients with Type I diabetes; it may also be the initial event in a patient with unrecognized Type I diabetes. HHNC occurs most often in patients with Type II diabetes. But HHNC may also occur in anyone whose insulin tolerance is stressed and in patients who've undergone certain therapeutic procedures—such as peritoneal dialysis, hemodialysis, tube feedings, or total parenteral nutrition.

Acute insulin deficiency (absolute in DKA; relative in HHNC) precipitates both conditions. Causes include:

- illness
- stress
- infection
- failure to take insulin (in a patient with DKA *only*).

Inadequate insulin hinders glucose uptake by fat and muscle cells. Since the cells can't take in glucose to convert to energy, glucose accumulates in the blood. At the same time, the liver responds to the demands of the energy-starved cells by converting glycogen to glucose and releasing glucose into the blood, *further* increasing the blood glucose level. When this level exceeds the renal threshold, excess glucose is excreted in the blood.

Still, the insulin-deprived cells can't utilize glucose. Their response? Rapid metabolism of protein, which results in loss of intracellular potassium and phosphorus and in excessive liberation of amino acids. The liver converts these amino acids into urea and glucose.

As a result of these processes, blood glucose levels grossly elevate. The result is increased serum osmolarity and glucosuria (higher in HHNC than in DKA, because blood glucose levels are higher in HHNC), leading to osmotic diuresis.

The massive fluid loss from osmotic diuresis causes fluid and electrolyte imbalances and dehydration. Water loss is greater than electrolyte loss, contributing to hyperosmolarity. This, in turn, perpetuates dehydration, decreasing the glomerular filtration rate and reducing the amount of glucose excreted in the urine. This leads to a vicious—and deadly—cycle: decreased glucose excretion *further* increases blood glucose levels, increasing hyperosmolarity and dehydration and finally causing shock, coma, and death.

All these steps hold true for both DKA and HHNC. But DKA has an additional simultaneous process that leads to metabolic acidosis. The *absolute* insulin deficiency causes cells to convert fats into glycerol and fatty acids for energy. The fatty acids can't be metabolized as quickly as they're released, so they accumulate in the liver, where they're converted into ketones (ketoacids). These ketones accumulate in the blood and urine and cause *acidosis*. Acidosis leads to more tissue breakdown, more ketosis, more acidosis, and, eventually, shock, coma, and death.

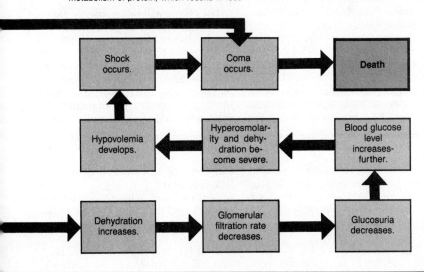

An I.V. was started for fluid and medication administration, a chest X-ray (using portable equipment) and a 12-lead EKG were taken, and cardiac monitoring was begun. If the patient was obtunded, an endotracheal tube and an NG tube were inserted to empty gastric contents and left in for continuous suctioning. Blood was drawn for a complete blood count (CBC), electrolytes, blood glucose, serum acetone, blood urea nitrogen (BUN), creatinine, serum amylase, lipase, and arterial blood gases (ABGs). A drop of the patient's blood was tested in the ED with a glucose reagent strip (such as Visidex II or Chemstrip bG) and with a nitroprusside reagent (such as Acetest) for serum ketones. His blood glucose and ketone levels were found to be elevated.

## Priorities

Your patient will have *decreased effective circulating volume*—a result of glycosuria and osmotic diuresis from his marked hyperglycemia. To stabilize him, your first priorities will be restoring his fluid volume and decreasing his hyperglycemia, in that order.

In addition to losing large amounts of water (up to 8 liters), your patient will lose electrolytes, particularly sodium (300 to 500 mEq), chloride, and potassium. Expect to administer normal saline solution rapidly. You may infuse as much as a liter in the first 30 minutes and give a total of 3 to 4 liters over the first 2 to 3 hours, using infusion rates of 1,000 ml/hour. The doctor may insert a central venous pressure (CVP) line to infuse fluid rapidly and to evaluate the relationship between the patient's volume status and his general heart function. This is especially likely if the patient is a child with long-standing diabetes or an elderly person, because these patients are most susceptible to fluid overload. Assist the doctor as necessary in placing the CVP line, and record the initial readings.

If your patient is severely dehydrated and has signs of hypovolemic shock, such as marked hypotension and weak pulses, expect to give plasma expanders (such as plasma, albumin, or other colloids) in addition to normal saline solution (see the "Hypovolemic Shock" entry in Chapter 14). Although you usually avoid inserting an indwelling (Foley) catheter in a diabetic patient because of the increased risk of infection, the doctor may have you insert one if your patient has minimal urine flow, doesn't urinate after he's received 500 ml of fluid I.V., or is comatose. This will allow you to measure his output accurately. Begin recording intake and output.

As soon as you've initiated fluid replacement, prepare to administer insulin to reduce your patient's hyperglycemia and to reverse the metabolic decompensation cycle. Usually, you'll administer the insulin I.V. or I.M. Why? Because the patient's probably hypotensive, and hypotension results in poor subcutaneous perfusion. So the insulin won't be absorbed if you give it subcutaneously. The method you use will depend on hospital protocols and the doctor's orders:

• constant I.V. infusion (after an initial 5- to 10-unit bolus)
• hourly I.V. boluses
• hourly I.M. injections (after an initial 10- to 20-unit bolus).

The doctor will determine the exact dosage based on the patient's body weight and on the severity of his hyperglycemia. Some doctors prefer continuous I.V. infusion because it seems to minimize the risks of rebound hypoglycemia and hypokalemia. And you'll give *regular* (rapid-acting) insulin only—long-acting insulins don't take effect immediately and can't be given I.V.

## Continuing assessment and intervention

Every 30 minutes, at least, monitor your patient's vital signs and CVP to assess the status of his hypovolemia and hypotension. The doctor may insert an arterial line to provide accurate, constant measurement of your patient's blood pressure and to make obtaining numerous blood samples easier and less upsetting for the patient. Every hour, draw blood for blood glucose, serum acetone, electrolytes, and ABG studies, and check the results to see how the patient's responding to fluid and insulin therapy—the doctor may order changes based on these results.

Assess your patient's mental status frequently. A decrease in his level of consciousness, no matter how slight, is a poor sign; so report this to the doctor *immediately*. Perform a total body assessment, too, to provide baseline data. In a patient with DKA, always suspect and check for infection, the second most common cause of DKA. (The most common cause, of course, is not taking insulin as prescribed.)

Obtain a urine sample from the patient and check it for cloudiness, foul smell, and mucus streaks—signs of a urinary tract infection. Poor urine output (below 30 ml/hour) despite fluid administration suggests that your patient may have underlying renal disease. Call the doctor; he'll have to reevaluate the patient's condition and, possibly, change the insulin dosage and the type or rate of fluid administration.

Assess your patient for respiratory infection, too. Auscultate his lungs, and listen for rhonchi or wheezes. (Rhonchi may signal pneumonia; wheezes may signal bronchitis.) Ask the patient if he's recently had a cough, a cold, or a sore throat, or if he simply hasn't felt well—he may be developing the flu or an upper respiratory tract infection.

Does your patient have any chronic condition? If he does, it may affect his medical treatment. For instance, if he has hyperthyroidism, he may need twice the normal insulin dosage. Or if he has renal disease, he'll need a reduced insulin dosage.

Inspect and palpate your patient's abdomen for signs of infection. You may note distention or tenderness, resulting from pancreatitis, appendicitis, or cholecystitis (any of these can precipitate DKA). When you palpate his abdomen, you may also note hepatomegaly (from fatty infiltration of the liver), common in patients who've had long periods of poorly controlled diabetes.

Be sure to inspect his extremities for areas of infection. Abscesses and ulcers on the legs and feet are common in patients with diabetes and may become ischemic or even gangrenous.

During your assessment and on a continuing basis, watch for signs of improved fluid balance. As your patient's dehydration and hyperglycemia are corrected, you should see:
• increased urine output
• increased CVP
• restored skin turgor
• improved mental status with an increase in alertness.

Of course, anytime you're giving large amounts of fluid you'll have to watch for signs of fluid overload and developing pulmonary edema, such as:
• steadily increasing CVP (an early sign)
• jugular venous distention
• frothy sputum
• rales.

Call the doctor *immediately* if you note any of these signs, and expect to decrease the fluid infusion rate. If you note increasing CVP early enough, you may prevent fluid overload from developing.

If your patient's blood glucose levels don't decrease within 1 to 2 hours, expect the doctor to increase the insulin dosage. If you're administering insulin by continuous infusion, he may ask you to double the hourly rate; if you're giving hourly I.M. or I.V. doses, he may ask you to double each dose or to switch to continuous I.V. infusion. The dosage adjustment will be based on your assessment findings and your patient's blood glucose levels. If the patient's clinical condition has deteriorated and his pH is very low, you may be asked to give bicarbonate and plasma expanders as well as additional insulin. In most patients, insulin and fluid replacement will correct acidosis. How-

## DIFFERENTIATING D.K.A. FROM H.H.N.C.

Your ability to distinguish diabetic ketoacidosis (DKA) from hyperglycemic hyperosmolar nonketotic coma (HHNC) could be crucial to your patient's survival. Although they're similar emergencies caused by hyperglycemia, they have important dissimilarities that require different interventions. For example, you'll give insulin to both DKA and HHNC patients to lower their blood glucose levels—but you'll usually have to give *less* insulin to HHNC patients (even though blood glucose levels are higher in HHNC than in DKA). Why? Because patients with HHNC are more sensitive to insulin and are more prone to insulin reaction.

The following chart, although not all-inclusive, provides some guidelines to help you make this critical differentiation.

| CLINICAL FEATURES | DKA | HHNC |
|---|---|---|
| **Onset** | Up to several days | Up to several days |
| **Acid-base balance and fluid status** | Acidosis, less dehydration | No acidosis, more dehydration |
| **Respiratory signs and symptoms** | Hyperventilation; Kussmaul's respirations | No hyperventilation; no Kussmaul's respirations |
| **Breath odor** | Fruity, acetone | No characteristic odor |
| **GI signs and symptoms** | Abdominal pain, anorexia, nausea, vomiting, diarrhea | Same, but rare |
| **Neurologic signs and symptoms** | Depressed sensorium | Depressed sensorium, hemiparesis, focal seizures, nystagmus, visual hallucinations |
| **Laboratory results** | | |
| *Blood:* | | |
| Glucose | High—but usually no greater than 800 mg/dl | Very high—greater than 800 mg/dl |

ever, if your patient's not improving, has an arterial blood pH of less than 7.1 or a serum bicarbonate level of less than 5 mEq/liter, or shows signs of shock, the doctor will ask you to administer bicarbonate. Usually, you'll give 44 mEq of sodium bicarbonate in 1 liter of 0.45 normal saline solution—use a hypotonic solution to prevent severe hypernatremia resulting from the additional sodium in the bicarbonate. (The sodium bicarbonate can also be given as an I.V. bolus.) After you've given the bicarbonate, watch your patient closely for signs of metabolic alkalosis, which may result from overcorrection (see *Understanding*

*Metabolic Acidosis,* page 465, and *Understanding Metabolic Alkalosis,* page 464). Check his next ABG results to determine if the dose was effective. And watch his cardiac monitor for dysrhythmias—bicarbonate therapy may cause severe hypokalemia as the decrease in acidosis allows potassium to move from the plasma back into the cells (see *EKG Changes in Electrolyte Imbalances,* pages 434 and 435).

Expect to give potassium, too, particularly if you've administered bicarbonate. This is because almost all patients with DKA have potassium deficits, due to the large quantities lost in their urine. Despite this, however, your

| CLINICAL FEATURES | DKA | HHNC |
|---|---|---|
| **Laboratory results** *(continued)* | | |
| *Blood: (continued)* | | |
| Ketones | Present | Absent |
| Sodium | Elevated, normal, or low | Elevated, normal, or low |
| Potassium | Elevated, normal, or low | Normal or elevated |
| Bicarbonate | Less than 10 mEq | Greater than 16 mEq |
| Osmolarity | Less than 330 mOsm/liter | Greater than 350 mOsm/liter |
| Blood urea nitrogen | Elevated | Elevated |
| Hematocrit | High | Normal to very high |
| $CO_2$ | Less than 10 mEq/liter | Normal |
| pH | Less than 7.25 | Normal |
| *Urine:* | | |
| Glucose | Elevated | Elevated |
| Ketones | Present | Absent |
| *Anion gap* | More than 12 mEq | 10 to 12 mEq |
| *Free fatty acids* | More than 1,500 mEq/liter | Less than 1,000 mEq/liter |
| **Age frequency** | All age-groups, but most often in childhood | Usually over age 40, but may occur in childhood |
| **Predisposing type of diabetes mellitus** | Type I (insulin-dependent diabetes mellitus) | Type II (non-insulin-dependent diabetes mellitus) |
| **Previous history of diabetes** | Almost always | In about 50% of patients |
| **Underlying renal or cardiovascular disease** | In about 15% of patients | In about 85% of patients |

patient's serum potassium level may initially be normal or even elevated, because his acidosis causes a shift in potassium ions from his cells to his plasma. As you administer fluids and insulin and the acidosis is corrected, his serum potassium levels may drop sharply.

Some doctors order initial potassium therapy at a low-dose level even if a patient's serum potassium level is normal or high; others wait until the level drops to normal or low. The doctor probably won't have you start potassium therapy until he determines that the patient's kidney function is adequate. He'll decide this by evaluating the patient's urine output or the results of his BUN and creatinine tests. Then he'll order a potassium dosage based on serum potassium levels—usually 10 to 20 mEq/hour. (You may also be asked to give oral potassium salts.) Check your patient's serial potassium level results so you can intervene to correct imbalances that may lead to dysrhythmias.

### Therapeutic care
Maintain a log of your patient's level of consciousness, reflexes, intake and output, CVP, and laboratory test results. Expect to administer antibiotics to treat specific infections—you *won't* give an-

tibiotics prophylactically until blood and urine cultures demonstrate infection. The doctor may also ask you to administer low-dose heparin if your patient is comatose, elderly, or severely volume depleted. This prevents venous thrombosis, a common consequence of the dehydration resulting from DKA.

Your patient's blood glucose level should decrease within a few hours if his insulin dosage is adequate. When it reaches a level of 250 to 300 mg/dl, the doctor may ask you to decrease the insulin dosage to 1 to 2 units/hour (to maintain a blood glucose level of 150 to 250 mg/dl), and you'll probably change the I.V. solution to $D_5W$ at 100 ml/hour (to avoid rebound hypoglycemia while insulin is administered to reduce ketone body production).

When your patient becomes more alert and his blood glucose and acidosis are stabilized, you'll remove your patient's NG tube, if present, and start him on an appropriate diet. You can also decrease blood glucose, serum acetone, ABG, and electrolyte studies to once every 2 to 4 hours. As soon as your patient's blood glucose level enters the normal range, the doctor will ask you to switch to administering subcutaneous insulin every 4 hours. He'll determine the patient's insulin dosage based on his blood glucose levels and a decrease in (or absence of) serum and urinary ketones. Soon after this (probably the next day), you'll start your patient on intermediate-acting insulin. Monitor him carefully for delayed hypoglycemia, which can occur when insulin dosage is being adjusted.

The doctor will remove your patient's CVP line when his volume status has returned to normal. If you inserted a Foley catheter earlier, remove it as soon as the patient's able to void. Encourage him to ambulate early.

Begin patient teaching right away by explaining how much easier preventing DKA is than treating it. Discuss the possible causes of his DKA with him, and suggest ways to avoid future episodes. Make sure you stress the importance of taking his insulin and maintaining food and fluid intake even when he's sick and doesn't want to eat. With recent events still fresh in his mind, his interest in your warnings should be high.

# Hyperglycemic Hyperosmolar Nonketotic Coma

## Prediagnosis summary
On initial assessment, the patient's signs and symptoms probably included:
• lethargy, stupor, or coma
• flat neck veins, decreased skin turgor, dry mucous membranes, and other indications of severe dehydration
• hypotension
• tachypnea
• tachycardia
• oliguria
• a history of polyuria, polydipsia, weight loss, and weakness
• indications of associated serious illness, such as infection or a renal or cerebrovascular disorder.

The patient was given supplemental oxygen (or was intubated if his respiratory status was poor). A large-bore I.V. was inserted for fluid administration, and blood samples were drawn for CBC, electrolytes, blood glucose, serum acetone, BUN, creatinine, and ABGs. He had a 12-lead EKG and a chest X-ray and was started on cardiac monitoring. To save time, the doctor tested his blood for blood glucose and ketones, using glucose reagent strips (such as Clinistix) and nitroprusside reagents (such as Acetest). These quick tests indicated that the patient's blood glucose level was severely elevated, with no serum ketones present.

## Priorities
Your patient with HHNC will have a severe fluid volume deficit—exceeding

## CLARIFYING THE TYPES OF DIABETES MELLITUS

As you may know, diabetes mellitus is actually four distinct types of diabetes, with different names and characteristics. To help you understand the current terminology as approved by the American Diabetes Association (ADA), here's a quick review of the two major types of diabetes, plus a description of the other two types, which are less common.

### TYPE I DIABETES MELLITUS, OR INSULIN-DEPENDENT DIABETES MELLITUS (IDDM)

**Characteristics**
The patient with Type I diabetes:
- has an absolute insulin deficiency
- is prone to ketosis
- most commonly develops the disease during childhood, although he may have developed it later
- *must* take insulin.

### TYPE II DIABETES MELLITUS, OR NON-INSULIN-DEPENDENT DIABETES MELLITUS (NIDDM)

**Characteristics**
The patient with Type II diabetes:
- has normal, elevated, or depressed insulin levels (relative insulin deficiency)
- is *not* prone to ketosis
- most commonly develops the disease after age 40, although he may have developed it during childhood
- usually *doesn't* need insulin except to correct occasional symptomatic or persistent hyperglycemia.

You should also be aware of two less common, usually temporary, types of diabetes. One type, which the ADA refers to as *other*, develops secondary to a preexisting condition or syndrome, such as pancreatic disease. The second type, *gestational diabetes*, develops during pregnancy.

---

that seen in patients with DKA (because of greater osmotic diuresis) and possibly as high as 10 liters or more. Your initial nursing priority, then, is to replace lost fluids over 12 to 48 hours and, if possible, to prevent hypovolemic shock.

Your patient's blood glucose levels may range from 800 mg/dl to 3,000 mg/dl, and his serum osmolarity may be 350 mEq/liter or more. You might think that the doctor would order a hypotonic solution to replace the patient's lost fluid volume and to dilute the osmolarity. But he probably won't. Instead, he'll probably ask you to rapidly infuse normal saline solution. Why? Because a hypotonic solution may increase *intra*cellular fluid volume rapidly at the expense of *extra*cellular fluid volume—increasing the patient's risk of hypovolemic shock. Normal saline solution, in contrast, helps correct the severe sodium deficit that accompanies your patient's fluid volume deficit and maintains extracellular fluid volume. By administering normal saline solution to your patient with HHNC, you'll help prevent hypovolemic shock and also avoid intracellular fluid overload that may lead to cerebral edema.

Expect to give normal saline solution very rapidly—1 liter/hour initially until the patient's blood pressure and pulse are stable and his urine output's increased. The doctor may insert an arterial line for blood pressure measurement and a CVP line for rapid fluid

## UNDERSTANDING OSMOLARITY

Osmolarity—it's an abstract concept that may seem more related to chemistry than to your ability to provide the best nursing care. But serum osmolarity levels do have a clinical application: they provide an accurate reflection of your patient's total body hydration.

Defined simply, osmolarity is the concentration of solutes in a solution, expressed in milliosmols (mOsm) per liter. Plasma proteins normally maintain osmolarity, but concentrations of both electrolytes and certain nonelectrolytes influence it. For example, if your patient has hyponatremia (decreased blood sodium), his blood is *hypo*osmolar: he has excess water relative to solute. If your patient has hyperglycemia, his blood is *hyper*osmolar: he has excess solute relative to water.

When your patient's blood is *hypo*osmolar, water is drawn *into* the cells, swelling them. When your patient's blood is *hyper*osmolar, water is drawn *out* of the cells, dehydrating and shrinking them.

These diagrams depict osmolar states. Note these states' laboratory values and corresponding signs and symptoms.

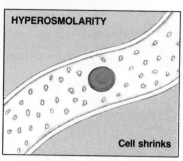

**HYPEROSMOLARITY**

Cell shrinks

- 350 to 375 mOsm/liter (restlessness, hyperirritability)
- 376 to 400 mOsm/liter (nystagmus, tremors, progressive lethargy)
- > 400 mOsm/liter (coma)

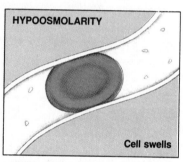

**HYPOOSMOLARITY**

Cell swells

- 260 to 275 mOsm/liter (restlessness, confusion)
- 240 to 259 mOsm/liter (muscle aches, twitches)
- < 240 mOsm/liter (seizures, water intoxication)

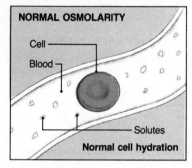

**NORMAL OSMOLARITY**

Cell

Blood

Solutes

**Normal cell hydration**

- 285 to 300 mOsm/liter

infusion. Assist the doctor as necessary, and document the initial readings. You may give 10 to 20 liters of fluid in the first 24 to 48 hours. If your patient's body fluid loss exceeds 25% and he has frank hypovolemic shock, you may also give plasma protein fraction (Plasmanate) and increase fluids to 4 to 5 liters during the first 12 hours. If your patient's comatose or has minimal urine output, you'll need to insert an indwelling (Foley) catheter to ac-

curately measure fluid output—even though he has an increased risk of infection because of his high blood glucose level.

Your patient's blood glucose levels should drop dramatically as you administer fluids. Fluid replacement will improve his renal perfusion, so his kidneys can eliminate glucose more readily. This improvement will also reduce stress hormone levels, which augment glucose production and elevate

when renal perfusion is decreased. If your patient's in shock or has a low initial level of serum sodium, the doctor probably won't order insulin initially—the patient's hyperglycemia will actually help maintain extracellular volume levels. Otherwise, expect to administer modest doses of insulin by continuous I.V. infusion (usually, about 0.05 to 0.1 unit/kg/hour) to correct hyperglycemia. Check your patient's blood glucose levels frequently, and report the values to the doctor—he'll adjust the insulin dosage so that the blood glucose level doesn't fall too rapidly.

Insulin has an additional benefit in the patient with HHNC: it allows insulin-dependent, starved tissues to metabolize glucose for energy. In a patient with DKA, insulin-dependent tissues can use serum ketones for fuel. But in a patient with HHNC, who has no serum ketones, glucose is the only fuel available, and the cells need insulin to metabolize it.

## Continuing assessment and intervention

Monitor your patient's vital signs and CVP every half hour (more frequently if he's in profound shock). Improvements in his blood pressure, pulse, and fluid volume status tell you you're providing effective fluid replacement. Check his urine output hourly—it should be at least 30 ml/hour. If it isn't, notify the doctor. He may ask you to increase the fluid infusion rate. He'll balance this against the need to lower the plasma osmolarity *slowly* once it reaches a level of about 320 mOsm/liter. (A slow reduction in osmolarity prevents overhydration and cerebral edema.) Expect to draw blood for blood glucose, electrolytes, and ABGs every hour to determine your patient's response to fluid and insulin therapy. Watch him for seizures, which may result from severe dehydration and hyperosmolarity. Pad the bed's side rails, and keep an airway at the head of the bed.

Take a detailed history from your patient (or from his family, if he's unconscious), and perform a thorough physical examination. In addition to providing baseline data, your assessment may help determine the underlying cause of the patient's HHNC. Remember, the extremely high mortality of this disorder (up to 50%) is due, in large part, to the acute major diseases that often precipitate HHNC.

Find out, first of all, whether your patient has a history of diabetes and, if he does, whether he's taking oral hypoglycemic agents rather than insulin (patients with Type II, non-insulin-dependent, diabetes are more likely to have HHNC than DKA). Also, ask if he has a history of renal disease, which is common in patients with HHNC. Check his urine—if it's cloudy, mucus-streaked, and foul-smelling, he may have a urinary tract infection.

Ask if the patient's had a recent upper respiratory infection, cough, or sore throat. Auscultate for rales and rhonchi, which may signal respiratory infection or pulmonary edema from CHF—CHF may have caused the episode of HHNC or may be a result of fluid overload. If your patient has these signs, don't forget to assess him for jugular venous distention and the presence of frothy sputum. Call the doctor *immediately* if you note these—he'll want you to adjust the patient's fluid infusion rate.

Find out if your patient's vomited or had diarrhea. Gently palpate his abdomen for areas of tenderness that may indicate infection sites. (Even if your patient's unconscious, he may flinch if the area hurts.)

Make sure you obtain a medication history, because certain drugs may precipitate HHNC. In particular, note if your patient's been taking:

● thiazide diuretics, such as hydrochlorothiazide (HydroDiuril) or chlorothiazide (Diuril), for hypertension or fluid retention

● glucocorticoids, such as dexamethasone (Decadron) or hydrocortisone (Cortef), for asthma, allergies, severe inflammation, adrenal insufficiency, or other disorders

• phenytoin (Dilantin) for a seizure disorder

• propranolol (Inderal) for dysrhythmias, angina, or hypertension

• diazoxide (Proglycem) for hypoglycemia.

If your patient developed HHNC while hospitalized for another disorder, note if he's undergone peritoneal lavage or received hyperalimentation therapy. These can precipitate HHNC even in nondiabetic patients. (You should also be aware that HHNC sometimes develops in patients with burns.)

Of course, as part of your assessment, you'll continue to check the patient for improvements in his fluid volume status. Look for:

• increased urine output

• increased CVP

• improved mental status

• improved skin turgor.

Continue to provide fluid replacement and insulin, and check his blood glucose and electrolyte levels hourly. Once your patient's urine output is satisfactory, expect to begin potassium therapy (usually, potassium chloride at 20 mEq/hour). However, if the patient's potassium levels are normal or low, the doctor may ask you to begin potassium at a reduced rate immediately. Watch for dysrhythmias, which can occur with hypokalemia.

### Therapeutic care
Check your patient's vital signs frequently. When his blood pressure's stable and his urine output's adequate (30 ml/hour), notify the doctor. With these signs that the patient's fluid balance is improving, the doctor will probably ask you to change the I.V. infusion—to continue rehydration and to correct the hyperosmolarity—to 0.45 saline solution at 250 to 500 ml/hour. Continue to monitor the patient's fluid balance carefully, and expect to give antibiotics if he has an underlying infection.

Your patient's blood glucose levels should decrease within a few hours in response to both fluid and insulin therapy. Check his blood glucose levels hourly, and document your findings. As his blood glucose level reaches the range of 300 mg/dl, expect to discontinue I.V. insulin and to start regular insulin subcutaneously at 4-hour intervals, followed the next day by intermediate-acting insulin, such as NPH or Lente. The doctor may ask you to add $D_5W$ to the I.V. infusion when the patient's blood glucose reaches a level of about 250 mg/dl, to prevent rebound hypoglycemia.

Continue to monitor his blood glucose and electrolytes every 2 to 4 hours (your patient may experience delayed hypoglycemia while his insulin doses are being adjusted). Remove his Foley catheter when he's stable; the doctor will remove his arterial and CVP lines. If your patient has an NG tube in place, expect to remove it and to start the patient on an appropriate diet. After his blood glucose has stabilized at normal, he probably won't need further insulin—expect to start him on his normal diet and oral hypoglycemic regimen if he's diabetic or to discontinue diabetic therapy altogether if some other cause precipitated his HHNC.

# Acute Hypoglycemia

### Prediagnosis summary
Initially, the patient had some combination of these signs and symptoms:

• altered level of consciousness (ranging from mild confusion and lethargy to coma)

• personality changes (for example, anxiety, depression, inappropriate behavior)

• visual disturbances (blurred vision, diplopia)

• tremors and palpitations

• uncoordinated body movements

• pallor

• diaphoresis

• hypothermia

- tachycardia
- muscular rigidity
- seizures
- depressed respirations.

An I.V. was inserted for fluid and medication administration, and the patient was connected to a cardiac monitor. A chest X-ray (using portable equipment) and 12-lead EKG were taken. If his respirations were severely depressed, he was intubated and started on mechanical ventilation. Blood was drawn for a CBC, blood glucose, electrolytes, BUN, creatinine, calcium, and ABGs. Additional blood was set aside for insulin and cortisol assays, and a drop of blood was tested with a glucose reagent strip, such as a Visidex II or a Chemstrip bG. If the initial blood glucose test results showed levels below 45 mg/dl, or if the patient was unconscious or severely lethargic, an I.V. bolus of 50 ml of 50% dextrose was given immediately.

**Priorities**
Because an extremely low blood glucose level can rapidly cause brain damage, your first priority is to assist with bringing your patient's glucose level back to normal. If he's *unconscious* and the initial dose of dextrose failed to awaken him, expect to give additional dextrose either as a bolus or as a continuous I.V. drip of 10% or 20% dextrose in water (D₁₀W or D₂₀W).

If your patient's *conscious* (or as soon as he regains consciousness), give him a fast-acting carbohydrate by mouth. You may give him sweetened orange juice, nondiet soda, candy, or warm tea or coffee sweetened with sugar.

**Continuing assessment and intervention**
Check your patient's vital signs frequently, especially his temperature—hypothermia may be due to hypoglycemia-induced increased peripheral vasodilation and diaphoresis. Keep your patient warm, and watch for signs that his blood glucose levels are returning to normal. As his blood glucose level rises, you should see dramatic improvement in his level of consciousness and a reduction in the signs and symptoms associated with hypoglycemia-induced catecholamine excess (diaphoresis, pallor, tremors, anxiety, tachycardia).

If your patient remains unconscious after the initial administration of dextrose, perform a neurologic assessment to determine if his hypoglycemia has resulted in coma (see the "Coma" entry in Chapter 6), and document your findings to provide a baseline. Expect to administer continuous I.V. dextrose (probably D₁₀W or D₂₀W) to maintain your patient's blood glucose level at 150 to 180 mg/dl. You may also give insulin to facilitate cellular glucose uptake. The doctor may ask you to give steroids or mannitol (Osmitrol) to reduce cerebral edema, and he'll order a computerized tomography scan to rule out other causes of coma.

Perform a thorough nursing assessment when your patient regains consciousness—or, if he's conscious, when his immediate signs and symptoms have subsided. Although hypoglycemia can be reversed promptly in most patients, determining the underlying cause will help prevent another episode.

Find out, first of all, if your patient's diabetic and, if he is, whether his diabetes is insulin-dependent (Type I) or non-insulin-dependent (Type II). (See *Clarifying the Types of Diabetes Mellitus,* page 445.) If he's insulin-dependent, find out when he last took his insulin and when he last ate, and ask him to recall the events leading up to the hypoglycemic episode. He may tell you, for instance, that he skipped a meal because he felt sick or that he was exercising particularly vigorously just before mealtime. If insulin shock caused his hypoglycemia, he usually won't need further treatment once his blood glucose level has returned to normal. You'll want to observe him for awhile to make sure he's stable, though, and you may want to set a time for him

# WHAT HAPPENS IN ACUTE HYPOGLYCEMIA

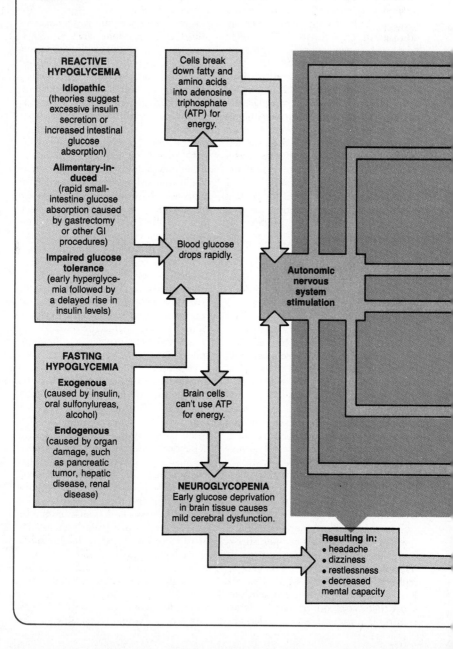

**REACTIVE HYPOGLYCEMIA**

**Idiopathic**
(theories suggest excessive insulin secretion or increased intestinal glucose absorption)

**Alimentary-induced**
(rapid small-intestine glucose absorption caused by gastrectomy or other GI procedures)

**Impaired glucose tolerance**
(early hyperglycemia followed by a delayed rise in insulin levels)

**FASTING HYPOGLYCEMIA**

**Exogenous**
(caused by insulin, oral sulfonylureas, alcohol)

**Endogenous**
(caused by organ damage, such as pancreatic tumor, hepatic disease, renal disease)

Cells break down fatty and amino acids into adenosine triphosphate (ATP) for energy.

Blood glucose drops rapidly.

Brain cells can't use ATP for energy.

**NEUROGLYCOPENIA**
Early glucose deprivation in brain tissue causes mild cerebral dysfunction.

**Autonomic nervous system stimulation**

**Resulting in:**
- headache
- dizziness
- restlessness
- decreased mental capacity

Normally, homeostatic mechanisms maintain blood glucose within narrow limits (60 to 120 mg/dl). The body burns available glucose and stores the rest as glycogen in the liver and muscles. When the glucose level drops, the liver converts glycogen back to glucose (glycogenolysis) or makes new glucose from noncarbohydrate sources, such as amino acids or fatty acids (gluconeogenesis). Hormones maintain the delicate balance between glucose production and use. *Insulin* prevents hyperglycemia; *epinephrine, glucogen, growth hormone,* and *cortisol* act as counterregulatory hormones to prevent hypoglycemia. But this balance is upset when your patient has either reactive or fasting hypoglycemia. Here's what happens:

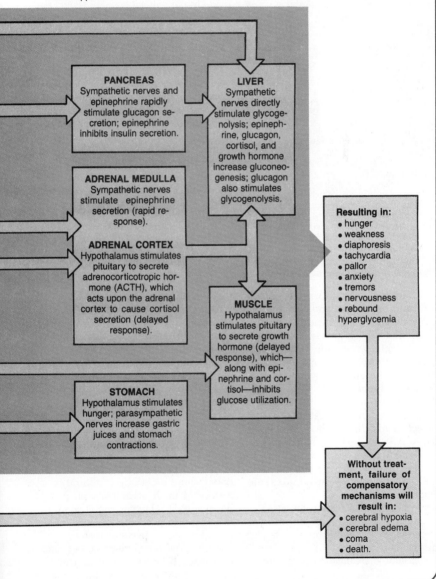

**PANCREAS**
Sympathetic nerves and epinephrine rapidly stimulate glucagon secretion; epinephrine inhibits insulin secretion.

**ADRENAL MEDULLA**
Sympathetic nerves stimulate epinephrine secretion (rapid response).

**ADRENAL CORTEX**
Hypothalamus stimulates pituitary to secrete adrenocorticotropic hormone (ACTH), which acts upon the adrenal cortex to cause cortisol secretion (delayed response).

**STOMACH**
Hypothalamus stimulates hunger; parasympathetic nerves increase gastric juices and stomach contractions.

**LIVER**
Sympathetic nerves directly stimulate glycogenolysis; epinephrine, glucagon, cortisol, and growth hormone increase gluconeogenesis; glucagon also stimulates glycogenolysis.

**MUSCLE**
Hypothalamus stimulates pituitary to secrete growth hormone (delayed response), which—along with epinephrine and cortisol—inhibits glucose utilization.

**Resulting in:**
- hunger
- weakness
- diaphoresis
- tachycardia
- pallor
- anxiety
- tremors
- nervousness
- rebound hyperglycemia

**Without treatment, failure of compensatory mechanisms will result in:**
- cerebral hypoxia
- cerebral edema
- coma
- death.

## EMERGENCY HYPOGLYCEMIA TREATMENT

Once you've brought your diabetic patient's hypoglycemic crisis under control, take some time to teach his family how to recognize the signs and symptoms of insulin shock (hunger, trembling, confusion) and how to intervene properly. Explain to the family that they must raise his blood glucose level *immediately* to prevent permanent brain damage and even death.

If he's conscious, someone should give him any one of the following:
• 4 oz of apple juice, orange juice, or ginger ale
• 3 oz of nondiet cola or other soda
• 2 oz of corn syrup, honey, or grape jelly
• 5 lifesavers, 6 jelly beans, or 10 gumdrops.

If he's *unconscious*, or if he has trouble swallowing, someone will have to administer glucagon subcutaneously.

Teach your patient's family how to prepare and administer a subcutaneous injection, and tell them to always keep a supply of glucagon at home.

to review his diet and insulin dosage with you, the doctor, and a dietitian.

If your patient's a Type II diabetic, ask if he's taking oral sulfonylureas, such as chlorpropamide (Diabinese), tolazamide (Tolinase), or tolbutamide (Orinase), because these drugs may also cause hypoglycemia. Take a complete medication history, as well, because many common drugs increase the hypoglycemic effect of the sulfonylurea drugs. Ask, in particular, if your patient's taking:
• sulfonamides, such as sulfamethoxazole (Gantanol) or co-trimoxazole (Bactrim)
• chloramphenicol (Chloromycetin)
• clonidine (Catapres), propranolol (Inderal), or guanethidine sulfate (Ismelin)
• monoamine oxidase (MAO) inhibitors

• warfarin sodium (Coumadin)
• phenylbutazone (Butazolidin)
• propoxyphene hydrochloride (Darvon), propoxyphene napsylate (Darvocet-N), or salicylates.

If oral sulfonylureas caused the patient's hypoglycemic episode, you'll have to observe him closely for several days or even weeks. This is because his hypoglycemia may persist or recur, especially if he's taking chlorpropamide, which has a long duration of action. Watch elderly patients and patients with compromised renal function particularly carefully, because they excrete chlorpropamide more slowly. Expect to administer continuous I.V. dextrose as $D_{10}W$ or $D_{20}W$ with additional boluses of 50% dextrose as necessary. Check your patient's blood glucose levels frequently, and make sure to provide an adequate diet. If your patient's blood glucose level isn't elevated after 4 to 6 hours of therapy, the doctor may ask you to add hydrocortisone hemisuccinate to the I.V. solution because of its hyperglycemic effects.

Ask your patient if he has an underlying endocrine disorder, such as hypoadrenalism or hypopituitarism, or renal or liver disease. Has he had GI surgery? All these conditions may precipitate hypoglycemia. Obtain a urine sample and note if his urine's concentrated, and palpate his abdomen for an enlarged liver.

Ask your patient if he's had nightmares, night sweats, or early morning headaches, which may indicate nocturnal hypoglycemia. Also ask if he's been eating more lately and has gained weight, because this could indicate chronic hypoglycemia from an insulinoma.

If your patient's not diabetic and doesn't have a chronic condition or a history of medication use that could have caused his hypoglycemia, ask him if he's experienced similar, less severe episodes before: periods of shakiness, sweating, tremors, nervousness, and confusion. If he has, see if he can remember how long after eating these episodes occurred. Note his answers carefully—repeated episodes of hypoglycemia 4 to 5 hours after eating may indicate reactive hypoglycemia, which requires ongoing medical treatment.

Finally, don't forget to consider the possibility that your patient has chronic alcoholism, so that alcohol, which inhibits glucose synthesis, may have caused his hypoglycemia. Find out when he last had a drink and when he ate last. And when you prepare to give him dextrose, expect that the doctor will also order I.V. thiamine *before* you give the dextrose, to prevent an acute episode of Wernicke-Korsakoff syndrome. If your patient with chronic alcoholism has this syndrome, thiamine may be life-saving—if he doesn't, the thiamine won't hurt him.

### Therapeutic care

Further care of your patient will depend on the cause of his hypoglycemia. If insulin shock caused it, he'll probably need only appropriate teaching regarding exercise, diet, and insulin therapy to make sure he understands how these factors interact. However, he'll need further care if other factors caused his hypoglycemia.

If overuse of sulfonylureas caused your patient's hypoglycemia, continue monitoring his blood glucose level closely, because his hypoglycemia may persist or recur for weeks. Continue I.V. dextrose infusion with boluses of 50% dextrose as necessary, with added hydrocortisone hemisuccinate if the doctor orders it. If the patient's hypoglycemia is particularly refractory, the doctor may also order oral diazoxide (Proglycem), which inhibits insulin release from the pancreas and decreases peripheral glucose utilization.

The patient may need further testing if overuse of insulin or oral sulfonylureas didn't cause his hypoglycemia. The doctor may order a fasting glucose tolerance test, liver function test, urinary or plasma cortisol measurement, plasma growth hormone measure-

ment, and other tests to determine the underlying cause. If these tests indicate that your patient's hypoglycemia is due to an underlying condition, such as certain types of previous GI surgery, an insulinoma, or renal failure, he'll receive treatment appropriate to the condition. The patient with hypoglycemia occurring after GI surgery may be treated with a diet of more frequent but smaller meals that also decreases his consumption of refined sugars; with drugs that delay gastric emptying; or with further surgery. If the patient has an insulinoma, it will be removed surgically, if possible; he may also be treated with oral diazoxide. The patient with hypoglycemia secondary to renal failure may need hemodialysis or peritoneal dialysis (see Chapter 13, GENITOURINARY EMERGENCIES).

If your patient has reactive (glucose-induced, postabsorptive) hypoglycemia, as determined by his response to a 5-hour glucose tolerance test, he (like the patient who's had GI surgery) may be started on a diet that emphasizes smaller, more frequent meals and reduced intake of refined sugars. Explain the rationale for this diet to your patient and, if necessary, arrange for him to meet with a dietitian.

# Thyrotoxic Crisis (Thyroid Storm)

### Prediagnosis summary

The patient was previously hyperthyroid, although this may not have been diagnosed. His signs and symptoms worsened suddenly so that, on initial assessment, he had some combination of the following signs and symptoms:

- irritability and restlessness, possibly progressing to delirium, psychosis, and coma
- tremors and weakness
- visual disturbances (for example, diplopia)

PATHOPHYSIOLOGY

## WHAT HAPPENS IN THYROTOXIC CRISIS

Thyrotoxic crisis, or thyroid storm, is an acute manifestation of hyperthyroidism, usually occurring in patients with preexisting (though often unrecognized) thyrotoxicosis. Left untreated, it's invariably fatal. Its onset is almost always abrupt, evoked by a stressful event, such as trauma, surgery, or infection. Other—less common—precipitating factors include:
• insulin-induced hypoglycemia or diabetic ketoacidosis
• cardiovascular accident
• myocardial infarction
• pulmonary embolism
• sudden discontinuation of antithyroid drug therapy

• initiation of radioiodine therapy
• preeclampsia
• subtotal thyroidectomy with accompanying excess intake of synthetic thyroid hormone.

The thyroid gland secretes the thyroid hormones thyroxine and triiodothyronine. When it overproduces these in response to any of the above-mentioned factors, systemic adrenergic activity increases. This results in epinephrine overproduction and severe hypermetabolism. These lead rapidly to cardiac, GI, and sympathetic nervous system decompensation. Signs include marked tachycardia, vomiting, and stupor that, untreated, progress to vascular collapse, hypotension, coma, and death.

---

• tachycardia, dysrhythmias, angina, and, possibly, signs of CHF
• warm, moist, flushed skin
• vomiting and diarrhea
• high fever that's insidious in onset and may rise *rapidly* to lethal levels (105° F., or 40.6° C.).

If the patient was elderly, his signs and symptoms may have been limited to cardiovascular disturbances, generalized muscle wasting, and depression or apathy progressing to coma. He may have had a slight, *slowly* increasing fever, or no fever at all.

An I.V. was inserted to administer fluid and medication, and a CVP line was inserted to monitor his fluid balance; he was also given supplemental oxygen. He was connected to a cardiac monitor, and a 12-lead EKG was taken. Blood was drawn for a CBC, electrolytes, lactic dehydrogenase (LDH), serum glutamic-oxaloacetic transaminase (SGOT), blood glucose, culture-and-sensitivity, serum triiodothyronine ($T_3$) and thyroxine ($T_4$), and a $T_3$ resin uptake. Urine was obtained for a urine culture.

### Priorities

Because thyrotoxic crisis may be rap-idly fatal, you'll need to do several things almost simultaneously. Your initial goals are to:
• correct your patient's fluid imbalance
• reduce his fever
• administer drug therapy to inhibit thyroid hormone release and synthesis and to decrease the effects of excess thyroid hormone on your patient's sympathetic nervous system.

Quickly start an I.V. infusion of normal saline solution, as ordered, to replace the fluid he's lost through increased respirations and profuse diaphoresis. Take your patient's temperature with a rectal probe (if available) or a rectal thermometer—if it's over 102° F. (38.9° C.), start general surface cooling measures immediately. Place the patient on a hypothermia blanket, and apply cold packs to his axillae and groin. Notify the doctor if the patient starts shivering—this elevates his metabolic rate and defeats the purpose of cooling. The doctor may order you to administer muscle relaxants to decrease it. If ordered, give an antipyretic, such as acetaminophen. (You *won't* give aspirin, because it increases free $T_4$ levels and would make his thyrotoxic crisis worse.)

You'll have to administer specific drug therapy to decrease your patient's hypermetabolism *before* you perform a thorough nursing assessment or evaluate laboratory test results. Expect to give a number of drugs that work in different ways to inhibit:

- thyroid hormone synthesis
- the effects of thyroid hormone on the sympathetic nervous system
- conversion of $T_4$ to $T_3$
- thyroid hormone release.

Expect to give propylthiouracil (PTU) or methimazole (Tapazole) first, orally or by NG tube. These drugs block thyroid hormone synthesis; PTU also impairs conversion of $T_4$ to $T_3$. At the same time, the doctor may ask you to administer a beta-blocking agent—probably propranolol (Inderal)—to decrease the effects of excess thyroid hormone on your patient's sympathetic nervous system, reducing his tachycardia, tachydysrhythmias, tremors, diaphoresis, and nervousness. However, the doctor will first want to determine if your patient has CHF—a serious complication in which propranolol use may be contraindicated (see the "Congestive Heart Failure" entry in Chapter 5). Look for edematous extremities, periorbital edema, and jugular venous distention, and listen for rales and an $S_3$ gallop. If you note these, report them to the doctor *before* you give propranolol. He may ask you to give the patient with CHF a low initial test dose, to see how he responds, and to administer digitalis and diuretics at the same time.

If your patient can't tolerate propranolol, the doctor may order reserpine or guanethidine—sympatholytics that don't aggravate CHF but also don't work as well as propranolol. These drugs also have serious side effects, including postural or resistant hypotension, somnolence, and diarrhea.

Propranolol also causes bronchoconstriction, so find out if your patient has asthma before you give it. If he does, inform the doctor—he may ask you to give an alternate beta-blocking agent, such as metoprolol or atenolol, which will cause less bronchoconstriction.

In addition to giving drugs that block thyroid hormone synthesis and sympathetic nervous system stimulation, expect to give a glucocorticoid, such as dexamethasone (Decadron) or hydrocortisone sodium succinate (Solu-Cortef), which will inhibit the conversion of $T_4$ to $T_3$ and also replace cortisol. (Thyrotoxic crisis may deplete cortisol, leading to adrenal crisis.)

## Continuing assessment and intervention

Assess your patient's vital signs every 15 minutes or as ordered, to see how he's responding to medication. Control his anxiety and restlessness by providing as quiet an environment as possible. Usually you *won't* administer a sedative, because this may mask signs of neurologic deterioration.

About 30 minutes to 2 hours after you give PTU or methimazole, expect to give an oral dose (or an I.V. drip, if the patient can't take medications orally) of a saturated solution of potassium iodide (SSKI). (Iodine therapy blocks the release of thyroid hormone.) If your patient's allergic to iodine, the doctor may order lithium instead, which also seems to block thyroid hormone release. If you give lithium, remember to check your patient's blood levels frequently—lithium has a very narrow margin of safety and may cause systemic toxicity. Other drugs the doctor may order include iopanoic acid (Telepaque) and ipodate sodium (Oragrafin), gallbladder dyes that, because they contain large quantities of iodine, also block thyroid hormone release.

Continue I.V. fluids, as ordered. Monitor your patient's intake and output carefully, and check his CVP readings. If your patient had signs of dehydration (for example, dry skin and mucous membranes, sunken eyes, decreased urine output, flat neck veins), these should improve as you correct his fluid balance. If your patient's fluid balance is precarious, the doctor may insert a Swan-Ganz catheter for hemo-dynamic monitoring.

Listen to your patient's bowel sounds and palpate his abdomen for areas of tenderness that may indicate infection. He'll probably vomit and have diarrhea as a result of his increased metabolic activity and peristalsis; if he's uncon-scious or stuporous, insert an NG tube to prevent aspiration. Check his vital signs for indications that cooling mea-sures have reduced his fever.

Take a quick history to identify any underlying chronic diseases (such as diabetes, asthma, or heart disease) and to determine what precipitated his thy-rotoxic crisis. Of course, ask if the pa-tient has a history of hyperthyroidism and, if he does, what medications he takes and if he takes them as ordered. Thyrotoxic crisis usually develops in *hyper*thyroid patients who:
• abruptly withdraw from an antithy-roid agent or iodine therapy
• have had X-ray dye studies
• have had surgery
• have trauma
• have an infection
• have DKA.

Thyrotoxic crisis can also occur in *hypo*thyroid patients who have taken improper doses of hypothyroid medi-cation.

What if your patient *hasn't* been di-agnosed as hyperthyroid before? Your patient's crisis may be the result of un-diagnosed and untreated hyperthy-roidism. Ask him if he's recently noticed any of these signs and symp-toms:
• weight loss
• heat intolerance
• visual disturbances
• diarrhea
• nocturia
• weakness and tremors
• emotional instability or anxiety
• insomnia.
Report your findings to the doctor.

Check the results of the laboratory tests initiated at the onset of your pa-tient's crisis. Expect to see an elevated blood glucose level, hypercalcemia, and an abnormal liver function test. Note these results, and use them as a baseline against which to measure your patient's progress. Draw additional samples after you've administered medications, and repeat the tests to de-termine how well your patient's re-sponding.

Check the $T_3$ and $T_4$ assays when they return from the laboratory—usually af-ter a day or more. Expect to see an elevated $T_4$ level and a normal or ele-vated $T_3$ level.

## Therapeutic care
Assess your patient's vital signs, car-diovascular status, and respiratory sta-tus frequently to determine how he's responding to therapy. He'll probably improve in 1 to 2 days and recover com-pletely within a week. Expect to wean him from iodine and steroids *gradually* to prevent a recurrence of thyrotoxic crisis; also expect to start an appro-priate drug regimen for managing his underlying hyperthyroidism. This may include a single dose of radioactive io-dine ($I^{131}$), which destroys some thy-roid cells and decreases thyroid hormone production, or continued treatment with PTU or methimazole to block thyroid hormone synthesis.

If your patient doesn't show signs of improvement within 24 to 48 hours, the doctor may start plasmapheresis or peritoneal lavage to remove circulating thyroid hormone from the patient's blood. These procedures sometimes help stop the progress of thyrotoxic cri-sis, although they don't necessarily im-prove the prognosis. Watch your patient closely after these procedures, because they can precipitate infection, hypo-tension, dehydration, or electrolyte im-balances.

Because infections and sepsis are the major precipitators of thyrotoxic crisis, check to make sure urine and blood cultures taken earlier are being pro-cessed, and take a sputum sample to send for culture-and-sensitivity test-ing. The doctor may ask you to give your patient broad-spectrum antibiotics after you've taken the cultures, even though the culture result won't be available immediately.

If your patient has DKA, remember that you may need to double his insulin dosage until he's euthyroid (see the "Diabetic Ketoacidosis" entry in this chapter). If your patient needs a thyroidectomy or any other surgical procedure, expect to administer PTU or methimazole until he's euthyroid; you'll also administer SSKI 10 days before surgery. Explain to the patient that he'll need continued medical treatment and that he should contact his doctor whenever he develops signs and symptoms of thyrotoxic crisis. Advise him to wear a Medic Alert bracelet, so his condition can be identified easily in an emergency.

# Myxedema Crisis

## Prediagnosis summary

The typical patient with myxedema crisis had a history of thyroid disease (either uncomplicated *hypo*thyroidism or *hyper*thyroidism, treated with surgery or I¹³¹) and some combination of these signs and symptoms:

- hypothermia (body temperature may be below 93° F., or 33.9° C.)
- hypoventilation
- hypotension
- hypoactive reflexes
- bradycardia
- facial (especially periorbital) and extremity edema
- dry, cool skin
- scant, coarse scalp and eyebrow hair
- pale, sallow, or yellow-orange complexion
- diminished level of consciousness, ranging from slow mentation to stupor and coma
- seizures.

The patient was given oxygen; if his hypoventilation was severe, he was ventilated by hand with an Ambu bag until he could be intubated. If he was comatose, an NG tube was inserted. A large-bore I.V. was inserted for fluid and medication administration, and a 12-lead EKG and a chest X-ray (using portable equipment) were taken. Cardiac monitoring was started. Blood was drawn for a CBC, electrolytes, blood glucose, BUN, creatinine, calcium, cortisol, creatine phosphokinase (CPK), LDH, SGOT, $T_4$, $T_3$, thyroid stimulating hormone, toxicology screen, and ABGs.

## Priorities

The doctor won't be able to diagnose myxedema crisis definitely until the patient's $T_4$ levels return from the laboratory. But he'll begin treatment immediately if he suspects this diagnosis, because any delay will worsen the patient's prognosis. You have three immediate priorities: to treat the patient's hypoventilation, to increase his cardiac output, and to administer thyroid hormone, as ordered.

Your patient will probably need to be intubated and started on mechanical ventilation to avoid the carbon dioxide retention and subsequent narcosis that accompany hypoventilation. Severe myxedema also decreases the respiratory center's response to hypoxemia and hypercapnia. Remember, your patient's myxedema crisis may have been precipitated by pneumonia or acutely exacerbated chronic obstructive pulmonary disease (COPD), which further compromises his respiratory status. Monitor your patient's ABGs frequently to determine if his respiratory status is improving; the doctor may decide to increase the percentage of oxygen. If your patient's hypoventilation is mild, so he doesn't need to be intubated, check his respirations and vital signs every 15 to 30 minutes. Especially note the depth and quality of his respirations.

Your patient will probably have severe hypotension and bradycardia—signs of reduced cardiac output and hypometabolism. The doctor may insert:

- a CVP line to monitor the relationship

PATHOPHYSIOLOGY

# WHAT HAPPENS IN MYXEDEMA CRISIS

Myxedema crisis (or myxedema coma) is the life-threatening final stage of severe, long-standing hypothyroidism. It occurs most commonly in elderly patients with pre-existing (although often undiagnosed) hypothyroidism who've experienced a stressful event, such as:
- infection
- exposure to cold
- cardiac disease
- thyroid gland surgery
- radiation therapy.

Other possible precipitating factors include:
- sedative or narcotic use
- overuse of antithyroid medications (such as propylthiouracil)
- abrupt discontinuation of thyroid hormone (thyroxine).

Thyroid hormone deficiency causes severe hypometabolism with a significant drop in respiratory rate, resulting in decreased pulmonary ventilation. This may lead to carbon dioxide narcosis and respiratory failure as myxedema crisis progresses. Thyroid hormone deficiency also prevents normal sympathetic responses in the myocardium, causing decreased heart rate and contractility. This results in decreased cardiac output, decreased blood pressure, and increased peripheral resistance.

Myxedema crisis affects other body systems, as well. Hypometabolism alters fluid and electrolyte balance, causing an increase in extracellular fluid and capillary permeability that leads to fluid retention, hyponatremia, and hypochloremia. Long-standing hypothyroidism results in characteristic nonpitting edema with thickened, puffy skin, coarsened facial features, and droopy eyelids (see the illustration). Edema also affects muscle and nerve fibers, leading to muscle weakness, apathy, and lethargy. In the GI tract, decreased peristalsis and absorption cause anorexia and constipation. Compromised renal function causes decreased urine output and proteinuria.

Severe hypothermia (possibly below 93° F., or 33.9° C.) develops as myxedema progresses. If the condition's not treated promptly, stupor, hypotension, shock, coma, and death ensue.

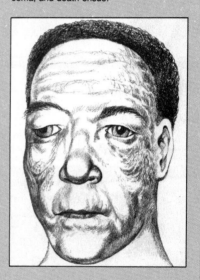

---

between the patient's fluid status and his heart function
- an arterial line for continual blood pressure measurement
- a Swan-Ganz catheter for hemodynamic status monitoring.

Insert an indwelling (Foley) catheter, as ordered, to accurately monitor the patient's fluid output, and start an intake and output record. Expect to infuse I.V. plasma expanders (probably colloids) to correct his decreased plasma volume. Chances are you *won't* give an adrenergic (pressor) agent, because:
- hypothyroid patients are relatively insensitive to adrenergic agents
- adrenergic agents can cause tachydysrhythmias if given with thyroid hormone
- adrenergic agents cause severe peripheral vasoconstriction. (Your patient already has this problem, so giving him an adrenergic agent will

make it worse.)

Expect to administer thyroid hormone I.V. to increase your patient's metabolism. (You won't be able to use an oral, I.M., or subcutaneous route, because the patient's decreased intestinal motility and circulation make absorption unpredictable.) The doctor will decide whether to give $T_4$ (as L-thyroxine) or $T_3$ (triiodothyronine). $T_3$ is metabolically active sooner than $T_4$, so you might expect the doctor to order it in preference to $T_4$. But $T_3$ is more difficult to obtain than $T_4$ (it's not commercially available and must be prepared in the hospital pharmacy), and its rapid action may lead to cardiac dysrhythmias. So the doctor will probably ask you to give $T_4$, which is commercially available and is converted to $T_3$ in the body. (When you give the patient $T_4$, his $T_4$ pool and $T_3$ serum concentration remain stable—his body

converts $T_4$ to $T_3$ as required.)

## Continuing assessment and intervention

Monitor your patient's vital signs and level of consciousness frequently, watching especially for improvements in his bradycardia, hypotension, and hypothermia. Remember that his temperature may be extremely low (below 93° F., or 33.9° C.). Use a rectal probe, if available, to measure his temperature accurately. If you don't have a rectal probe, use a glass thermometer to take his temperature rectally every half hour or so. Make sure you shake the thermometer all the way down—otherwise, because the patient's hypothermia is so severe, you risk a false reading. Start a temperature chart to detect improvement or deterioration in your patient's condition. (Remember, the degree of your patient's hypothermia

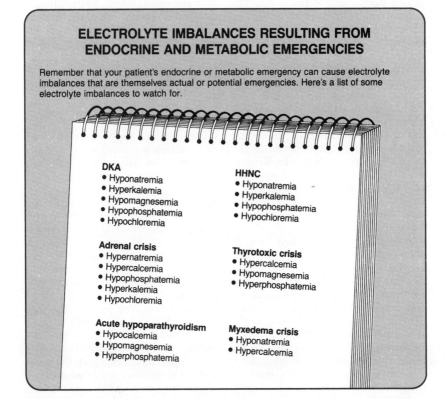

## ELECTROLYTE IMBALANCES RESULTING FROM ENDOCRINE AND METABOLIC EMERGENCIES

Remember that your patient's endocrine or metabolic emergency can cause electrolyte imbalances that are themselves actual or potential emergencies. Here's a list of some electrolyte imbalances to watch for.

**DKA**
- Hyponatremia
- Hyperkalemia
- Hypomagnesemia
- Hypophosphatemia
- Hypochloremia

**Adrenal crisis**
- Hypernatremia
- Hypercalcemia
- Hypophosphatemia
- Hyperkalemia
- Hypochloremia

**Acute hypoparathyroidism**
- Hypocalcemia
- Hypomagnesemia
- Hyperphosphatemia

**HHNC**
- Hyponatremia
- Hyperkalemia
- Hypophosphatemia
- Hypochloremia

**Thyrotoxic crisis**
- Hypercalcemia
- Hypomagnesemia
- Hyperphosphatemia

**Myxedema crisis**
- Hyponatremia
- Hypercalcemia

may correlate with his chances of survival. Remember, too, that a "normal" temperature may actually indicate infection in this patient.)

Thyroid hormone administration should restore your patient's temperature to normal within 24 hours. Until then, cover him with a blanket to prevent further heat loss, but *don't* start active rewarming. Why? Because the peripheral vasodilation this causes may lead to vascular collapse, divert blood from his vital organs, and induce shock.

Perform a quick assessment to establish a baseline and to help determine the precipitating cause of your patient's myxedema crisis—expect to find out that it was an infection. (Don't forget, however, that your patient's hypometabolism may be masking signs of infection, such as increased temperature, diaphoresis, and tachycardia.) Ask the patient (or his family) whether he has a history of thyroid disease and, if he does, whether he takes any medication to control it. Look for the facial and extremity edema characteristic of myxedema. Auscultate his lungs for rales or rhonchi, which may signal pneumonia, and for wheezes, which may signal aggravated COPD. Auscultate his bowel sounds in all four quadrants— they may be decreased or absent due to decreased peristalsis. Palpate the patient's abdomen for areas of tenderness, which may indicate infection sites. Obtain a urine sample and check it for a foul odor and for mucus streaks, cloudiness, and sediment; these may indicate a urinary tract infection.

Your patient's diminished cardiac output will correspondingly diminish his renal blood flow, decreasing glomerular filtration and impairing his ability to excrete water. As a result, he may develop dilutional hyponatremia. Restrict fluids as ordered, and slowly administer an I.V. solution of hypertonic saline or normal saline and dextrose. This will correct his hyponatremia and any hypoglycemia he may develop. Monitor his electrolyte levels and

fluid balance frequently, and adjust the infusion rate as necessary (and as ordered).

Expect to administer corticosteroids (usually I.V. hydrocortisone), because:
• endogenous corticosteroid production decreases in a patient with myxedema crisis and will be insufficient as administration of fluid and thyroid hormone increases his metabolism.
• if he has an underlying infection or coexisting illness, this will increase his need for corticosteroids.
• thyroid hormone administration may increase his body's metabolism of corticosteroids.

Draw blood for laboratory tests, as ordered, so you can compare the values to those from his initial tests and measure his improvement. His CPK, SGOT, and LDH values, initially elevated because of his decreased metabolic clearance, should decrease as his metabolism increases. His $T_4$ levels, initially decreased, should approach normal with therapy. Don't forget to check his hemoglobin and hematocrit levels— hypothyroid patients often have anemia, and you may have to transfuse blood if his hematocrit level is below 25 to 30 ml/100 ml.

## Therapeutic care

Continue to monitor your patient's level of consciousness, vital signs, and hydration status frequently. If your patient remains comatose, keep his NG tube in to prevent aspiration, and keep his Foley catheter in to prevent urinary retention. Turn him frequently to prevent pressure sores. Listen for bowel sounds—your patient may develop an adynamic ileus as a result of his decreased metabolism. Administer a mild laxative, as ordered, to prevent fecal impaction.

Your patient may need mechanical ventilation for up to 2 weeks because of intercostal muscle and diaphragm weakness, atelectasis, and (if he has it) pneumonia. As his condition improves and his respiratory status approaches normal, expect to begin weaning him from the ventilator and to provide respiratory therapy as necessary.

If your patient's serum $T_4$ level is still decreased after 48 hours and he's still comatose, expect to give a repeat bolus of $T_4$—especially important if the patient also has an infection. Obtain blood, urine, and sputum samples for culture, and arrange for the patient to have another chest X-ray. If an infection's identified, administer antibiotics as ordered.

As your patient's serum $T_4$ level returns to normal and his condition improves, expect to switch him to oral thyroid hormone and to begin weaning him from hydrocortisone. Start a program of patient teaching regarding long-term management of hypothyroidism to help prevent further emergency episodes. Remind him that he needs to continue taking his oral thyroid hormone medication even when he feels better, and advise him to wear a Medic Alert bracelet.

# Adrenal Crisis

## Prediagnosis summary

On initial assessment, the patient had a history of:
- progressive weakness
- irritability
- lack of appetite
- headache
- nausea and vomiting
- diarrhea
- abdominal pain
- fever.

If he wasn't seen within 8 to 12 hours of the onset of his signs and symptoms, extracellular volume depletion (up to 20%) may have led to circulatory collapse. The patient had these signs and symptoms:
- hypotension
- tachycardia and thready pulse
- oliguria
- cool, clammy skin

- flaccid extremities
- lethargy
- confusion, restlessness, and progressively decreasing level of consciousness
- hyperpyrexia.

If he's had Addison's disease (the major cause of adrenal crisis) for some time, he may have hyperpigmented skin and mucous membranes.

The patient was given supplemental oxygen by nasal cannula or mask. A 12-lead EKG and a chest X-ray were taken (using portable equipment), and he was connected to a cardiac monitor. A large-bore I.V. was inserted for fluid and medication administration. Blood was drawn for a CBC, electrolytes, BUN, creatinine, glucose, calcium, ABGs, and cortisol.

## Priorities

Because adrenal crisis may be rapidly fatal, the doctor won't wait for the results of laboratory studies. He'll make a tentative diagnosis on the basis of the patient's history and signs and symptoms and begin treatment immediately.

Your immediate priorities are to correct your patient's overwhelming fluid deficit and to replace glucocorticoids. The doctor will insert a CVP line to infuse large amounts of fluid and to monitor the patient's fluid balance. If your patient has limited cardiac reserve as a result of cardiac disease, the doctor may also insert a Swan-Ganz catheter. Expect to rapidly infuse 5% dextrose in normal saline solution to correct your patient's sodium and water deficit and to prevent hypoglycemia. The doctor will ask you to give the first liter of fluid over ½ to 2½ hours. Then, he'll use CVP measurements to determine continuing replacement. Your patient will probably need 3 to 4 liters over the first 24 hours. If he's in profound shock and doesn't respond to fluid administration, you may need to give colloids, such as albumin, but you probably *won't* need to give a vasopressor. Insert an indwelling (Foley) catheter as ordered for accurate output measurement, and start an intake and output record.

# WHAT HAPPENS IN ADRENAL CRISIS

Adrenal crisis is either primary or secondary. *Primary* adrenal crisis, the most prevalent form, results from the absence or deficiency of glucocorticoids (principally cortisol) and mineralocorticoids (principally aldosterone) following atrophy or destruction of the adrenal cortex. This

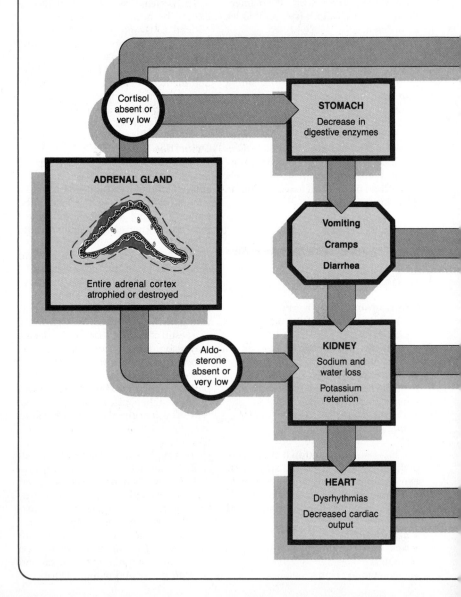

deficiency may stem from a number of causes—for example, Addison's disease (chronic adrenal insufficiency), adrenal vein thrombosis, or destruction or surgical removal of the adrenal gland. *Secondary* adrenal crisis results from destruction or surgical removal of the pituitary gland or from sudden discontinuation of corticosteroid therapy.

No matter what its underlying cause may be, the precipitating factor in primary adrenal crisis is usually stress associated with trauma, surgery, or infection. Such stress demands increased cortisol output from the adrenal gland. Inability to meet this demand sets off the sequence of events highlighted in this flowchart.

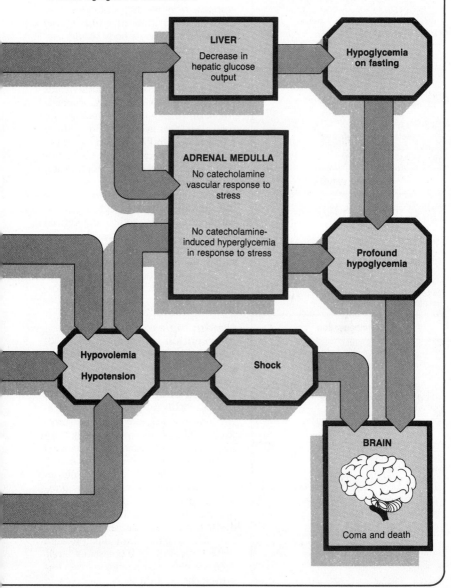

**LIVER**

Decrease in hepatic glucose output

**Hypoglycemia on fasting**

**ADRENAL MEDULLA**

No catecholamine vascular response to stress

No catecholamine-induced hyperglycemia in response to stress

**Profound hypoglycemia**

**Hypovolemia**

**Hypotension**

**Shock**

**BRAIN**

Coma and death

## UNDERSTANDING METABOLIC ALKALOSIS

In contrast to metabolic acidosis, metabolic alkalosis is a state of *decreased* acid and *increased* bicarbonate (base) in the blood, resulting from conditions that cause:
• severe acid loss
• decreased serum potassium and chloride
• excessive bicarbonate intake.
Arterial pH level is above 7.45; $HCO_3$ is above 29 mEq/liter.

### Predisposing factors

• Vomiting
• GI suctioning
• Diuretic therapy
• Corticosteroid therapy
• Cushing's syndrome
• Excessive bicarbonate intake
• Hypokalemia
• Hypercalcemia

### Signs and symptoms

• Neuromuscular irritability
• Tetany
• Twitching
• Seizures
• Central nervous system depression that may progress to coma
• Cardiac dysrhythmias
• Nausea and vomiting
• Hypoventilation (a sign that respiratory compensation's beginning)

### Compensation

In the presence of high $HCO_3$, the respiratory system compensates with *hypoventilation* to *increase* $H_2CO_3$ (as reflected in $Pco_2$) and to bring pH to normal by adjusting the ratio of $HCO_3$ to $H_2CO_3$ to 20:1 (normal).

### Interventions

• Give the patient normal saline solution and potassium I.V.
• Evaluate and correct his electrolyte imbalances.
• If his alkalosis is severe, give ammonium chloride I.V.
• Observe precautions to prevent seizures.
• Monitor his vital signs and fluid balance.
• Discontinue diuretics, if previously given.
• Treat the underlying cause, as ordered.

Expect to replace glucocorticoids by giving repeated I.V. boluses or a continuous I.V. infusion of hydrocortisone (as hemisuccinate, phosphate, or succinate). Why is replacing glucocorticoids so important? Because glucocorticoids stimulate gluconeogenesis, inhibit the inflammatory response, and increase the body's response to stress. Expect to give, over 24 hours, an amount equal to the amount the patient's body would normally produce under stress—100 to 300 mg. If primary adrenal hypofunction caused your patient's adrenal crisis, he'll have a lack of mineralocorticoids (aldosterone) as well as glucocorticoids. However, even though mineralocorticoids are necessary for sodium reabsorption and potassium excretion, you *won't* replace this hormone initially. This is because, in high doses, mineralocorticoids may cause excessive salt retention. (The hydrocortisone you administer has enough mineralocorticoid effect to produce the desired degree of sodium retention. This is one reason why you give hydrocortisone rather than synthetic corticosteroids, such as dexamethasone [Decadron] or prednisone, which lack mineralocorticoid effects.)

### Continuing assessment and intervention

Take your patient's vital signs every 10 to 15 minutes and monitor his CVP readings to assess his fluid status. You may need to adjust the I.V. infusion rate. Watch his cardiac monitor for dysrhythmias, which may arise from electrolyte imbalances—particularly from his hyperkalemia. You may see peaked T waves, decreased P-wave amplitude, a prolonged PR interval, low voltage, or a widened QRS complex—*a dangerous sign* that may indicate impending cardiac standstill. Report any dysrhythmia you observe to the doctor *immediately.* Then draw blood to send to the laboratory for a potassium level.

Observe your patient for signs of improvement. Within a few hours, you

should see:
- increased blood pressure
- decreased heart rate
- increased urine output
- improved level of consciousness
- decreased fever.

As he responds to fluid, dextrose, and glucocorticoid administration, you should note corresponding correction of his hyperkalemia, hyponatremia, and hypercalcemia.

Perform a baseline assessment to look for the underlying cause of your patient's adrenal crisis—it's probably an infection. Obtain samples for blood, urine, and sputum cultures, and send them to the laboratory. Note if his urine is cloudy or mucus-streaked. Ask the patient if he's recently had a cold, the flu, or a productive cough. Listen to his lungs for rales or rhonchi, which may indicate a respiratory tract infection. Ask if he's had nausea, vomiting, or diarrhea recently, and palpate his abdomen for areas of infection.

Remember, your patient will have a decreased ability to respond to stress because of his decreased glucocorticoid level. You can help reduce his *psychological stress* by explaining the therapy you're administering and the procedures you're performing. By providing a quiet environment, keeping him on bed rest, and scheduling rest periods between nursing care procedures, you can also help reduce his *physical stress.*

If, despite fluid and sodium replacement, your patient's blood pressure is still decreased and he still has hyperkalemia, the doctor may then ask you to give mineralocorticoids in addition to glucocorticoids.

### Therapeutic care
Continue to assess your patient's vital signs and fluid status frequently. Maintain accurate intake and output records, and check your patient's weight and electrolyte levels daily. Report your findings to the doctor—he'll reduce the I.V. infusion to a keep-vein-open rate when your patient's fluid deficit is cor-

## UNDERSTANDING METABOLIC ACIDOSIS

Metabolic acidosis is a state of *excess* acid accumulation and *deficient* bicarbonate (base) in the blood, resulting from conditions that cause:
- excessive fat metabolism in the absence of carbohydrates
- anaerobic metabolism
- underexcretion of metabolized acids or inability to conserve base
- loss of sodium bicarbonate from the intestines.

Arterial pH level is below 7.35; $HCO_3$ is below 22 mEq/liter.

### Predisposing factors

- DKA
- Addison's disease
- Renal failure
- Starvation
- Ethanol intoxication
- Tissue hypoxia
- Diarrhea
- Intestinal malabsorption
- Salicylate poisoning
- Low-carbohydrate, high-fat diet

### Signs and symptoms

- Headache and lethargy
- Central nervous system depression that may progress to coma
- Cardiac dysrhythmias
- Nausea and vomiting
- Anorexia
- Dehydration
- Kussmaul's respirations (a sign that respiratory compensation's beginning)

### Compensation

In the presence of low $HCO_3$, the respiratory system compensates with *hyperventilation* to *decrease* $H_2CO_3$ (as reflected in $Pco_2$) and to bring pH to normal by adjusting the ratio of $HCO_3$ to $H_2CO_3$ to 20:1 (normal).

### Interventions

- Give the patient sodium bicarbonate I.V.
- Evaluate and correct his electrolyte imbalances.
- Observe precautions to prevent seizures.
- Monitor his vital signs and fluid balance.
- Treat the underlying cause, as ordered.

rected. He'll also remove the CVP line. If your patient has an infection, expect to give antibiotics specific for the causative organism.

Your patient's crisis should subside in a few days. As his condition improves, expect to taper the dosage of hydrocortisone and to switch him to an oral maintenance dosage. When the hydrocortisone dosage has been tapered to below 100 mg/day, the doctor will ask you to begin administering mineralocorticoids—probably oral fludrocortisone acetate (Florinef) or I.M. desoxycorticosterone acetate (Percorten Acetate, Doca Acetate) or desoxycorticosterone pivalate (Percorten Pivalate). Your patient will continue oral glucocorticoid and mineralocorticoid therapy after discharge.

Continue to provide a quiet environment to reduce your patient's stress. Begin patient teaching by explaining why he's taking corticosteroid medications and what effects they have. Make sure he understands that he'll need an increased dosage if he's ill or stressed. Remind him that if his food and fluid intake decreases (for example, during illness) or his fluid loss increases (for example, if he's vomiting, has diarrhea, or is sweating excessively), he should go to the hospital for evaluation to avoid another crisis.

Teach the patient and his family how to give I.M. corticosteroids—typically, 100 mg of hydrocortisone sodium succinate—in an emergency. And tell him to wear a Medic Alert bracelet identifying his condition and to carry a card in his wallet describing his current therapy.

# Acute Hypoparathyroidism

## Prediagnosis summary
On initial assessment, the patient had signs of neuromuscular excitability:

- mild paresthesias (numbness in feet and hands, circumoral tingling)
- muscle cramps
- carpopedal spasm
- positive Chvostek's and Trousseau's signs
- urinary retention
- laryngeal spasm (causing stridor, dyspnea, and cyanosis)
- severe tetany
- convulsions *without* incontinence or loss of consciousness.

He also had alterations in his mental status—irritability, paranoia, confusion, or depression.

An I.V. was inserted for fluid and medication administration. A 12-lead EKG was taken, and the patient was connected to a cardiac monitor. He was given supplemental oxygen—or, if he had severe laryngeal spasms, he was intubated. Blood was drawn for a CBC, BUN, creatinine, blood glucose, serum calcium, serum magnesium, and serum phosphate.

## Priorities
Your patient's hypoparathyroidism will cause severe hypocalcemia, so your first priority is to reestablish his normal serum calcium levels. Expect to administer I.V. calcium—10 to 20 ml of 10% calcium gluconate in $D_5W$—over 5 to 10 minutes. (You *won't* give calcium in saline, because this causes calcium excretion and worsens hypocalcemia.) Avoid infiltration, and give the solution slowly to prevent hypotension and cardiac arrest. Monitor the patient's blood pressure during the infusion, and watch the cardiac monitor to detect EKG changes characteristic of hypocalcemia: a prolonged QT interval without ST segment or QRS complex changes. Keep in mind that a prolonged QT interval predisposes your patient to ventricular tachycardia.

I.V. calcium acts rapidly but also has a short half-life, so you may need to repeat the dose to maintain appropriate serum calcium levels. Or the doctor may ask you to give a continuous infusion over 4 to 6 hours. Draw blood

## WHAT HAPPENS IN ACUTE HYPOPARATHYROIDISM

Hypoparathyroidism is a deficiency of parathyroid hormone (PTH). Causes of acute hypoparathyroidism include:
• injury to the parathyroid glands
• accidental removal of the parathyroid glands during thyroidectomy or other neck surgery.
  Other, less common, causes include:
• autoimmune disease
• tumor
• tuberculosis
• sarcoidosis
• hemochromatosis
• severe magnesium deficiency associated with alcoholism and intestinal malabsorption (causes a reversible form of hypoparathyroidism).
  Normally, PTH (with the aid of vitamin D) maintains serum calcium and phosphate

levels by:
• balancing calcium levels in bone, blood, kidneys, intestines, and soft tissues
• maintaining an inverse relationship between serum calcium and serum phosphate (this means that if the level of one begins to fall, the other rises, because the product of the two is constant).
  Diminished or absent PTH levels disrupt this balance, however, causing:
• excessive reabsorption of phosphate by the renal tubules
• decreased release of calcium from bone
• decreased renal calcium reabsorption
• decreased intestinal calcium absorption.
  The result? Severe hypocalcemia and hyperphosphatemia, which can lead to seizures, tetany, laryngospasm, and central nervous system abnormalities.

periodically to monitor the patient's serum calcium levels.

If calcium doesn't alleviate your patient's signs and symptoms, this may mean that your patient's hypoparathyroidism is due to hypomagnesemia (as in a patient with chronic alcoholism or malabsorption syndrome), which decreases parathyroid hormone (PTH) release. If the doctor suspects this, he'll ask you to give I.V. magnesium (as magnesium sulfate solution), instead of calcium, to alleviate the patient's signs and symptoms. Magnesium administration has three main benefits: it will relieve the patient's tetany, increase his PTH secretion, and improve his target organ response to PTH.

## Continuing assessment and intervention

Your patient's signs and symptoms of neuromuscular irritability should disappear soon after you administer I.V. calcium. Perform a baseline assessment and look for signs of improvement. Check his extremities for reduced tetany, paresthesias, and muscle cramps, and assess his breathing rate

and rhythm. Note improvements in his mental status—his irritability and confusion should decrease as his serum calcium levels return to normal. If your patient had laryngeal spasms, they will subside once his serum calcium level returns to normal. At that time, he'll be removed from the ventilator and extubated.

Take a history to help determine the underlying cause of his hypoparathyroidism. Ask if he's had thyroid or other neck surgery, and look for any neck scars; his parathyroid glands may have been accidentally removed or injured during thyroid surgery. Determine if he has a history of intestinal malabsorption, alcoholism, renal failure, or laxative abuse. These conditions cause vitamin D resistance or deficiency, which decreases the effect of PTH on target tissues. Determine what medications your patient is taking: phenytoin (Dilantin), barbiturates (especially phenobarbital), and some laxatives cause vitamin D resistance. Although decreased vitamin D levels cause a compensatory *increase* in PTH levels, your patient will be hypocalcemic in the absence of vitamin D, because target tissues can't respond to PTH without it. This isn't true hypoparathyroidism—your patient is producing PTH. But because he can't effectively use the PTH, the *effect* is the same—hypocalcemia. Under any of the circumstances described, he'll need long-term vitamin D therapy.

### Therapeutic care

Monitor your patient's serum calcium level to determine if it's being maintained at a normal level. As you may know, calcium therapy is rapidly effective. However, if *magnesium deficiency* caused the patient's hypoparathyroidism, expect to give magnesium for up to 5 days before his calcium level returns to normal. If your patient has *chronic hypoparathyroidism*, expect to switch him from I.V. to oral calcium (this may involve changing his diet or giving him supplemental calcium). If his chronic hypoparathyroidism is the result of parathyroid gland removal or destruction, your patient will need to ingest approximately 1 g of calcium/day for the rest of his life.

To increase calcium in your patient's diet, give him calcium-rich foods, such as dairy products (cheese, ice cream, milk, yogurt), spinach, and almonds. If he can't eat dairy products because he can't tolerate lactose or if he has an aversion to calcium-rich foods, give him oral calcium supplements, such as calcium carbonate or calcium glubionate.

You'll also need to administer vitamin D orally to increase the patient's calcium absorption and target-organ use of PTH. Initially, you may give vitamin $D_3$, which acts quickly and has a short half-life. You may be asked to administer vitamin $D_2$, along with vi-

---

## ELICITING SIGNS OF LATENT TETANY

Tetany, a serious manifestation of acute hypocalcemia, often accompanies hypoparathyroidism. If not discovered and treated, tetany can rapidly progress to convulsions and laryngeal spasm. You can check for latent tetany by looking for these two characteristic signs when assessing your patient:

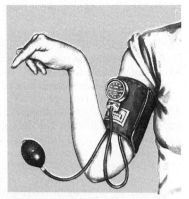

**Trousseau's sign:** a carpopedal spasm causing the patient simultaneously to flex his wrist, to adduct his thumb, and to extend one or more fingers. To attempt to elicit this sign, occlude the arm's blood flow for 3 minutes by applying and inflating a blood pressure cuff.

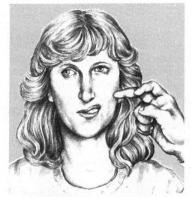

**Chvostek's sign:** a facial muscle spasm you can attempt to elicit by lightly tapping your patient's facial nerve adjacent to her ear.

# CASE IN POINT: FAILING TO READ THE LABEL

Judy Samuels, age 16, is a patient with brittle diabetes on your medical-surgical unit. Because her condition's so unstable, her insulin dosages vary each day. When you check her chart this time, you find an order to administer isophane insulin suspension (NPH) 40 units S.C. You go to the refrigerator to get the insulin. Then, just as you're about to grasp the bottle, a student nurse interrupts—can you help her with an urgent problem? Telling her you'll be right there, you take down the insulin bottle and administer the dose to Judy.

A few minutes later, when you check on Judy, she's going into shock. You call the doctor quickly and administer I.V. dextrose, as ordered. Within minutes, Judy's condition stabilizes, but she'll need additional treatment.

You know, of course, that Judy's reaction means something went wrong. So you take the responsibility for following up. First, you check Judy's chart to see if she ate breakfast; she did. Then you check the bottle you used to prepare the insulin—and find it's labeled *regular* insulin, not NPH. When Judy's parents ask what happened and learn of the mishap, they're very upset. So upset, in fact, that they intend to sue you for negligence.

Suppose this incident really happened. Would you be liable for Judy's prolonged hospitalization?

In a case involving a similar situation *(Habuda v. Trustees of Rex Hospital,* 1968), the nurse was found liable. Why? The court ruled that she breached her duty to read a drug label and so gave her patient the wrong medication. Her patient required further treatment for injuries from the wrong drug.

How can you avoid liability in situations like this? Remember this rule of thumb: Read all drug labels *three* times. *First,* read the label as soon as you take the drug out of the cabinet or refrigerator. *Second,* read it when you prepare the dose. *Third,* read it when you put the drug bottle back. Following this rule will always protect you from giving the wrong medication; adhere to it even if your unit's extremely busy. And remember this: A doctor may not be legally responsible for rechecking a drug you hand to him for administration to a patient. In fact, your duty to read drug labels carefully is so widely accepted that a doctor can avoid liability if evidence at a trial shows he relied on you to hand him the correct drug.

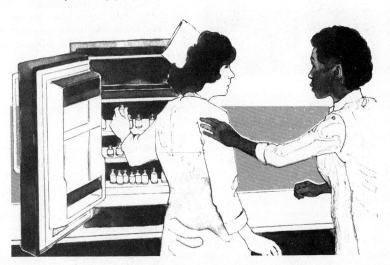

*Habuda v. Trustees of Rex Hospital,* 164 S.E. 2d 17 (N.C., 1968).

tamin D$_3$, to maintain a normal calcium level during the first few weeks of your patient's treatment. This is because vitamin D$_2$ acts more slowly and will have its maximum effect after about 30 days, when the vitamin D$_3$ will no longer be effective. The doctor will probably switch the patient to oral vitamin D$_2$ for long-term therapy. This change will be made because vitamin D$_3$ is very expensive.

If your patient's taking glucocorticoids, the doctor may need to *increase* his vitamin D dosage because glucocorticoids inhibit vitamin D's action. However, if the patient's taking thiazide diuretics, the doctor will *decrease* the dose of vitamin D. Why? Because thiazide diuretics cause reduced renal clearance of calcium, and this may cause *hyper*calcemia.

Advise your patient with chronic hypoparathyroidism that he'll need to take calcium and vitamin D for the rest of his life. Remind him, too, that he should be alert to symptoms of developing hypocalcemia, such as muscle spasms and tingling in his extremities.

# A FINAL WORD

Endocrine emergencies have always perplexed health-care professionals. Why? Because:
• they're difficult to diagnose, mimicking many other disorders.
• they're difficult to treat because hormones affect so many body systems.
• they're difficult to understand. (Even today, scientists don't completely understand the pathophysiology of many endocrine emergencies.)

As a nurse, you may sometimes feel that the knowledge you need to care for patients during and after endocrine emergencies is overwhelming. But take heart—endocrine research has expanded rapidly in recent years, and new technologies continue to appear that make caring for these patients easier.

As you know, rapid, correct diagnosis of endocrine emergencies depends in part on accurate laboratory testing of patients' hormone levels. Many of these tests are now performed by *radioimmunoassay*—a type of laboratory test that wasn't commonly available even a decade ago. These tests allow you to monitor your patient's blood hormone levels frequently and more accurately than in years past. So you can more closely determine how he's responding to therapy.

Other developments help *prevent* endocrine emergencies by increasing patients'—and doctors'—control over chronic endocrine conditions. For instance, in the last few years, three new products have become available that can help your diabetic patient avoid the hazards of DKA and hypoglycemia. One such group of products are *home blood glucose monitoring systems,* which allow your patient to test his blood glucose levels visually at home; this helps him avoid extremes of hypo- and hyperglycemia. *Glycosylated hemoglobin tests* are another important advance; these tests allow the doctor to monitor your patient's average blood glucose levels accurately over a period of several months, encouraging better compliance. And *insulin pumps,* although still under development, offer new hope for diabetic patients whose blood glucose levels are unstable despite careful management. Be sure to stay informed about these and other new products and developments: they can help you provide patient teaching that may prevent endocrine emergencies.

No matter what type of endocrine condition a patient of yours has, chances are he'll have to live with it indefinitely. By helping him understand his condition and control it, you'll help him avoid complications and keep control of his life.

# Selected References

Borg, Nan, ed. *Core Curriculum for Critical Care Nurses.* American Association of Critical Care Nurses. Philadelphia: W.B. Saunders Co., 1981.

Brunner, Lillian S., and Suddarth, Doris S. *Textbook of Medical-Surgical Nursing,* 4th ed. Philadelphia: J.B. Lippincott Co., 1980.

Cavalier, J.P. "Crucial Decisions in Diabetic Emergencies," *RN* 43:32-7, November 1980.

DeGroot, Leslie J., ed. *Endocrinology,* vol. 1. New York: Grune & Stratton, 1979.

Evangelisti, J.T., and Thorpe, C.J. "Thyroid Storm—A Nursing Crisis," *Heart and Lung* 12(2):184-94, March 1983.

Felig, P., et al. *Endocrinology and Metabolism.* New York: McGraw-Hill Book Co., 1981.

Johanson, B.C., et al. *Standards for Critical Care.* St. Louis: C.V. Mosby Co., 1981.

Kinney, Marguerite, et al. *AACN's Clinical Reference for Critical Care Nursing.* New York: McGraw-Hill Book Co., 1981.

Koppers, L.E. "Pheochromocytoma—Critical Care," *Critical Care Quarterly* 3:93-7, September 1980.

Krieger, Dorothy T., and Bardin, C. Wayne, eds. *Current Therapy in Endocrinology 1983-84.* St. Louis: C.V. Mosby Co., 1983.

Luckmann, Joan, and Sorenson, Karen C. *Medical-Surgical Nursing: A Psychophysiologic Approach.* Philadelphia: W.B. Saunders Co., 1980.

Niedringhaus, L. "A Nursing Emergency... Acute Adrenal Crisis," *Focus on Critical Care* 10(1):30-6, February 1983.

Preedy, J.R.K. "Emergency: Acute Adrenocortical Failure," *Hospital Medicine* 19(7):90-102, July 1983.

Rabin, David, and McKenna, Terence, eds. *Clinical Endocrinology and Metabolism.* Science and Practice of Clinical Medicine Series. New York: Grune & Stratton, 1982.

Rush, D.R., et al. "Drugs Used in Endocrine Metabolic Emergencies," *Critical Care Quarterly* 3:1-9, September 1980.

Sneid, D. "Hyperosmolar Hyperglycemic Nonketotic Coma," *Critical Care Quarterly* 3:29-43, September 1980.

Sommers, M.S. "Nonketotic Hyperosmolar Coma (Care Plan)," *Critical Care Nurse* 3(1):58-61, January/February 1983.

Walter, R.M., Jr., and Warsaw, T. "Diabetic Ketoacidosis—A Treatment Appraisal," *Heart and Lung* 10:112-3, January/February 1981.

Williams, Robert H. *Textbook of Endocrinology,* 6th ed. Philadelphia: W.B. Saunders Co., 1981.

Winters, B. "Nursing Implications of Hyperosmolar Coma," *Heart and Lung* 12:439-46, July 1983.

Zschoche, Donna A. *Mosby's Comprehensive Review of Critical Care,* 2nd ed. St. Louis: C.V. Mosby Co., 1980.

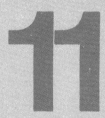

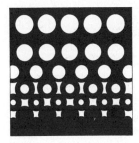

# Hematologic Emergencies

## Introduction

You're on the medical-surgical unit, checking your patients one last time before your shift's scheduled to end, when you see a call light rapidly flashing. It's Mrs. Rita Bowen, age 60, who was admitted for treatment of a pulmonary embolism shortly after your shift began. She's been receiving a maintenance dose of heparin through a continual I.V. infusion drip, to prevent new clots from forming. Her last laboratory tests showed that her partial thromboplastin time (PTT) was two and one half times normal—well within the acceptable therapeutic range. She had drifted off to sleep when you looked in on her half an hour ago. Now, as you head for her room, you wonder what the problem could be.

"I'm so glad you're here!" says Mrs. Bowen. She's lying on her side, holding a wad of tissues to her nose and trying unsuccessfully to stop it from bleeding. "I guess I must've dozed off. I woke up when I felt the blood coming out of my nose. I can't seem to stop it. What's happening to me?"

You're immediately concerned that Mrs. Bowen's nosebleed may mean she's receiving an anticoagulant overdose. But before you can be sure, you know you'll have to see if you can stop the bleeding and do a rapid emergency assessment.

First, you help Mrs. Bowen sit up.

Then, you tell her to tilt her head forward to prevent blood from running down the back of her throat, and you show her how to try to control the bleeding—by gently pinching her nostrils with a sterile gauze pad.

While she's doing this, you check her vital signs. Blood pressure? Low/normal. Pulse? Rapid. As you take her pulse, you notice several petechiae and ecchymoses on her hands and arms.

Meanwhile, Mrs. Bowen's renewed efforts to control her nosebleed still aren't working. You check the infusion pump quickly, but the dials are still where you set them, so you know Mrs. Bowen's heparin dosage hasn't been altered. Nevertheless, her signs and symptoms have reinforced your first, instinctive impression: possible anticoagulant overdose.

You notify the doctor, who orders a *stat* PTT and tells you to stop the heparin infusion immediately. Just to be on the safe side, you prepare to administer protamine sulfate to neutralize the heparin already in Mrs. Bowen's circulation. Her diagnosis isn't certain, but you've done all you can to care for her emergency condition.

Sure enough, when the laboratory results come in 10 minutes later, Mrs. Bowen's PTT is severely prolonged. She does have an anticoagulant overdose. Your nursing assessment skills proba-

# A NEW ADVANCE IN BLOOD REPLACEMENT

Within the next few years, you may see widespread use—particularly in emergencies—of perfluorochemical (Fluosol-DA), a blood substitute that's being tested in some centers now. When it's approved, you can expect to give Fluosol in many emergency situations. Here's why:
• It's easy to use. It can provide *immediate* treatment for bleeding emergencies without being refrigerated, typed, or cross-matched. So rescue personnel can carry it and administer it at the scene of an emergency or in the ambulance.
• It's versatile. It can treat almost any condition related to acute ischemia.
• It can increase the survival rate of patients with emergencies. Because it can replace lost blood quickly, with no advance preparation, it can save time—and lives.

Fluosol works by performing two essential blood functions: plasma expansion and oxygen transport. It's not an artificial blood, however, so it can't provide clotting factors, platelets, or other blood products.

Researchers are clinically testing Fluosol now. Currently, the Food and Drug Administration's protocol allows use of this experimental blood substitute for:
• Jehovah's Witnesses with severe anemia who refuse blood transfusions on religious grounds

• patients with embolic, basilar ischemic, or vasospastic strokes. (All test subjects must have normal hepatic, renal, and pulmonary functions, and must not receive more than two doses of Fluosol.)

Before receiving Fluosol, each patient must be pretreated with corticosteroids to prevent such reactions as:
• mild chest pain
• shortness of breath
• a drop in white blood cell count.

After pretreatment, researchers slowly infuse 20 ml/kg of Fluosol. (Even without desensitization, side effects usually correct themselves in minutes.)

When a patient receives it without supplemental oxygen, Fluosol acts mostly as a volume expander. If it's administered with high concentrations of oxygen, however, Fluosol carries an increased amount of oxygen to the patient's tissues without using the oxygen contained in his hemoglobin.

Fluosol can also restrict tissue hypoxia, reduce the size of brain infarcts, and treat sickle cell anemia, because its oxygen-carrying particles—70 times smaller than red blood cells (RBCs)—infiltrate ischemic tissues better than RBCs do.

Here's a chart to show you how Fluosol compares with blood.

| BLOOD | FLUOSOL |
|---|---|
| • Expands the patient's circulating volume | • Expands the patient's circulating volume |
| • Has RBCs and hemoglobin that carry oxygen to ischemic tissues | • Has particles 70 times smaller than RBCs, which can infiltrate and carry more oxygen to ischemic tissues |
| • Carries 95% of the blood's oxygen no matter how much supplemental oxygen is given | • Can carry extra oxygen when administered with high concentrations of supplemental oxygen |
| • Provides clotting factors and platelets | • Doesn't provide clotting factors or platelets |
| • Must be refrigerated, typed, and cross-matched | • Doesn't need to be refrigerated, typed, or cross-matched |
| • Usually requires no pretreatment | • Requires pretreatment with corticosteroids to prevent reactions |
| • Is readily available | • Is available only for experimental use pending FDA approval |

bly prevented an even more serious emergency.

This time, you knew what to do for a patient with a hematologic emergency. But do you feel confident that you could recognize even subtle signs and symptoms in such a patient—particularly one who has a traumatic bleeding injury—and intervene appropriately?

Hematologic disorders are usually chronic conditions with periodic crises, which can be emergencies. But a hematologic emergency can also arise as a complication of a preexisting condition or of treatment (as in Mrs. Bowen's situation). This chapter will help you become familiar with possible causes of hematologic emergencies and the interventions that must follow.

# INITIAL CARE

## Prehospital Care: What's Been Done

Rescue personnel's goal was to get the patient with a hematologic emergency to the ED as quickly as possible. In the meantime, they attempted to stabilize the patient's airway, breathing, and circulation. If necessary, they suctioned blood and accumulated secretions from the patient's airway. If he appeared anemic and his breathing was labored, they provided supplemental oxygen to prevent hypoxemia. If he was known to have hemophilia and was bleeding uncontrollably, they inserted an I.V. and began fluid replacement. Their objective was to avoid compromising his circulatory status until the blood factor he needed could be transfused in the hospital.

# What to Do First

Your first goal is to rapidly assess and stabilize your patient's airway, breathing, and—especially—circulation. You'll need critical thinking and rapid responses to prevent your patient's hematologic emergency from compromising his hemodynamic status.

Patients with chronic hematologic disorders generally know what to expect and how to proceed when a crisis strikes. If the patient's experiencing such a crisis for the first time, however, you'll need to make a special effort to alleviate his anxiety.

### Airway
Assess and intervene appropriately to ensure that your patient's airway is patent and remains so. (See the "Life Support" section in Chapter 3.) A hematologic emergency doesn't usually compromise a patient's airway. But when hemoptysis or hematemesis results from his underlying condition, airway obstruction can easily occur. Try to clear his mouth with finger sweeps first. If his airway's still occluded, suction it with a tonsil-tip catheter. (Set the suction pressure as low as possible, to minimize mucosal trauma.)

### Breathing
If your patient's suffering from anemia or massive hemorrhage, he may have tachypnea. You'll have to act quickly to restore adequate breathing. Tachypnea is a sign of increased respiratory effort to overcome an oxygen deficit, possibly from hemoglobin deficiency—a direct result of loss or destruction of red blood cells (RBCs). (As you probably know, a hemoglobin deficiency decreases the blood's oxygen-carrying capacity and can cause hypoxia.) If rescue personnel didn't initiate supplemental oxygen, do so now. Insert a large-gauge I.V. to facilitate fluid and/or blood replacement.

# INITIAL ASSESSMENT CHECKLIST

**Assess the ABCs first and intervene appropriately.**

**Check for:**
• petechiae, ecchymoses, hematoma, or uncontrolled bleeding, indicating a coagulation disorder
• fever, chills, subnormal body temperature, or signs of dehydration, possibly indicating sepsis
• progressively deteriorating mental status, possibly indicating cerebral ischemia due to red blood cell sickling
• shortness of breath, tachypnea, or cyanosis, indicating hypoxemia from decreased red blood cells.

**Intervene by:**
• inserting a large-gauge I.V. for fluid or blood component therapy
• applying thrombin-soaked gauze or Gelfoam to bleeding sites to promote coagulation and hemostasis.

**Prepare for:**
• blood or component transfusion or factor replacement
• reverse isolation.

Blood will be drawn for hemoglobin and hematocrit levels, arterial blood gases (ABGs), platelet count, typing and cross matching, PT, and PTT. Monitor his ABGs frequently, and observe him closely for signs of respiratory compromise (increasingly shallow respirations, drowsiness, restlessness, cyanosis). Be prepared to assist the doctor with intubation and mechanical ventilation, if necessary.

## Circulation

Most of your initial assessment and interventions will be focused on stabilizing your patient's circulation. Your goal is to control bleeding and to prevent hypovolemic shock.

First, assess your patient for external

and internal hemorrhage. Look for obvious signs of trauma—bruises, open wounds, lacerations. If your patient doesn't have a history of trauma, then a hematologic disorder, such as a platelet or clotting deficiency, may be causing the hemorrhage. (See *Understanding Normal Blood Clotting*, pages 478 and 479.) Do you see bleeding from body orifices or trauma sites, or blood oozing from needle-puncture or I.V. infusion sites? These could indicate that your patient has a coagulation disorder that's preventing the formation of hemostatic plugs.

Signs and symptoms that may occur with internal hemorrhage include:
• abdominal distention, rigidity, and pain
• an enlarged, ecchymotic joint or flank
• occult or frank blood in urine, feces, vomitus, or sputum
• Grey Turner's or Cullen's sign
• dyspnea and/or tachypnea.

Quickly take your patient's baseline vital signs. Then, try to stop any external bleeding by applying direct pressure to the site for at least 5 minutes. If the bleeding's secondary to an underlying hematologic disorder, such as thrombocytopenia or hemophilia, direct pressure won't stop it. Your next step is to elevate the bleeding site, if possible, and apply a thrombin-soaked gauze pad to promote coagulation. Cover this with a pressure dressing and ice pack. (Check your patient's peripheral pulse below the pressure dressing to make sure the dressing isn't compromising his peripheral circulation.) Notify the doctor and continue monitoring your patient's vital signs, noting any trends (such as an increasingly faint and rapid pulse or dropping blood pressure) that indicate impending hypovolemic shock.

If your patient appears to be going into shock, your goal will be to maintain or restore adequate blood volume and tissue perfusion via fluid replacement and blood transfusion. (See *Administering Blood Transfusions*, page 493.) Prepare to help the doctor insert a central venous pressure line, for massive fluid replacement, and an arterial line to provide easy access for serial blood samples. (Of course, these procedures won't be done if the patient has a clotting disorder, because they may exacerbate bleeding.)

If your patient has sickle cell crisis, he'll have ischemia from sickling (clumping) blood cells. Expect to administer large amounts of fluid through a large-bore I.V. to increase his blood volume and decrease his blood's viscosity. If he has a history of hemophilia and is bleeding (internally or externally), prepare to administer cryoprecipitate or plasma to replace the needed clotting factor (VIII or IX).

In a patient who's receiving a blood or blood component transfusion, be alert for signs and symptoms indicating a transfusion reaction. (See *Recognizing Transfusion Reactions*, page 494.) If your patient has sudden onset of headache, fever, chills, or back pain, *stop the transfusion immediately and notify the doctor*. Obtain blood and urine samples for detection of free hemoglobin and for further testing.

### General appearance

When you're assessing your patient for signs and symptoms of hemorrhage, remember to note indications of multiple bleeding sites in his skin and mucous membranes. Look for petechiae and purpuric skin lesions, especially in the conjunctivae and inside his mouth. Observe your patient's general appearance for signs of hypoxemia, such as cyanosis and pallor, from excessive blood loss. Also note indications of infection—such as fever, chills, redness, or localized inflammatory response. You may not see the traditional signs of infection if your patient has an accompanying white blood cell (WBC) deficiency (granulocytopenia). Why? Because a patient with granulocytopenia can't produce the inflammatory response that usually accompanies an infection. For example, his skin may be pale instead of red.

### Mental status

Check your patient frequently for changes in his level of consciousness. As a nurse, you know that these are often the first observable signs of decreased perfusion to the brain and may result from hypovolemia, hypoxia, or sepsis. If your patient seems restless or disoriented, ensure his safety by keeping his bed in a low position with the side rails up. Have someone else notify the doctor—don't leave your patient alone. The doctor may order fluid resuscitation, supplemental oxygen, and medications, such as vasopressors.

If your patient is in sickle cell crisis, he may have cerebral ischemia, which can cause his mental status to deteriorate. When you administer fluid, as ordered, to clear the sickled cells, this will allow normal RBCs to function. The oxygen they supply should relieve the cerebral ischemia.

# What to Do Next

Now that you've completed your emergency assessment and intervened as necessary, follow up by taking your patient's history and performing a physical examination to discover the nature and extent of his chief complaint.

If your patient has *excessive bleeding,* try to determine how long he's been bleeding and how much blood he's lost. Find out whether the bleeding was caused by trauma or precipitated by a preexisting hematologic disorder. Ask your patient about previous bleeding episodes, too—particularly whether any occurred following medical or dental procedures.

If your patient complains of a *swollen, painful joint,* it may indicate hemarthrosis (bleeding into the joint).

When you assess your patient for *pallor or cyanosis,* look for signs and symptoms of hypoxemia secondary to anemia. If your patient has hemolytic anemia, he may have pallor with ac-

# UNDERSTANDING NORMAL BLOOD CLOTTING

Normal blood clotting, as you know, is an essential physiologic mechanism designed to prevent excessive bleeding by plugging ruptured or torn blood vessels. You need to understand this mechanism to see how any disruption in its delicate balance can cause a potentially fatal bleeding emergency. Here's how it works:
   A tissue or vascular injury triggers vasoconstriction and causes platelet plug formation to

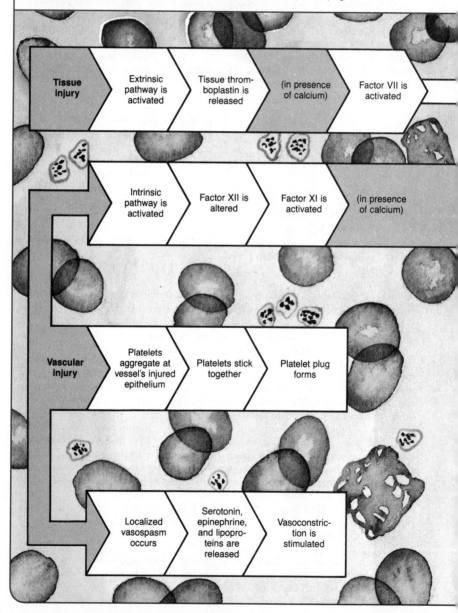

**Tissue injury** → Extrinsic pathway is activated → Tissue thromboplastin is released → (in presence of calcium) → Factor VII is activated →

Intrinsic pathway is activated → Factor XII is altered → Factor XI is activated → (in presence of calcium)

**Vascular injury** → Platelets aggregate at vessel's injured epithelium → Platelets stick together → Platelet plug forms

Localized vasospasm occurs → Serotonin, epinephrine, and lipoproteins are released → Vasoconstriction is stimulated

create a first line of defense against bleeding. These effects slow the bleeding until a permanent fibrin clot forms. (Fibrin clot formation is the most effective and most important part of normal blood clotting.)

This flowchart outlines the sequence of events in normal clotting from the initial injury to adequate clot formation.

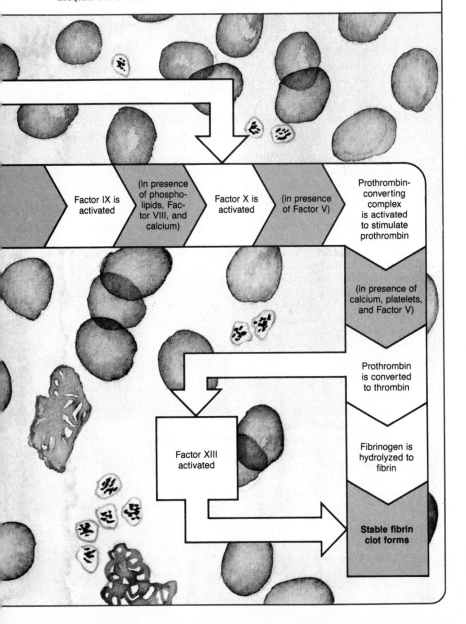

Factor IX is activated

(in presence of phospholipids, Factor VIII, and calcium)

Factor X is activated

(in presence of Factor V)

Prothrombin-converting complex is activated to stimulate prothrombin

(in presence of calcium, platelets, and Factor V)

Prothrombin is converted to thrombin

Factor XIII activated

Fibrinogen is hydrolyzed to fibrin

**Stable fibrin clot forms**

companying *jaundice*—signs that destruction of RBCs is exceeding the rate at which his liver can convert heme particles to bilirubin. *Pale or cyanotic nail beds* may mean your patient has decreased peripheral oxygenation. If he's *cyanotic* and complains of *sharp pain*, these may indicate prolonged tissue hypoxia, even impending tissue necrosis and infarction.

Ask your patient or a family member whether the family has any history of inherited hematologic diseases (such as sickle cell anemia) or clotting factor deficiencies (such as hemophilia). If the answer's positive, find out if the patient's been tested for these disorders. If he hasn't been tested, genetic karyotyping (chromosomal) studies will be needed to see if an underlying hematologic disorder may be causing his signs and symptoms. Remember to ask about your patient's general medical history, too. Liver disease, for example, can impair hemostasis and cause a hematologic emergency.

Find out if your patient's been taking anticoagulants, steroids, or antibiotics, or receiving chemotherapy. Any of these can alter his hematologic status or influence his signs and symptoms. For example, if he's bleeding, ask:
• when chemotherapeutic drugs were last administered to him. Why? Because some chemotherapeutic agents have delayed (up to 4 weeks) hematologic effects, such as WBC suppression.
• if he's taking an anticoagulant. The drug he's taking may have exceeded the therapeutic level, causing an overdose and resulting in excessive anticoagulation and bleeding.
• if he's taking an antibiotic, which may have produced a blood dyscrasia as a side effect.
• if he's taking a corticosteroid, which could be masking signs and symptoms of systemic infection.

Remember, your patient with WBC deficiency is at high risk for systemic infection. But, because his defense system is weakened, he may not exhibit the typical signs and symptoms. So look for subtle signs and symptoms of infection, especially infection of his lungs, urinary tract, perirectal abscesses, skin, or mucous membranes. For example:
• A *productive cough* may mean he has a respiratory infection secondary to granulocytopenia.
• Complaints of *dysuria* or *frequent urination* may indicate a urinary tract infection.
• *Perianal pain and edema* may indicate perirectal abcesses.

Look for signs of opportunistic infections if your patient is immunologically suppressed from corticosteroid therapy or granulocytopenia. If you see such signs and symptoms as *white, patchy lesions* in your patient's mouth or *moist, red rashes* in large skin folds, he may have a yeast infection caused by *Candida albicans*. Be sure to observe him for areas of *purulent drainage* or *pus formation*, too. But remember: If your patient has granulocytopenia, his neutrophils are immature and limited in number, so the usual inflammatory responses (such as purulent drainage, pus formation, and leukocytosis) may be absent.

# CARE AFTER DIAGNOSIS

## Sickle Cell Crisis

**Prediagnosis summary**
The patient had a history of sickle cell anemia, and an initial assessment revealed some or all of the following signs and symptoms of sickle cell crisis:
• sudden, severe pain in his chest, abdomen, back, hand, or foot
• aching joint pain
• increased weakness

# RECOGNIZING SICKLE CELL CRISIS SYNDROMES

You're already familiar with the generalized painful crisis of sickle cell anemia. But do you know that other groups of signs and symptoms can signal sickle cell crisis, too? Some of these signs and symptoms are similar to those associated with sepsis and meningitis. Others may indicate different sickle cell crisis syndromes, such as head-foot syndrome or acute chest syndrome. So be alert for signs of sickle cell crisis syndromes—recognizing them early will allow you to intervene before the complications become life-threatening emergencies.

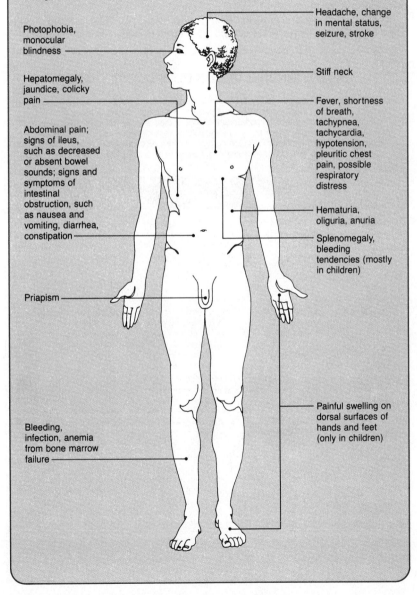

Photophobia, monocular blindness

Hepatomegaly, jaundice, colicky pain

Abdominal pain; signs of ileus, such as decreased or absent bowel sounds; signs and symptoms of intestinal obstruction, such as nausea and vomiting, diarrhea, constipation

Priapism

Bleeding, infection, anemia from bone marrow failure

Headache, change in mental status, seizure, stroke

Stiff neck

Fever, shortness of breath, tachypnea, tachycardia, hypotension, pleuritic chest pain, possible respiratory distress

Hematuria, oliguria, anuria

Splenomegaly, bleeding tendencies (mostly in children)

Painful swelling on dorsal surfaces of hands and feet (only in children)

- dyspnea
- scleral icterus.

He may also have had some combination of the following signs and symptoms of infection, which may have precipitated his crisis:
- fever
- productive cough
- dyspnea and tachypnea
- a draining leg ulcer.

Blood was drawn for testing to detect the cause of the patient's sickle cell crisis. Laboratory results revealed some or all of the following factors and conditions:
- increased WBC count (indicating infection and possible sepsis)
- trace hemoglobin in urine and increased bilirubin and reticulocyte count (indicating hemolysis)
- decreased $O_2$ (indicating hypoxemia)
- decreased pH and decreased $CO_2$ and electrolyte levels (indicating acidosis).

---

## UNDERSTANDING BLOOD COMPONENT THERAPY

All blood component products are extracted from whole blood, but each has different characteristics. So some blood components treat certain hematologic disorders better than others. The doctor will choose a blood component product based on how well it will treat your patient's condition. For example, if your patient needs volume replenishment quickly, he'll receive a volume expander. If his blood isn't clotting properly, he'll receive a product with clotting factors.

Here's a chart to help you learn more about blood component products and their uses.

| TYPE | CONTENTS | USES | NURSING CONSIDERATIONS |
|---|---|---|---|
| **Whole blood** | • Red blood cells (RBCs), white blood cells (WBCs), platelets, plasma, and plasma clotting factors | • To restore blood volume and to replenish oxygen-carrying capacity in a patient with massive hemorrhage | • Administer through a large-gauge I.V. over 2 to 4 hours, or as ordered. |
| **Packed cells** | • RBCs and 20% plasma<br>• Less sodium and potassium than whole blood | • To replenish blood's oxygen-carrying capacity while minimizing risk of fluid overload in patients with severe anemia, slow blood loss, or congestive heart failure | Administer more slowly than whole blood (unless diluted with saline solution). |
| **Washed cells** | • RBCs and 20% plasma<br>• Fewer WBCs and platelets than packed cells | • To replenish blood's oxygen-carrying capacity in patients previously sensitized by transfusions | • Administer at a slower rate than whole blood (unless diluted with saline solution). |
| **Granulocytes** | • WBCs and 20% plasma | • To treat life-threatening granulocytopenia ($<500/mm^3$) | • Administer rapidly.<br>• Expect the patient to develop fever, chills, hypertension, or disorientation during transfusion; these are considered to be transfusion reactions. |

## Priorities

Your first priority is to begin hydrating your patient to minimize the risk of vaso-occlusive complications.

Expect to insert a large-gauge I.V. catheter and to begin infusing normal saline solution at double the normal rate. For example, normal fluid management for an average adult is 125 ml/ hour; you'll need to administer 250 ml/ hour while the patient's in sickle cell crisis. This will increase his hydration, decrease his blood viscosity, and prevent additional cell sickling.

Quickly assess your patient for signs and symptoms of dehydration, such as poor skin turgor and dry mucous membranes, and ask whether he's had any illness recently that caused fluid loss through diarrhea or vomiting. If dehydration triggered your patient's sickle cell crisis, he'll need even more aggressive fluid replacement, because his decreased fluid volume makes his

| TYPE | CONTENTS | USES | NURSING CONSIDERATIONS |
|---|---|---|---|
| **Plasma (fresh-frozen)** | • Clotting Factors II, III, V, VII, IX, X, and XIII; fibrinogen; prothrombin; albumin; and globulins | • To treat patients with clotting factor deficiencies (the only treatment for Factor V deficiency) <br> • To expand volume | • Fresh-frozen plasma takes 20 minutes to thaw, so call the blood bank ahead of time. <br> • Administer 1 unit over 1 hour. |
| **Platelets** | • Platelets, WBCs, and plasma | • To correct low platelet counts ($<10,000/mm^3$) | • Administer 1 unit over 10 minutes. |
| **Cryoprecipitate** | • Factors VIII and XIII and fibrinogen | • To replace clotting factors in patients with disseminated intravascular coagulation, hemophilia A, von Willebrand's disease, fibrinogen deficiency, or Factor XIII deficiency | • Administer rapidly *immediately after thawing,* to ensure factor activation. |
| **Albumin (5% and 25%)** | • 5% and 25% albumin from plasma | • To replace volume in patients suffering from shock, burns, hypoproteinemia, or hypoalbuminemia | • Administer 1 ml/minute or, *if the patient's in shock,* administer rapidly. <br> • May administer with dextrose 5% in water. |
| **Plasma protein fraction** | • 5% albumin and globulin solution in saline solution | • To expand volume in patients with burns, hemorrhage, or hypoproteinemia | • Administer 1 ml/ minute. <br> • Risk of hepatitis or sensitization is low. |
| **Prothrombin** | • Factors II, VII, IX, and X | • To replace clotting factors in patients with hemophilia B or bleeding secondary to severe liver disease | • Prothrombin is used infrequently because of increased hepatitis risk. |

blood more viscous and increases the incidence of sickling.

## Continuing assessment and intervention

After you've intervened to increase your patient's hydration, give a narcotic analgesic (such as morphine or Demerol I.M.), as ordered, to relieve his severe pain. Insert an indwelling (Foley) catheter to monitor your patient's urine output accurately. Perform a complete physical assessment, and take his history. Your goals are to discover the extent of his disease and to identify what precipitated his sickle cell crisis, so you and the doctor can intervene appropriately to correct it.

While you take your patient's vital signs, ask him to describe the events that preceded his crisis. For example, was he exposed to extreme changes in temperature? This could have constricted his peripheral vessels and started a sickling cycle. Also ask him about any past crises. How frequent were they, and how long did each last? This information may help explain the present crisis.

Check your patient's peripheral pulses. If they're diminished or absent, he may have vascular compromise from extensive sickling. Keep your patient warm with blankets and local heat applications to dilate his peripheral vessels and to help prevent additional sickling. If your patient has an increased pulse rate and fever, he may have an infection. Blood cultures will be taken to determine if the infection has spread into his systemic circulation and caused sepsis.

Because his peripheral circulation's impaired, your patient is susceptible to leg ulcers. If he has a localized infection from an open wound, culture the wound drainage. Then clean the wound with an antimicrobial solution and apply antiseptic ointment and a sterile dressing. Be prepared to begin antibiotic therapy, as ordered.

If your patient has a productive cough, check the color of his sputum.

(As you probably know, yellow or green sputum indicates a respiratory infection. Expect to administer supplemental oxygen. Culture the sputum to determine the causative organism.) Then listen to his breath sounds. If they're diminished, or if your patient has rhonchi, ask him whether he also has shortness of breath or pain on inspiration—additional indications of possible respiratory infection. Prepare your patient for a chest X-ray to determine whether he has pneumonia. Remember: *Pneumonia can be catastrophic for a patient with sickle cell anemia,* because decreased oxygen can cause additional sickling and precipitate sickle cell crisis. If he has pneumonia, your patient will need aggressive I.V. antibiotic therapy.

If your patient's a postpubescent female, ask when she had her last menstrual period and whether any possibility exists that she's pregnant. If so, blood and urine should be obtained for pregnancy testing.

If your patient is pregnant, she'll need special care. Why? Because massive cell sickling occurs in the placenta as a result of increased blood flow to that area. Packed RBCs will be transfused at regular intervals throughout her pregnancy to replenish the supply of normal RBCs in the placenta—and the fetus.

If your patient has complications, such as cerebral ischemia, heart failure, respiratory distress, or priapism, anticipate administering exchange transfusions. (See *Administering Blood Transfusions,* page 493, and the "Priapism" entry in Chapter 13.) Remember: The purpose of transfusing blood in a patient with sickle cell crisis isn't to raise his hemoglobin or hematocrit levels—it's to prevent increased blood viscosity by simultaneously *transfusing* healthy blood and *phlebotomizing* sickling blood cells. If your patient suddenly develops fever or chills, indicating a transfusion reaction, *immediately stop the transfusion and notify the doctor.* (See *Recognizing Transfusion*

# WHAT HAPPENS IN SICKLE CELL CRISIS

Sickle cell crisis occurs when a patient with sickle cell anemia experiences cellular oxygen deprivation—for example, from an infection, from exposure to cold or to high altitude, or from overexertion.

Sickle cell anemia results from an alteration in the molecular structure of hemoglobin: one amino acid is substituted for another. This deprives the red blood cells of needed oxygen; in response, their altered hemoglobin molecules aggregate, sickling the cells and causing cellular, vascular, and tissue damage. The result is disabling pain and—ultimately—tissue necrosis. This flowchart outlines the sequence of events in sickle cell crisis.

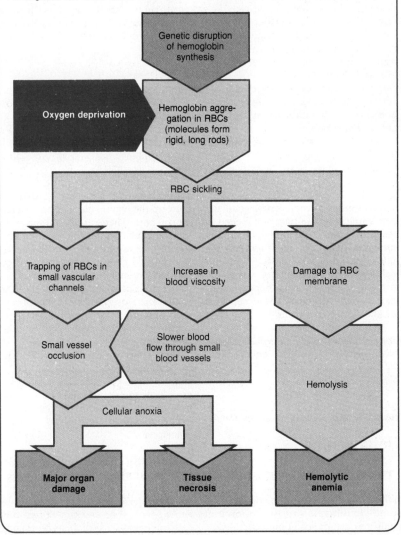

*Reactions,* page 494.)

## Therapeutic care

The goal of therapy is to stop your patient's intensified sickling cycle. You'll know that the emergency is over when your patient's signs and symptoms of crisis are resolved—for example, when his pain subsides and his infection clears.

In the meantime, monitor your patient's reactions to therapy.

Because your patient's being hydrated at double the normal rate, he's susceptible to fluid overload. Monitor his intake and output frequently, and reassess him to detect early signs of hypervolemia, such as edema, increased dyspnea and tachypnea, or rales. This way, you and the doctor can correct fluid overload before it progresses to pulmonary edema or congestive heart failure.

If the doctor suspects that your patient has fluid overload, he'll readjust the I.V. infusion rate to a level that will return your patient's volume status to normal.

In addition to monitoring your patient's intake and output, you'll need to carefully observe his reactions to narcotic analgesics. This is important because patients who suffer frequent sickle cell crises can develop iatrogenic addiction. If this may be happening in your patient, the doctor will consider an alternative treatment.

Finally, your patient may have a folate deficiency, which often accompanies anemia. If your patient has this deficiency, expect to administer folate prophylactically.

# Hemophilia

## Prediagnosis summary

The patient had a history of hemophilia. On initial assessment, he had some combination of the following signs and symptoms of an acute bleeding episode:

- swollen, painful joints
- local, persistent bleeding disproportionate to the severity of his injury
- subcutaneous bleeding
- bleeding from mucous membranes
- abdominal pain and distention
- hematemesis or melena.

The patient's PTT was prolonged, and his PT and bleeding time were normal. Blood drawn for a complete blood count (CBC) showed decreased hemoglobin and hematocrit levels and confirmed significant blood loss. A large-gauge I.V. catheter was inserted for fluid replacement and medication access.

## Priorities

Your first priority is controlling your patient's bleeding, to prevent hemorrhage and hypovolemic shock.

If your patient has bleeding into a joint, elevate the affected limb with pillows, apply ice packs, and immobilize the joint in slight flexion.

If your patient is bleeding from an accessible site, first elevate the area and soak up the oozing blood with a sterile gauze pad. Then, apply a thrombin-soaked gauze pad to the bleeding site, to promote coagulation, and cover the pad with a pressure dressing and an ice pack. Remember to check your patient's peripheral pulses below the joint or dressing, to make sure that joint capsule distention or the dressing isn't compromising his peripheral circulation.

Next, check your patient's vital signs to establish baseline values and to assess for signs of shock, such as an increasingly faint and rapid pulse. If you note these signs, notify the doctor and expect to adjust the rate of fluid replacement.

## Continuing assessment and intervention

Now that you've intervened to control hemorrhage and to prevent hypovolemic shock, your assessment and further interventions will focus on raising

## WHAT HAPPENS IN HEMOPHILIA

Hemophilia A and B are genetically transmitted clotting disorders caused by coagulation-factor deficiencies. Hemophilia A (classic hemophilia) is more common and results from a Factor VIII deficiency; hemophilia B results from Factor IX deficiency. Normal amounts of these factors circulate in both types of hemophilia, but they're functionally inadequate.

Once an injury occurs, the clotting factor deficiency disrupts normal clotting by prohibiting Factor X activation, prothrombin-thrombin conversion, and fibrinogen-fibrin conversion. The end result: impaired clot formation and continued bleeding at the injury site.

Hemophilia A and B are sex-linked (X chromosome), recessive traits. Males with the abnormal chromosome have the disorder and can transmit the gene. Females can be carriers but don't have the characteristic effects. Each daughter of a *carrier* has a 50% chance of being a carrier; each son of a carrier has a 50% chance of having the disorder. If a *hemophiliac* has children, all of his daughters will be carriers, but none of his sons will have the disorder.

your patient's blood factor levels until hemostasis is achieved.

Take your patient's history to find out what caused his bleeding episode and to determine which factor replacement therapy he needs. Find out whether he's a Type A or Type B hemophiliac; then tell the blood bank the blood component you'll need for transfusion. (See *Understanding Blood Component Therapy*, pages 482 and 483.)

To determine the extent of your patient's bleeding, ask him what precipitated the episode. If it's the result of penetrating trauma, he'll probably have only local bleeding (at the site). But a patient who's bleeding from a fall injury may have other bleeding sites that aren't apparent, so look for associated injuries. If he's suffered blunt trauma to his head, perform a complete neurologic assessment. This is important, because intracerebral bleeding can cause hematoma. (See the hematoma entries in Chapter 6.)

Now, begin factor replacement therapy. If your patient's a Type A hemophiliac, he'll require Factor VIII replacement; expect to infuse cryoprecipitated antihemophilic factor (AHF) or lyophilized AHF or both, in a dose large enough to raise his clotting factor

level above 25% of normal. If he's a Type B hemophiliac, he'll require Factor IX replacement; follow the same dosage guidelines to infuse fresh-frozen plasma or Factor IX concentrate. (See *Administering Blood Transfusions*, page 493, and *Understanding Blood Component Therapy*, pages 482 and 483.)

As in any blood component transfusion, monitor your patient closely for signs and symptoms of a transfusion reaction, and be prepared to intervene (see *Recognizing Transfusion Reactions*, page 494). You'll also need to reassess him frequently throughout the factor replacement procedure for possible indications of spontaneous bleeding, such as hematuria or increased joint pain or swelling.

### Therapeutic care

Blood will be drawn at regular intervals to test your patient's hematocrit and hemoglobin levels and PTT. Monitor these laboratory results closely to assess how factor replacement is affecting your patient's clotting ability.

To relieve your patient's pain, the doctor will order analgesics to be administered by mouth; this will avoid the possibility of hematoma formation at I.M. injection sites.

If your patient complains of *new* joint pain, inform the doctor before you administer any analgesic; this pain may indicate fresh internal bleeding. The doctor will reassess your patient and adjust his therapy as necessary.

Finally, warn your patient to be alert for signs and symptoms of posttransfusion hepatitis—such as anorexia, jaundice, or scleral icterus—which may occur several weeks after factor replacement. This warning is especially necessary if your patient received blood factor concentrates, which are prepared from plasma drawn from multiple donors.

# Hemorrhage Secondary to Thrombocytopenia

## Prediagnosis summary

During his initial emergency assessment, the patient indicated he had a history of thrombocytopenia. He also had some combination of the following signs and symptoms of hemorrhage secondary to his condition:
- sudden onset of petechiae or ecchymoses
- mucosal and submucosal bleeding
- malaise
- general weakness
- dyspnea
- tachycardia
- changes in his level of consciousness.

An emergency physical examination was performed to detect the location of the patient's hemorrhage. Blood was drawn for typing and cross matching and for coagulation testing. A large-gauge I.V. catheter was inserted for fluid replacement and medication access. Laboratory test results showed a severely diminished platelet count and a prolonged bleeding time. The patient's PT and PTT were normal. He was placed on bed rest.

## Priorities

Your first priority is to take your patient's vital signs quickly, looking for fever (which increases platelet destruction) and the combination of decreased blood pressure and faint, rapid pulse (which indicates hypovolemic shock).

Your next priority is to control any bleeding and to prevent hypovolemic shock. Apply direct pressure to external bleeding sites, but don't remove any clots. Cover the sites with thrombin-soaked gauze pads, pressure dressings, and ice packs.

Replace fluids using crystalloids, volume expanders, whole blood, and/or platelet concentrate. (See *Understanding Blood Component Therapy*, pages 482 and 483.) You'll initially infuse crystalloids and volume expanders, to increase your patient's depleted fluid volume. Then you'll infuse whole blood, to restore lost blood cells, and platelet concentrate to correct your patient's critically low platelet count, to control bleeding, and to prevent cerebral hemorrhage. When you're transfusing either platelet concentrate or whole blood to compensate for extensive blood loss, you'll need to replace fluid as rapidly as possible. Rapid infusion is necessary to prevent hypovolemic shock and to keep fragile platelets from lysing. When you're transfusing whole blood, you may need to use a pressure cuff to facilitate rapid infusion.

### Continuing assessment and intervention

When blood's infused rapidly, a transfusion reaction can develop within minutes (see *Recognizing Transfusion Reactions*, page 494). If your patient's receiving a rapid blood transfusion, assess him closely throughout, and be prepared to intervene quickly. If you see urticaria and your patient complains of pruritis, he may be having a sensitivity reaction. Fever, vomiting, or headache indicates a febrile reaction. If you observe any of these signs in your patient, *stop the transfusion immediately and notify the doctor.* He'll ask

## ABO AND RH BLOOD COMPATIBILITY

As you know, administering incompatible blood to a patient can cause a potentially fatal hemolytic reaction.

If you can't obtain blood that's identical to your patient's, remember that anyone can receive O⁻ (the "universal donor"), and that anyone with Rh⁺ blood can receive Rh⁻ blood as long as it's ABO-compatible.

This chart shows you which types of blood are compatible with others. Use it to help ensure that your patient's receiving compatible blood. For example, a patient who's A⁺ can receive blood that's O⁻, O⁺, A⁻, or A⁺.

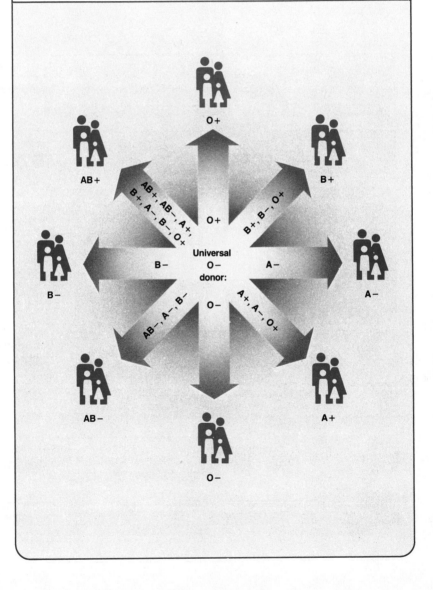

you to administer antihistamines, if your patient's having a sensitivity reaction, or corticosteroids to suppress the immune response that's causing a febrile reaction. You may also need to administer antipyretics to prevent destruction of platelets when the transfusion resumes.

While your patient's being transfused and you're watching for a pos-

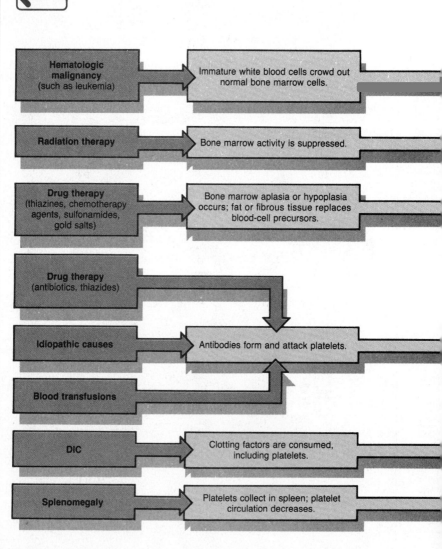

## WHAT HAPPENS IN THROMBOCYTOPENIA

| | |
|---|---|
| **Hematologic malignancy** (such as leukemia) | Immature white blood cells crowd out normal bone marrow cells. |
| **Radiation therapy** | Bone marrow activity is suppressed. |
| **Drug therapy** (thiazines, chemotherapy agents, sulfonamides, gold salts) | Bone marrow aplasia or hypoplasia occurs; fat or fibrous tissue replaces blood-cell precursors. |
| **Drug therapy** (antibiotics, thiazides) | Antibodies form and attack platelets. |
| **Idiopathic causes** | |
| **Blood transfusions** | |
| **DIC** | Clotting factors are consumed, including platelets. |
| **Splenomegaly** | Platelets collect in spleen; platelet circulation decreases. |

sible transfusion reaction, take his history to identify what precipitated his hemorrhage. Has your patient had any recent illnesses? Certain viral infections, such as measles or mononucle-osis, can accelerate platelet destruction. Has he been taking any medications? Some medications, such as antibiotics, chemotherapeutic agents, quinidine sulfate, thiazides, and gold salts, stim-

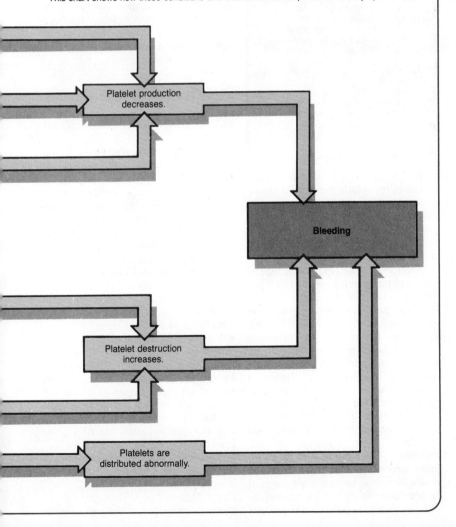

Thrombocytopenia is the most common cause of bleeding disorders. It's characterized by a severe decrease in platelets that can result from hematologic malignancy, radiation or drug therapy, idiopathic causes, blood transfusions, disseminated intravascular coagulation (DIC), or splenomegaly. If your patient has one of these conditions or receives any of these therapies, be especially alert for occult signs and symptoms of bleeding. The excessive hemorrhaging that thrombocytopenia causes can lead to shock if you don't intervene quickly.

This chart shows how these conditions and treatments develop into thrombocytopenia.

Platelet production decreases.

Bleeding

Platelet destruction increases.

Platelets are distributed abnormally.

## BRUSHING UP ON SAFETY

When you're caring for a patient with a bleeding disorder, take a moment to look around his room. Have you done everything you can to protect him from injury? Of course, you've padded his side rails and removed obstacles—such as the wastebasket and the overbed table—from his path. But what about less obvious but equally dangerous safety hazards? Here's a surprising example: that seemingly harmless toothbrush. It poses a real threat to this patient if it has sharp bristles that could cause his gums to bleed. To reduce this risk, wrap the toothbrush bristles with gauze or provide a soft-bristle or special foam toothbrush (Toothette).

Keep an eye out for any object the patient uses that may cause a bleeding injury. You may help prevent catastrophic bleeding.

ulate the production of platelet antibodies in the spleen. Inform the doctor of your findings. He'll change the patient's drug treatment if necessary. You may be asked to administer corticosteroids, too, to prevent additional platelet antibodies from forming.

Throughout your continuing assessment and intervention, protect your patient from trauma, which could cause bleeding. Keep his side rails up, and encourage him to use an electric razor and a soft toothbrush. You generally won't perform invasive procedures, such as urinary catheterization or venipuncture. If venipuncture becomes necessary, apply pressure on the puncture site until the bleeding stops.

Because your patient will need to avoid strain, which could exacerbate bleeding, expect to administer stool softeners. Test your patient's stool, urine, and vomitus for blood. If he has occult bleeding, he may have internal hemorrhage. Notify the doctor, and expect to transfuse additional platelet

concentrate to control the bleeding.

### Therapeutic care

The goal of therapy is to raise your patient's platelet count so hemostasis can occur. To gauge your patient's progress, peripheral blood smears will be tested regularly. Expect platelet replacement to be discontinued once your patient's platelet count returns to normal.

After hemostasis has been achieved, your patient may need a splenectomy to remove the site of platelet sequestration and to prevent future hemorrhage secondary to thrombocytopenia. In the meantime, continue to administer corticosteroids as ordered. Begin preoperative teaching if the patient's scheduled for surgery.

# Anticoagulant Overdose

### Prediagnosis summary

The patient was receiving therapeutic Coumadin (warfarin) or heparin to treat a thromboembolic disease or to prevent thrombus formation after surgery or during prolonged bed rest. On initial emergency assessment, he revealed some combination of the following signs and symptoms:
• persistent mucosal bleeding
• persistent epistaxis
• frank or occult bleeding in stool, urine, vomitus, or sputum
• ecchymoses and petechiae
• deteriorating mental status.

The patient's baseline vital signs were taken and checked for signs of hypovolemic shock. Blood was drawn for *stat* typing and cross matching, for coagulation testing, and for determining the severity of his blood loss. If he was taking Coumadin, his PT was at least three times normal; if he was receiving heparin, his PTT was also at least three times normal.

### Priorities

Your first priority for your patient with

# YOUR ROLE IN AN EMERGENCY

## ADMINISTERING BLOOD TRANSFUSIONS

As you know, if a blood transfusion's administered improperly, the patient may develop a transfusion reaction. To minimize the risk of reaction and subsequent complications when you transfuse blood, review the procedure outlined here.

### Equipment
• Blood administration set with filter and drip chamber
• 250 ml normal saline solution
• whole blood or selected blood component
• I.V. pole, venipuncture equipment, and 20G—or larger—angiocatheter (if the patient doesn't already have an I.V. line)

### Before the procedure
• Explain the procedure to the patient.
• Make sure he's signed a consent form. If the patient's religious beliefs prohibit blood transfusions, make sure you follow your hospital's protocols.
• Take the patient's vital signs to serve as baseline values.
• Check that the blood type ordered is compatible with the patient's blood type.
• Check the doctor's order for specific directions concerning how many units to administer and over how much time.
• Check the patient's history to see if he's had a reaction to a previous transfusion. If so, he has a greater chance of developing a reaction again, so watch him carefully.
• If the patient doesn't have an I.V. line established, see that one is started. Infuse normal saline solution to keep the vein open. Blood is viscous, so avoid using an existing line if the needle or angiocatheter is smaller than 19G.
• Obtain the blood from the blood bank or blood refrigerator *just before administering it.* Remember, red blood cells (RBCs) deteriorate at room temperature.
• Compare chart information—the patient's identification number—with his compatibility record. Also compare the patient's name and identification number on his wristband with the information on the compatibility record and blood bag. If the patient can speak, ask him to identify himself by his full name.
• Check the expiration date on the blood bag and observe the blood for abnormal color, RBC clumping, gas bubbles, and abnormal cloudiness. If you see any of these, return the blood; it may be contaminated or hemolyzed.
• Check your hospital's policy for transfusion protocol on how often to take the patient's vital signs during the transfusion and how to dispose of the empty blood bag. Follow this policy to the letter.
• If you're giving whole blood, gently invert the bag several times to mix the cells.
• Prepare for transfusion by letting the blood run through the administration set to expel air from the tubing.

### During the procedure
• Keep the patient warm.
• Hang the blood 3′ to 4′ (about 1 m) above the level of the patient's heart.
• Plug the blood tubing into the port closest to the patient, turn the saline solution off, and begin transfusing the blood slowly, 25 to 30 drops/minute. (He should receive only 50 ml over the first 30 minutes.)
• Remain with the patient and take his vital signs periodically. Watch him for signs of transfusion reaction for the first 15 to 30 minutes. If no signs of reaction appear within that time, adjust the flow clamp to the ordered infusion rate.
• Check the patient after another 15 minutes, then check the patient hourly or according to specific protocol.

### After the procedure
• Flush the filter and tubing with normal saline solution if the manufacturer recommends this.
• If you have to give another transfusion, disconnect the set that's hanging and use another set with the next unit.
• If you don't have to give another transfusion, disconnect the blood line and flush the main line with normal saline solution.
• Reconnect the original I.V. or discontinue the saline as ordered.
• Record the date and time of the transfusion, the type and amount of blood transfused, the patient's vital signs during the transfusion, and any transfusion reaction and subsequent interventions.

WARNING

# RECOGNIZING TRANSFUSION REACTIONS

During a blood transfusion, your patient's at risk for developing any of five types of reactions. To learn to recognize them and to intervene appropriately, study this chart.

If your patient develops any sign or symptom of a reaction, immediately follow this procedure:
• Stop the transfusion.
• Change the I.V. tubing to prevent infusing any more blood. Save the tubing and blood bag for analysis.
• Administer saline solution I.V. to keep the vein open.
• Take the patient's vital signs.
• Notify the doctor.
• Obtain urine and blood samples from the patient and send them to the laboratory.
• Prepare for further treatment.

| REACTION | SIGNS AND SYMPTOMS | NURSING CONSIDERATIONS |
|---|---|---|
| **Hemolytic** | Include chills, fever, low back pain, headache, chest pain, tachycardia, dyspnea, hypotension, nausea and vomiting, restlessness, anxiety, shock | • Expect to place the patient in a supine position, with his legs elevated 20° to 30°, and to administer oxygen, fluids, and epinephrine to correct shock.<br>• Expect to administer mannitol to maintain the patient's renal circulation.<br>• Expect to insert an indwelling (Foley) catheter to monitor the patient's urinary output (should be about 100 ml/hr).<br>• Expect to administer antipyretics to lower the patient's fever. If his fever persists, expect to apply a hypothermia blanket or to give tepid sponge or alcohol baths. |
| **Plasma protein incompatibility** | Include chills, fever, flushing, abdominal pain, diarrhea, dyspnea, hypotension | • Expect to place the patient in a supine position, with his legs elevated 20° to 30°, and to administer oxygen, fluids, and epinephrine to correct shock.<br>• Expect to administer corticosteroids. |
| **Blood contamination** | Include chills, fever, abdominal pain, nausea and vomiting, bloody diarrhea, hypotension | • Expect to administer fluids, antibiotics, corticosteroids, vasopressors, and a fresh transfusion. |
| **Febrile** | Range from mild chills, flushing, and fever to extreme signs and symptoms resembling a hemolytic reaction | • Expect to administer an antipyretic and an antihistamine for a *mild* reaction.<br>• Expect to treat a *severe* reaction the same as a hemolytic reaction. |
| **Allergic** | Range from pruritus, urticaria, hives, facial swelling, chills, fever, nausea and vomiting, headache, and wheezing to laryngeal edema, respiratory distress, and shock | • Expect to administer parenteral antihistamines or, for a severe reaction, epinephrine or corticosteroids.<br>• If the patient's only sign of reaction is hives, expect to restart the infusion, as ordered, at a slower rate. |

severe anticoagulant overdose is to stop anticoagulant administration and to begin slowly infusing the appropriate antidote, as ordered, to neutralize the anticoagulant circulating in your patient's body.

If your patient's suffering from a *Coumadin-induced* clotting disorder, expect to administer fresh-frozen plasma for immediate factor replacement and vitamin $K_1$ at a rate of 1 mg/minute. If your patient's suffering from a *heparin-induced* clotting disorder, expect to administer protamine sulfate slowly, not exceeding a rate of 50 mg/10 minutes.

### Continuing assessment and intervention
Now that you've intervened to counteract the anticoagulant overdose, attempt to control your patient's bleeding. To aid vasoconstriction, apply pressure dressings and ice packs to external bleeding sites. Expect to assist the doctor with iced saline lavage for internal bleeding.

Next, take your patient's medication history. (Certain drugs, such as antibiotics, can inhibit clotting mechanisms and may potentiate an anticoagulant overdose.)

While you take your patient's history, check his vital signs frequently. If you note a decreasing blood pressure and an increasingly faint, rapid pulse, indicating hypovolemic shock, *notify the doctor immediately.* As ordered, insert a second I.V. catheter and begin rapid fluid replacement with crystalloids and volume expanders until fresh whole blood and fresh-frozen plasma are available. Place your patient in a modified Trendelenburg position and apply medical antishock trousers (a MAST suit) to increase perfusion to major organ tissues.

To assess your patient's reaction to fluid replacement, connect him to a cardiac monitor and check his vital signs every 5 minutes. If his status isn't improving at a satisfactory rate, and he had a Coumadin overdose, the doctor

may ask you to administer Konyne—a plasma concentrate of vitamin K-dependent factors—to trigger coagulation, even though this will increase the patient's risk of hepatitis.

### Therapeutic care
After the antidote's been infused, blood will be drawn to retest your patient's clotting time. Closely monitor his PT or PTT. When it returns to the therapeutic range, your patient's hemodynamic status should stabilize. Then his anticoagulant therapy can be resumed.

Once anticoagulant therapy is started again, you'll need to continue monitoring your patient's PT or PTT closely to make sure it stays within the established therapeutic range. And, of course, be prepared to intervene if overdose occurs again.

# Disseminated Intravascular Coagulation

### Prediagnosis summary
The patient had abnormal bleeding despite no known history of hemorrhagic disorder. Initially, he showed some combination of the following signs and symptoms:
- petechiae and ecchymoses
- continuous bleeding from mucous membranes, orifices, or venipuncture sites
- blood in urine, stool, vomitus, or sputum
- altered level of consciousness
- cool, mottled extremities
- cyanosis.

The patient's orthostatic vital signs were taken to establish baseline values and volume status quickly. Blood was drawn for coagulation testing and for a CBC. Laboratory results revealed that the patient's thrombin time, PT, and PTT were prolonged; his hemoglobin, hematocrit, platelet count, and fibrin-

PATHOPHYSIOLOGY _____

# WHAT HAPPENS IN DISSEMINATED INTRAVASCULAR COAGULATION

Disseminated intravascular coagulation (DIC) paradoxically produces clotting *and* hemorrhaging. This coagulopathy occurs secondary to overactivation of the normal clotting cascade, especially in patients with gram-negative sepsis, abruptio placentae or missed abortion, burns, heat stroke, shock, adult respiratory distress syndrome, and transfusion reactions. It *rarely* occurs as a primary disorder; it's almost always a complication of another disease process, and this accounts for its high mortality.

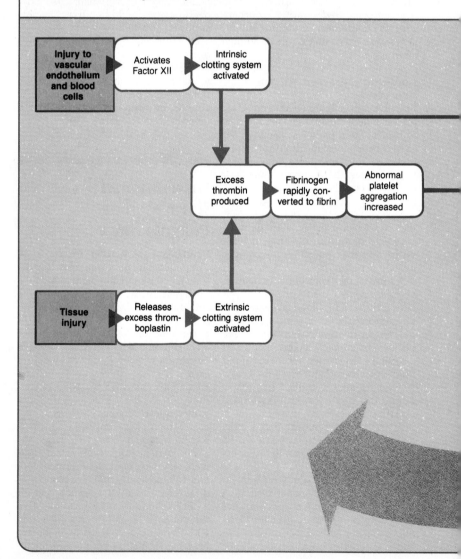

DIC's abnormal clotting can develop in three ways:
- extensive activation of the clotting mechanism's extrinsic pathway
- extensive vascular endothelium alterations, which activate the clotting mechanism's intrinsic pathway
- blood cell damage, which can also trigger the clotting mechanism's intrinsic pathway.

No matter how it begins, DIC can lead to a destructive cycle. It can cause shock, which perpetuates DIC, which again results in shock, and so on.

Obviously, DIC represents a serious threat to your patient. His condition depends on the severity of his primary problem and the amount and speed of coagulation.

Knowing the conditions that predispose a patient to DIC and being alert for early signs and symptoms of DIC will facilitate early treatment and increase his chances of survival.

Review the chart below to understand the paradoxic path of DIC.

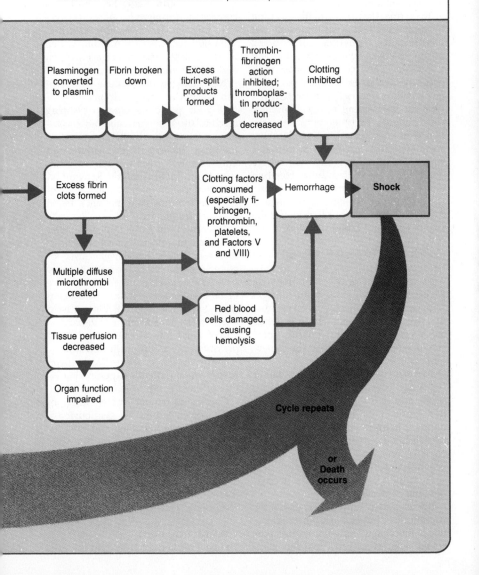

ogen levels were decreased; and his fibrinogen-splitting products were increased. An I.V. was inserted for fluid and medication access.

## Priorities

Because your patient's using up coagulation factors and platelets faster than his clotting mechanism can produce new ones, your first priority is to prevent his bleeding from compromising his hemodynamic status.

To do this, try to control his bleeding by applying direct pressure to external bleeding sites, if possible, and by using thrombin-soaked gauze to promote clot formation. Then cover the sites with pressure dressings and ice packs. If he's bleeding internally, expect to assist with an iced saline lavage. Maintain your patient's body temperature with blankets, to decrease his peripheral vasoconstriction. Expect to administer supplemental oxygen; this will relieve hypoxemia associated with bleeding and decrease ischemia in thrombotic tissues. If your patient's hypovolemic, the doctor may ask you to increase the rate of fluid and blood infusion.

## Continuing assessment and intervention

After you've intervened to stabilize your patient's hemodynamic status, try to find out what initially triggered his massive intravascular clotting. Then focus your subsequent nursing interventions on helping to treat the underlying cause.

For example, if your patient has a history of infection, culture his blood, urine, and sputum to discover whether he's septic. If he is, the bacterial endotoxins in his bloodstream could have caused his disseminated intravascular coagulation (DIC). Expect to administer antibiotic therapy, as ordered, and sodium bicarbonate to reverse accompanying acidosis.

If your patient's pregnant, assess for vaginal bleeding or back pain indicating hemorrhage from premature placental separation. This, too, increases

the risk of DIC by releasing thromboplastins into the patient's general circulation. Be prepared to assist with an emergency cesarean section.

If your patient's received multiple packed-cell transfusions to treat a preexisting condition, his blood cells may have been replaced *but not his clotting factors*, and this may have triggered DIC. Anticipate transfusing plasma to replace his clotting factors.

Expect to administer heparin I.V. to control the initial event of the DIC cycle—massive intravascular clotting. This will neutralize thrombin, which is being generated in large amounts, and inhibit additional clotting.

Next, expect to transfuse fresh-frozen plasma or cryoprecipitate to activate your patient's normal clotting mechanism. If heparin and blood component therapy are ineffective, the doctor may have you administer an antifibrinolytic agent (such as Amicar), to inhibit fibrinolysis. Remember, this medication may cause hypotension, so monitor your patient's blood pressure frequently.

Insert an indwelling (Foley) catheter and begin monitoring your patient's intake and output hourly, checking for oliguria—which may indicate that your patient's hypovolemic from massive blood loss. Reassess your patient's vital signs, looking for signs of a transfusion reaction (such as fever or tachycardia) and of shock (such as decreased blood pressure and a faint, rapid pulse).

*Notify the doctor immediately* if you suspect your patient's experiencing either of these conditions.

Check your patient for bleeding from his gastrointestinal or genitourinary tract. Hematest his urine and stool for occult blood. If you suspect that your patient has intraabdominal bleeding, take a baseline measurement of his abdominal girth to monitor for distention—which would indicate his condition's worsening.

## Therapeutic care

The goal of therapy is to treat the precipitating condition so that your patient's clotting mechanism returns to normal. To gauge the effectiveness of his therapy, monitor the results of his serial blood studies—especially of his hematocrit and hemoglobin levels and coagulation times.

In the meantime, your therapeutic care will focus on preventing another DIC cycle from starting. Protect your patient from injury by keeping him on complete bed rest, and assess him for early signs of DIC, such as hematomas, easy bruising, and blood oozing at I.V. insertion sites.

Finally, keep your patient's family informed of his progress, and prepare them to accept his appearance (bruises, dried blood). Provide emotional support for your patient and his family.

## TAKE THE TIME

Your patient in reverse isolation never sees a friendly face. Why? Because all his visitors, nurses, and doctors must wear gowns, caps, gloves, and masks. He may end up feeling physically *and* emotionally isolated.

To ease his loneliness and anxiety, help him understand why he's in reverse isolation. Explain that it protects *him* from the outside world. He's not contaminated; everyone else is! Set up a regular schedule for visiting him. Encourage him to talk about how he feels, and provide emotional support. Ask him if there's anything you can bring him. And before you leave, remind him that you'll be back.

# Infection Secondary to Granulocytopenia

## Prediagnosis summary

The patient had a history of granulocytopenia. On initial assessment, he showed some combination of the following signs and symptoms of infection secondary to his condition:
• sore throat or mouth ulceration
• cervical adenopathy
• dyspnea
• progressive weakness and fatigue.
After his baseline vital signs were taken—revealing fever and tachycardia—the patient was placed on bed rest.

## Priorities

Your first priority is to assist with isolation of the microorganism that's causing your patient's infection. Obtain urine, blood, sputum, and throat cultures. Then insert an I.V. catheter and begin infusing broad-spectrum antibiotics, as ordered, to fight the infection. Because your patient has granulocytopenia, he's extremely vul-

nerable to further infection, so be sure to keep him in reverse isolation.

## Continuing assessment and intervention

After you've intervened to combat your patient's infection, administer analgesics as ordered to relieve pain at the infection site. Then take his history to discover what precipitated his infection. Has he been taking medications? Certain drugs, including some chemotherapeutic agents, can impair production of WBCs. Of course, this will make your patient even more susceptible to infection. The same problem exists if your patient's been receiving radiation treatments. Inform the doctor of your findings. He'll reassess your patient and adjust his drug therapy if necessary.

When your patient's laboratory tests are returned, make sure the causative organism is sensitive to the broad-spectrum antibiotic your patient's receiving. If it isn't, notify the doctor, who'll change his order accordingly. Administer antibiotics promptly at the ordered intervals, to maintain therapeutic levels. If you note signs of infection at the I.V. insertion site, discontinue the I.V., culture the inser-

PATHOPHYSIOLOGY

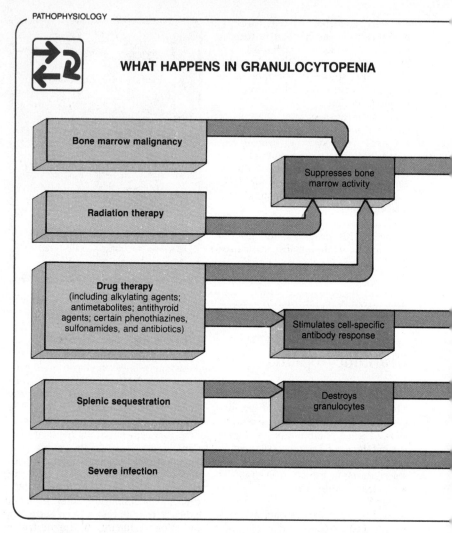

## WHAT HAPPENS IN GRANULOCYTOPENIA

Bone marrow malignancy

Radiation therapy

Drug therapy
(including alkylating agents;
antimetabolites; antithyroid
agents; certain phenothiazines,
sulfonamides, and antibiotics)

Splenic sequestration

Severe infection

Suppresses bone
marrow activity

Stimulates cell-specific
antibody response

Destroys
granulocytes

tion site, and reinsert the I.V. at another site using strict aseptic technique.

Anticipate administering antipyretics to reduce your patient's fever and to control his fever-induced hypermetabolic state. If his fever's extreme, you may also need to give him a cool sponge bath and to place a hypothermic blanket underneath him.

Monitor your patient's intake and output frequently to gauge his hemodynamic status. To prevent introducing infection-causing bacteria, avoid indwelling (Foley) catheterization—un-

less your patient's in septic shock, when you'll need to accurately measure his urine output every hour. (See the "Septic Shock" entry in Chapter 14.)

Because septic shock's a serious threat to your patient, monitor his vital signs carefully for decreasing blood pressure and increasingly rapid, faint pulse. (As you know, these signs can indicate septic shock.) If you note these signs, connect your patient to a cardiac monitor and intervene as needed to prevent hypoxemia, to perfuse vital organs, and to correct acidosis. Be

Granulocytopenia's primary characteristic is a severe decrease in the number of circulating neutrophils (granulocytes), which constitute the majority of white blood cells——the infection-fighting cells that the bone marrow produces. When these aren't produced in sufficient numbers (or are destroyed faster than they can be produced), the patient's defense against infection is severely compromised. Untreated granulocytopenia may be fatal if it results in overwhelming infection and septic shock. Here's a flowchart to help you understand this life-threatening disorder.

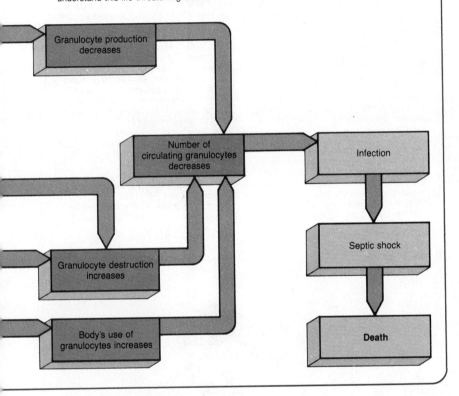

prepared to administer supplemental oxygen by nasal cannula, mask, or mechanical ventilation. As ordered, begin massive fluid replacement and—if necessary—administer a vasopressor to restore adequate blood pressure and to perfuse vital organs. Insert a Foley catheter so you can accurately monitor your patient's intake and output, and his perfusion status, hourly. Also expect to administer sodium bicarbonate I.V., to correct acidosis, and corticosteroids, to improve your patient's blood perfusion and to increase his cardiac output.

### Therapeutic care

The goal of therapy is to combat your patient's infection successfully; this will include increasing the number of infection-fighting WBCs in his circulation. Expect to transfuse granulocytes, as ordered.

While your patient's infection is being cleared, your care will focus on preventing additional infections. To do this, you'll need to:

• keep your patient on bed rest, in re-

# CASE IN POINT: MISTAKEN IDENTITY

Jim Smith, age 34, who was admitted to the hospital for hematologic testing, is now a patient on your floor. His initial test results show decreased hemoglobin and hematocrit levels, so the doctor orders a blood transfusion.

Your floor's short-staffed, so you rush to obtain the blood Jim needs and to start the tranfusion. Within 15 minutes he's become hypotensive and tachycardic, with low back pain and a temperature of 102° F. (38.9 C.) Recognizing these as possible signs and symptoms of a hemolytic transfusion reaction, you stop the transfusion immediately and call the doctor. Jim goes into shock. At first, you're not sure why Jim's having a reaction—but the reason soon becomes clear.

You pull your patient's chart to compare his compatibility slip with his blood bag's information. The name and Rh factor match, but the patient numbers and blood types *don't*. No wonder he's having a reaction... you gave him the wrong blood!

As you close his chart, you see a name alert—there's *another* Jim Smith on the unit. Distracted and hurried, you missed it earlier.

Later, your patient develops acute renal failure that requires hemodialysis. Does he have a case if he files suit against you, the doctor, and the hospital?

A similar real-life incident, *Necolayeff v. Genesee Hospital* (1946), involved mistaken identity. A nurse and an intern gave a blood transfusion to Mrs. Necolayeff, whose doctor never ordered it. The transfusion was ordered for another patient on the same floor. In the lawsuit that followed, the nurse and the intern were found negligent.

The lesson here is, clearly, that you must always follow your hospital's transfusion protocols. These additional guidelines will also help you avoid liability:

• Remember that you're responsible for making sure every requisition for blood has the patient's full name and hospital identification number on it.

• Before the transfusion, compare the patient's identification number and blood type on his chart with his compatibility record. Also compare the patient's name and ID number on his wristband with the information on the compatibility record and blood bag. If the patient can speak, ask him to identify himself by his full name.

• Always ask a co-worker to verify this information.

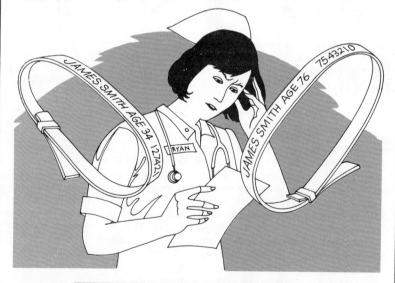

*Necolayeff v. Genesee Hospital, 61 N.Y.S. 2d 832 (N.Y., 1946)*

verse isolation, and maintain meticulous skin care. Turn your patient every 2 hours to relieve pressure on bony prominences, and watch for pressure sores—potential infection sites. Use a sheepskin or an egg-crate mattress on your patient's bed to help prevent formation of pressure sores.

• keep your patient on a diet high in calories, protein, and vitamins, to build up his nutritional reserves. Encourage him to drink lots of fluids, to minimize bacteria proliferation in the bladder, and to prevent the dehydration that may accompany infection.

• maintain oral hygiene and destroy bacteria in your patient's mouth by having him gargle with a 1:1 hydrogen peroxide and water solution after every meal. If he has ulcerative mouth lesions, gargling will also help remove necrotic tissue.

• keep your patient on a routine of prophylactic pulmonary hygiene that includes regular coughing, turning, and deep breathing. This will help remove bronchial secretions, which provide a favorable growth medium for microorganisms.

## A FINAL WORD

As you may know, recent technologic developments have improved the outlook for patients with hematologic emergencies. For example, advances in genetic counseling now help identify persons with inherited hematologic disorders. And the creation of synthetic blood components, such as Fluosol-DA, can mean the difference between life and death for patients who can't—or won't—tolerate blood transfusions.

As a nurse, you're in an important position to *prevent* some hematologic emergencies. Why? Because hematologic emergencies so frequently occur right on the medical-surgical unit, as complications of patients' preexisting medical problems or treatment. Knowing which of your patients are at high risk, and being on the alert for iatrogenic complications, are your keys to prevention. For example, any patient who's suffered trauma, is acutely ill, or has had surgery can develop DIC. And patients who've received blood transfusions or anticoagulant drugs, such as heparin, are at high risk for developing adverse tranfusion reactions or anticoagulant overdose.

You can also help keep a patient's chronic hematologic disorder from becoming a hematologic emergency by making him aware of the special risk he faces. Teach him to avoid behavior that can precipitate crises and to recognize signs and symptoms of impending crises. Then you'll know you're doing all you can to protect and care for this uniquely vulnerable patient.

## Selected References

Cohen, Alan S., and Combes, John R., eds. *Medical Emergencies: Diagnostic Management Procedures from the Boston City Hospital,* 2nd ed. Boston: Little, Brown & Co., 1983.
Franco, L.M. "Acute Disseminated Intravascular Coagulation," *Critical Care Update* 8:17-20, January 1981.
Rapaport, Samuel I. *Introduction to Hematology.* New York: Harper & Row Publishers, 1971.

Sullivan, D. "The Crises of Sickle Cells," *Emergency Medicine* 13:28-31, November 30, 1981.
Vogelpohl, R.A. "Disseminated Intravascular Coagulation... a Review of the Diagnostic Tests and the Medical and Nursing Interventions," *Critical Care Nurse* 1:38-43, May/June 1981.
Williams, William J., et al. *Hematology,* 3rd ed. New York: McGraw-Hill Book Co., 1983.

# 12

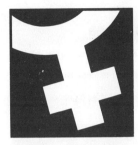

# Obstetric and Gynecologic Emergencies

## Introduction

You hurry over to cubicle four in the ED and find yourself looking into the frightened eyes of Mary Jorgenson, age 15. Brought in by her parents because of her heavy vaginal bleeding, she's lying on her side, her legs drawn up, her arms holding her abdomen.

As you walk toward her, you're already beginning your assessment. You note that her respirations are rapid—probably 40 per minute—her skin's pale, and her face glistens with sweat.

According to Mary's parents, she started complaining of abdominal pain about 2 hours ago; she also told them that her period was "real heavy." During the 20-minute drive to the hospital, she bled heavily enough to soak through a perineal pad and her clothing. Could she be pregnant—suffering from a spontaneous abortion or an incomplete induced abortion? Was she the victim of rape—afraid to tell her parents? Or could her problem simply be a heavy menstrual period with dysmenorrhea? Mary's distress, profuse bleeding, and rapid pulse push the hope of simple dysmenorrhea from your mind. You know she's got a more serious problem and that you have to stabilize her condition quickly.

Would you know how to assess and intervene for a patient like Mary? Her vaginal bleeding makes an obstetric/gynecologic (OB/GYN) emergency

obvious. However, in other such patients (those who have abdominal pain *without* vaginal bleeding, for example), the source of the emergency won't be so obvious. And, if the emergency involves a pregnant woman, you need to know how to assess and support the fetus as well as the woman.

Particularly in OB/GYN emergencies, you also need to know how to provide emotional support. This is because any condition that affects a woman's reproductive system carries a possible threat to her future fertility. This may cause great emotional stress.

As a nurse, you know that life-threatening OB/GYN emergencies can arise in any setting—on a gynecology unit, on a medical-surgical unit, or in a walk-in clinic, as well as in the ED. In fact, you should be aware of the possibility of an OB/GYN emergency in any woman between ages 14 and 60 who has a chief complaint of abdominal pain.

Whatever her age, the woman with an OB/GYN emergency needs fast, expert care. That means you must be prepared to conduct a rapid emergency assessment, to institute life-support measures as needed, to assist the doctor with diagnostic and treatment procedures, and to monitor changes in the patient's condition. This chapter tells you the procedures to follow.

# IDENTIFYING HIGH-RISK PREGNANCIES

Your pregnant patient's depending on you to help her have a healthy baby. One way to do this is to identify and manage any factors that place her at high risk. Then, if an emergency does arise, you'll be able to make a quick, accurate assessment and to focus your interventions appropriately.

Use this chart to gather data that may indicate your patient's at risk for a pregnancy-related emergency.

## MEDICAL HISTORY

**General medical history**
- Hypertension
- Diabetes
- Cancer (within the past 5 years)
- Cardiovascular disease
- Lupus erythematosus
- Infectious disease

**Family history of:**
- Tay-Sachs
- Sickle cell anemia
- Cystic fibrosis
- Hereditary disorders

## PREVIOUS PREGNANCIES

**Medical complications**
- Toxemia
- Bleeding
- Rubella
- Anemia

**Length of labor**
- Prolonged
- Precipitous

**Delivery methods**
- Cesarean section
- Mid-to-high forceps extraction
- Vacuum extraction
- Breech extraction

**Outcomes**
- Two or more pregnancies terminated before 28 weeks
- One or more pregnancies terminated after 28 weeks
- Two or more births yielding live premature neonates, weighing under 2,500 g
- One or more neonatal deaths within 7 days of birth
- One or more births yielding a neonate weighing 4,000 g or more
- One or more neonates traumatized during delivery, born alive or not

## CURRENT STATUS

**Age**
- Under 18 at time of conception
- Over 35 at time of conception

**Weight**
- Under 100 lb
- More than 20% overweight
- Over 30-lb weight gain during pregnancy
- Under 15-lb weight gain during pregnancy

**Health habits**
- Poor nutrition
- Crash dieting or fasting
- Drug addiction or abuse
- Alcoholism
- Smoking more than two packs of cigarettes daily

**Emotional status**
- Fearful
- Anxious
- Hostile
- Ambivalent
- Family problems
- Few emotional supports

**Economic status**
- Low income
- Inadequate housing

10

# INITIAL CARE

## Prehospital Care: What's Been Done

If a rescue team brought your patient to the hospital, they took steps to stabilize her airway, breathing, and circulation—putting in an oral airway or an esophageal obturator airway, if necessary, and providing oxygen by nasal cannula or mask. If paramedics responded, they may have started an I.V. of dextrose 5% in water at a keep-vein-open rate and placed the patient on a cardiac monitor.

If the patient had heavy vaginal bleeding and showed signs of hypovolemic shock, rescue personnel may have applied medical antishock trousers (a MAST suit). They noted how long it took her to saturate a perineal pad and whether her clothing was saturated with blood. If they needed to apply additional perineal pads, they saved all saturated pads. They also collected any clots or tissue she passed, so the doctor could determine if she had a spontaneous abortion and whether it was complete. If qualified to do so, they inserted a large-bore I.V. catheter and began a rapid infusion of Ringer's lactate, to increase the woman's fluid volume and to allow access to a vein for blood transfusions. If the patient was obviously pregnant, rescue personnel probably positioned her on her left side with a wedge under her right hip, to relieve uterine pressure on the vena cava.

If the patient reported that she'd been raped, rescue personnel discouraged her from washing or changing her clothes before they transported her. They also assessed her for other trauma she may have suffered during the rape.

## What to Do First

Rapid assessment, recognition of acute and potential OB/GYN problems, recognition of the need to support two lives if the woman's pregnant, and initiation of lifesaving measures are the keys to providing proper care for patients with OB/GYN emergencies.

As is true for any patient with a life-threatening emergency, your first priority is to assess and stabilize the woman's airway, breathing, and cir-

PRIORITIES

### INITIAL ASSESSMENT CHECKLIST

**Assess the ABCs first and intervene appropriately.**

**Check for:**
• tachycardia; cool, clammy, pale skin; and restlessness, indicating occult bleeding and shock
• fetal bradycardia or tachycardia, indicating fetal distress
• hypertension, edema of face and hands, proteinuria, apprehension, and vertigo, indicating preeclampsia
• generalized edema, tonic-clonic convulsions, and coma, indicating eclampsia.

**Intervene by:**
• starting an I.V. with a large-bore catheter
• administering oxygen by mask or nasal cannula
• placing the woman on her left side or in a supine position, if needed
• sending blood to the laboratory for typing and cross matching, coagulation times, and indirect Coombs' test.

**Prepare for:**
• blood transfusions
• RhoGam administration
• magnesium sulfate administration
• emergency delivery
• surgery.

culation. If she's obviously pregnant, remember that the anatomic and physiologic changes of pregnancy may alter her response to physical insults and to your interventions (see *Assessing the Pregnant Patient*). Keep in mind, too, that the fetus may respond *differently* to the same insult or intervention. (Of course, you can't always tell if your patient's pregnant; if it's not obvious, you'll have to wait until after you've secured her airway, breathing, and circulation to take a menstrual history and to perform a pregnancy test.) Your secondary assessment must include both the mother and the fetus, but you have to concentrate on the mother during your *initial* assessment. If you don't attend to *her* vital functions first in an emergency, neither she nor the fetus may survive.

## Airway

As in any life-threatening emergency, start by making sure air is moving in and out of your patient's upper airway. Although few OB/GYN emergencies directly affect a patient's airway, the complications of these conditions may. A patient with eclampsia, for example, will have seizures, which may cause her tongue to occlude her airway. If this

## ASSESSING THE PREGNANT PATIENT

As you know, a pregnant woman's body undergoes obvious changes, such as swelling and tenderness of the breasts, amenorrhea, and increasing uterine size. You don't have any trouble assessing these changes. But some others aren't quite so obvious and may *look* like potential problems, even though they're normal. Reviewing this list will help you recognize the range of normal physiologic changes of pregnancy. You'll also learn how to adjust your nursing care to prevent pregnancy-related problems.

| NORMAL PHYSIO-LOGIC CHANGES | NURSING CONSIDERATIONS |
|---|---|
| Maternal blood volume increases by 30% to 50%. | • Watch your patient for *hypo*tension (even stable vital signs may indicate hemorrhage and fetal compromise). Be alert for other signs of hypovolemic shock, and administer fluids and oxygen (as ordered) to support the fetus.<br>• Expect her blood pressure to increase in the third trimester, although it will still be below her antepartal level.<br>• Watch her for a mean arterial blood pressure of 105 mm Hg or more, which may indicate a problem. |
| Maternal cardiac output increases by as much as 35%. | • Expect the maternal pulse to be faster than the antepartal baseline—8 beats faster per minute by her 13th week and 15 beats faster per minute by term. |
| The maternal heart enlarges, moves up and to the left, and rotates anteriorly. | • Don't adjust your hand placement for cardiac compressions if your patient arrests.<br>• Adjust your stethoscope placement to auscultate the maternal apical pulse and heart sounds. |
| Maternal gastric motility decreases. | • Expect maternal stomach-emptying time to increase to 6 or 7 hours by term.<br>• Insert a nasogastric tube if vomiting occurs and aspiration is a danger. |
| The gravid uterus crowds the maternal diaphragm; sensitivity of the maternal respiratory center to $PCO_2$ increases. | • Expect that your patient will be short of breath, with an increased respiratory rate.<br>• Assess her for dizziness, lightheadedness, or headache.<br>• Place her in a semi-Fowler position for maximal lung expansion. |

happens, insert an oral airway to keep the patient's airway open and to protect her from injury. Have someone notify the doctor *immediately* and don't leave the patient alone *at any time*. If she's unconscious, assist the doctor with endotracheal intubation, if ordered.

Patients with other OB/GYN emergencies may vomit and aspirate their vomitus. Protect such a patient's airway by positioning her on her left side, clearing her oropharynx with a finger sweep and suctioning, and inserting a nasogastric (NG) tube to evacuate her stomach contents and to prevent further vomiting.

## Breathing

After you've made sure your patient's airway is clear, assess the rate, depth, and pattern of her respirations. But remember—mild shortness of breath in a pregnant patient is most likely associated with crowding of her diaphragm by the gravid uterus, so it probably isn't serious (see *Assessing the Pregnant Patient*). Explain this to her, and, if her condition allows, put her in a semi-Fowler position to relieve pressure on her diaphragm.

If her breathing's rapid, determine whether it's tachypnea or hyperventilation. The difference can be critical. Hyperventilation is typically a sign of anxiety, but tachypnea may be a sign of a life-threatening problem:

• Tachypnea may be one of the first signs that your patient's hemorrhaging: when bleeding becomes severe, her respirations increase as a result of sympathetic adrenal stimulation.

• Tachypnea (accompanied by dyspnea and apprehension) may be an early sign of thromboembolic or amniotic fluid pulmonary embolus (see the "Pulmonary Embolism" entry in Chapter 4).

To relieve your patient's breathing difficulty, provide oxygen by mask or nasal cannula.

If your patient has hyperventilation rather than tachypnea and she also complains of light-headedness and tingling in her arms and legs and around her mouth, anxiety is the most likely cause. If she's pregnant, her anxiety can stress the fetus. Calm her by slowly and quietly directing her attention to her breathing and helping her slow it down. If this doesn't work, have her breathe into a paper bag to reestablish normal respirations. Provide emotional support, and keep her informed. Before each procedure, explain what you're doing and why.

## Circulation

The most common threat to your patient with an OB/GYN emergency is hypovolemic shock. Take her pulse and blood pressure, to provide baseline values. Remember that if your patient's pregnant, her body position may significantly influence her pulse rate and blood pressure. If her condition permits, perform a tilt test (see *Using the Tilt Test to Evaluate Hypovolemia*, page 302). A positive tilt test indicates internal bleeding, such as may occur with placenta previa or abruptio placentae. If you suspect internal bleeding or if your patient's bleeding vaginally, expect to start at least one I.V. with a large-bore catheter *immediately*. Infuse fluids rapidly, as ordered. Remember, though—if your patient's obviously pregnant, you'll begin replacing fluids long *before* her blood pressure indicates a substantial fluid loss. Why? Because a pregnant woman is normally *hyper*volemic, so she may show no signs of hypovolemia until she's lost about 30% of her circulating blood (see *Assessing the Pregnant Patient*). Compensatory mechanisms in the mother's body shunt her circulation from the placenta to her vital organs to protect her from shock; this may cause uterine blood flow to fall by about 20% before the mother's blood pressure drops. By that time, her fetus may be dead.

If your patient has a thready pulse, an increasingly rapid pulse, or a drop in blood pressure, suspect heavy bleeding with a large loss of circulating blood volume. If you note a significant

## POSITIONING YOUR PREGNANT PATIENT

When your pregnant patient lies on her back, her uterus presses the vena cava against her vertebral column. This decreases venous return and cardiac output, causing supine hypotensive syndrome. These actions combine to reduce placental perfusion and may result in fetal distress.

To prevent supine hypotensive syndrome, place your patient on her left side with a pillow under her right hip. This will move the uterus away from the vena cava and help everyone rest a little easier.

change—or a clear trend—in either pulse or blood pressure, call the doctor *immediately*, increase the I.V. infusion rate as ordered, and anticipate blood transfusions. Draw blood for a complete blood count (CBC), typing and cross matching, coagulation times, and arterial blood gases. If the woman's pregnant, anticipate termination of the pregnancy or cesarean section delivery, and send blood for antibody screening with the indirect Coombs' test.

If your patient has profuse vaginal bleeding and she doesn't appear to be pregnant, put her in a supine position with her feet elevated 20° to 30° to enhance venous return to her vital organs. If she's obviously pregnant, lower the head of the bed and put her on her left side with a pillow under her right hip to displace her uterus laterally and to increase placental perfusion (see *Positioning Your Pregnant Patient*).

Remember that *hyper*tension in a pregnant patient is also a danger sign. Extremely high blood pressure or a trend toward increasing blood pressure may signal preeclampsia. Notify the doctor *immediately*, and watch your patient closely—she's at high risk for having a seizure.

### General appearance

Assess your patient's appearance for further clues to the cause of her emergency condition.

Check her skin for cyanosis, pallor, coldness, and clamminess. These signs, accompanying hypotension, indicate shock. Check her face and hands for edema, which may be the first sign of preeclampsia.

Check for lacerations or bruises in her abdominal and genital area—these may indicate rape or abuse that the patient's afraid or ashamed to report.

### Mental status

Most OB/GYN patients are awake and alert. If your patient is confused, agitated, or restless, suspect decreased cerebral perfusion from severe blood loss or preeclampsia. Give her supplemental oxygen by cannula or mask, protect her from injuring herself, and assess her level of consciousness frequently.

Many patients with OB/GYN emergencies are thoroughly frightened and embarrassed. Don't overlook your patient's need for ongoing emotional support and for privacy.

# What to Do Next

Once you've assessed your patient's airway, breathing, and circulation and intervene appropriately, you can continue your assessment by determining if your patient is pregnant, because this will affect the care you give. You won't administer certain drugs to a pregnant woman, for example, even if she's in pain. And the doctor probably won't perform a vaginal examination if she has vaginal bleeding, nor will he order abdominal X-rays.

You may note her pregnancy immediately, or she may tell you she's had a positive pregnancy test. If she doesn't know if she's pregnant, ask her about the date and nature of her last menstrual period. This will help you evaluate the possibility that she's pregnant—and, if she may be, this information will also help you calculate an expected date of confinement (EDC) if pregnancy's likely. (See *When Is She Due?*) Ask if she's sexually active and if she uses any form of birth control. (If she uses an intrauterine device, be alert for signs of infection, spontaneous abortion, or ectopic pregnancy.) If you determine that she may be pregnant, obtain a urine sample for a 2-minute urine immunologic pregnancy test, and draw blood for a serum test of human chorionic gonadotropin (HCG).

If your patient's obviously pregnant, quickly obtain some information about her current pregnancy before you move on to assess her chief complaints. Ask questions like these:

• Has she felt fetal movement? When was the last time? The sudden and continued absence of fetal movement for several days may indicate that the fetus has died. Violent fetal activity indicates fetal distress, possibly from a prolapsed cord. If you have any reason to suspect this condition, *call the doctor immediately* and follow the steps outlined in *Danger: Prolapsed Cord,* page 514.

• Have her membranes ruptured? If so, what was the appearance of the amniotic fluid? Normal amniotic fluid is clear and odorless, whereas brown or green fluid is an indication of meconium. (If you note meconium, report it to the doctor *immediately.* He'll want to evaluate the fetus for intrauterine hypoxia. And, after delivery, he'll evaluate the neonate for meconium aspiration syndrome—a serious neonatal respiratory distress disorder.) Test any fluid to make sure it *is* amniotic fluid by holding a strip of litmus paper at your patient's vaginal opening. If the paper turns dark blue, the leaking fluid is probably amniotic. Remember, however, that the presence of blood in a fluid will also turn a strip blue.

Quickly evaluate fetal well-being by checking fetal heart tones (see *Monitoring Fetal Heart Rate,* pages 512 and 513). Call the doctor *immediately* if heart tones are absent, bradycardic

(slower than 120 beats/minute), or tachycardic (more than 160 beats/minute); these findings indicate fetal distress, so the doctor may want to perform an immediate cesarean section.

If your patient hasn't been sent for surgery, your next step is to assess her chief complaints. She may have *pain, bleeding, nausea and vomiting, vaginal discharge,* or *swollen face and extremities.* Or she may have been *raped.* Remember to assess her complaints in light of whether she's pregnant.

Ask, first, if she has any *abdominal pain.* If she does, note the type, quality, and duration of the pain:

• Sudden, knifelike pain may indicate abruptio placentae or impending uterine rupture, whereas gradual, generalized abdominal cramping is more likely to indicate spontaneous abortion.

• Sharp continuing pain may indicate abruptio placentae or impending uterine rupture; crampy pain is more characteristic of abortion.

• Pain starting on one side of the lower abdomen may indicate ectopic pregnancy or a ruptured ovarian cyst, particularly if it radiates to one shoulder.

• Abdominal pain and backache may indicate abruptio placentae.

• Excruciating abdominal pain may indicate a ruptured ectopic pregnancy or impending uterine rupture.

Palpate your patient's abdomen

### WHEN IS SHE DUE?

Whatever the nature of your pregnant patient's emergency, you need to know her estimated date of confinement (EDC), or "due date." If she doesn't know this date, you can approximate it using a technique known as Nägele's rule:

Ask her the starting date of her last menstrual period (LMP). Subtract 3 months from this date, then add 7 days. For example, if her LMP started March 13, subtract 3 months (December 13) and add 7 days—for a December 20 EDC.

## MONITORING FETAL HEART RATE

Any maternal emergency, such as bleeding, trauma, or induction of labor, can quickly cause an emergency for the fetus by depriving it of oxygen. You can prevent this by monitoring the fetus for prolonged or inappropriate bradycardia and intervening as needed.

Use one of these three methods to monitor the fetus for distress: monitoring by fetoscope, external electronic fetal monitoring (ultrasound), or internal electronic fetal monitoring.

Normally, when your patient has a contraction, the fetal heart rate (FHR) will decelerate until the contraction's over and then return to baseline. Check the FHR 30 to 45 seconds after a contraction ends. (If you're using electronic monitoring, you'll see the relationship between the uterine contraction and the FHR at the same time.) If the FHR hasn't returned to within 4 to 6 beats/minute of its baseline, the fetus' life may be in danger. Alert the doctor *immediately*.

During any maternal emergency, monitor the FHR *at least* every 15 minutes. Check it before, during, and after a contraction—this is the time when

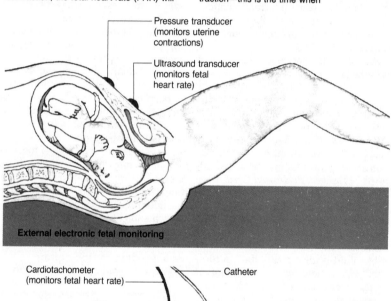

Pressure transducer (monitors uterine contractions)

Ultrasound transducer (monitors fetal heart rate)

**External electronic fetal monitoring**

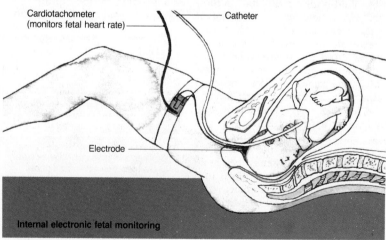

Cardiotachometer (monitors fetal heart rate)

Catheter

Electrode

**Internal electronic fetal monitoring**

interruption of oxygen delivery to the fetus is commonly detected.

**Monitoring by fetoscope** is the simplest method of fetal monitoring. Place the fetoscope over the mother's lower right abdomen. Listen for the fetal heartbeat, which sounds like a watch ticking under a pillow. You'll also hear a uterine souffle— the swooshing sound of the uterine blood flow. If the FHR is the same as the mother's pulse (80 to 100 beats/minute), you're listening to the souffle. FHR should be between 120 and 160 beats/minute. You can amplify the heart sounds with a Doppler device. First lubricate the Doppler's transducer, then use it like a fetoscope to monitor the FHR.

**External electronic fetal monitoring** (ultrasound) is a noninvasive technique for monitoring contractions and FHR *before* or *after* the membranes rupture. To prepare your patient for ultrasound monitoring, lubricate her abdomen and place the pressure transducer on the area of the fundus where the contractions are strongest. Adjust the transducer strap to fit snugly around the patient's abdomen. (This transducer converts the uterine contraction's pressure into an electronic signal and records it on graph paper.) To measure the FHR, reposition the ultrasound transducer over the spot where the fetal heart sounds are clearest. Remember that, though ultrasound's the easiest method to use, it needs frequent adjustments.

**Internal electronic fetal monitoring** monitors contractions and FHR when the mother has ruptured membranes and a dilated cervix (2 to 3 cm), with the fetus' presenting part positioned at its opening. To perform this procedure, first help the doctor insert a saline-filled catheter into the mother's uterus, then connect the catheter to an external transducer. As contractions raise the catheter's fluid pressure, the transducer converts the pressure into an electronic signal recorded on graph paper as a curved line. Next, to measure the FHR, assist the doctor in inserting a spiral electrode into the skin of the fetus' presenting part. This will chart the heart rate instantly via a cardiotachometer and record it on graph paper. Internal fetal monitoring is the most accurate way to check FHR and uterine contractions, because the mother's movements don't affect it. However, it's an invasive procedure requiring sterile conditions and caution when placing the electrode.

gently, noting rigidity, tenderness, or any mass that may indicate bleeding. If she's pregnant, monitor the intensity, duration, and interval of any contractions, and measure the height of the fundus, to provide a baseline for assessing possible intrauterine bleeding (see *Measuring Fundal Height,* page 533). Continue to check fundal height every 15 minutes. If you can't palpate the fundus, measure the patient's abdominal girth, which—if it's increasing—also indicates internal bleeding.

The doctor may ask you to assist with a vaginal examination unless the patient's obviously pregnant and bleeding vaginally. If she is, he may suspect placenta previa and defer the examination until he can arrange for a double setup in the operating room. The reason? If your patient's bleeding is from placenta previa, vaginal examination may precipitate massive hemorrhage and, therefore, delivery of a premature infant; with the double setup, the doctor will be prepared for this possibility.

If your patient complains of *vaginal bleeding* and *isn't* pregnant, find out what her menstrual periods are usually like. How quickly does she saturate a pad or tampon? Are they painless or accompanied by cramping? This will help you evaluate her current bleeding episode. Assess the amount of blood lost by counting the number of perineal pads she's saturated in a measured period of time. If possible, weigh the pads to estimate her blood loss. If her bleeding is uncontrollable, the doctor may do a dilatation and curettage (D&C). Prepare her for surgery as necessary. (Keep in mind that her bleeding may be the aftermath of an induced abortion. If this seems likely, obtain as much history information as possible and alert the doctor—he'll take precautions against infection.)

If she complains of *vaginal bleeding* and *is* pregnant, you must also consider the condition of her fetus. Check fetal heart tones again; if they indicate fetal distress and the patient's close to term, the doctor may do an immediate ce-

## DANGER: PROLAPSED CORD

A prolapsed umbilical cord is one of the most common—and most frightening—birth complications you'll ever witness. If it's not corrected within 5 minutes, expect fetal hypoxia, central nervous system damage, and possibly death. Fortunately, your quick assessment and intervention can help both mother and fetus survive this traumatic birth event.

A prolapsed cord is an umbilical cord that's displaced below the fetus' presenting part. It's common in women whose amniotic membranes rupture early in labor, carrying the long, loose cord below the unengaged presenting part in a sudden gush of fluid. The cord may even slip through the mother's cervix into her vagina. But the most serious damage is done when the fetus compresses the cord, interrupting the blood flow from the placenta.

Watch for these signs and symptoms of prolapsed cord:
• The mother feels the cord "slither" down after the membranes rupture.
• The umbilical cord is visible or palpable in the birth canal.
• Fetal activity is violent.

• Fetal bradycardia occurs with variable deceleration during contractions.

Your first priority's to relieve the pressure on the cord until the doctor can perform an emergency cesarean section (or, for a patient with a fully dilated cervix, a forceps delivery). Here's how to proceed:
• Place your patient in the knee-chest position, to shift fetal weight off the cord.
• Using two gloved fingers, push the fetus' presenting part off the cord. Don't push the cord back into the uterus—this may traumatize the cord and stop blood flow to the fetus. You may also cause an intrauterine infection.
• Notify the doctor and continue to relieve the pressure while the operating room's being prepared.
• Ask another nurse to give supplemental oxygen, to start a large-gauge I.V., to send blood for typing and cross matching, and to insert a nasogastric tube, as ordered.
• Accompany the patient to the operating room, keeping pressure off the cord and watching for signs of maternal and fetal distress.

---

sarean section. If the fetus is in no distress, the doctor may ask you to give the patient oxytocin (Pitocin), to induce labor (see *Highlighting Oxytocin*, page 541). Remember that even scant bleeding may indicate a serious complication. Check her perineal pads for tissue or clots, and if you find either, place the material in a labeled specimen container for the laboratory. The doctor may order a D&C in the event of an inevitable or incomplete abortion. If your patient's bleeding heavily, she's at risk for shock and for disseminated intravascular coagulation (see the "Disseminated Intravascular Coagulation" entry in Chapter 11). Prepare her for blood transfusion, if necessary.

Your pregnant patient may complain of *nausea* or *vomiting*. Both are common in patients with abruptio placentae, ectopic pregnancy, preeclampsia, or impending uterine rupture. If she's vomiting, insert an NG tube as ordered, if you haven't already done so.

Ask your patient if she's had a *vag-inal discharge*. A foul-smelling discharge is common in septic abortion and missed abortion. It may also indicate sepsis associated with foreign objects, such as tampons or condoms, retained in the vagina.

Your patient may complain of *swollen hands and face*. This may be the presenting sign of preeclampsia, so report it to the doctor *immediately*. Why is this important? Because preeclampsia may progress to eclampsia with little warning. Assess the degree of edema and whether it's pitting or nonpitting, and monitor your patient's blood pressure closely.

If your patient reports that she's been *raped*, provide a calm, quiet environment and comfort her emotionally before the examination begins.

After you've assessed your patient's chief complaints, ask her whether she has any chronic diseases—such as cardiac disease, diabetes, anemia, or renal disease—that you know will identify her as a high-risk patient. Find out about any allergies and about any medications the patient's taking; then take an obstetric history. How many times has she been pregnant? What were the outcomes of the pregnancies? Ask if she's ever had a cesarean section or spontaneous abortion and whether she knows if she's Rh negative.

Whatever the nature of your elderly patient's OB/GYN emergency, anticipate that she may have one or more chronic conditions and that these may complicate her care. Be particularly careful not to injure your patient during your physical examination; the doctor may use a nasal or pediatric speculum for the vaginal examination.

## Special Considerations

### Pediatric
When your patient's an infant, a child, or a teenager with severe vaginal trauma or bleeding, consider the possibility of sexual abuse. Calm the child by keeping your voice calm and by starting your examination at a distance from the injured area, such as the patient's head, and working down. If the child is very frightened by your examination, notify the doctor. He may order sedation or general anesthesia so that he can perform a thorough pelvic examination without traumatizing the patient further. If you find evidence of possible abuse, follow your hospital's protocol about notifying authorities.

An adolescent who's pregnant requires special consideration, because both she and her fetus are high-risk patients. She may have received little or no prenatal care; she may not even know, or may not admit, that she's pregnant. This means that, in addition to assessing her emergency condition, you may also have to help her come to grips with her pregnancy. When you're taking her history, be alert for possible drug use, preeclampsia, and infection. She'll probably have prolonged labor, and she may need a cesarean section.

### Geriatric
Because they're less able to defend themselves than younger adults, elderly women are highly vulnerable to sexual assault. And, of course, because of their age, they're more likely to sustain serious injury from assault.

# CARE AFTER DIAGNOSIS

## Spontaneous Abortion

### Prediagnosis summary
The patient with a spontaneous abortion has a history of one or more missed menstrual periods and a negative or weakly positive pregnancy test, depending on the length of gestation.

If the patient has a *threatened* abortion, initial findings included:
- vaginal bleeding
- mild or no contractions
- a closed cervix
- appropriate uterine size for length of pregnancy.

The process of a threatened abortion may stop on its own within a few days, or it may continue through uterine contractions to partial or complete expulsion of the products of conception (incomplete or complete abortion).

If the patient has an *inevitable* abortion, initial findings included:
- an unremarkable amount of bleeding (comparable to a normal menstrual period), with no tissue or clots passed
- moderately severe contractions with possible amniotic sac rupture
- an opened cervix
- appropriate uterine size for length of pregnancy.

An inevitable abortion is just what the term describes: an irreversible process of uterine expulsion.

PROCEDURES

## YOUR ROLE IN AN EMERGENCY

## PERFORMING AN EMERGENCY DELIVERY

If you were asked to help a woman in precipitous labor, with no time to transport her to a hospital or to wait for a doctor, are you confident you'd know what to do? (As a nurse, you probably know that precipitous labor means birth takes place less than 2 hours after labor begins, with the baby's head crowning very quickly.) Here's how you can assist with an emergency delivery.

### Priorities
Remember three priorities as you prepare for the delivery:
• *Prevent maternal and fetal infection.* You probably won't have time to wash the perineum. But if clean water's available, take time to wash your hands and to put a clean towel or coat under the mother. Be careful, during the delivery, to keep your hands out of the mother's vagina.
• *Keep the delivery slow.* The baby's likely to be born headfirst, without any major difficulty. The most important thing you can do is to control the speed of the delivery, because this will help prevent stress on the fetus and hemorrhage-causing lacerations of the mother's perineum.
• *Protect the newborn baby from cold stress* by keeping him warm and dry after birth.

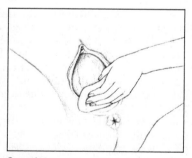

### Crowning
If the baby's head is showing, birth is imminent. *Don't move the mother.* Instead:
• Keep the delivery slow by helping her establish a breathing rhythm. Tell her quietly and calmly, "Pant, pant, pant, as if

you're blowing out candles." Set the pace by breathing with her.
• Don't let the head pop out or exert any pressure to pull it out. Gently press a folded towel, clean cloth, or your hand against the baby's crowning head, to slow delivery and to prevent cranial hemorrhages and vaginal or perineal tears.
• As the head emerges, continue to exert gentle counterpressure on it. At the same time, see if the membrane has broken. (The baby's head will be crowning against it.) If it hasn't, tear it or pinch it with your fingernail to keep the baby from aspirating amniotic fluid with his first breath. Assess the fluid, too: clear, odorless fluid is normal; brown or green fluid indicates the presence of meconium. Be sure to report this finding to the doctor later, as it may indicate that the baby experienced a hypoxic episode.

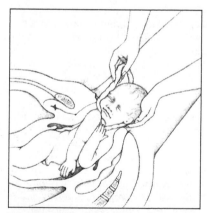

### Releasing the cord
• As the baby's head emerges, slip your fingers under it, feeling for the umbilical cord. If it's wrapped loosely around his neck, gently lift it over his head. If it's tight, tie the cord tightly in two places, cut between the ties, and release the cord before continuing.

### Cleaning the airway
• When the baby's head has emerged, support it with both hands and allow it to rotate to one side; gently stroke the baby's nose downward to expel amniotic fluid and mucus. Stroke the baby's throat from the neck to the chin, then sweep your finger into the baby's mouth to clear it of any mucus. Wipe any remaining mucus from the baby's face and remove any remnant of the amniotic sac at the base of his neck.

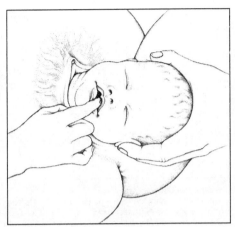

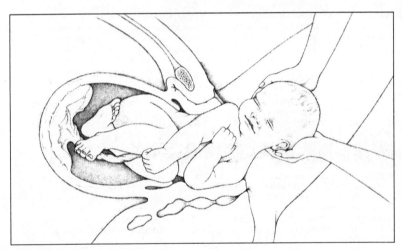

### Delivering the shoulders
• Deliver the shoulders with the next contraction. Tell the mother to breathe quickly four times, exhaling as if she's blowing out a candle, then to push hard. Place a hand on either side of the baby's head for support and, as the contraction begins, exert downward pressure to deliver the anterior shoulder under the symphysis pubis. Then, at the next contraction, apply steady upward pressure to deliver the posterior shoulder. Be careful not to force the baby when you exert upward pressure—you risk damaging the spinal cord.

• Tell the mother to push hard once more to deliver the rest of the baby. The baby will be very slippery, so support him with one hand cupped around his head, grasping his buttocks or feet with the other as they emerge. Supporting the baby with one arm, hold him securely with his head down to drain mucus from his mouth and nose, then gently rub his back or the soles of his feet until he starts to cry.

*(continued)*

## PERFORMING AN EMERGENCY DELIVERY *(continued)*

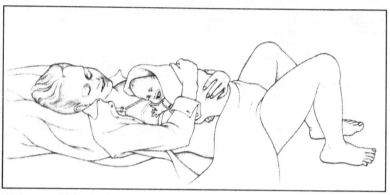

### Keeping the baby warm

Even a healthy baby can die if he isn't kept warm. Here's how to protect him:

• Quickly dry the baby with a towel or clean cloth, then place him stomach-down, with his head to one side, on his mother's bare stomach. The baby will stay warm and his weight on the fundus will stimulate uterine contractions.

• Immediately cover the entire baby—including his head—leaving just his face exposed. If he has to work to stay warm, he may require more oxygen than he can get from ambient air. When he doesn't get it, he can develop severe respiratory problems. External warming will help prevent this situation.

• Get a baseline Apgar score (see below).

• Tie the cord tightly when it stops pulsating, to prevent the baby's blood from leaking back into the placenta and causing anemia or shock. You can use shoestrings or strips of torn clothing to tie the cord. But don't use wire: it might cut the cord and cause bleeding. Make the first tie about 3″ (7.6 cm) from the baby's abdomen, the second about 5″ (12.7 cm) from the abdomen. If you don't have anything handy for tying the cord, don't worry—it'll clot naturally, and this should suffice for a while. Cover the cord with a towel to keep it clean, and wait for the doctor to cut it. Don't use nonsterile scissors or a nonsterile knife to cut the cord—this exposes the baby to a risk of tetanus.

• Assess the mother: Put a fresh towel or cloth under her so you can assess bleeding. Expect some lochia (blood mixed with uterine secretions), but if you see bright red bleeding, suspect a tear in the perineum or vagina. Using a towel as a pressure dressing, tell the mother to press her thighs together to hold it tightly in place. Assess her abdomen every 5 minutes, and massage her fundus if it feels soft. If bleeding continues or the uterus begins to feel soft and boggy, begin uterine massage again, let the baby suckle, or have the mother massage her breast. This releases oxytocin and stimulates contractions.

• Reassess the baby—get another Apgar score about 5 minutes after delivery.

### Assessment criteria for Apgar scoring

• *Heart rate:* Score 0 if absent, 1 if less than 100 beats/minute, 2 if over 100. Slip your hand under the baby's chest to check the heart rate. Start immediate CPR, if necessary.

• *Respiratory effort:* Score 0 if absent, 1 if slow or irregular, 2 if good or if the baby's crying. Again, start CPR if needed.

• *Muscle tone:* Score 0 if flaccid, 1 if you note some flexion of extremities, 2 if you note active motion.

• *Reflex irritability:* Score 0 if no response, 1 if the baby cries weakly or grimaces, 2 if the baby coughs, sneezes, or cries vigorously.

• *Color:* Score 0 if the baby's blue, 1 if he has a pink body with blue extremities, 2 if he's completely pink.

### Delivering the placenta

The placenta may not be delivered for up to 30 minutes after the baby's delivered, so don't wait for it. Get the mother and baby to the hospital as soon as possible. If you can't get to the hospital within that time, here's what to do:
• Watch for advance signs of placental delivery—cord lengthening, a slight gush of vaginal blood, or changes in the shape of the uterus (the fundus rises in the abdomen and becomes globe-shaped).
• When you see these signs, tell the mother to push hard once more while you apply downward pressure on the fundus with one hand. (Don't pull the cord, or you'll tear it from the placenta and cause hemorrhage.)

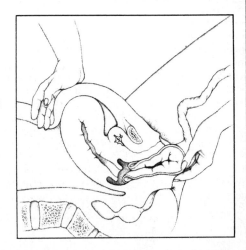

### Positioning the placenta

• After the placenta's delivered, put it in a towel or other clean material. Place it on the mother's abdomen slightly above the baby's level if you had nothing to tie the cord with. This will prevent backflow of fetal blood to the placenta.
• Check the fundus—it should be starting to firm up. Massage it until it becomes firm, if necessary.
• Transport mother and baby to the hospital as soon as possible.

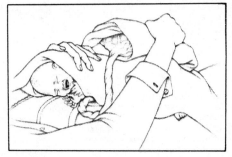

### Finishing up

• Reassure the mother, when appropriate, that the baby's well and that she did a good job.
• Do your best to remember—for later recording—the time of the birth, the manner of presentation, the cord position (around the baby's neck or not), 1-minute and 5-minute Apgar scores, the baby's sex, the placenta's appearance and intactness, and the mother's condition.
• Also, make sure you or someone in the ED accurately identifies the mother and baby.

### Warning

Don't try to deliver a baby—inside the hospital or out—whose foot, arm, or shoulder presents first. Get the mother to the hospital *immediately*. Managing foot, arm, and particularly shoulder presentations

in a vaginal delivery is difficult even for experienced obstetricians. At worst, nonmedical attempts can be fatal to mother and baby.

Sometimes, in a breech presentation, the baby's body will come out easily, leaving the head in the uterus. When this happens, you can't wait to get the mother to the hospital to complete the delivery, because the baby's oxygen supply will be interrupted until the head is delivered. Reach into the vagina with one hand, crook your finger in the baby's mouth, and exert light maxillary pressure while you press over the bladder area with the other hand. This should enable you to complete the delivery quickly when the next contraction begins. (This is one time when putting your hand in the mother's vagina, usually contraindicated, is permissible, to save the baby.)

If the patient has an *incomplete* abortion, initial findings included:
• possibly heavy bleeding, with clots and tissue
• severe uterine contractions
• an open cervix, with tissue visible
• small uterine size for length of pregnancy
• hypotension and a blood hemoglobin level that may be less than 11 g/100 ml.
Your patient with an incomplete abortion has expelled some, but not all, of the products of conception.

If the patient has a *complete* abortion, initial findings included:
• minimal or no bleeding, following a history of profuse bleeding with passage of tissue and clots

• continuing mild contractions
• an open cervix
• small uterine size for length of pregnancy
• hypotension and a blood hemoglobin level that may be less than 11 g/100 ml.
A complete abortion, of course, is one in which all the products of conception have been expelled.

If the patient has a *missed* abortion, initial findings included:
• a possible history of bleeding without cramping
• amenorrhea
• a history of weight loss.
In a missed abortion, the fetus has died, but after 8 weeks or longer, neither it nor any other products of conception

---

DRUGS

## HIGHLIGHTING RhoGam

An Rh-negative mother whose fetus is Rh-positive will become sensitized to Rh-positive blood and develop anti-Rh-positive antibodies when her blood is exposed to fetal blood. Exposure occurs when the placenta separates from the uterine wall, or during:
• delivery of an Rh-positive infant
• elective or spontaneous abortion
• ectopic pregnancy.
Then, during each future pregnancy, these antibodies will enter the fetal circulation, attach to the Rh-positive red blood cells, and hemolyze them. This condition, known as erythroblastosis fetalis, causes severe anemia and elevated bilirubin levels, and it can cause fetal death.

To prevent these antibodies from forming and to protect the mother's later pregnancies, expect to give RhoGam, an $Rh_0$ (D) immune globulin. You'll give RhoGam to a previously unsensitized Rh-negative woman *within 72 hours* of exposure of maternal blood to fetal blood. Use the following nursing guidelines for patients who may receive RhoGam:

**Before administration**
• Check your patient's Rh blood group when you get her laboratory report. If her blood is Rh-negative, and refined testing methods are available, check for the presence of the $D^u$ antigen. If she has it, she won't develop Rh antibodies. If she

doesn't have it, she'll probably receive RhoGam.
• Check the results of her indirect Coombs' test. As you know, this test detects the presence of Rh-positive antibodies in the blood. RhoGam is contraindicated if the Coombs' test is positive, because a positive test indicates that the mother has already formed the antibodies.
• Send a sample of blood from the infant's cord after your patient delivers or miscarries. If the infant's blood is the same as the mother's, the mother won't develop the antibodies from the mixing of their blood, and she won't need RhoGam.
• Explain to her that RhoGam will prevent her from developing antibodies that might endanger her fetus in future pregnancies.

**After administration**
• Complete the patient form on the dosage packet and attach it to the patient's records immediately after administering the injection.
• Monitor your patient's reaction. Adverse reactions are uncommon, but she may develop a slight fever and discomfort at the injection site. If this happens, administer an analgesic, as ordered, and apply a heating pad or warm soak (as ordered) to the affected area.
• Tell her to expect to receive RhoGam after each potentially sensitizing event, such as delivery or abortion.

## WHAT HAPPENS IN SPONTANEOUS ABORTION

A spontaneous abortion occurs when a pregnancy terminates naturally and the fetus isn't viable—able to live outside the uterus. Fetal weight's usually less than 500 g (17⅝ oz), with gestational age less than 20 weeks.

The cause of spontaneous abortion is the embryo's death or failure to implant and develop normally. Several factors predispose women to spontaneous abortion:
• abnormal embryonic development, such as chromosomal aberrations and placental abnormalities
• maternal diseases and infections, such as syphilis and influenza
• problems related to the uterus—for example, poor hormonal development of the endometrium, bicornate uterus, incompetent cervix, and use of an intrauterine device
• other causes, such as aged or defective

sperm, trauma, psychogenic or immunologic factors, or use of certain drugs.

When the embryo dies, the mother's estrogen and progesterone levels decrease. This triggers the uterus to contract, causing it to expel its contents.

Types of spontaneous abortion include:
• *incomplete abortion,* when the uterine contents aren't completely expelled
• *inevitable abortion,* when the embryo or fetus can't be saved
• *threatened abortion,* when the pregnancy may be saved and the embryo or fetus may be able to live
• *missed abortion,* when the embryo or fetus is dead, but not expelled
• *septic abortion,* when the embryo or endometrial lining's infected, usually resulting from attempted termination of early pregnancy.

---

have been expelled.

If the patient has a *septic* abortion, initial findings included:
• fever, elevated white blood cell count, and elevated sedimentation rate
• some discharge or bleeding, with or without tissue passage
• constant lower abdominal pain
• an open cervix
• small or appropriate uterine size for length of pregnancy.
Infection is, of course, the overriding problem in a septic abortion, which may be from a nonmedical attempt to induce abortion.

Whatever her abortion type, the patient was given supplementary oxygen and I.V. fluids (probably Ringer's lactate) via a large-bore catheter. Blood was drawn for CBC, electrolytes, blood glucose, clotting profile, blood urea nitrogen (BUN), creatinine, and typing and cross matching.

### Priorities
You have four possible priorities for a patient with a spontaneous abortion (depending on the type):

• replacing fluids
• giving medication to stimulate contractions
• culturing an infectious organism
• maintaining her on bed rest.

If your patient has an *inevitable, incomplete, complete,* or *threatened* abortion and is bleeding heavily, your first priority is replacing fluids, as ordered, to avert the threat of hypovolemic shock.

Then the doctor may ask you to start an I.V. infusion of oxytocin (Pitocin) if your patient's abortion is *inevitable, incomplete, complete,* or *missed* (see *Highlighting Oxytocin,* page 541). Oxytocin reduces bleeding after a complete abortion by constricting blood vessels and by helping the uterus contract and clamp down on the vessels. In a patient with an inevitable, incomplete, or missed abortion, oxytocin initiates uterine contractions and promotes expulsion of the products of conception. (The doctor may alternatively ask you to give prostaglandin suppositories, such as dinoprostone [Prostin $E_2$], which have a similar effect.)

If your patient has a *septic* abortion, obtain a culture immediately and start antibiotics, as ordered, to reduce the risk of septic shock. Replace fluids or blood as necessary.

If the patient has a *threatened* abortion and is bleeding heavily, she'll be admitted and placed on bed rest to try to save her pregnancy. If she isn't bleeding heavily, the doctor may ask you to discharge her with instructions to stay in bed, to avoid sexual intercourse for 2 weeks after the bleeding stops, to call her own doctor when she gets home to arrange a visit, and to return to the ED if she has further signs and symptoms.

## Continuing assessment and intervention

As soon as possible, perform a thorough assessment of your patient to collect baseline information. Ask about previous gynecologic problems and about her menstrual history. Find out the outcome of previous pregnancies. Monitor her fluid status: she's likely to be hypovolemic from the vaginal bleeding and the oxytocin (if she received this drug), which acts as an antidiuretic. (See *Highlighting Oxytocin,* page 541.) Start an intake and output record, and measure your patient's blood pressure and pulse rate frequently to make sure she doesn't go from *hypo*volemic to *hyper*volemic.

Monitor the progress of your patient's abortion: her contractions should be effective but not severe enough to cause uterine rupture. Note the amount of her bleeding, and keep any tissue she passes so that the pathologist can determine whether the abortion is complete and, perhaps, determine the cause of the abortion. If her bleeding becomes profuse, increase the rate of the I.V. infusion and call the doctor *immediately.*

Check her hematocrit and hemoglobin levels, and continue assessing her fluid status. Watch for bleeding from the nose, gums, or puncture wounds, such as I.V. insertion sites—this may indicate that your patient's developing disseminated intravascular coagulation (see the "Disseminated Intravascular Coagulation" entry in Chapter 11). Be sure to time the frequency, duration, and intensity of your patient's contractions and to note uterine tenderness and firmness during a contraction. Stop the infusion and call the doctor *immediately* if her contractions become too rapid or hard, because these may cause uterine rupture. (See *Preventing Uterine Rupture,* page 538.)

If your patient's receiving oxytocin, her contractions are likely to be quite painful. Be sure to give her sufficient doses of analgesics, as ordered, to reduce her discomfort. If she's in her first trimester or her early second trimester and you've administered oxytocin to facilitate an *inevitable* or *incomplete* abortion, the doctor may perform a D&C to make sure all the products of conception are removed. If the patient received oxytocin later in her second trimester, she may not need a D&C.

Your patient with a *threatened* abortion may have been admitted for observation. Watch her for continued bleeding, because she may progress to an inevitable abortion. The doctor will check the patient's cervical os if she continues to bleed. If it's open, he may give oxytocin or a prostaglandin suppository, and he may perform a D&C or use suction to facilitate the abortion.

If your patient had a *septic* abortion, watch for rising temperature, rapid pulse, hypotension, and tachypnea. These may indicate septic shock, so report these findings to the doctor *immediately,* and give antibiotics as ordered. The doctor may perform a D&C after the patient's been given antibiotics.

Continue to monitor your patient's intake and output. If she had a D&C, she should have only scant bleeding after curettage. If the amount of bleeding increases, try massaging her uterus. If this fails to cause her uterus to contract, so the bleeding doesn't stop, notify the doctor. He'll probably order an oral oxytocic, such as ergonovine maleate.

If your patient had an *inevitable, incomplete, complete, missed,* or *septic* abortion, the doctor will ask you to give RhoGam (Rh₀ [D] immune globulin) if she's Rh negative and had a negative indirect Coombs' test (see *Highlighting RhoGam,* page 520).

### Therapeutic care

As soon as your patient's vital signs are stable, her bleeding's controlled, and the doctor's sure she has expelled all the products of conception, she'll probably be discharged. But even if she's on your unit only a few hours, you'll have time to provide some of the emotional and psychological support she and her family need. A terminated pregnancy produces a feeling of great loss in most women. Your patient may also feel that the abortion was a punishment for negative feelings about the pregnancy or for some other presumed wrongdoing. Losing the baby may even make her feel abnormal or inferior.

You can help her by listening empathetically and then encouraging her and her family to talk about their feelings and to grieve openly. Help your patient handle the long-term implications of the abortion by referring her for psychological counseling, if her reaction seems extreme, or for obstetrical counseling if she has a history of repeated abortions.

# Ectopic Pregnancy

### Prediagnosis summary

The patient with an ectopic pregnancy probably had a history of one or two missed menstrual periods. She may not have known she was pregnant. If she was initially examined *before the ectopic pregnancy ruptured,* she had some of these signs and symptoms:

• scant, dark red vaginal bleeding
• lower abdominal pain, which might be sharp or dull, constant or intermittent, or referred to the right shoulder

• the usual signs of early pregnancy (amenorrhea; swollen, tender breasts; enlarged uterus; soft, blue cervix)
• a palpable crepitant mass in one of the lower quandrants on pelvic examination
• severe abdominal pain in response to any movement of the cervix during a pelvic examination.

If she was initially examined *after the pregnancy ruptured,* she probably had most of the above signs and symptoms plus profuse vaginal bleeding following an intense, unilateral, tearing pain in the left or right lower abdominal quadrant. She may have been pale and dizzy and may have had other signs and symptoms of profound blood loss.

One or more I.V.s were started with large-bore catheters, supplemental oxygen was given by mask or nasal cannula, and food and fluid by mouth were restricted. Blood was drawn for a CBC, electrolytes, blood glucose, Venereal Disease Research Laboratory test, sedimentation rate, indirect Coombs' test, serum HCG, and typing and cross matching. A blood transfusion may have been started. Urine was obtained for a 2-minute urine immunologic pregnancy test. An indwelling (Foley) catheter was inserted, and intake and output measurements were started. Culdocentesis or laparoscopy confirmed an ectopic pregnancy (see *Understanding Culdocentesis,* page 525).

### Priorities

Surgery is the only treatment for an ectopic pregnancy, so your initial priority is to stabilize your patient until the operating room is ready. Replace lost blood volume with I.V. fluids or blood, as ordered, and titrate the I.V. infusion to her urine output. Monitor her pulse and blood pressure carefully, particularly if her vaginal bleeding is profuse. If her pulse rate increases and her blood pressure decreases, notify the doctor *immediately.* He may ask you to increase the I.V. infusion rate or to begin transfusing blood if you haven't

PATHOPHYSIOLOGY

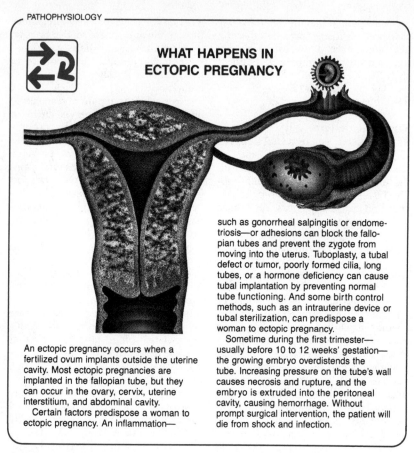

### WHAT HAPPENS IN ECTOPIC PREGNANCY

An ectopic pregnancy occurs when a fertilized ovum implants outside the uterine cavity. Most ectopic pregnancies are implanted in the fallopian tube, but they can occur in the ovary, cervix, uterine interstitium, and abdominal cavity.

Certain factors predispose a woman to ectopic pregnancy. An inflammation— such as gonorrheal salpingitis or endometriosis—or adhesions can block the fallopian tubes and prevent the zygote from moving into the uterus. Tuboplasty, a tubal defect or tumor, poorly formed cilia, long tubes, or a hormone deficiency can cause tubal implantation by preventing normal tube functioning. And some birth control methods, such as an intrauterine device or tubal sterilization, can predispose a woman to ectopic pregnancy.

Sometime during the first trimester— usually before 10 to 12 weeks' gestation— the growing embryo overdistends the tube. Increasing pressure on the tube's wall causes necrosis and rupture, and the embryo is extruded into the peritoneal cavity, causing hemorrhage. Without prompt surgical intervention, the patient will die from shock and infection.

done so already.

Prepare your patient for surgery as ordered. Expect to give preoperative pain medications and to insert an NG tube (and—if you haven't yet inserted one—a Foley catheter, as ordered).

### Continuing assessment and intervention

When your patient returns from surgery, monitor her vital signs every 15 minutes and assess her for bleeding at the incision site and from her vagina. Because the pregnancy was ectopic, her uterus won't be enlarged, but you'll need to record the amount and type of vaginal discharge by recording the number of perineal pads saturated and the interval of time involved. Check for possible internal bleeding, as well, by palpating her abdomen and by measuring her abdominal girth for a baseline value; then take repeated measurements. Continue to check intake and output, to monitor her fluid status. If she hasn't been catheterized and she's unable to void within 8 to 10 hours after surgery, you'll have to catheterize her. Before you do this, however, try encouraging her to void.

Check her hemoglobin and hematocrit levels frequently to assess the amount of blood she's lost and her need for fluid replacement. Her hematocrit level will drop if she's hemorrhaging internally, so report a lowered hematocrit level to the doctor *immediately*.

Take a careful history, including a menstrual and an obstetric history. Ask if she uses any form of birth control and, if so, what form. Find out how many times she's been pregnant before and the outcome of those pregnancies. (See *Identifying High-Risk Pregnancies,* page 506.) Of course, you'll also want to ask her about any chronic diseases and about any food or drug allergies.

### Therapeutic care

Continue to check your patient's hemoglobin and hematocrit levels, to detect internal hemorrhage. She may develop anemia if she's had slow blood loss, so expect to administer an oral iron supplement, as ordered. Apply antiembolism stockings, such as TEDS, to reduce her risk of thrombophlebitis from venous stasis. If possible, encourage early ambulation, because this also reduces the risk of thrombophlebitis and helps prevent pulmonary complications. Check her legs periodically for reddened or tender calves and for a positive Homans' sign; notify the doctor *immediately* if you see any of these signs. He may ask you to give an anticoagulant, such as heparin.

---

## UNDERSTANDING CULDOCENTESIS

If your patient has a positive pregnancy test and severe abdominal pain, she may have an ectopic pregnancy. The best way to confirm this is by culdocentesis—a simple diagnostic procedure. If her culdocentesis shows bleeding into the cul-de-sac of Douglas, expect to prepare her for an *immediate* exploratory laparotomy.

Assist the doctor and give your patient emotional support during this short (but painful) procedure. Help her relax by explaining what's being done and why. Then place her in the lithotomy position,

drape her, and assemble the equipment. The doctor will insert a sterile speculum and forceps into the vagina to visualize the cul-de-sac of Douglas. Then he'll prepare her vagina with povidone-iodine and insert an 18G spinal needle through the vaginal wall behind the cervix and into the cul-de-sac. If the syringe fills with nonclotted blood, the test is positive for a ruptured ectopic pregnancy. If it fills with clotted blood or straw-colored fluid, or fails to withdraw any fluid, the patient will need a laparoscopy before laparotomy.

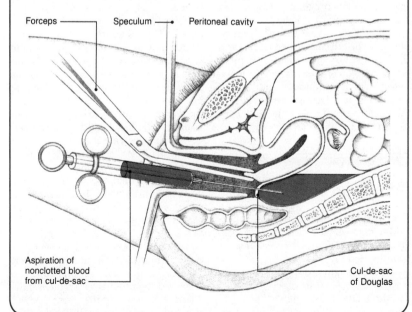

Forceps — Speculum —• Peritoneal cavity —

Aspiration of nonclotted blood from cul-de-sac —

Cul-de-sac of Douglas

Check your patient's incision for signs of infection; also check for a malodorous vaginal discharge. If appropriate, obtain a wound culture and administer antibiotics, as ordered. Expect to administer RhoGam (Rh$_o$ [D] immune globulin) if your patient is Rh negative and had a negative indirect Coombs' test (see *Highlighting RhoGam*, page 520).

Continue I.V. fluids until your patient's bowel sounds return; then expect to start her on oral fluids and food. Encourage adequate diet and fluid intake, and give her analgesics, as ordered, to keep her comfortable.

Your patient's likely to be physically stable soon after she returns from surgery, but she may experience a profound postoperative depression. She'll not only grieve for the fetus she has lost, but she'll also be frightened about the possible effects of the ectopic pregnancy and the surgery on her ability to become pregnant and to deliver a healthy child in the future. As you know, surgeons make every effort to leave a normal tube, ovary, and uterus when they're repairing the rupture from an ectopic pregnancy. (Make sure the doctor explains to the patient exactly what was done during surgery, and that he discusses her chances of having a subsequent successful pregnancy.) Listen supportively if your patient wants to talk, and encourage her to express her feelings—especially if the doctor *wasn't* able to leave her reproductive organs intact.

---

# Acute Placenta Previa

## Prediagnosis summary
Initial assessment of the patient with an acute placenta previa revealed some combination of:
- painless, bright red vaginal bleeding
- third-trimester pregnancy
- audible fetal heart tones
- maternal hypotension and fetal bra-

dycardia or tachycardia
- a soft, nontender, noncontracting uterus
- possibly an abnormal (oblique or transverse) fetal presentation.

An I.V. and supplemental oxygen were started, and blood was drawn for CBC, electrolyte, and blood glucose levels, clotting profile, and typing and cross matching.

## Priorities
If your patient's hemorrhage is severe and fetal age is more than 37 weeks, your patient will be transferred to surgery, where the doctor will perform a vaginal examination using a "double setup": the operating room will be prepared so that either a vaginal delivery *or* a cesarean section can be performed. The doctor will examine the position of the placenta and, if it doesn't cover the cervical os, he may rupture the patient's membranes and induce labor. If the placenta *does* cover the os, the doctor will perform a cesarean section to deliver the fetus. Prior to surgery, insert an I.V. line and an indwelling (Foley) catheter, and prepare the patient as ordered.

If your patient's bleeding isn't severe and fetal age is less than 37 weeks, the doctor may ask you to give the patient supplemental oxygen and I.V. fluids and to place her on bed rest so the fetus has more time to mature. (If the bleeding becomes severe and can't be stopped, the doctor will perform a cesarean section, and the baby will be maintained in the intensive-care nursery.) Monitor fetal heart tones (see *Monitoring Fetal Heart Rate*, pages 512 and 513). If the fetus isn't in distress, the doctor may ask you to administer betamethasone, which may improve the fetus' chance of survival (see *Highlighting Betamethasone*, page 528). After you give betamethasone, monitor fetal heart tones every 5 minutes. At the first sign of fetal distress, notify the doctor *immediately*.

Record the number of perineal pads the patient uses and the time required to saturate them, and roll your patient

PATHOPHYSIOLOGY

## WHAT HAPPENS IN PLACENTA PREVIA

Placenta previa's the most common cause of bleeding during the last months of pregnancy. It happens when the placenta develops in the lowest part of the uterus, on or near the cervical opening. As the illustrations show, placenta previa can vary in severity from total to partial to low placental implantation.

Placenta previa's exact cause isn't known, but certain factors may increase a pregnant patient's risk:
• age 35 or older
• high parity
• a scar on the lower uterus, such as from a previous cesarean section
• a history of placenta previa
• an enlarged placenta due to fetal erythroblastosis or multiple gestation.

These factors may contribute to defective vascularization of the decidua basalis in the fundus. This forces the placenta to spread over a wider area in the lower uterine segment to provide an adequate fetal blood supply, so that it approaches or covers the cervical os.

In the last weeks of pregnancy, when the lower uterus contracts and the cervix dilates, placenta previa causes the placental villi to tear away from the uterine wall, exposing the uterine sinuses. Depending on the number of sinuses exposed, bleeding will be profuse, scanty, or nonexistent until labor begins.

If placenta previa isn't detected in time, and if the child isn't delivered by cesarean section (or by vaginal delivery if the placenta doesn't completely obstruct the birth canal), severe maternal bleeding and shock may occur, together with fetal hypoxia and death.

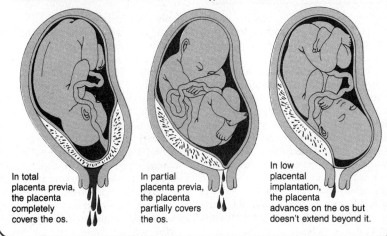

In total placenta previa, the placenta completely covers the os.

In partial placenta previa, the placenta partially covers the os.

In low placental implantation, the placenta advances on the os but doesn't extend beyond it.

over occasionally to check whether blood has pooled under her. (If it has, try to estimate its contribution to her blood loss.)

Monitor your patient's vital signs closely, watching for any indicator of internal hemorrhage or impending shock, such as:
• diaphoresis and pallor
• increasing pulse rate
• decreasing blood pressure
• restlessness and thirst

• rising fundal height (see *Measuring Fundal Height,* page 533).

If she develops any of these signs or symptoms, call the doctor *immediately.* At the first sign of fetal or maternal distress, the doctor will transfer her for an emergency cesarean section.

## Continuing assessment and intervention

If your patient is *on bed rest* and is being monitored in an attempt to allow

DRUGS

## HIGHLIGHTING BETAMETHASONE

Normally, the adrenal cortex secretes glucocorticoids that promote fetal lung maturation and surfactant synthesis. But when your pregnant patient has premature labor or a pregnancy that must be terminated before term, betamethasone (a synthetic steroidlike hormone) can provide the lung maturity stimulation her fetus needs to avoid respiratory distress syndrome.

To get the best results with betamethasone, your patient must be 28 to 32 weeks pregnant and be able to continue the pregnancy *safely* for another 24 to 48 hours. You'll probably give her betamethasone (Celestone Soluspan) 2 ml (12 mg) I.M. once daily for 1 or 2 days before delivery or cesarean section—or as ordered.

If your patient's had a *cesarean section* or a *vaginal delivery*, direct your care toward preventing postpartum complications. Monitor her vital signs and inspect her perineal pads every 15 minutes. Check her dressing, too, if she's had a cesarean section. Check the position and firmness of her uterus by palpating gently for the fundus. If it's boggy, massage it gently until it contracts. Call the doctor if it remains soft—he may have to order I.V. oxytocin or oral ergonovine to contract the uterus and to control bleeding (see *Highlighting Oxytocin,* page 541). Infuse I.V. fluids as ordered, and maintain intake and output records.

Take your patient's medical and obstetric history and find out what events preceded the emergency. Also ask about any chronic diseases that might slow your patient's recovery.

the fetus to mature further, the doctor will probably do additional testing to determine the position of the placental implant. The doctor will commonly perform sonography or a radioisotope scan. These tests will show the position of the vascular areas of the placenta, including the implantation site. Explain these procedures to your patient.

As soon as possible, do a thorough assessment for baseline information you can use to assess any changes in your patient's condition.

Continue to monitor the patient's vital signs and perineal pads for indication of severe bleeding; check fetal movement and heart rate for signs of distress. Measure the height of the uterine fundus (see *Measuring Fundal Height,* page 533). Check her uterus frequently for the onset of any contractions. Notify the doctor *immediately* if contractions begin, if the bleeding increases, or if the fetus shows signs of distress. If your patient begins to have contractions, the doctor may order ritodrine (a drug that inhibits smooth muscle contractility) to try to stop them. Monitor the duration, interval, and intensity of any contractions.

## Therapeutic care

If your patient is on *bed rest,* continue to monitor her vital signs, amount of vaginal bleeding, and fetal heart tones frequently. If she stops bleeding, the doctor may discharge her with instructions to remain on bed rest and to return to the hospital if bleeding occurs.

If your patient had a *cesarean section* or *vaginal delivery,* continue to monitor her vital signs frequently until stable. Monitor her hemoglobin and hematocrit levels to detect anemia related to blood loss. Give oral iron supplements, if ordered. Continue oxytocin or oral ergonovine, as ordered, to stimulate uterine contractions. Notify the doctor if bleeding increases: increased bleeding may indicate retained placenta or abnormal involution of the placental site, and a D&C may be necessary.

Give your patient who's had a cesarean section pain medications, as needed, and prophylactic antibiotics, if ordered.

Encourage progressive ambulation within 24 hours to help prevent pulmonary complications and thrombophlebitis and to enhance return of bowel function. Auscultate her bowel sounds frequently—they may be absent for 24 to 36 hours after surgery. When her bowel sounds return, expect to discontinue your patient's I.V. and to start her on oral food and fluids. If ordered, apply antiembolism stockings, such as TEDS, to help prevent thrombophlebitis. Have her cough and deep-breathe every 2 hours for 24 hours to help prevent pulmonary complications.

Expect your patient to need emotional support and reassurance even if her baby survived, because emergency treatment for placenta previa can be a terrifying and depressing ordeal for a mother anticipating a normal delivery. If she went through Lamaze classes in anticipation of a vaginal delivery, she may feel depressed about the cesarean delivery. Clearly, if her baby suffered central nervous system damage or died, she needs even more support from you.

---

# Abruptio Placentae

### Prediagnosis summary
The patient with abruptio placentae is in the third trimester of pregnancy and may have had a history of chronic hypertension or preeclampsia. Signs and symptoms during initial assessment depended on the severity of her condition.

If she had *moderate abruptio,* assessment findings may include:
• moderate (100 to 500 ml), dark red vaginal bleeding
• moderate abdominal pain
• uterine contractions, with failure of the uterus to relax completely between contractions
• an irritable uterus that's tender on palpation
• signs and symptoms of mild hypovolemic shock
• fetal bradycardia or tachycardia
• increased uterine size.

If she had *severe abruptio,* assessment findings may include:
• profuse (more than 500 ml), dark red

vaginal bleeding
• sudden onset of severe, sharp, unremitting abdominal pain
• backache
• nausea or vomiting
• a rigid (boardlike), irritable uterus that's very tender on palpation
• signs and symptoms of moderate to profound hypovolemic shock
• possible cessation of fetal movement
• absent or faint bradycardic or tachycardic fetal heart tones
• increased uterine size.

A large-bore I.V. was inserted, and Ringer's lactate was infused to replace fluids. Blood was drawn for CBC, electrolytes, blood glucose, clotting profile, fibrinogen levels, fibrin-split products, Rh factor, and typing and cross matching. Oxygen was started to increase fetal oxygenation. The doctor performed ultrasonography to locate the placenta, to rule out placenta previa, and to visualize the degree of placental separation and the presence of clots.

### Priorities
Your priorities are to prevent maternal complications, such as shock and disseminated intravascular coagulation (DIC), while your patient's being prepared for an emergency cesarean section or induced vaginal delivery. The doctor will attempt delivery within 6 hours after the onset of your patient's signs and symptoms, because coagulation defects are time-related and prompt delivery reduces maternal risk.

Quickly assess the mother's vital signs. If her bleeding is profuse, the doctor may insert a central venous pressure (CVP) line so you can monitor her fluid status quickly and accurately. If you find typical signs of shock— thready pulse; decreased blood pressure; cold, clammy skin; tachycardia— call the doctor *immediately* and increase the fluid infusion rate or begin transfusing blood as ordered (see the "Hypovolemic Shock" entry in Chapter 14). If your patient isn't in shock, assess her vital signs every 15 minutes for impending shock.

PATHOPHYSIOLOGY

# WHAT HAPPENS IN ABRUPTIO PLACENTAE

Abruptio placentae—premature separation of the placenta from the uterine wall—typically occurs sometime after 20 weeks' gestation. It can range in severity from mild partial abruptio (less than 30% placental separation) to severe abruptio (more than 50% placental separation). Abruptio placentae may be so slight that it's diagnosed only after delivery—or it can be so extensive that it causes fetal death and severe maternal complications.

Unlike placenta previa, the risk of abruptio placentae doesn't increase with age. But other factors can increase a woman's risk:
• maternal hypertension
• high parity
• previous abruptio placentae
• abdominal trauma
• amniocentesis
• sudden uterine decompression, such as occurs in membrane rupture due to hydramnios (excessive amniotic fluid).

Abruptio placentae begins when small arteries in the uterine wall degenerate, rupture, and hemorrhage into the decidua basalis, forming clots. If this causes a severe decrease in the blood flow to the placenta, its affected part pulls away from the decidua and dies. Distended by pregnancy, the uterus can't contract and compress the torn vessels effectively, so the hemorrhage continues. Blood accumulates in the uterus and beneath the placenta, causing the uterus to become firm, even more distended, and very tender.

In severe abruptio, the placenta traps the hemorrhage behind it; the hemorrhage has no place to escape, so the blood invades the myometrial tissue. This turns the uterine muscle blue (Couvelaire uterus) and irritates the uterus, causing weak contractions. Even after delivery, the presence of blood in the myometrial tissue may make the uterus contract poorly, so bleeding may continue unless the doctor performs a hysterectomy. The severe bleeding, retroperitoneal clotting, and significant uterine wall damage can also result in disseminated intravascular coagulation, shock, and maternal and fetal death.

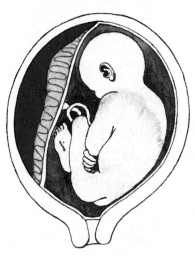

**SEVERE ABRUPTIO PLACENTAE**

Assess the mother's blood loss by determining how fast she's saturating perineal pads—weigh them, if possible. Have blood ready in case she needs a transfusion. Don't forget to assess the height of her fundus: A rising fundus indicates a concealed hemorrhage that may be rapidly fatal (see *Measuring Fundal Height,* page 533). Watch for external bleeding from her gums, nose, and I.V. sites, too, especially if your patient has severe abruptio. Such bleeding indicates DIC—a rare condition that's fatal unless treated *immediately.*

Call the doctor if you note these signs (see the "Disseminated Intravascular Coagulation" entry in Chapter 11).

You have priorities related to the fetus, too. Assess the fetus for baseline data, then monitor the fetal heart rate with an external monitor. Notify the doctor of any changes or signs of fetal distress (see *Monitoring Fetal Heart Rate,* pages 512 and 513). Check fetal position and the degree of fetal engagement, too, and assess the timing of any contractions.

Monitor your patient's urine output

closely. If it drops below 30 ml/hour, she may have poor kidney perfusion secondary to depleted intravascular volume, so notify the doctor. If the patient's bleeding moderately or heavily and can't void on her own, get orders to insert an indwelling (Foley) catheter.

Make sure arrangements have been made for infant resuscitation in the delivery or operating room. Prepare your patient for surgery, as ordered, and assemble her laboratory tests and available assessment and history data.

## Continuing assessment and intervention

If the fetus is *alive and in no distress,* the doctor may induce labor and deliver the baby vaginally. If the fetus is *alive but in distress,* he may perform a rapid cesarean section. If the fetus is *dead or very immature,* he may induce labor with oxytocin (Pitocin). (See *Highlighting Oxytocin,* page 541.)

After surgery or delivery, your patient's still not out of danger. If she has severe abruptio, she may develop coagulation defects. And, if her uterus won't contract after delivery, bleeding may continue into the uterine muscle—producing a Couvelaire uterus. Notify the doctor *immediately* if your patient's vital signs show a trend consistent with shock or if her abdominal girth increases. He may take the patient back to the operating room for a hysterectomy, which also reduces the chance that she will develop DIC (because the damaged uterus is removed).

Once your patient's condition is stable, perform a thorough assessment while you continue monitoring her vital signs and measuring any blood loss. Gently palpate her abdomen, noting any uterine rigidity, irritability, or tenderness. If she's had a *vaginal delivery,* check her uterus to make sure it's not boggy and soft; if it is, massage it gently until it contracts. If it stays soft, notify the doctor and prepare to administer a drug such as oxytocin. If she's had a *cesarean section,* inspect her dressing and perineal pads frequently. Check the position and firmness of her uterus by palpating gently for the fundus. Massage her uterus if it's soft. She may need I.V. oxytocin or oral ergonovine to contract the uterus and to control bleeding.

Maintain your patient's I.V. infusion, as ordered, and an accurate intake and output record. Check her hematocrit and hemoglobin levels after surgery or delivery, to detect anemia. Check her clotting times hourly (or as ordered). If a stable clot forms in 6 minutes or less, your patient's fibrinogen level is adequate. But if blood fails to clot within 15 to 20 minutes, her fibrinogen level is critically low and you must notify the doctor *immediately.* He may ask you to administer fibrinogen replacement along with analgesics and antibiotics.

## Therapeutic care

If your patient had a *cesarean section* or an *emergency hysterectomy,* provide postoperative care by:
• checking her incision site frequently for signs of bleeding or infection
• turning her frequently
• encouraging her to cough and deep-breathe every 2 hours
• encouraging early ambulation
• auscultating her bowel sounds to note when they return. (At that time, you'll probably discontinue her I.V. infusion and start her on oral food and fluids.)

If she had a *vaginal delivery,* provide perineal care by washing her and applying fresh pads as needed. Check her episiotomy site frequently to make sure the incision's healing properly.

Don't forget to provide emotional support, as well. If the baby survives but needs intensive care, your patient may feel bewildered and frightened because she can't have her baby with her. Explain what's being done for her baby and why. If her baby didn't survive, or if she needed an emergency hysterectomy, she'll need even more intensive emotional support. Give her the chance to express her feelings, and offer to call the chaplain and others who can support her.

# Preeclampsia/ Eclampsia

## Prediagnosis summary

Initial assessment findings for the patient with *preeclampsia* included some combination of the following:
- rapid weight gain
- edema of the face, fingers, and abdomen, especially in the morning
- hypertension
- proteinuria.

If she had *severe preeclampsia*, she had these additional signs and symptoms:
- blood pressure above 160/110 mm Hg at rest
- weight gain greater than 3 lb (1.4 kg) per week during the third trimester
- edema after 12 hours of bed rest
- a history of proteinuria of 5 g/24 hours or 3 + to 4 + on a single qualitative evaluation
- oliguria or a history of less than 500 ml of urine output per 24 hours
- severe headache
- blurred or double vision
- epigastric pain
- nausea and vomiting
- irritability and emotional tension
- possible pulmonary edema
- hyperreflexia
- possible cyanosis.

If she had *eclampsia*, she had all the signs and symptoms of severe preeclampsia plus tonic and clonic seizures and one or more of the following:
- postseizure coma
- rapid postseizure respirations with possible cyanosis
- oliguria that may progress to anuria.

An I.V. was started for fluid and medication administration. Supplemental oxygen was given, and cardiac monitoring was initiated. Blood was drawn for CBC, electrolytes, blood glucose, platelet count, uric acid, BUN, creatinine, liver enzymes, fibrinogen, fibrin-split products, clotting profile, magnesium levels, and typing and cross matching. A urine sample was obtained via catheter and tested for protein.

## Priorities

You have three priorities with this patient:
- to prevent seizures from developing or to control them if present
- to reduce maternal blood pressure
- to prolong the pregnancy as long as you can safely do so.

To prevent or control seizures, the doctor will ask you to give your patient magnesium sulfate or diazepam (see *Highlighting Magnesium Sulfate*, page 536). Both drugs decrease hyperreflexia, relieve cerebral vasospasm, decrease blood pressure, and increase urine output. Keep her on complete bed rest and decrease stimuli—bright lights, noises, drafts. As a precaution, raise the bed's padded side rails, and keep the following emergency and seizure equipment nearby:
- an oral airway
- oxygen
- intubation and respiratory equipment
- suction equipment
- diazepam (Valium)
- magnesium sulfate (and its antidote calcium gluconate) plus other emergency medications
- I.V. equipment.

Complete bed rest will reduce your patient's blood pressure and cardiac work load, enhancing the effect of the magnesium sulfate or diazepam. If your patient's diastolic pressure stays above 110 mm Hg, the doctor may order an antihypertensive such as hydralazine.

Monitor her blood pressure, and remember that *changes* in blood pressure, indicating a trend, are more significant than individual readings. Monitor her intake and output, and obtain a urine sample for an albumin test and for a complete urinalysis to rule out other causes of proteinuria (for example, infection).

Reducing your patient's blood pressure and keeping her calm and quiet will help you meet your third priority—to stabilize the fetus. Check fetal heart tones, using an external monitor (see *Monitoring Fetal Heart Rate,* pages 512 and 513). At the first sign of fetal distress *notify the doctor* and prepare to send the patient for an emergency cesarean section.

## Continuing assessment and intervention

After you've intervened to reduce the patient's blood pressure and to prevent seizures (and if she didn't need a cesarean section), do a thorough assessment.

Begin with an assessment of fetal status. Palpate the patient's abdomen gently to determine the position of the

### YOUR ROLE IN AN EMERGENCY

### MEASURING FUNDAL HEIGHT

You usually measure a pregnant woman's fundal height to estimate the number of weeks of gestation. The fundus reaches the umbilicus at around 20 weeks' gestation, and from then on the number of centimeters of fundal height roughly equals the number of weeks of gestation.

Here's another way to use fundal height: as an aid in assessing OB/GYN emergencies—for example, to detect severe uterine bleeding in a woman who's at least 13 weeks pregnant. If the patient isn't having contractions, a rapid increase in fundal height can alert you to a developing emergency—internal hemorrhage, abruptio placentae, or trauma, for example. Because you can see this early warning signal before a change in the mother's vital signs occurs, you may be able to prevent these life-threatening complications.

### Equipment
• Flexible (not stretch) metric tape measure
• Ballpoint pen.

### Before the procedure
• Have your patient empty her bladder.
• Help her lie on her back. If her condition permits, elevate her head and knees to relax her abdominal muscles.

### During the procedure
• Place your hands along her sides and move them toward her head, gently pressing on the abdomen until you've located the fundus.
• Draw a line with a ballpoint pen, marking the top of the fundus.
• Measure the distance from the top of the symphysis pubis to the top of the fundus. This is the fundal height.

### Nursing considerations
• Measure and record the fundal height every 15 minutes.
• Notify the doctor *immediately* if fundal height increases while the patient's abdomen is relaxed.

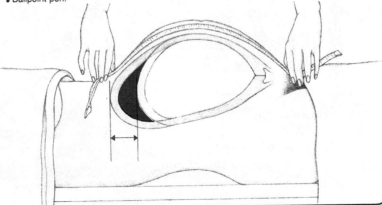

# WHAT HAPPENS IN PREECLAMPSIA AND ECLAMPSIA

Preeclampsia's a syndrome that can occur anytime after 20 weeks' gestation. Signs of preeclampsia include hypertension, weight gain, edema, and proteinuria. Eclampsia is preeclampsia plus convulsions, which may be followed by coma, hypertensive crisis, or shock. Eclampsia's

most common in first pregnancies of women predisposed to preeclampsia by multiple gestation, a hydatidiform mole, diabetes mellitus, renal disease, hypertension, hydramnios, a family history of preeclampsia, or poor nutrition.

Preeclampsia's exact pathophysiologic

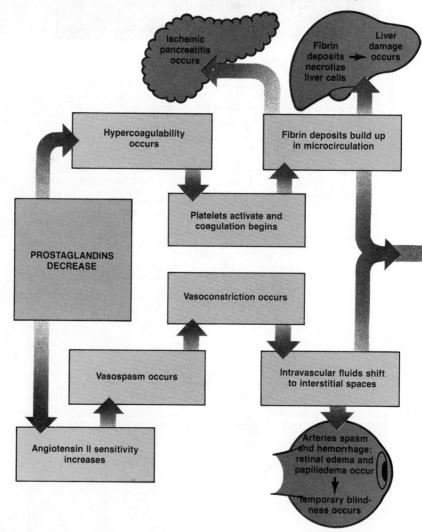

mechanism isn't known. Theories cite:
- inadequate sodium or protein intake
- uterine ischemia due to circulatory impairment from uterine distention
- a prostaglandin deficiency (the current theory).

This chart explains the prostaglandin deficiency theory. Normally, a pregnant woman is resistant to angiotensin II's pressor effects during her pregnancy. (Why? Because adequate levels of prostaglandins maintain resistance to angiotensin II.) A *prostaglandin deficiency* will lead to increased sensitivity and these changes:
- vasospasm, vasoconstriction, and increased peripheral vascular resistance, with intravascular fluid shifts to the interstitium
- hypercoagulability with fibrin deposits.

Without intervention (immediate delivery or cesarean section), this combination can be fatal.

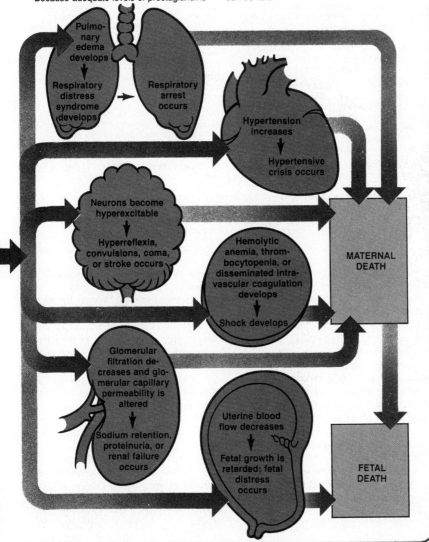

Pulmonary edema develops → Respiratory distress syndrome develops → Respiratory arrest occurs

Hypertension increases → Hypertensive crisis occurs

Neurons become hyperexcitable → Hyperreflexia, convulsions, coma, or stroke occurs

Hemolytic anemia, thrombocytopenia, or disseminated intravascular coagulation develops → Shock develops

Glomerular filtration decreases and glomerular capillary permeability is altered → Sodium retention, proteinuria, or renal failure occurs

Uterine blood flow decreases → Fetal growth is retarded; fetal distress occurs

MATERNAL DEATH

FETAL DEATH

## HIGHLIGHTING MAGNESIUM SULFATE

To prevent seizures in your preeclamptic patient, the doctor may order magnesium sulfate—an effective sedative, anticonvulsant, and antihypertensive. You'll prepare and administer the dose as an I.M. injection with lidocaine or as a continuous I.V. infusion, as ordered. But you'll have to be extra alert to make sure your patient gets the drug's benefits without potentially life-threatening side effects: central nervous system depression, respiratory paralysis, and circulatory collapse. Here are guidelines for safely administering magnesium sulfate to your patient:

• Monitor her vital signs before and after each I.M. dose (every 15 minutes with I.V. administration). Notify the doctor and withhold magnesium sulfate if the patient's respirations are below 12/minute, if she has decreased blood pressure or pulse, or if you note any signs of fetal distress.

• Check her knee jerk and patellar reflexes before each I.M. dose (hourly if you're infusing the drug). Loss of these reflexes may be the first sign of toxicity, so withhold the next dose (or stop the infusion) and notify the doctor if these reflexes are absent.

• Pay close attention to your patient's physical complaints, assessing which ones may be related to her preeclampsia and which to the drug therapy. Some early signs and symptoms of magnesium toxicity are a hot, flushed feeling, thirst, diaphoresis, hypotension, and muscular flaccidity. Later signs and symptoms result from central nervous system, renal, respiratory, and cardiac depression.

• Insert an indwelling (Foley) catheter, if needed, and monitor the patient's intake, output, and urine specific gravity. If your patient voids less than 30 ml/hour, withhold the next drug dose (or stop the infusion) and notify the doctor.

• Keep calcium gluconate, magnesium sulfate's antidote, at your patient's bedside. If she develops respiratory or cardiac depression, give her 20 ml of 10% calcium gluconate over a 3-minute period per the doctor's standing order. Notify the doctor *immediately,* and resuscitate the patient as needed. Give calcium gluconate every hour as ordered (not exceeding eight doses in 24 hours) until you've relieved her cardiac, respiratory, renal, and/or neurologic depression.

fetus. Time the duration and frequency of any uterine contractions. If your patient's developed eclampsia, reassess fetal status after every seizure. Arrange for continuous external fetal monitoring (see *Monitoring Fetal Heart Rate,* pages 512 and 513).

Check your patient's fluid status frequently. Insert an indwelling (Foley) catheter to get an accurate assessment of urine output, and assess her face, hands, and abdomen for edema. Auscultate her lungs, checking for rales, wheezes, and other signs of pulmonary edema.

As you assess your patient, check for signs and symptoms that may herald a progression from preeclampsia to eclampsia:
• severe and continuous headache
• dim or blurred vision.

If your patient has a seizure, record a description of the circumstances of its onset, precipitating factors, the type of seizure, its duration, and its aftermath. If the patient remains *unconscious* after the seizure, record the depth and duration of the postseizure coma; if she's *conscious,* describe her level of consciousness. Call the doctor for orders for repeated doses of anticonvulsant medication, and be alert for further seizures. Always keep an airway at your patient's bedside, and keep the side rails up and padded.

Watch for bleeding from the patient's gums, nose, or I.V. sites, because the generalized vasospasm that accompanies preeclampsia and eclampsia may precipitate DIC (see the "Disseminated Intravascular Coagulation" entry in Chapter 11). *Immediately* report any unusual bleeding to the doctor.

Get a thorough history, paying particular attention to information that will affect the care your patient needs: a history of hypertension, of previous pregnancies, and of the current pregnancy—including the EDC, last fetal movement, and such problems as abdominal pain and bleeding.

### Therapeutic care

Check your patient's blood pressure at least every 4 hours, and screen her urine daily for protein. Monitor creatinine clearance to evaluate her kidney function, and evaluate her urinary or blood estriol level to determine fetal well-being. Expect to continue giving her magnesium sulfate and, possibly, antihypertensive medication. Don't forget to support her emotionally.

If your patient has (or develops) eclampsia, the doctor will induce labor or perform a cesarean section within 6 to 12 hours after she's stabilized.

After delivery, remember that the danger of convulsions from eclampsia doesn't pass for 48 hours. Maintain seizure precautions, and be alert for signs that a seizure's developing. Obtain an order for a sedative, too, and keep your patient calm and quiet. Monitor her blood pressure carefully, and continue checking the protein level in her urine. The protein—and her edema—should disappear within 5 days after delivery.

Give your patient analgesics and antibiotics as ordered, assess her surgical incision if she had a cesarean section, and continue monitoring her vital signs. She'll stay in the hospital several days longer than most new mothers.

---

# Uterine Rupture

### Prediagnosis summary

The patient with *complete uterine rupture* experienced sudden, intense, and sharp tearing or lacerating pain in her lower abdomen, followed by dissipat-
ing pain. Most likely, this occurred during labor, particularly if:
- labor was prolonged, obstructed, or traumatic
- the fetus was excessively large
- oxytocin (Pitocin) was injudiciously used to stimulate labor.

However, your patient's uterus may also have ruptured during late pregnancy. She probably had a history of a previous cesarean section or of multiple previous pregnancies that weakened the uterine wall. Or she may have had previous surgery involving the myometrium.

On initial assessment, she had a combination of these signs and symptoms:
- vaginal bleeding
- fetal bradycardia or absent fetal heart tones
- absence of fetal movement or of uterine contractions
- a palpable fetus in the abdominal cavity; a palpable uterus (a hard mass) next to the fetus
- signs and symptoms of shock.

If her rupture was *impending* or *incomplete,* she showed some of these signs and symptoms:
- severe abdominal pain with restlessness and anxiety
- a ridge or ballooning-out of the uterus around the symphysis pubis
- an indentation across her lower abdominal wall, dividing the upper and lower uterine segments, with acute tenderness around the symphysis pubis
- tetanic contractions lasting more than 90 seconds
- nausea and vomiting
- fetal bradycardia or tachycardia.

One or more I.V.s were started with large-bore catheters, and blood was drawn for CBC, electrolytes, blood glucose, and typing and cross matching. Oxygen was given by mask or nasal cannula, and the patient was positioned on her left side to increase blood flow to the fetus. Food and fluid by mouth were restricted, an indwelling (Foley) catheter was inserted, and a urine specimen was sent for testing.

## PREVENTING UTERINE RUPTURE

Anytime you note that your patient's contractions are extremely strong and prolonged, with little or no relaxation between them, your patient may be in danger of uterine rupture—a condition that's potentially fatal to both mother and child.

To assess for excessively hard contractions quickly, just feel your patient's abdomen. With a Braxton Hicks contraction (the mild, intermittent contractions that normally occur during the course of pregnancy), the abdomen feels as spongy as the end of your nose; with a medium-hard contraction, the abdomen feels about as hard as your chin; and with a full contraction, the abdomen feels as hard as your forehead.

Be sure to alert the doctor immediately and prepare the patient for cesarean section if your patient's having unrelenting hard contractions.

### Priorities

Immediate surgery is the only hope for your patient and her fetus—your patient will die without treatment, and even with treatment, fetal mortality is 50% to 75%. While the operating room is being prepared, your first priority for your patient is to institute aggressive fluid replacement with I.V. fluids, to prevent irreversible shock. Start replacement with Ringer's lactate, as ordered, and be prepared to administer plasma, plasma expanders, and blood. The doctor may insert a CVP line to infuse fluids rapidly and to allow you to monitor your patient's fluid status accurately. Continue giving oxygen by mask or nasal cannula to improve fetal and maternal oxygenation. Prepare the patient for a laparotomy, get a quick history (including allergies and current medications), give preoperative medication as ordered, and assist with her transfer to surgery. If the patient's rupture is *complete,* the doctor will open her abdomen and remove the uterus and the fetus (some doctors will repair a smooth uterine tear, and leave the uterus intact, if bleeding is controllable). If the rupture's *impending,* he'll perform a cesarean section.

### Continuing assessment and intervention

Following surgery, monitor your patient's vital signs every 5 to 15 minutes until she's stable. Continue fluid replacement as ordered—she'll typically need blood. Monitor her CVP values, which should be in the range of 6 to 12 cm $H_2O$. If they're higher or lower, report your findings to the doctor and expect to adjust the fluid or blood infusion rate. Keep an accurate record of her fluid intake and output, and record the number of perineal pads the patient saturates and the intervals of time involved. Report any increase of bleeding, passage of large clots, or purulent discharge. To detect anemia related to blood loss, assess your patient's serial hematocrit and hemoglobin levels.

Check her abdomen and surgical incision for swelling and tenderness. Note the number of dressing changes. Give an analgesic such as Demerol (meperidine), as ordered, for pain.

Also assess your patient for pulmonary complications. Auscultate her lungs for rales, wheezes, or other signs of congestion. Tender or red calves may indicate thrombophlebitis.

Watch for signs of infection, such as increased temperature or pulse rate and decreased blood pressure. If you note any of these, notify the doctor and give antibiotics as ordered.

When your patient's condition is stable, take a medical and obstetric history to help determine the cause of her uterine rupture and to identify any chronic diseases or allergies.

### Therapeutic care

Using the patient's baseline values to guide you, continue to assess her condition frequently and carefully, watching for increased bleeding, infection at the incision site, and pulmonary complications. Auscultate for bowel sounds, too; these may be absent for 24 to 36 hours after surgery. When they return, expect to start your patient on oral food and fluids and to decrease her I.V. fluids. Help her reestablish optimum bowel function by encouraging early ambulation, adequate diet, and adequate fluid intake. (Early ambulation will also help prevent thrombophlebitis and pulmonary emboli.) Continue to give your patient analgesics (if necessary), as ordered.

One of your most important interventions for this patient is providing information and emotional support to start her working through her postoperative depression. If her baby died during or after the rupture, she'll have to work through her grief over the loss. Even if her baby survived, your patient will still have to adjust to the effects of the uterine rupture and surgery; if the doctor performed a hysterectomy, for example, she won't be able to bear another child. Even if he was able to repair the torn uterus or to perform a cesarean section, the doctor may advise her not to become pregnant again because of the danger of repeated rupture.

Encourage your patient to talk about her feelings, and listen supportively. Arrange for additional counseling, if indicated.

---

# Postpartum Hemorrhage

## Prediagnosis summary
On initial assessment, this patient's signs and symptoms included:
- excessive bleeding after delivery, probably a continuous trickle.
- possibly a large, soft, boggy uterus
- pallor and restlessness
- chills
- dyspnea and air hunger
- diaphoresis
- decreased blood pressure
- thready pulse.

An I.V. was started for fluid and blood replacement, and supplemental oxygen was given. Blood was drawn for CBC, electrolytes, clotting profile, glucose, and typing and cross matching.

## Priorities
Your most important priority for this patient is to begin uterine massage *immediately* (see *Massaging the Postpartum Uterus*, page 540). While you massage her uterus, have someone call the doctor to examine the patient and to decide if the hemorrhage is due to *uterine atony*, to *lacerations*, or to *retained placental fragments*.

Begin fluid replacement, as ordered, and watch for such early signs and symptoms of shock as increased restlessness, thirst, dizziness or lightheadedness, pallor, and increased diaphoresis. These may precede ominous changes in her blood pressure and pulse, especially if blood is oozing out in a continuous trickle. Notify the doctor of *any* changes in vital signs, even seemingly insignificant ones, *immediately*. If signs and symptoms of shock appear, increase the patient's infusion rate as ordered, start oxygen by mask or nasal cannula, put the head of her bed down, and raise her feet.

Keep track of how much blood your patient's losing—she can lose a large volume within a few hours. Keep an accurate count of the number of perineal pads she saturates in a given period of time. Be sure to check underneath her, as well, for blood that may have pooled there. If you have any reason to think she's losing a life-threatening volume of blood, call the doctor *immediately*.

Check the fundus for texture, position, and tenderness. The uterus should feel hard after you massage it, and the height of the fundus should be about level with the patient's umbilicus. (See *Measuring Fundal Height*, page 533.) If your patient's fundus is high, suspect a full bladder. If she can't urinate and

## MASSAGING THE POSTPARTUM UTERUS

If vaginal bleeding is heavier than it should be for your postpartum patient, stimulate uterine contractions by massaging her uterus. Simply place one hand just above her symphysis pubis, to support the bottom of her uterus, and cup your other hand around the fundus. Use a gentle but firm circular motion to massage the fundus.

The uterus should respond quickly; stop massaging when it becomes apple-shaped and hard as wood. Be careful not to overdo the massage—this encourages muscle fatigue that can cause uterine relaxation and hemorrhage. It's uncomfortable for the patient, too.

Reassess her uterus every 15 minutes for the first hour after it's contracted. If it starts to feel soft and boggy, like a very ripe tomato, begin massaging again.

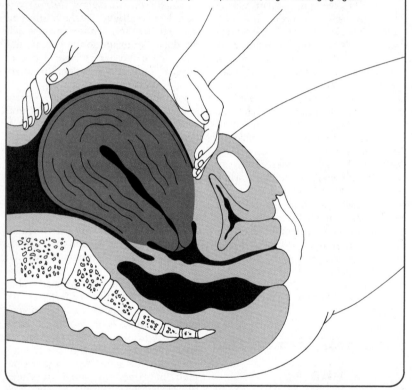

her bladder seems distended, catheterize her as ordered. (Catheterization may return as much as 2,000 to 3,000 ml of urine.) Internal bleeding may be the cause if the fundus remains elevated after catheterization and palpation is painful. Call the doctor *immediately*.

A uterus that continues to feel boggy and soft may indicate that the patient has retained placental fragments that prevent her uterus from contracting firmly. Or, if her uterus assumes the shape of an apple and has a woody hardness, and she still continues to bleed profusely, she probably has a laceration of the cervix, the vagina, or the perineum. In both these situations, surgery is indicated. The doctor will have to take the patient back to the operating room or the delivery room to evacuate her uterus or to repair the laceration. Prepare her for surgery as ordered.

## Continuing assessment and intervention

If your patient's hemorrhage is due to *uterine atony*, massage should be effective in contracting her uterus—so she shouldn't need to return to the operating room. Massage her uterus until it feels hard and woody; every 15 minutes, stop massaging and reassess the fundus and uterus. Be prepared to begin massaging again if the uterus shows the slightest relaxation—evidenced by a soft, boggy feeling or by recurrent bleeding. But be careful not to *over*-massage once the uterus is contracted: this contributes to muscle fatigue, which encourages uterine relaxation—so her uterus may become soft and boggy again. Remember, too, that massage can be painful and tiring to the patient—she may only want to relax and sleep. Explain why you need to perform this procedure, and that you'll do it only as long as necessary.

_____ DRUGS

### HIGHLIGHTING OXYTOCIN

If your patient has an incomplete or inevitable abortion, life-threatening complications of pregnancy, abnormally prolonged labor, or uncontrolled postpartum bleeding, the doctor may order oxytocin (Pitocin), a uterine muscle stimulant.

Oxytocin produces uterine contractions that resemble labor by increasing myofibril cells' permeability to sodium. This enhances the uterine muscle's ability to contract. Unfortunately, this potent drug's effects are unpredictable—it can cause uterine rupture, decreased uteroplacental perfusion, even fetal death. To prevent such adverse effects, follow these guidelines:
• Take your patient's complete obstetric and gynecologic history. She has a higher risk of uterine rupture—and needs close monitoring—if she's older than 34 or has had cervical or uterine surgery, uterine sepsis, a previous traumatic delivery, or multiple births.
• Obtain a history of her current pregnancy, too. If you find any indication that her pelvis isn't adequate for a vaginal delivery, withhold oxytocin until you've talked to the doctor.
• Check the medication sheet for possible drug interactions. Administer oxytocin cautiously if the patient's receiving another cytoxic agent, cyclopropane, or thiopental anesthesia.
• When mixing the solution, make sure you know the concentrations and dosages that are used for different purposes, and select the correct one for your patient.
• When you're giving oxytocin to induce labor, stay with the patient at all times, and make sure a doctor is available for immediate intervention, if necessary.
• Always piggyback oxytocin with a 5% dextrose or 0.9% sodium chloride solution in case you need to stop the medication quickly.
• Increase the I.V. flow rate, as ordered, every 15 to 30 minutes (up to 20 milliunits/minute) until it produces three to four contractions every 10 minutes.
• Decrease the I.V. flow rate, as ordered, once you've established a normal contraction pattern.
• Every 15 minutes, monitor and record fetal heart rate (preferably via internal monitor), maternal vital signs, and the contractions' frequency, intensity, and duration, as well as the duration of the resting period between contractions.
• *Stop the infusion immediately,* open up the main I.V. line, turn the patient on her left side, administer oxygen, and *notify the doctor* if contractions occur less than 2 minutes apart or last more than 90 seconds. Also alert the doctor if your patient develops nausea, vomiting, extreme restlessness, or an hourglass-shaped uterus (signaling imminent uterine rupture), or if you detect signs of fetal hypoxia.
• Monitor maternal intake and output (you may need to insert an indwelling [Foley] catheter). Water intoxication may occur with long-term infusion, because oxytocin has an antidiuretic effect.
• When giving oxytocin to prevent postpartum bleeding, wait until the placenta's delivered to begin the infusion. Otherwise, the uterus will clamp down, and the placenta won't be delivered.

Continue to check your patient's vital signs every 5 to 15 minutes, and report any changes to the doctor. Keep an accurate count of saturated perineal pads, and monitor her urine output. If your patient's unable to void, reports that her bladder feels full, and reports increasing pelvic and perineal pain, notify the doctor. If her bladder's not distended, these signs and symptoms may mean that, although she's no longer bleeding externally, she has a hematoma that's collecting blood.

When her uterus has contracted and her bleeding has stopped, obtain a complete medical and obstetric history from her.

What if her uterus won't contract on its own, and the bleeding continues? Then the doctor will probably order an oxytoxic drug such as oxytocin or ergonovine (see *Highlighting Oxytocin,* page 541); as a last resort, he may perform a hysterectomy.

### Therapeutic care

After your patient's stabilized (or when she returns from surgery), watch her vital signs to be sure that her pulse and blood pressure return to their baseline values after fluid replacement. (This will also indicate that her fluid replacement is adequate.) Check her serial hematocrit and hemoglobin levels, too— these may indicate anemia due to blood loss. Monitor her temperature carefully, and watch for other signs of puerperal infection: anemia increases susceptibility to this complication.

If your patient went to the operating room for *repair of minor lacerations,* assess her vital signs and vaginal bleeding when she returns from surgery. Watch for purulent discharge and other signs of infection, and provide analgesics as necessary. She'll probably be discharged within a day or two after surgery.

If she required *more extensive surgery* (removal of placental fragments, repair of a major cervical laceration, or a hysterectomy), she'll need more extensive care afterward. Assess her

regularly for pallor, diaphoresis, restlessness, and other signs and symptoms of shock. Give prophylactic antibiotics, as ordered, and check the wound site. Watch for purulent wound drainage that indicates a developing infection, and follow your hospital's protocol to obtain a wound culture and CBC at the first sign of infection.

Encourage early ambulation to diminish the risks of thrombophlebitis and pulmonary complications and to help reestablish your patient's bowel function. When her bowel sounds return, discontinue I.V. fluids as ordered, and start her on oral food and fluids. Give analgesics as necessary to keep her comfortable.

# Ruptured Ovarian Cyst

## Prediagnosis summary

The patient with a ruptured ovarian cyst may have had a history of menstrual irregularities and chronic pelvic pain. She reported sudden onset of sharp or dull pain on one side of her abdomen. She also had some of these signs and symptoms:

• abdominal pain with guarding and unilateral tenderness during pelvic examination

• scant to profuse vaginal bleeding

• tachycardia

• diaphoresis

• mild to severe hypotension, depending on her degree of blood loss.

A large-bore I.V. catheter was inserted, and fluid or blood replacement was provided as necessary. Supplemental oxygen was given by mask or nasal cannula. A complete menstrual history was obtained, and she was examined for signs of pregnancy or acute abdominal emergency (because a ruptured ovarian cyst may be easily confused with an ectopic pregnancy or with appendicitis). Blood was drawn for CBC, clotting profile, electrolytes, blood glucose, serum test for HCG, and a 2-minute urine immunologic pregnancy test. Pregnancy tests were negative.

## Priorities

Your immediate priority is to monitor your patient's vital signs and to continue fluid replacement until surgery can be performed. Continue infusing Ringer's lactate, but prepare for transfusions of whole blood, plasma, or plasma components, depending on your patient's hematocrit values. (See *Understanding Colloid and Crystalloid Solutions* in the Appendix.) Insert an indwelling (Foley) catheter, and keep accurate intake and output records. Report *immediately* any change in your patient's vital signs that may indicate she's going into shock.

After you've taken your patient's vital signs, administer pain medication as ordered. If the doctor orders sonography or an emergency laparotomy, prepare her for the procedure. If these diagnostic procedures indicate a ruptured cyst, the doctor will perform surgery to remove or drain it. If necessary, he'll remove the affected ovary, as well.

## Continuing assessment and intervention

Following your patient's surgery, your priorities will be the same as for any postoperative patient: Monitor her vital signs, fluid status, and mental status, reporting any changes that may signal developing complications.

After your patient's stabilized, perform a thorough nursing assessment. Begin by checking for vaginal bleeding and for pulse and blood pressure changes, which may indicate continued bleeding from a cyst. Report any significant findings to the doctor *immediately.*

If your assessment doesn't reveal any complications, take your patient's history, following these guidelines:
- Obtain a description of how her illness began.
- Take a thorough menstrual history to find out whether she's had amenor-

---

### UNDERSTANDING RUPTURED OVARIAN CYSTS

An ovarian cyst is a nonneoplastic sac on an ovary, containing fluid or semisolid material. Cysts can form in many different ways. The most common are:
- *growth of endometrial tissue in the ovary.* This tissue bleeds during the menstrual period and forms a blood- and clot-filled cyst.
- *a mature corpus luteum hemorrhaging into its cavity.* This can create a blood-filled cyst in the ovarian wall.
- *overdistention of the ovarian follicle.* This occurs when a follicle fills with serous fluid.

Although ovarian cysts differ in their development, size, and composition, any of them can grow and spontaneously rupture into the peritoneum. When this happens, the ruptured cyst releases fluids that irritate the peritoneum. Blood vessels in the ovarian capsule tear, causing hemorrhage. If this surgical emergency isn't corrected quickly, the patient may go into shock.

---

rhea, oligomenorrhea, or dysmenorrhea—because these indicate the possibility of polycystic ovarian disease.
- Ask about other gynecologic problems, such as pelvic inflammatory disease, previous episodes of bleeding, or miscarriages, which may indicate the need for further diagnostic studies.

### Therapeutic care

The need for pain control, bed rest, and emotional support is ongoing for the patient with a ruptured ovarian cyst. Watch her for signs of peritonitis (severe, generalized abdominal pain; rebound tenderness; fever), which may develop if the ruptured cyst leaks into and irritates the peritoneum. (See *Danger: Peritonitis*, page 332.)

Help your patient feel comfortable expressing any fears that the cyst is a sign of cancer or that the surgery has affected her fertility. If you know that her fears are groundless, reassure her. Otherwise, be sure her doctor is aware of her fears so that he can discuss them with her.

# Rape

## Prediagnosis summary

Rape—unlawful sexual intercourse without consent—is a legal term, not a medical diagnosis. And rape itself seldom creates a medical emergency. (When a rape-related medical emergency exists, it's typically a stab wound, fracture, laceration, or a combination of these injuries.)

However, rape and its aftermath are a *personal* emergency for the victim, and she's likely to come to the hospital looking for help. She may have an assortment of lacerations, bruises, and fractures. She may have vaginal bleeding and vaginal, abdominal, and rectal pain. She almost certainly will have a severe emotional reaction ranging from feelings of shame and worthlessness to hysteria and terror, with such accompanying physical signs as tachycardia, tachypnea, and diaphoresis.

## Priorities, assessment, and intervention

Your first priority is to give your patient a private room and continuous emotional support during your assessment and emergency interventions. If you can't stay with her, find someone who can. If she's physically unstable from trauma associated with the rape, start an I.V. line and provide oxygen, as ordered. Cover any severely bleeding wounds with pressure dressings, immobilize any fractures, and get X-rays. Then, with your patient's physical stability ensured, begin a thorough assessment and examination, following your state's laws for collecting evidence and your hospital's protocol for caring for a rape victim. Remember, although your patient may not initially want to prosecute her attacker, she may change her mind. Unless you've collected objective evidence of sexual intercourse and a history of force, prosecution will be impossible.

Before you begin your assessment, ask someone to bring you a sterile speculum and a rape collection kit containing such items as capped and labeled laboratory tubes, glass slides, a clean comb, a nail scraper, and paper bags for clothing.

Make your patient feel as safe and comfortable as possible by explaining the examination that you and the doctor will conduct and by assuring her that you'll stay with her. Encourage her to ask questions about anything she doesn't understand. Start by taking a history of the incident, recording the patient's own words whenever possible. She's likely to be ashamed to tell you what has happened and even more ashamed to have you write it down. To ease her embarrassment, ensure complete privacy during this time, and explain that you need the information to plan her care. Offer nonjudgmental emotional support during the history, and let her vent her feelings as she tries to relate the incident.

After you've recorded a history of the incident, collect a sexual history, including what birth control measures, if any, she uses (if she's sexually active), and the date of her last menstrual period. Take a medical history, including any medications she's taking and any allergies or chronic diseases she has. Before the physical examination begins, assist the doctor with obtaining necessary consent, and witness the patient's signature.

Help your patient remove her clothing, and save it to be analyzed for semen and bloodstains. Circle any suspected blood or semen stains on the clothing with a laundry marker, and place each piece of clothing in a paper bag. (Don't use plastic bags: an airtight bag will stimulate bacterial action that may alter the evidence.) Record any bruises, scratches, and other injuries on your patient's body.

Collect scrapings from underneath your patient's fingernails, because these may contain skin or blood specimens that will help identify the attacker. Put specimens in capped laboratory tubes, and label each tube with your initials, the date, and the patient's name and hospital number.

During the doctor's examination, hold your patient's hand, talk to her, and comfort her. Assist the doctor in the following procedures:

• Collect an aspirated or scraped specimen from any of the patient's orifices that may contain sperm or seminal fluid (pharynx, vagina, rectum, or urethra). These specimens will also be cultured for gonorrhea. (Remember that use of a lubricant may make analysis of specimens impossible; so use only water or saline on the speculum.) Semen specimens will dry out quickly, so have someone take the properly labeled specimens to the laboratory immediately and wait for them while the laboratory technician records the number of sperm per high-power field. (For permanent smears, the doctor will order a Pap smear, methylene blue test, or Gram stain.)

• Comb your patient's pubic hair to collect foreign hairs—or let her do this herself. Place all the hairs collected in a labeled container. Then ask your patient's permission to clip a few of her pubic hairs for comparison. Put these in a labeled container, as well.

• Draw blood for syphilis testing.

• Send blood and urine samples for pregnancy testing, a toxicology screen, and a blood alcohol level. Remember that failure to label and seal specimens will break the chain of evidence necessary to use the specimens in a trial. *Don't* let any specimen leave the examination room without a label, the initials of someone present during the examination, and a sealed lid. *Don't* leave the room until the next person in the chain collects the evidence and until you've both signed for each item.

### Therapeutic care

Assist the doctor in cleaning and treating any injuries, in explaining the purpose of prophylactic medications, and in administering them. The doctor will probably ask you to administer four kinds of prophylactic treatment:

• tetanus prophylaxis for any open wounds (see *Guidelines for Tetanus Prophylaxis*, pages 66 and 67)

• antibiotics, if the wounds are contaminated

• venereal disease prophylaxis

• pregnancy prophylaxis (if the patient isn't using a reliable contraceptive).

Inform the patient that she may have contracted venereal disease through any mucous membrane (oral, genital, or anal), and advise her that she should have prophylactic treatment. If she chooses to be treated, expect to give her probenecid orally, followed by penicillin I.M., as ordered. If she's allergic to penicillin, the doctor may order tetracycline to be given orally.

Advise her, too, about her risk of becoming pregnant. You'll need her signed consent before you administer the first dose of pregnancy prophylaxis (diethylstilbestrol [DES] or another estrogen, which many women call the "morning-after pill"). The doctor should explain the risks—such as danger to the fetus (if she was pregnant before the rape) and danger to the fetus if the DES is ineffective in stopping a pregnancy caused by the rape. He should also explain the possible side effects of DES—such as nausea and vomiting, vaginal spotting, rash, and insomnia during the 5-day treatment.

If your hospital doesn't offer pregnancy prophylaxis, you or the doctor can refer your patient to another hospital. If your patient is too upset to make a decision about taking DES, don't pressure her. Tell her she has time to make her decision. If she decides to wait, discuss her options:

• She can make up her mind, any time within 24 hours after the attack, to start taking DES.

• She can wait to find out whether she's pregnant. (But make sure she understands that having intercourse *before* she learns whether she's pregnant will make it impossible to know which encounter caused the pregnancy.) If she

# CASE IN POINT: FAILING TO MONITOR CONTRACTIONS

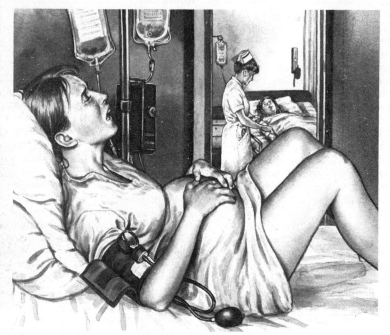

Paula Kelly, age 41, is admitted to your labor room in labor with her ninth child. Three hours after rupture of her amniotic membrane, her cervix hasn't dilated beyond 4 cm, so her doctor orders I.V. oxytocin (Pitocin) to accelerate her labor. You start the oxytocin, as ordered.

The patient in the next labor room needs an emergency cesarean section, so you spend the next 40 minutes preparing her for the operating room: starting an I.V., getting her chart ready, inserting an indwelling (Foley) catheter, and reassuring her and her nervous husband. You're too busy to monitor Paula's contractions, but you ask her frequently how she's doing and tell her to let you know of any problems. Suddenly, Paula cries out in pain, and in a glance you see that her abdomen has taken on an hourglass shape.

You tell the doctor immediately, but before he can deliver the baby by cesarean section, her uterus ruptures and the baby dies. You're named as a defendant in the resulting lawsuit.

Unfortunately, incidents like this really happen. In the case of *Long v. Johnson* (1978), the jury found the nurse liable for failing to monitor a woman's contractions continuously during oxytocin administration.

To reduce your risk of liability when administering an oxytocic drug to a patient in labor, follow these guidelines:
• Stay with the patient at all times, and record the frequency, intensity, and duration of her contractions every 15 minutes. Monitor the fetal heart rate, the maternal vital signs, and the resting period between contractions every 15 minutes, too.
• If you see signs of maternal or fetal distress during oxytocin administration, immediately shut off the infusion and open the main line solution. *Then* call the doctor.
• Support the patient's vital systems and institute resuscitation as needed.

---

*Long v. Johnson*, 381 N.E. 2d 93 (Ind. 1978)

learns she is pregnant, she can decide whether to have an abortion, to keep the child, or to put it up for adoption.

Help your patient and any family members present decide what they'd like to do, offering nonjudgmental support for their decisions.

When you're sure all examinations are completed, offer your patient a shower, a toothbrush and some mouthwash, and a change of clothing if possible. If a relative or friend is coming to the hospital to get her, stay with her until the person arrives. With her permission, call a women's crisis center if one's nearby. Many of these organizations have volunteers who can provide counseling and help guide rape victims through the legal system.

Before your patient leaves, make sure she has an appointment with her doctor, to check again for venereal disease and pregnancy.

## A FINAL WORD

Today, your *clinical* role in managing obstetric and gynecologic emergencies is complex. And your responsibilities to these patients will probably continue to grow in line with advances in obstetric and gynecologic care and related technology.

But your *supportive* role as a nurse also gets a workout with these patients. Picture the typical situation of a woman with an obstetric or gynecologic emergency: She's feeling frightened and threatened not only as a mother (or future mother) but also as a woman. Her doctor is probably male. So she's more likely than other patients to make you her confidant, to tell you *how* and *what* she's feeling.

Of course, you'll give her support. In turn, her reliance on you may mean that she tells you things she hesitates to tell her doctor, out of embarrassment. In this way, you may uncover important information about her condition. Be sure to stay alert for this possibility—your quick action in response to something your patient tells you could be lifesaving.

What does this added dimension of care mean to you? It may mean that while you're coping with the expected clinical challenges involved in caring for these patients, you'll also gain some unexpected—and uniquely satisfying—professional rewards.

## Selected References

Butnarescu, Glenda F., and Tillotson, Delight M. *Maternity Nursing: Theory to Practice.* New York: John Wiley & Sons, 1983.

Clark, Ann L., et al. *Childbearing: A Nursing Perspective,* 2nd ed. Philadelphia: F.A. Davis Co., 1979.

Dionne, Kathleen E. "If You Must Deliver A Baby," *RN* 44(9): 36-41, September 1981.

Jensen, Margaret D., et al. *Maternity Care: The Nurse and the Family,* 2nd ed. St. Louis: C.V. Mosby Co., 1981.

Moore, Mary Lou. *Realities in Childbearing,* 2nd ed. Philadelphia: W.B. Saunders Co., 1983.

Olds, Sally. *Obstetric Nursing.* Reading, Mass.: Addison-Wesley Publishing Co., 1980.

Reeder, Sharon R., and Mastroianni, Luigi, Jr. *Maternity Nursing,* 15th ed. Philadelphia: J.B. Lippincott Co., 1983.

Royko, M.A. "An Obstetric Emergency: Abruptio Placentae Vs Ruptured Uterus... Case Review," *Journal of Emergency Nursing* 8(1): 4-5, January/February 1982.

# EMERGENCY!
## Atlas of
## Major Injuries

In the pages of this full-color atlas, you'll discover dozens of illustrations and photographs of emergencies you can expect to encounter during your nursing career.

The first section illustrates *patterns of injury* for patients injured in auto accidents and falls and *mechanisms of injury* for patients with:
- blunt trauma to the spine
- blunt trauma to the head
- blunt trauma to the chest
- blunt trauma to the abdomen
- penetrating trauma to the head
- penetrating trauma to the chest
- penetrating trauma to the abdomen.

Photographs in the second section show exactly what you can expect to see when patients come into your ED with:
- thermal, electrical, or chemical burns
- frostbite
- dog bites
- snake or spider bites
- gunshot wounds
- eye injuries.

Understanding these injury patterns and mechanisms, and recognizing these types of injuries, may make the difference between life and death for some of your patients with emergencies.

When you must manage emergencies, be sure that your nursing knowledge is as well focused and comprehensive as you can make it. This special atlas will help.

## PATTERNS OF INJURY

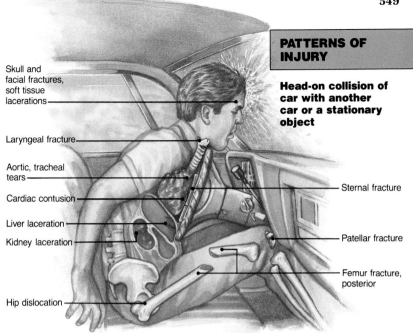

### Head-on collision of car with another car or a stationary object

Skull and facial fractures, soft tissue lacerations

Laryngeal fracture

Aortic, tracheal tears

Cardiac contusion

Liver laceration

Kidney laceration

Hip dislocation

Sternal fracture

Patellar fracture

Femur fracture, posterior

Driver strikes windshield, dashboard, and steering wheel, sustaining multiple injuries from direct force (fractures), compression (organ contusions and lacerations), excess stress (structural tears at points of attachment), and transmission of force (dislocations).

### Head-on collision of car with pedestrian (Waddell's triad)

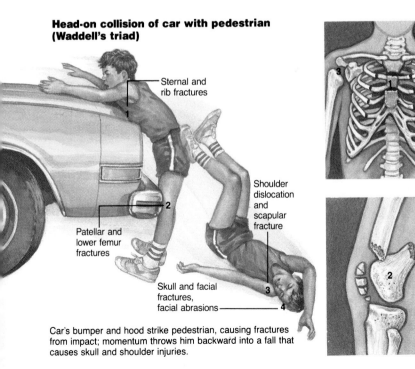

Sternal and rib fractures

Shoulder dislocation and scapular fracture

Patellar and lower femur fractures

Skull and facial fractures, facial abrasions

Car's bumper and hood strike pedestrian, causing fractures from impact; momentum throws him backward into a fall that causes skull and shoulder injuries.

## PATTERNS OF INJURY

### Lateral collision of car with pedestrian

Car's bumper and hood cause fractures from impact; excessive stress tears ligaments in both knees.

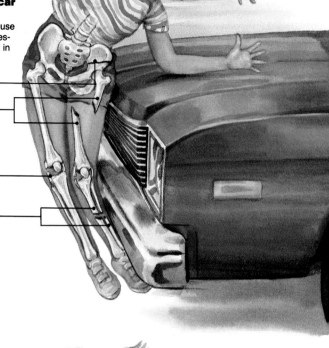

Pelvic fracture —

Femur fracture —

Knee ligament tears (both knees) —

Tibia and fibula fractures —

### Fall onto buttocks

Compression force causes spinal injuries.

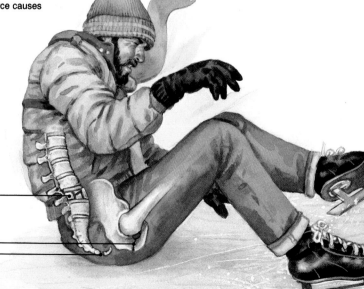

Compression fractures of the lumbar vertebrae —

Pelvic fracture —
Coccyx fracture —

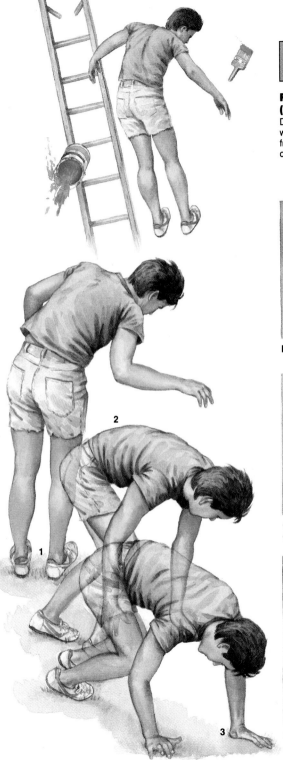

## PATTERNS OF INJURY

### Fall from a height (Don Juan syndrome)
Direct force causes heel and wrist fractures; acute flexion from forward momentum causes spinal injuries.

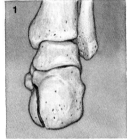

**Bilateral heel fractures**

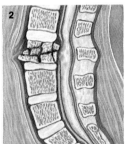

**Compression fractures of vertebrae**

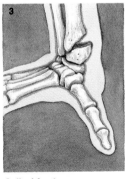

**Colles' fractures**

## BLUNT TRAUMA TO THE HEAD

### Person's head strikes a stationary object

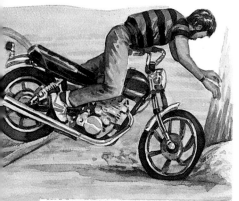

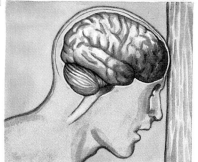

**Coup injury.** Sudden stopping of the head's momentum flings the brain against the inside of the skull; bruises occur at the point of impact.

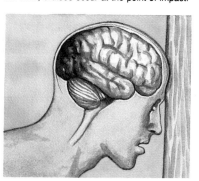

**Contrecoup injury.** The brain rebounds, striking the skull's opposite wall; contusions and lacerations occur opposite the point of impact.

### Person's head strikes a stationary object

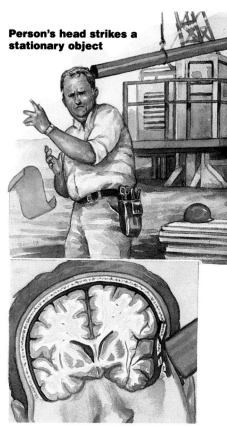

**Depressed fracture.** Depressed bone fragments from a blow to the skull cause cerebral hematoma, contusions, and lacerations.

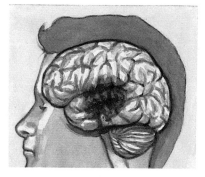

**Acute epidural hemorrhage.** A temporal or parietal skull fracture lacerates the middle meningeal artery; acute epidural hematoma results.

## BLUNT TRAUMA TO THE SPINE

**Person's cervical spine injured by moving object**

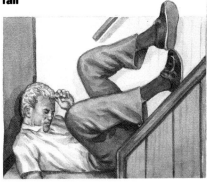

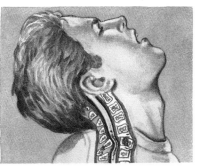

**Acute cervical hyperextension.** Resulting vertebral fracture or ruptured disk causes intradural hemorrhage, edema, and cord compression.

**Person's cervical spine injured in a fall**

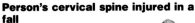

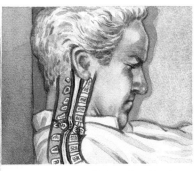

**Acute cervical hyperflexion.** Resulting fracture and dislocation of cervical vertebrae cause cord compression.

**Person's cervical spine crushed in headfirst fall**

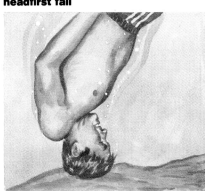

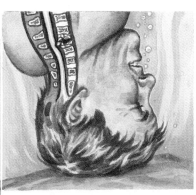

**Forceful cervical compression.** Vertebral bone fragments project into spinal canal.

## BLUNT TRAUMA TO THE CHEST

**Moving object strikes a person's chest**

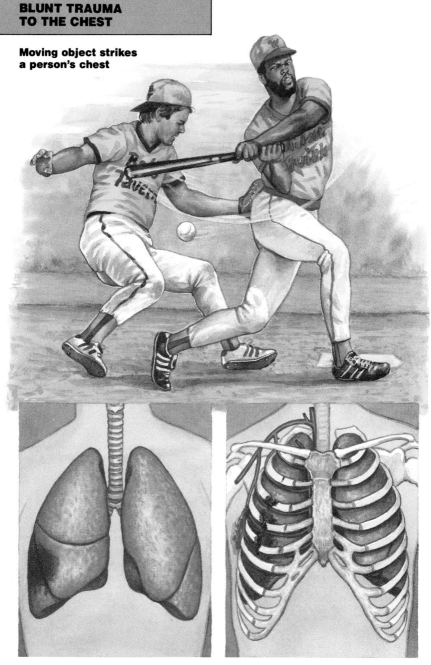

**Pulmonary contusion.** A forceful impact bruises lung tissue without lacerating it; edema, hemorrhage, and atelectasis result.

**Hemothorax.** Blunt chest trauma fractures the ribs and lacerates the intercostal or thoracic arteries; blood collects in the pleural cavity.

**Person's chest strikes a stationary object**

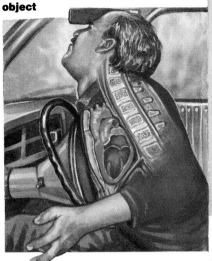

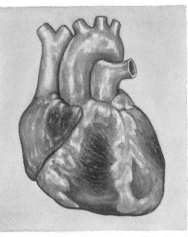

**Cardiac contusion.** Compression of the heart between the sternum and vertebrae bruises the myocardium.

**Massive object crushes a person's chest**

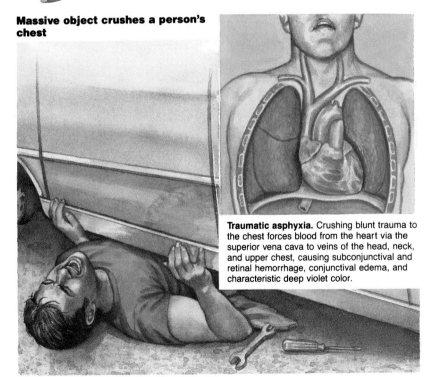

**Traumatic asphyxia.** Crushing blunt trauma to the chest forces blood from the heart via the superior vena cava to veins of the head, neck, and upper chest, causing subconjunctival and retinal hemorrhage, conjunctival edema, and characteristic deep violet color.

## BLUNT TRAUMA TO THE ABDOMEN

### Moving object strikes a person's abdomen

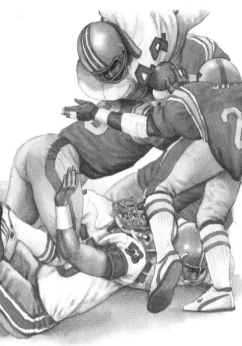

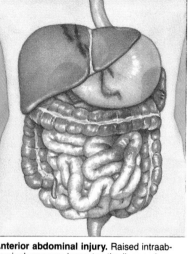

**Anterior abdominal injury.** Raised intraabdominal pressure lacerates the liver and spleen, ruptures the stomach, and bruises the duodenum.

### Moving object strikes a person's posterior abdomen

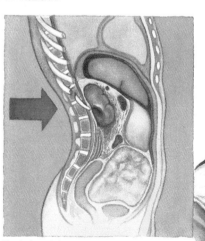

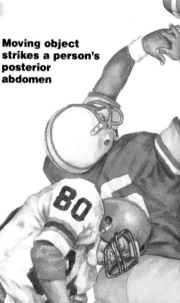

**Posterior abdominal injury.** Twelfth-rib fracture and kidney laceration cause urine extravasation and perinephric hematoma.

**Moving object penetrates a person's head**

**Path of bullet entering and exiting brain.** A high-velocity bullet creates a small entrance wound, a path of pulped tissue and bone and metal fragments, and a larger exit wound.

**Path of bullet entering and lodging in brain.** After it creates an initial path, the bullet ricochets off the inside of the skull and causes another path of pulped brain tissue.

## PENETRATING TRAUMA TO THE CHEST

### Moving object penetrates a person's chest

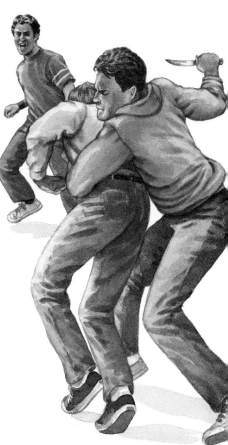

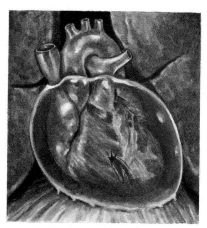

**Cardiac tamponade.** A penetrating heart wound causes bleeding into the pericardial sac; blood accumulation constricts the heart and impairs its function.

**Tension pneumothorax.** A penetrating chest wound punctures the lung and creates a valvelike opening in the chest wall. Intrapleural pressure, which increases as air's trapped in the pleural space, causes a mediastinal shift; cardiac output decreases, and the opposite lung is compressed.

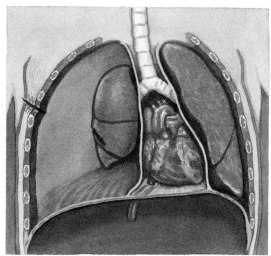

**Moving object penetrates a person's abdomen**

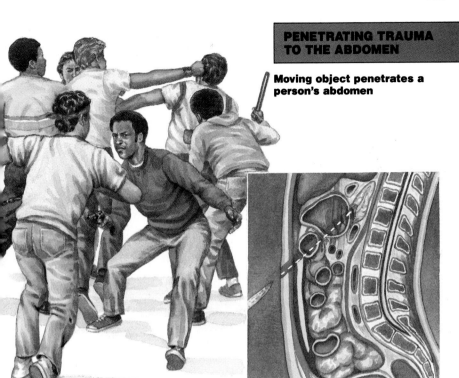

**Knife wound.** A single stab may penetrate the omentum, stomach, large intestine, pancreas, aorta, and inferior vena cava.

**Bullet wound.** Before lodging in the back, a bullet ricocheting through the abdomen may injure the liver, intestines, and kidney.

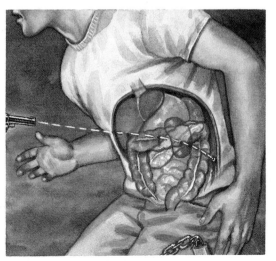

**BURNS**

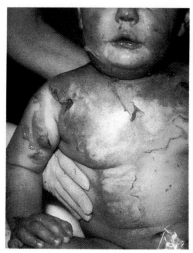

**1.** A partial-thickness (second-degree) burn. Note blisters.

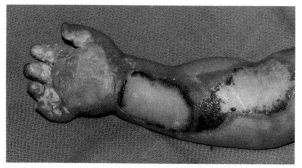

**2.** A full-thickness (third-degree) burn. Note leathery skin.

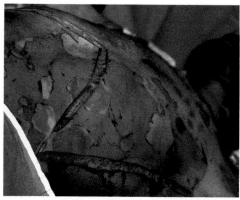

**3.** A full-thickness thoracic burn. Note escharotomy.

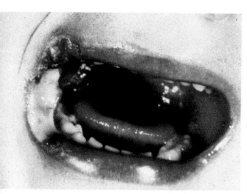

**4.** Electrical burn of mouth from chewing on electrical cord.

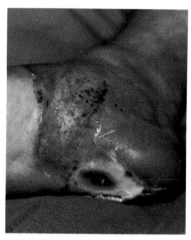

**5.** Electrical burn exit wound.

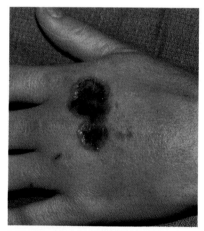

**6.** Chemical burn from nitrofluoric acid.

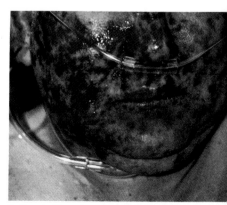

**7.** Chemical burn from hydrofluoric acid.

**ENVIRONMENTAL INJURIES**

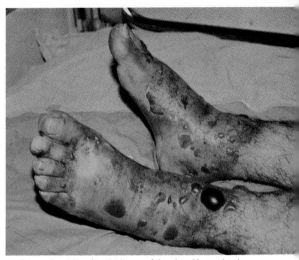

**8.** Severe frostbite after 24 hours of thawing. Hemorrhagic blebs have formed.

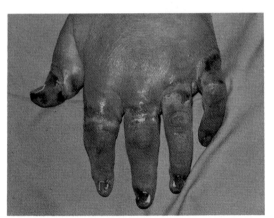

**9.** Final stage of frostbite. Fingers are necrotic.

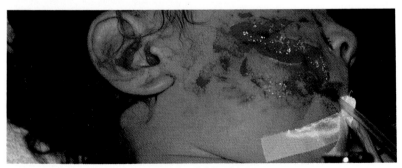

**10.** Dog bite. Note laceration of cheek and underlying tissues.

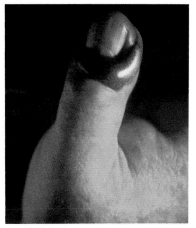

**11.** Bite from copperhead snake after 10 minutes.

**12.** Bite from copperhead snake after 2 hours. Note swelling and hemorrhagic bleb.

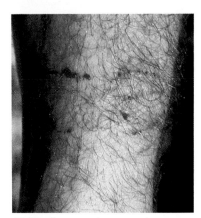

**13.** Bites from nonpoisonous snake.

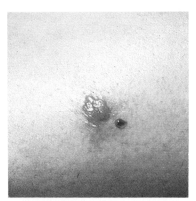

**14.** Bite from brown recluse spider. Note early "bull's eye" appearance.

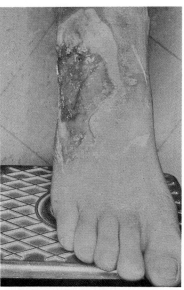

**15.** Bite from brown recluse spider: necrosis and sloughing 4 weeks after bite.

## GUNSHOT WOUNDS

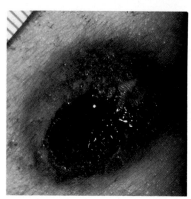

**16.** Bullet wound from gun fired at close range. Note black and brown powder burns.

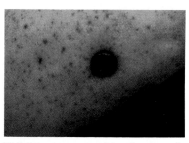

**17.** Bullet entrance wound (small and round) from gun fired at a distance.

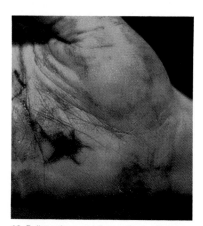

**18.** Bullet exit wound (larger than entrance wound; irregular shape).

## EYE INJURIES

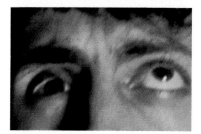

**19.** Blow-out orbital fracture. Note restricted upward gaze.

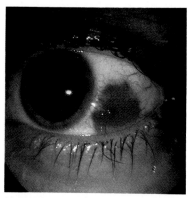

**20.** Subconjunctival hemorrhage from a penetrating piece of metal.

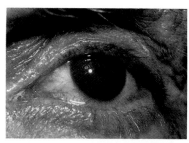

**21.** Hyphema (accumulation of blood in anterior chamber of the eye, due to blunt trauma).

# COMPARING ACCIDENTAL DEATHS

**Transportation**

| | |
|---|---|
| AGE *Under 15* | 4,053 |
| *15 to 29* | 25,136 |
| *30 to 44* | 10,966 |
| *45 to 59* | 6,799 |
| *Over 60* | 7,994 |

**Falls**

| | |
|---|---|
| AGE *Under 15* | 241 |
| *15 to 29* | 715 |
| *30 to 44* | 749 |
| *45 to 59* | 1,253 |
| *Over 60* | 9,662 |

**Fire-related**

| | |
|---|---|
| AGE *Under 15* | 1,344 |
| *15 to 29* | 827 |
| *30 to 44* | 687 |
| *45 to 59* | 870 |
| *Over 60* | 1,967 |

**Drowning**

| | |
|---|---|
| AGE *Under 15* | 1,441 |
| *15 to 29* | 2,034 |
| *30 to 44* | 772 |
| *45 to 59* | 468 |
| *Over 60* | 495 |

**Inhalation/ aspiration**

| | |
|---|---|
| AGE *Under 15* | 410 |
| *15 to 29* | 211 |
| *30 to 44* | 308 |
| *45 to 59* | 471 |
| *Over 60* | 1,927 |

**Firearms**

| | |
|---|---|
| AGE *Under 15* | 298 |
| *15 to 29* | 847 |
| *30 to 44* | 348 |
| *45 to 59* | 222 |
| *Over 60* | 154 |

**Poisonings**

| | |
|---|---|
| AGE *Under 15* | 169 |
| *15 to 29* | 1,447 |
| *30 to 44* | 1,258 |
| *45 to 59* | 810 |
| *Over 60* | 835 |

**Electrical current/lightning**

| | |
|---|---|
| AGE *Under 15* | 78 |
| *15 to 29* | 508 |
| *30 to 44* | 274 |
| *45 to 59* | 138 |
| *Over 60* | 97 |

Adapted from latest available statistics (1981) supplied by the National Center for Health Statistics.

Note: Figures don't include accident victims of unknown ages.

# 13

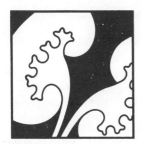

# Genitourinary Emergencies

## Introduction

After a busy night in the ED, you're enjoying a temporary lull in the activity when a rescue team brings teenaged Jim Chamness through the door on a stretcher. "He stopped his car at a red light and got rear-ended. The steering wheel hit him in the stomach," one of the rescue team members calls to you as you rush to the boy's side.

You're glad to note that Jim's conscious and has no obvious fractures. Rapidly, you assess his airway, breathing, and circulation; then you ask him how he feels. "It hurts all through here," Jim answers as he gestures toward his lower right rib and across his abdomen. "My back hurts, too," he adds.

He looks pale, and his skin feels cool and clammy when you check his vital signs. Gently, you palpate his abdomen—it's rigid, possibly due to internal bleeding. You ask a rescue team member to help you turn Jim on his side so you can inspect his back. When you remove his shirt, you note a purplish bruise over his right flank.

Quickly, you report your findings to the doctor. He tells you to start an I.V. for fluid replacement and to insert an indwelling (Foley) catheter to monitor Jim's urine output. In the course of performing these procedures, you discover that Jim has blood in his urine.

You're not sure exactly what's wrong with Jim, but you suspect that he has genitourinary (GU) injuries. His problem could be anything from a simple renal contusion to a shattered kidney. You know you'll have to act quickly and expertly to manage his genitourinary emergency and to forestall possibly serious complications.

Do you feel confident about caring for a patient like Jim?

Any emergency, of course, requires that you recognize the patient's problem quickly and intervene immediately *and* appropriately. But a patient with a GU emergency can be particularly challenging. Why? Because early detection of his serious GU problem can make a critical difference in the outcome of his care. For example, the time between injury and the onset of shock or sepsis can be frighteningly short, and loss of function is common. What's more, a patient who's sustained severe kidney damage or male genital trauma may risk losing the affected organ if transplantation or replantation isn't possible. This patient will need your understanding and emotional support, in addition to your expert nursing care.

So you can see how important your nursing skills are in managing these challenging patients. Reading this chapter will help you acquire the confidence—and nursing know-how—that you need.

# INITIAL CARE

## Prehospital Care: What's Been Done

As in all emergencies, rescue personnel's first goal was to stabilize the patient's airway, breathing, and circulation. If his airway was blocked with vomitus or blood, they attempted to clear it with suction or finger sweeps (see the "Life Support" section in Chapter 3). If he was bleeding externally, they applied direct pressure to the bleeding site. If the patient's condition was unstable, rescuers may also have inserted a large-gauge I.V. catheter for fluid replacement.

If the patient's penile or scrotal skin was avulsed, rescue personnel covered the denuded area with saline compresses. If his penis was amputated, they wrapped the severed part in dressings soaked in cool, sterile saline solution and placed it in a plastic bag on ice. They also covered the trauma site with saline compresses, and they may have applied a tourniquet if the penis was amputated below the penile-scrotal junction. If the patient had signs and symptoms of shock (such as cool, clammy skin and a steep drop in blood pressure), rescue personnel probably put him in a modified Trendelenburg position; they also may have applied medical antishock trousers (a MAST suit) to keep blood circulating to his vital organs.

If the patient had a nontraumatic GU emergency—such as acute renal failure or a renal calculus—rescue personnel probably took a brief initial history. They may also have started an I.V. with a large-bore catheter to try to restore the patient's electrolyte balance.

## What to Do First

Your first priority, as always, is to assess your patient's airway, breathing, and circulation. If rescue personnel started life-support measures, quickly reassess the patient and, if necessary, continue the measures they initiated. (Be prepared to intervene appropriately, of course, if your patient's status changes.)

### Airway

Make sure his airway's clear—use suction or a finger sweep to clear it, if necessary—and turn his head to one side. Keep airway adjuncts close at hand in case swelling from an associated chest injury compromises your patient's airway.

### Breathing

Assess your patient's breathing for depth, rate, and pattern. If tissue hypoxia from septic shock compromises his breathing, provide supplemental oxygen with a nasal cannula or mask. Be prepared to assist with endotracheal intubation or mechanical ventilation, if needed.

A GU emergency probably won't directly compromise your patient's airway or breathing—unless he's sustained GU trauma associated with chest or abdominal trauma. In this situation, assess the patient for paradoxical chest wall movement (indicating flail chest), and splint his chest wall with sandbags, if necessary. Obtain blood for arterial blood gases (ABGs), and be prepared to assist with chest tube insertion if signs of pneumothorax or hemothorax are present.

### Circulation

Hemorrhage from a traumatic GU emergency or associated trauma can readily compromise your patient's circulation. Watch him closely for signs and symptoms of shock from excessive

## NEW ADVANCES IN TREATING RENAL CALCULI

When a patient comes into your ED with a painful renal calculus, what treatment options come to your mind? You probably expect to:
• monitor the patient closely for 24 hours or longer to see if he passes the calculus
• prepare him for major surgery if he doesn't pass the calculus.

Now, however, some centers are offering two more methods to remove renal calculi: extracorporeal shock wave lithotripsy (ESWL) and percutaneous ultrasonic lithotripsy (PUL). Both methods require *little or no surgery* and reduce patients' risk of postoperative hemorrhage and other complications.

ESWL uses timed, spark-induced shock waves to break up calculi into fine particles. First the calculus is visualized by X-ray while the patient's placed on a cardiac monitor and given an epidural anesthetic. (The patient and attending staff must wear ear plugs because the spark makes a loud noise.) Then he's placed in a warm-water tank with the site of his calculus positioned at the point where two special X-ray systems cross—this is where the shock waves are focused. (To avoid disrupting the patient's cardiac rhythm, the

system emits high-energy shock waves, synchronized to his EKG's R waves.) The treatment lasts for 30 to 60 minutes, as shock waves move painlessly through water and flesh, breaking up the calculus. Within a few days, the calculus particles are excreted in the patient's urine.

PUL requires minor surgery to create a nephrostomy tract. Using a rigid nephroscope, the doctor visualizes the calculus then inserts an ultrasound device until it contacts the calculus. Silent sound waves gradually shatter the stone into fragments, which are removed through the ultrasonic device by continuous suction.

Each of these treatments has its advantages and disadvantages. PUL offers a relatively low cost, low risk of complications, and a short recovery period—but it's painful and requires some surgery. ESWL's a *totally* noninvasive procedure with an even lower risk of complications and an even shorter recovery time, but it's expensive and can be used only on radiopaque calculi. However, both methods are safe, effective alternatives to traditional methods of treating this extremely painful condition.

blood loss. If he's lost over 1,000 ml of blood—from renal pedicle trauma or pelvic fracture, for example—his pulse rate will significantly increase, and his blood pressure will drop steeply. Check his vital signs often, and assess him for hypovolemia using the tilt test. (See *Using the Tilt Test to Evaluate Hypovolemia,* page 302.)

If you think your patient's going into shock, elevate his feet by placing a pillow beneath them or by raising the foot of his bed, keeping the head of his bed flat. Immediately start rapid I.V. fluid replacement with volume expanders and crystalloids. Obtain blood for typing and cross matching, complete blood count (CBC), electrolytes, blood urea nitrogen (BUN), serum amylase, hemoglobin and hematocrit, and coagulation testing. Prepare to transfuse blood, if needed. You may also assist the doctor with inserting arterial and central venous pressure (CVP) lines, to

replace fluids more aggressively and to assess the patient's fluid status accurately.

Inspect his abdomen, back, and flanks for abrasions and discolorations. These could be signs of internal bleeding. If his flanks have a bluish cast, for example, he may have retroperitoneal bleeding (usually this bleeding occurs in Gerota's fascia—the covering of the kidney). Similar discoloration in the pelvic area or perineum could mean bleeding from pelvic trauma. Butterfly ecchymoses on his buttocks may indicate bleeding within the pelvic floor. If the doctor orders emergency surgery, continue to give your patient fluids and/ or blood while you prepare him for surgery.

Start recording the patient's intake and output so you can monitor his fluid balance. Normally you'd insert a Foley catheter to do this. But *don't* catheterize him if he has blood at the tip of his urethral meatus or if he sustained a pelvic fracture and now is unable to void. Why? Because these are signs of urethral injury, and the passage of the catheter could cause further trauma—possibly converting a partial urethral tear to a complete one. If urethral trauma is suspected, prepare the patient for an emergency retrograde urethrogram, as ordered. The doctor may insert an indwelling suprapubic catheter, to drain the bladder continuously, or he may aspirate the patient's urine with a suprapubic needle.

## General appearance
A patient with a GU emergency will probably be noticeably ill-at-ease and

PRIORITIES

# INITIAL ASSESSMENT CHECKLIST

**Assess the ABCs first and intervene appropriately.**

**Check for:**
• ecchymoses in the flank area, indicating retroperitoneal bleeding
• a suprapubic mass or perineal mass, indicating urine extravasation
• severe, colicky flank pain, indicating renal calculi.

**Intervene by:**
• checking the patient's urine for blood with a urine testing strip, straining it for kidney stones, and sending the specimen to the laboratory for urinalysis and culture-and-sensitivity testing
• starting I.V. fluids to maintain the patient's fluid volume and to provide access to blood, if needed
• giving narcotics and analgesics, as ordered, to control pain.

**Prepare for:**
• intravenous pyelography
• a retrograde urethrogram
• suprapubic catheter insertion
• transfer of the patient to a replantation center.

in pain. He may also be nauseated, dehydrated, or in shock, and he may have sustained blunt or penetrating trauma to the abdomen, lower rib area, or flank.

You'll be able to recognize some GU emergencies immediately on the basis of the patient's physical appearance. For example, in a patient with priapism, the corpus cavernosa will be erect while his glans penis and corpus spongiosum are flaccid. Other GU emergencies, such as a urinary tract infection (UTI), will be less obvious.

Observe the general condition of the patient's skin. If it's dry, with poor turgor, he may be dehydrated—possibly from excessive vomiting or renal insufficiency. If it's pale, cool, and clammy, he may be going into shock—possibly from dehydration, blood loss, or sepsis.

In a patient who's suffered blunt or penetrating trauma, be alert to the possibility of GU injury even when you have no apparent reason to suspect it. Look for ecchymoses, hematomas, or swelling on his abdomen, flanks, and pelvic area. If he has a penetrating abdominal wound, find out when he had his last tetanus shot. If it was over 5 years ago, give tetanus prophylaxis and prophylactic antibiotics, as ordered (see *Guidelines for Tetanus Prophylaxis,* pages 66 and 67).

## Mental status
A patient with a GU emergency that affects urination, such as a urethral trauma, will be anxious because of the extreme discomfort and stress this type of emergency causes.

Be alert if your patient becomes increasingly confused, lethargic, or disoriented; he may be experiencing renal failure or going into shock from extreme fluid loss or sepsis (see the "Septic Shock" entry in Chapter 14).

Remember, a male patient with a genital emergency will probably feel extremely anxious and frightened because of the threat to his sexual functioning. Encourage him to verbalize his fears. Provide emotional support and try to alleviate his anxiety.

# What to Do Next

Now that you've stabilized your patient's airway, breathing, and circulation, perform a thorough nursing assessment to identify his chief complaints and to evaluate his GU status. Remember, your patient may be reluctant to discuss a voiding problem—especially in the ED, with its lack of privacy. Make an effort to gain his trust in the short time you have for gathering information. Allow him to take the lead by telling you the problem as he perceives it. Then follow up with specific questions that will help you clarify and evaluate his emergency.

As a nurse, you know that many GU emergencies can quickly lead to renal failure or septic shock. Consider these possibilities throughout your assessment, and continue to monitor his vital signs. If his condition deteriorates, be prepared to stop your assessment immediately and to intervene as needed.

If your patient complains of *pain* in his abdomen, genitals, flanks, or pelvis, find out whether he's felt this pain before. Was the pain's onset sudden or gradual? Where is the pain located? This information can help you evaluate your patient's GU emergency. For example, pain in the flank and groin may indicate epididymitis or testicular torsion. With epididymitis, the discomfort builds gradually. With testicular torsion, your patient will probably be able to tell you the exact moment his pain began.

If he points to a specific site when you ask him where his pain's located, you'll know that his pain's *localized*. If he gestures toward an area, his pain's *generalized*.

Localized pain in the lower rib area may suggest renal trauma. Generalized pain in the upper or lower abdominal quadrants, flank, and costovertebral angle region indicates possible GU tract trauma. While you examine his abdomen, assess, too, for *referred* or *radiating pain*—common in patients with GU emergencies. Pain that's referred to the scrotum or labia may have originated in the lower ureter—possibly from distention due to a ureteral calculus.

Ask your patient to describe the severity and character of his pain—these may suggest the cause of his GU emergency. For example, if the patient complains of feeling as if he's on "pins and needles," with cramps that seem to build to a peak and then subside, he may have colicky pain—possibly from an obstruction in his GU tract. You can also differentiate your patient's pain by observing his reaction to it. For example, if he's restless or can't seem to sit still, his pain's probably colicky. If he's doubled over, clutching his stomach, his pain's probably severe, suggesting associated internal injuries.

Find out whether your patient was in an accident that caused blunt trauma to his abdomen. If so, find out when, where, and how the accident occurred. If he was in a motor vehicle accident, for example, was he the driver or a passenger? How many cars were involved, and at what speeds were they traveling? Was the patient thrown from his car? Ask him to describe the blow's location and force.

(Watch him closely while you continue your assessment. Remember, he may have internal bleeding and could go into hypovolemic shock very quickly.)

If your patient complains of *oliguria,* or *frequency* or *urgency* of urination, his lower urinary tract may be inflamed. Gently palpate and percuss his bladder, asking how long he's had these complaints and if he's ever experienced them before. To gather clues to the severity of his problem, find out whether he has any associated signs or symptoms. For example, if, besides urgency, he reports *suprapubic pain* and a *feeling of fullness,* you'll probably find that his bladder's distended from urinary retention, possibly due to a urinary tract obstruction or infection. If your patient's bladder is distended, call the doctor *immediately*. He may ask you to catheterize your patient to drain his bladder. If so, be sure to clamp the catheter after 1,000 ml of urine have been drained, to prevent mucosal damage from too-rapid drainage.

Has your patient noticed any blood in his urine? If so, when does the blood appear? Blood that appears at the beginning or end of urination is classified as *initial* or *terminal hematuria*, respectively, and indicates bleeding from

---

WARNING

# NEPHROTOXIN ALERT

As part of your drug history assessment, use this quick checklist to find out if your patient's been exposed to any of the most common nephrotoxic substances. As you know, nephrotoxins can cause renal damage and even renal failure if you don't intervene quickly. And they're particularly dangerous to a patient with a history of genitourinary problems. Here's what to do if your patient's come in contact with a nephrotoxic substance:

• Notify his doctor.
• Document your findings.
• Be prepared to perform emergency dialysis or gastric lavage and to administer drugs, as ordered.
• Be alert for signs and symptoms of renal damage.

## NEPHROTOXIN CHECKLIST

Ask your patient or his family if he's ingested, been exposed to, or been injected with any of the following substances:

**Chemicals**

☐ Antifreeze (such as ethylene glycol)

☐ Solvents (such as carbon tetrachloride)

☐ Insecticides (such as chlorinated hydrocarbons and organophosphates)

☐ Mercuric chloride

☐ Lead

☐ Arsenic

☐ Creosol

**Biological products**

☐ Horse serum

☐ Vaccines

☐ Poisonous mushrooms

**Drugs**

☐ Aminoglycosides (such as gentamicin, kanamycin, amikacin)

☐ Amphotericin B

☐ Polymyxin B

☐ Bacitracin

☐ Colistin

☐ Combination nonnarcotic analgesics

☐ Iodine-containing dye used in X-rays

☐ Gold salts

☐ Nonsteroidal anti-inflammatory agents (such as indomethacin, ibuprofen)

the urethra or bladder outlet. If there's blood throughout his urine stream, he has *total hematuria,* indicating disease of (or injury to) his bladder, ureters, or kidneys.

Ask him, if he can, to describe the color of his urine. If it's dark brown, he may have upper urinary tract bleeding. Lower urinary tract bleeding may make his urine pink or red, depending on the amount of blood. You'll need to obtain a urine specimen for analysis soon, but right now continue assessing for your patient's chief complaints.

If he complains of *nausea* or *vomiting,* ask when it started and how often it occurs. Auscultate his abdomen for bowel sounds—if they're hypoactive, he may have an ileus, accompanied by renal or ureteral colic. Listen for bruits over his abdominal aorta and iliac vessels, especially if he's an elderly man. An abdominal aortic aneurysm, renal artery thrombosis, or renal artery embolism may be causing his bowel symptoms. If his vomiting's severe, you may have to stop your assessment and insert a nasogastric (NG) tube to decompress his stomach and to keep him from aspirating gastric contents.

While you're examining your patient, remember that the kidneys, ureters, and bladder *cannot* be felt in their normal states. Some abnormal findings—such as a distended bladder or kidney mass—should be obvious on palpation. Others—such as ureteral distention—won't be palpable and can only be detected on X-rays.

Gently palpate his abdomen, being especially alert for rigidity and tenderness. If his abdomen's rigid and tender, *immediately* stop your examination and call the doctor: your patient may have internal bleeding. If his abdomen's not rigid, assess him for palpable masses—usually the result of extravasated blood or urine secondary to trauma. If you detect a flank mass, he may have a renal injury. A mass in the perineum or groin may indicate bladder, ureteral, or urethral trauma. A retroperitoneal mass may be due to renal

capsule distention or renal ischemia—either may result from bleeding.

If your patient has suspected urethral trauma, instruct him *not* to void, and don't catheterize him until urethral trauma's been ruled out. If urethral trauma isn't suspected, and the patient's able to void, obtain a clean-catch, midstream urine sample. (If he can't void, catheterize him, as ordered.) Even if his urine appears normal, check it for the presense of occult blood with a multipurpose urine testing strip. Save a specimen for the doctor to observe, and send the rest to the laboratory for urinalysis.

Ask your patient if he has any chronic GU disorders, such as renal failure, UTI, or renal calculi. If so, he may be experiencing an acute exacerbation of his chronic problem or a flare-up of its signs and symptoms. Also ask whether he has any other chronic diseases, such as diabetes, leukemia, or sickle cell anemia—these can precipitate such GU emergencies as UTI, renal calculus, or priapism. And, of course, the presence of a chronic illness will affect your patient's care.

Has he had surgery for any GU condition? If he had surgery to repair a torn ureter, for example, a stricture may have formed while his ureter was healing, so that now it's blocking his urine flow. Ask, too, if he's had abdominal surgery for any other condition. If your patient's a woman, be sure to ask if she's had any obstetric or gynecologic surgery, such as a hysterectomy; sometimes a ureter's nicked during this type of procedure.

Ask your patient if he's currently taking any medications. Be alert if he's taking any nephrotoxic agents, such as tetracycline or gentamicin: as you may know, nephrotoxins can trigger GU emergencies—for example, acute renal failure. (See *Nephrotoxin Alert.*) Keep in mind that certain drugs can change the color of urine so that it mimics hematuria. Phenazopyridine, for example, colors urine a bright reddish orange. Also, ask whether he's allergic to any medications, and record your findings.

# Special Considerations

## Pediatric

Because their kidneys are proportionately larger and are protected by a minimal layer of fat, children are more susceptible to renal injuries than adults. What's more, Gerota's fascia—the tissue that surrounds the kidneys—isn't fully developed until a child reaches age 10.

When you're evaluating genital injury in a child, be alert for signs of child abuse. Document your findings carefully. Remember: You're obligated by law to report suspected child abuse.

## Geriatric

Prostatic hypertrophy is a common cause of urinary tract obstruction and acute urinary retention in elderly males.

An elderly patient's more susceptible to infection from common procedures, such as urethral catheterization, especially if he's had an indwelling catheter for a long time. So be particularly alert for signs of infection, which can easily progress to sepsis and shock.

# CARE AFTER DIAGNOSIS

# Acute Renal Failure

## Prediagnosis summary

Initially, the patient had some combination of these signs and symptoms:
- nausea, vomiting, anorexia
- fluctuations in body weight
- poor skin turgor
- dry mucous membranes

- decreased urine output
- Kussmaul's respirations
- uremic breath
- muscular twitching
- deteriorating mental status
- tachycardia.

A large-bore I.V. catheter was inserted to administer fluid and medication. The patient was connected to a cardiac monitor, and an EKG was taken. Radiographic studies such as kidney-ureter-bladder (KUB), ultrasound, or intravenous pyelogram (IVP) were done. A straight urethral catheter was inserted, and a urine specimen was obtained for analysis to detect proteinuria, casts, cellular debris, and red and white blood cells and to measure specific gravity. Blood was drawn for a CBC, electrolytes, BUN, creatinine, calcium, phosphorus, ABGs, and typing and cross matching.

## Priorities

Your first priority is to assist with reinstating the patient's normal renal function. If his IVP revealed decreased renal perfusion, and his signs and symptoms included dehydration, sudden oliguria, and increased BUN and creatinine levels, the doctor will assume that a *prerenal* process caused the kidney failure. Expect to assist with insertion of a CVP line to gauge your patient's circulating fluid volume. If it's low, the doctor will ask you to give your patient a fluid challenge with normal saline solution. He may also ask you to administer diuretics and catecholamines. These will increase renal blood flow by drawing interstitial fluid into the patient's bloodstream.

If X-rays revealed a GU tract obstruction, the doctor will recognize that a *postrenal* process caused the patient's problem, which originated in the kidney. Again, expect to hydrate your patient—this time, the reason is to try to flush out the obstruction. Strain your patient's urine with a gauze mesh filter. Reserve any stones or sandy granules trapped in the filter for laboratory analysis. If the obstruction's too large to

## WHAT HAPPENS IN ACUTE RENAL FAILURE

Acute renal failure is the *sudden* failure of your patient's kidney function, most often from acute tubular necrosis. Urine output typically drops to less than 400 ml/day. Underlying causes of acute renal failure fall into three categories:

• *Prerenal causes* are factors occurring outside the kidneys that impair renal blood flow and lead to ischemia and decreased glomerular filtration. Examples include hypovolemia (from hemorrhage or dehydration), circulatory insufficiency (from shock or congestive heart failure), and increased renal vascular resistance (from bilateral renal vascular obstruction caused by thrombosis or embolism). Because prolonged renal ischemia can lead to tubular necrosis, prerenal causes of acute renal failure can lead to intrarenal disease.

• *Postrenal causes* may obstruct urinary outflow at any point from the kidneys to the urethra. Examples include renal calculi, blood clots, and benign prostatic hypertrophy. The results are hydronephrosis, tubular ischemia, and atrophy—all can lead to irreversible renal failure.

• *Intrarenal causes* are disorders that damage the kidneys themselves, causing the nephrons to malfunction. The disorder may be a primary kidney disease, such as acute glomerulonephritis or acute

pyelonephritis, but most often it's acute tubular necrosis. The exact pathophysiology of acute tubular necrosis is unknown, but several theories explain how it may cause renal failure:
– by decreasing renal blood flow and profoundly reducing the glomerular filtration rate
– by necrotizing tubular epithelial cells, which then slough off and obstruct the tubules
– by "back-leaking" tubular fluid into the renal interstitium and obstructing nephrons
– by altering the glomerular structure, reducing the glomerular filtration rate and permeability.

Depending on the duration and severity of the renal failure, hyperkalemia, hyperphosphatemia, and hypocalcemia will occur. If his fluid status and electrolyte imbalances aren't corrected, acute renal failure will become irreversible and lead to cardiac or respiratory complications that can result in death.

---

pass through the GU tract, the doctor may order cystoscopic surgery to break up the stone and remove it. Or, if the obstruction's a neoplasm, a nephrectomy may be performed. Prepare your patient for surgery, as ordered.

If radiographic studies showed that your patient's kidneys are enlarged, the doctor will suspect that he's retaining too much fluid in his nephrons (hydronephrosis). (See *Danger: Hydronephrosis,* page 599.) This, too, probably means that his kidney failure's due to a *postrenal* process. Expect to prepare your patient for surgical insertion of a nephrostomy tube to drain metabolic wastes from his kidneys.

If X-rays and laboratory studies revealed an intrinsic renal disorder, such as may result from acute pyelonephritis or exposure to nephrotoxic drugs, the

doctor will suspect that an *intrarenal* process caused the patient's renal failure. Your priority will be specific to the underlying cause. For example, you may give antibiotics or discontinue the causative drug, as ordered.

### Continuing assessment and intervention
First, check your patient's vital signs to assess his current hemodynamic status.

Assess your patient's respiratory status for signs of hypervolemia (jugular vein distention, tachycardia, moist rales, and breathing abnormalities), especially if he received massive hydration to perfuse his kidneys. During the diuretic stage of recovery or following removal of an obstruction, check for rapid pulse rate, poor skin turgor,

PROCEDURES

# YOUR ROLE IN AN EMERGENCY

## ASSISTING WITH PERITONEAL DIALYSIS

Expect to perform emergency peritoneal dialysis, as ordered, on patients with acute renal failure and patients who've ingested poison or a drug overdose. A patient with any of these acute emergency problems may need 36 to 72 hours of continuous peritoneal dialysis, which is the safest and simplest way to remove toxins from the patient's body.

### Equipment
• Dialysate solution in 2-liter bottles or bags
• Warmer, heating pad, or water bath
• Three surgical masks
• Dialysis administration set with drainage bag
• I.V. pole
• Dialysis kit or tray with:
  3-ml syringe with needle
  lidocaine (1% or 2%)
  sterile drape
  scalpel
  peritoneal catheter
  peritoneal stylet
  sutures
  precut drain sponges
  4″ x 4″ gauze pads
  povidone-iodine solution
• Nonallergenic tape
• Specimen container

### Before the procedure
• Gather the equipment, then warm the first bottle of dialysate to body temperature, using the warmer, heating pad, or water bath.
• Explain the procedure to the patient, and record her vital signs.
• Have the patient empty her bladder. If she can't urinate, obtain an order for straight catheterization.
• Weigh the patient and record her weight.
• Place her in a supine position and give her a surgical mask to wear.
• Check the warmed dialysate—it should be clear and colorless.
• Add medication—such as heparin, potassium chloride, or antibiotics—to the dialysate, as ordered. Be careful to prevent contamination.
• Put on a surgical mask and set up the dialysis administration set.

### During the procedure
• Assist the doctor in cleaning and draping the patient's abdomen, anesthetizing the insertion site, and inserting the catheter. Then connect it to the administration set.

• After the doctor's sutured and secured the catheter, place the precut drain sponges around it. Cover them with gauze pads, and tape them in place.
• Test the catheter's patency by instilling 500 ml of dialysate, as ordered, into the patient's peritoneal cavity and then draining it into the bag. Outflow should be brisk. (If the catheter isn't patent, as evidenced by slow outflow, assist the doctor in repositioning or replacing it.)
• If the catheter's patent, clamp the outflow line and infuse the prescribed volume of dialysate over a period of 5 to 10 minutes. Then clamp the inflow line.
• Let the dialysate dwell in the patient's peritoneal cavity for the prescribed time (usually 10 to 45 minutes) while you warm the next bottle of dialysate.
• Drain the peritoneal cavity contents into the bag for the prescribed amount of time, or until the flow stops (usually 10 to 30 minutes).
• Repeat this infusion-dwell-drain cycle with new bottles of dialysate, as prescribed.
• Check the patient's vital signs every 15 minutes during the first cycle and hourly thereafter. Monitor her heart rate and rhythm for dysrhythmias.
• Notify the doctor *immediately* if the patient's condition or vital signs change suddenly—this may indicate impending shock or circulatory overload.

### Nursing considerations
• Change the patient's dressing daily, using sterile technique.
• Check her catheter insertion site for signs of infection.
• If the patient has abdominal cramps during the infusion, slow it down, check that the dialysate's warm, and check the tube for air. Encourage the patient to change her position, as needed, to relieve the cramps.
• Weigh the patient daily at the same time and in the same stage of the dialysis cycle.

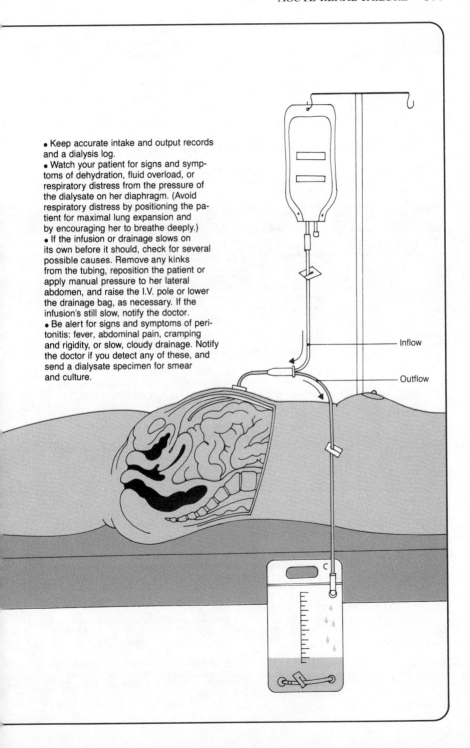

- Keep accurate intake and output records and a dialysis log.
- Watch your patient for signs and symptoms of dehydration, fluid overload, or respiratory distress from the pressure of the dialysate on her diaphragm. (Avoid respiratory distress by positioning the patient for maximal lung expansion and by encouraging her to breathe deeply.)
- If the infusion or drainage slows on its own before it should, check for several possible causes. Remove any kinks from the tubing, reposition the patient or apply manual pressure to her lateral abdomen, and raise the I.V. pole or lower the drainage bag, as necessary. If the infusion's still slow, notify the doctor.
- Be alert for signs and symptoms of peritonitis: fever, abdominal pain, cramping and rigidity, or slow, cloudy drainage. Notify the doctor if you detect any of these, and send a dialysate specimen for smear and culture.

Inflow

Outflow

and soft, sunken eyeballs, possibly indicating hypovolemia.

Notify the doctor *immediately* if you suspect fluid imbalance. He'll quickly reassess your patient. Then, if your patient has hypervolemia, the doctor will probably order a decrease in fluid intake, or a diuretic, to correct hypervolemia before it progresses to congestive heart failure and pulmonary edema. If your patient has hypovolemia, try to correct it before it progresses to shock. Expect to increase your patient's fluid intake with colloids or crystalloids.

## COMPARING HEMODIALYSIS AND PERITONEAL DIALYSIS

When one of your patients needs dialysis, you need to know exactly what's happening and what complications to expect. Hemodialysis and peritoneal dialysis share a common purpose: to remove toxic wastes from a patient's blood when renal failure prevents his

|  | INDICATIONS | PROCESSES |
|---|---|---|
| **Hemodialysis** | Your patient with renal failure will receive hemodialysis when he has:<br>• hypercatabolism<br>• hyperkalemia<br>• severe respiratory insufficiency<br>• a large, draining abdominal wound<br>• intraabdominal adhesions<br>• a diffusely infected abdominal wall<br>• critical volume excess. | In hemodialysis, a synthetic semipermeable membrane separates the blood and dialysate compartments in the dialyzer and permits water and solutes to move to and from the blood:<br>• The doctor will create an arteriovenous access (AV shunt or fistula).<br>• The patient will need heparin to prevent clotting.<br>• Blood moves from the patient's artery, through the arterial lines, and into the dialyzer, where diffusion, osmosis, and ultrafiltration occur. The dialysate draws wastes, excess fluids, and electrolytes across the semipermeable membrane.<br>• Detoxified blood leaves the dialyzer, undergoes filtering and monitoring for bubbles, and returns to the patient's veins through the venous lines.<br>• Dialyzer pressure adjustments can increase or decrease the rate of ultrafiltration to make it more efficient and better suited to the patient's needs. |
| **Peritoneal dialysis** | Your patient with renal failure will receive peritoneal dialysis when he's refused blood transfusions or has:<br>• a severe blood-clotting disorder<br>• cardiovascular disease<br>• exhausted circulatory access sites<br>• atherosclerotic veins. | In peritoneal dialysis, the patient's peritoneal membrane acts as the semipermeable membrane and transmits body wastes to the dialysate from the peritoneal fluid.<br>• The doctor will insert a peritoneal catheter for access to the peritoneal cavity.<br>• The patient may need medications, such as antibiotics, potassium, or heparin, added to the dialysate, as ordered.<br>• The dialysate is instilled into the peritoneal cavity, where it will dwell and draw the wastes, excess fluids, and electrolytes across the peritoneal membrane by osmosis and diffusion. The waste-laden dialysate is drained into a collection bag.<br>• The instill-dwell-drain cycle is repeated until all wastes and excess fluid are removed and the patient's acid-base balance is restored. |

Now, take a detailed patient history to help determine what precipitated his acute renal failure. Ask whether your patient's had any recent illnesses, with accompanying vomiting or diarrhea, or recent surgery that required anesthesia. Any of these conditions may have dehydrated him and decreased his renal blood flow by precipitating renal vasoconstriction from diminished blood volume or release of antidiuretic hormone.

Find out about your patient's medication history—especially if he's now

kidneys from functioning normally. These procedures also purify the blood of patients with certain types of drug overdoses or acute poisoning. But that's where the similarities stop. The indications, processes, advantages, and disadvantages for each procedure are quite different, as shown in the chart below.

| ADVANTAGES | DISADVANTAGES |
|---|---|
| Hemodialysis is:<br>• relatively quick—it takes only 3 to 8 hours to complete and provides fast results in acute emergencies.<br>• effective—most patients need fewer than three treatments per week.<br>• more efficient at removing low-molecular-weight substances from the patient's blood. | Hemodialysis:<br>• requires expensive equipment and a specially trained nurse.<br>• requires surgery to create a circulatory access.<br>• may cause complications, such as internal or external hemorrhage, anemia, hepatitis, cardiovascular problems, air emboli, rapid fluid and electrolyte shifts (dialysis disequilibrium syndrome), muscle cramps, intracranial bleeding from excess heparin, and shunt or fistula complications. |
| Peritoneal dialysis is:<br>• immediate—it can be performed right away in most patients.<br>• low-risk, with few life-threatening complications.<br>• less stressful to the patient's cardiovascular system, causing no blood loss.<br>• less risky for patients with bleeding problems, because they receive less heparin (if any at all) than they would with hemodialysis.<br>• more gradual in shifting the patient's fluid and electrolyte levels.<br>• more efficient at removing middle-weight molecular substances from the patient's system.<br>• simpler, requiring less-complex equipment and little training to perform.<br>• performed via peritoneal catheter instead of circulatory access. | Peritoneal dialysis:<br>• can take 10 to 72 hours to complete.<br>• may need to be done more than three times a week.<br>• carries a high risk of peritonitis.<br>• may cause protein depletion, respiratory distress, and extreme fluid and electrolyte imbalances in the patient.<br>• may not be used for patients who've had recent abdominal surgery or extensive abdominal trauma. |

taking or has recently taken any nephrotoxic drugs (any of the penicillins, gentamicin, or tobramycin). Remember, high concentrations of nephrotoxic agents can damage renal tubules. (See *Nephrotoxin Alert*, page 572.)

### Therapeutic care

To assess your patient's fluid status, weigh him daily. For consistent weight readings, use the same scale, schedule the weigh-ins at the same time each day, and have him wear the same type of clothing.

Document anything that is different about each weigh-in. To evaluate his fluid status further, use his daily weight and intake and output records to validate each other. Here's how: 1 ml of water weighs 1 g, so if your patient's intake exceeds his output by 1,000 ml in 24 hours, you should see a weight increase of about 1 kg. If his output exceeds his intake, negative fluid balance should produce weight loss. (Remember, because of your patient's high risk of infection, you probably won't insert an indwelling [Foley] catheter. Be sure to remind your patient to save his urine after voiding.)

You'll need to check your patient's serial blood tests frequently, because the specific therapeutic care he'll require depends on whether his serum laboratory values are abnormal after initial fluid replacement or surgery.

If your patient's ABGs show an abnormally low pH (< 7.35), expect to correct his acidosis by administering sodium bicarbonate and calcium through I.V. push and/or I.V. additive. Reassess his ABGs after treatment to see if his acid-base balance is restored. If it isn't, inform the doctor: he may want to adjust the amount of sodium bicarbonate and calcium your patient's receiving.

If your patient's electrolytes include an increased potassium or decreased sodium level, expect to correct hyperkalemia by administering dextrose and insulin I.V. and Kayexalate (sodium polystyrene sulfonate) orally (or rec-

tally, if he's on fluid restriction). To correct hyponatremia, expect to replace your patient's I.V. fluid with one higher in sodium. Reassess your patient's electrolytes after treatment; if his electrolyte balance isn't restored, inform the doctor.

In a patient whose serum calcium level is decreased (< 8.0 mg/dl) and whose serum phosphate level is elevated (> 4.5 mg/dl), expect to administer calcium gluconate I.V. to correct his hypocalcemia. To correct his serum phosphate elevation, expect to administer a phosphate-binding antacid, such as aluminum hydroxide gel (Amphojel). Afterward, reassess his serum calcium and phosphate levels. If they haven't returned to normal, inform the doctor.

If your patient's BUN and serum creatinine levels steadily increase, his vital signs become unstable, and his mental status deteriorates, his hemodynamic status is probably compromised. You may be asked to prepare your patient for surgery, where an arteriovenous shunt will be inserted for hemodialysis access. (See *Comparing Hemodialysis and Peritoneal Dialysis*, pages 578 and 579.) Or, more likely, you'll be asked to assist with peritoneal dialysis to remove accumulated metabolic wastes from your patient's kidneys. (See *Assisting with Peritoneal Dialysis*, pages 576 and 577.) Take your patient's vital signs before and after the procedure, to detect hypotension from too-rapid fluid loss.

A decrease in your patient's hematocrit and hemoglobin levels may indicate his kidneys aren't able to produce erythropoietin, a hormone that stimulates red blood cell production. Expect to transfuse blood, as ordered, to prevent anemia. (See *Administering Blood Transfusions*, page 493.)

Your patient with acute renal failure will require total parenteral nutrition—a high-carbohydrate, high-calorie, low-protein I.V. fluid—to prevent tissue catabolism, which increases metabolic waste production.

To avoid stomatitis, encourage your patient to maintain oral hygiene by rinsing frequently with a fluoridated mouthwash.

Remember, your patient has decreased resistance to infection and septic shock. (See the "Septic Shock" entry in Chapter 14.) Check all wounds and I.V. insertion sites frequently for signs of infection. If you see any, call the doctor *immediately*. To avoid skin breakdown and bed sores, keep your patient on an egg-crate mattress, and turn him every 2 hours. Culture any drainage from the infection site and expect to administer broad-spectrum antibiotics. When culture-and-sensitivity test results are returned, check that the causative organism's sensitive to the antibiotic your patient's receiving.

To help decrease the risk of respiratory complications, encourage your patient to breathe deeply and to cough frequently. You may also assist with incentive spirometry, as ordered.

Finally, don't forget to provide emotional support. The prospect of losing kidney function or becoming dependent on dialysis can be frightening to your patient. Encourage him to verbalize his fears. He'll need your reassurance and understanding in addition to your best nursing care to help him through this crisis.

# Renal Trauma

## Prediagnosis summary
The patient had a history of blunt or penetrating trauma to the abdomen or flank. In addition, he may have had:
- associated injuries
- costovertebral, flank, or abdominal pain
- pain radiating to his groin
- hematuria
- oliguria
- signs of shock
- ileus
- a visible or palpable flank mass

- a hematoma or ecchymoses over his upper abdomen or flank (Grey Turner's sign)
- nausea and vomiting.

A large-bore I.V. catheter was immediately inserted to administer fluid and medication. Tetanus prophylaxis was given, if indicated. If the patient showed signs of hypovolemic shock, rapid fluid replacement with normal saline solution, colloids, or blood was started to increase blood volume and to ensure renal perfusion. In addition, a MAST suit may have been applied to help stabilize his hemodynamic status. (See the "Hypovolemic Shock" entry in Chapter 14.) An indwelling (Foley) catheter was inserted, and a urine specimen was obtained for urinalysis to detect microscopic hematuria. Unless the patient was unstable, a computerized tomography (CT) scan, IVP, renal arteriogram, or KUB X-ray was taken to determine whether he sustained a renal laceration, fracture, or pedicle injury. Blood was drawn for typing and cross matching, CBC, and electrolytes.

## Priorities
Because of the danger of hemorrhage and permanent loss of kidney function, your first priority is to prepare your patient for emergency surgery. The doctor will attempt to control renal bleeding and to repair the damaged kidney, but if your patient's injuries are too extensive for repair, the doctor will do an emergency nephrectomy.

## Continuing assessment and intervention
After your patient returns from surgery, expect to administer analgesics and broad-spectrum antibiotics, as ordered. Blood will be drawn for serial testing (BUN and creatinine to detect renal failure and CBC to detect blood loss and infection). Check these laboratory results frequently—along with your patient's vital signs, fluid balance, and physical appearance—for signs and symptoms of renal complications.

Assess your patient's abdomen to detect kidney enlargement, tenderness, distention, or rigidity. If you detect any of these signs, and your patient has accompanying nausea, vomiting, and decreased or absent bowel sounds, he may have a paralytic ileus or peritonitis. (See *Danger: Peritonitis*, page 332.) The doctor will order a flat-plate X-ray of your patient's abdomen to detect free air under the diaphragm. Expect to insert an NG tube to remove gastric acids and enzymes until peristalsis returns.

Check your patient's surgical dressings for drainage. If you see excessive bloody drainage, and your patient's hematocrit and hemoglobin levels are decreasing, these findings indicate that significant blood loss is occurring at the incision site. He may also be bleeding internally. If you see purulent drainage with localized redness and swelling, and your patient has fever, tachycardia, increased pain, and chills,

PATHOPHYSIOLOGY

## WHAT HAPPENS IN RENAL TRAUMA

Overlooking the presence of renal trauma is surprisingly easy. True, the kidneys are very mobile (fixed only at the renal pedicle) and are surrounded and protected by the back musculature, abdominal wall, and viscera, so kidney trauma is rarer than it might otherwise be. But you can't afford to ignore the fact that blunt or penetrating trauma to a patient's flank, back, or upper abdomen *can* cause renal contusions, lacerations, fractures, and pedicle injuries.

Your patient's treatment will depend on which type of injury he's sustained. To help you act quickly and expertly when caring for a patient with renal trauma, here's information

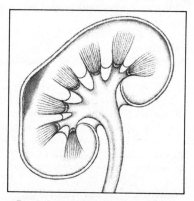

Renal *contusions* are the least traumatic and most common renal injuries. You may see flank soreness and hematuria from a small hematoma or bruise of the patient's kidney. These problems are relatively minor, but the patient will be treated with bed rest to prevent additional injury or complications.

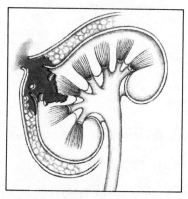

Renal *lacerations* damage the renal parenchyma. Depending on its depth and severity, a renal laceration may or may not bleed into the renal collecting system. If the renal capsule ruptures, you may see signs and symptoms of retroperitoneal bleeding, such as an expanding flank mass, increasing pain, fever, abdominal distention, ileus, nausea, vomiting, and shock. *Retroperitoneal bleeding can also lead to rapid exsanguination.* This patient requires immediate surgery to repair the lacerations and to control the bleeding.

he may have a perinephric abscess. Culture the drainage, and notify the doctor.

Expect to transfuse blood if your patient is hemorrhaging; afterward, closely monitor his hematocrit and hemoglobin levels. If they continue to drop, your patient may need surgery to control his bleeding. If your patient has a perinephric abscess, you may be asked to prepare him for surgery for insertion of a drain. The doctor will reevaluate your patient's antibiotic therapy and may change his medication order. If the infection is so severe that your patient becomes septic and shows signs of shock, expect to administer supplemental oxygen and vasopressors and to start fluid replacement for restoration of your patient's hemodynamic status.

Watch for signs of decreased renal function—electrolyte imbalance, acidosis, or decreased urine output. If you to explain the types of renal trauma, their signs and symptoms, their nursing implications, and the complications they can cause.

Complications of renal trauma are usually related to extravasation, vascular disruption, or delaying surgery beyond 5 days. But some complications—such as rebleeding, progressive renal failure, and sepsis—can occur up to 6 weeks after the injury. Keep in mind that these complications are emergencies, too.

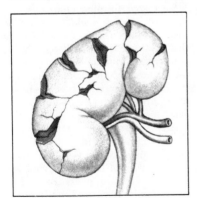

Renal *fractures*, also referred to as shattered or pulped kidney, are deep lacerations throughout the kidney. They disrupt the renal collecting system and can cause severe urine extravasation, renal fragmentation, massive bleeding, and rapid exsanguination. This patient will probably already be in shock when you see him. He'll need immediate surgery to repair the lacerations (or to remove the kidney) and to control his massive bleeding.

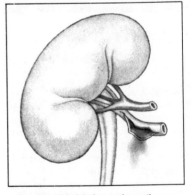

Renal *pedicle injuries* are lacerations or disruptions of vessels and arterial intima tears of the pedicle. They can lead to massive bleeding and shock or to vascular thrombosis and ischemic renal necrosis. You'll see such signs and symptoms as palpable flank mass, shock, and evidence of multiple injuries. This patient also needs immediate surgery; the kidney is probably unsalvageable.

see these signs, notify the doctor *immediately* and anticipate the need for dialysis (see *Assisting with Peritoneal Dialysis*, pages 576 and 577).

### Therapeutic care
Continue monitoring your patient's blood chemistries, urinalysis, vital signs, and intake and output for delayed onset of renal complications. As with all postoperative patients, you'll also need to provide pulmonary care. Encourage your patient to perform deep-breathing and coughing exercises every hour. Keep him on strict bed rest, and reposition him at least every 2 hours.

To prevent wound contamination and UTI, use strict aseptic technique. Change dressings as needed. To prevent reflux of urine, keep catheters below your patient's bladder level and keep drainage tubing unkinked. Expect to continue your patient's antibiotic therapy, as ordered.

# Bladder Trauma (Ruptured Bladder)

### Prediagnosis summary
The patient had a history of blunt or penetrating abdominal trauma. Initial assessment revealed some combination of the following signs and symptoms:
• lower abdominal pain over the pelvic or suprapubic regions
• a strong urge to void, but inability to do so
• doughy swelling above the symphysis pubis
• swelling of his scrotum, buttocks, or perineum
• abdominal rigidity
• decreased or absent bowel sounds
• hematuria
• signs and symptoms of shock.

A retrograde urethrogram was taken; if the patient's urethra was intact, an indwelling (Foley) catheter was

inserted, and a cystogram was performed. A rectal examination was also performed to quickly determine the extent of bladder injury.

### Priorities
Your first priorities are to stabilize your patient and to prepare him for immediate surgery. If an I.V. catheter hasn't already been inserted, do so now to administer fluid and medication. If he shows signs of shock, immediately begin fluid replacement, as ordered. Also start tetanus prophylaxis, if indicated. During surgery, the doctor will insert a suprapubic cystostomy tube to drain extravasated blood and urine and to divert urine from the urethra. He'll also attempt to repair bladder tears.

### Continuing assessment and intervention
Concentrate your nursing assessment on detecting complications early so you can intervene before your patient's renal function is compromised.

Start by performing a thorough baseline examination, including a detailed history. Find out what caused your patient's injury. If he's suffered blunt or penetrating trauma, how and when did the accident occur? Remember, bladder injuries can be iatrogenic—be sure to inquire about recent abdominal surgery.

Assess your patient's vital signs frequently. Because of his potential to develop sepsis, be especially alert for trends, such as fever occurring with decreased blood pressure and increased pulse rate—and check your patient often for other signs of infection. If he has flank pain, decreased output, and cloudy or foul smelling urine, he may have a UTI. If you note localized redness, tenderness, abdominal pain, and purulent wound drainage, your patient may have an abscess. Faint or absent bowel sounds, peritoneal pain, nausea, and vomiting could accompany peritoneal necrosis from undrained extravasated urine. If you suspect that your patient has an infec-

# CASE IN POINT:
# FAILURE TO ASSESS THE PATIENT PROPERLY

You're caring for Jon Chen, age 42, who's had surgery for removal of a renal calculus. During the surgery, the surgeon inserted a nephrostomy tube. Over the first 10 days of recovery, Jon complained about the tube continually and expressed concern about whether it was working properly. Today the surgeon removed the tube, so you (and the other nurses on your floor) hope that Jon's complaining will stop.

As soon as you begin your shift, however, Jon complains again, this time telling you he has severe pain where the tube was. Irritated, you nevertheless check his chart and find an order to give Tylenol #3 for pain. So you quickly assess the tube site and administer the medication.

Jon continues to complain off and on during the next several hours. With each complaint, you explain that the medication will take effect soon, but you don't reassess the tube site. Finally, Jon falls asleep; later, he awakens writhing in agony. This time, you call the surgeon, who examines Jon and finds that a mass has formed at the tube site. This means that Jon must have another nephrostomy tube inserted and must remain in the hospital much longer than he'd anticipated. Needless to say, he's very upset. And when he learns that, if you or another nurse had reassessed the site of his pain and called the doctor sooner, this additional physical and emotional stress might possibly have been avoided, he announces he's suing for

negligence.

If you were really involved in this situation, could you be found negligent? A similar case, *Kolakowski v. Voris* (1979), involved nurses who noted Mr. Kolakowski's complaints but failed to properly assess the severity of his condition. The court's ruling: the nurses should have known that his signs and symptoms were unusual and that they required notifying the doctor immediately.

To avoid placing yourself in such a situation, follow these guidelines when you assess a patient who's in pain:

• Always obtain a baseline assessment of your patient's pain when you begin caring for him; reassess him against this baseline often.

• Don't disregard *any* patient's complaint of pain—no matter how often he complains, reassess his pain each time.

• *Thoroughly* assess the pain site. Check under any wound dressing for blood or drainage, and, unless the doctor specifically ordered you not to, remove the dressing and look for swelling or inflammation.

• Of course, *always* inform the doctor of any change in your patient's condition that you think is significant.

• Give pain medication promptly and monitor its effectiveness. Remember, you're responsible for determining whether a pain medication is effecitve. If it isn't, notify the doctor so he can increase the patient's dosage or order a stronger medication.

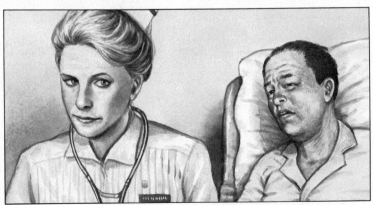

*Kolakowski v. Voris*, 395 N.E. 2d 6 (Ill. App. Ct. 1979)

tion, culture the site, if possible. Inform the doctor, and expect to administer antibiotics.

Monitor your patient's intake and output every hour, and inform the doctor *immediately* if urine output drops below 30 ml/hour (oliguria may be an early sign of impending renal failure). Obtain blood for electrolyte, BUN, and creatinine testing to determine if renal failure's occurring. Anticipate administering fluids to increase the patient's urine output. If he develops acute renal failure, expect that dialysis will be started. (See *Assisting with Peritoneal Dialysis,* pages 576 and 577.)

### Therapeutic care

Keep your patient on strict bed rest and administer analgesics as ordered to re-

---

## CARING FOR URINARY DRAINAGE TUBES

Genitourinary trauma, disease, or surgery can obstruct your patient's normal urine flow or necessitate diverting it. In either situation, you or a doctor will insert a drain, catheter, or tube into the patient's urinary tract to keep his urine flowing.

| TYPE AND LOCATION | DESCRIPTION |
|---|---|
| **Nephrostomy tube** 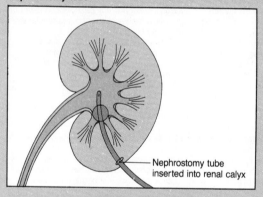 Nephrostomy tube inserted into renal calyx | Balloon- or mushroom-shaped tube inserted directly into the renal pelvis or calyx, surgically or percutaneously, and connected to a closed drainage system |
| **Ureteral stent** 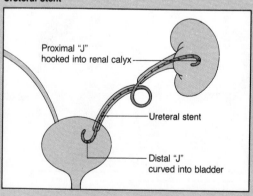 Proximal "J" hooked into renal calyx — Ureteral stent — Distal "J" curved into bladder | Small tube placed inside the ureter via cystoscope, nephrostomy tube, or surgery, and either taped to a urethral catheter or connected to a drainage bag at the nephrostomy tube site |

lieve his pain. Your further care will center on preventing postoperative complications.

For example, to prevent postoperative respiratory infection, maintain pulmonary hygiene by turning your patient at least every 2 hours. Encourage him to breathe deeply and to cough frequently.

Initially, maintain your patient's nu-tritional status by infusing supplemental I.V. fluids. When he's able to tolerate oral fluid, encourage him to drink lots of fluids to prevent UTI.

Use strict aseptic technique when you care for his catheters and drains. Clean the insertion sites with povidone-iodine solution, and apply antiseptic ointment. To prevent skin breakdown and irritation, keep your

---

When you're caring for this type of patient, give special care to his drainage tube, as shown in this chart.

| PURPOSE | NURSING CONSIDERATIONS |
|---|---|
| • To drain urine directly from the kidney after surgery or when an obstruction blocks urine flow<br>• To allow renal tissue to regenerate after trauma<br>• To provide permanent drainage when the ureter no longer functions | • Check tube patency frequently to prevent urine flow obstruction and possible kidney damage.<br>• Tape the tube to the patient's skin to keep it from being dislodged. If it becomes dislodged, call the doctor immediately.<br>• Clean the tube site twice a day with antimicrobial ointment or hydrogen peroxide, and cover it with sterile gauze.<br>• Watch for bleeding or urine leaks at the nephrostomy site. Expect hematuria for 24 to 48 hours after percutaneous tube placement.<br>• Maintain a closed drainage system to prevent kidney infection.<br>• Make sure the tube doesn't kink when your patient lies on his side. Never clamp the tube.<br>• Keep separate output records for each kidney if both have tubes.<br>• Never irrigate the nephrostomy tube unless the doctor orders irrigation, and never use more than 10 ml of warm sterile saline solution. |
| • To maintain urine flow through the ureter, especially in patients with ureteral obstructions<br>• To restore renal function<br>• To promote healing<br>• To maintain ureter size and patency after surgery | • If an indwelling (Foley) catheter is used with the stent, tape it to the patient's thigh and make a note on his chart that this is a *ureteral stent* catheter.<br>• Care for the tube site (as described above).<br>• Watch for bleeding and signs of infection.<br>• Observe for signs of stent dislodgement, such as colicky pain and decreased urine output. The double "J" stent prevents dislodgement by hooking into the renal calyx and curving into the bladder, as shown in illustration.<br>• Measure and record intake and output.<br>• If the doctor orders irrigation, irrigate the ureteral stent *slowly*, and never use more than 4 ml of warm saline solution. |

*(continued)*

## CARING FOR URINARY DRAINAGE TUBES *(continued)*

| TYPE AND LOCATION | DESCRIPTION |
|---|---|

### Cystostomy tube (suprapubic catheter)

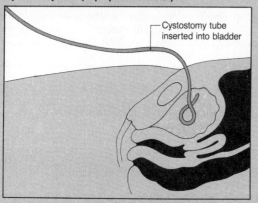

Cystostomy tube inserted into bladder

Tube inserted into the bladder, via incision or puncture in the suprapubic area, and attached to a closed drainage system

### Urethral catheter (indwelling, Foley)

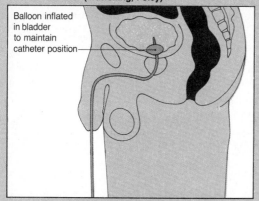

Balloon inflated in bladder to maintain catheter position

Catheter inserted through the urethra to the bladder and attached to a closed drainage system

---

patient's abdomen dry. Change his dressings when they become moist, and replace his suprapubic drainage bag if the seal breaks and leakage occurs.

# Ureteral Injuries

### Prediagnosis summary
The patient had a history of penetrating or severe blunt trauma or recent abdominal surgery. On initial assessment, he also had some of these signs and symptoms:
• hematuria
• an obvious wound
• extravasated urine
• leakage of urine from the vagina or from a surgical incision
• flank or abdominal pain, or both (in the lower quadrant on the affected side)
• fever

| PURPOSE | NURSING CONSIDERATIONS |
|---|---|
| • To drain the bladder after gynecologic or bladder surgery or when the patient has a fractured pelvis<br>• To divert urine flow from the urethra, usually when urethral strictures or injuries block the urethra<br>• To provide more comfortable drainage than an indwelling urethral catheter does and to reduce chances of bladder infection | • Check catheter patency frequently. Avoid kinks in the tubing that could block urine flow.<br>• Notify the doctor if the catheter won't drain properly. Expect to pull out the catheter 1″ (2.5 cm) at a time until the urine flows, and be prepared to irrigate the catheter as ordered (usually with 50 ml of sterile normal saline solution).<br>• Tape the drainage tube to the side of the patient's abdomen.<br>• Cover the catheter area with a sterile dressing.<br>• Change the incision dressings at least every 24 hours, noting the color, character, and amount of drainage.<br>• Clean the incision site with povidone-iodine solution, as ordered.<br>• Inspect the incision for redness, warmth, swelling, or purulent drainage.<br>• If required, perform a voiding trial by clamping the catheter for 4 hours, having the patient try to urinate, unclamping the catheter, and measuring the residual urine. |
| • To drain the bladder after surgery or GU trauma (including urethral trauma in some patients), and when the patient can't void adequately | • Make sure the system is draining constantly and that urine doesn't collect in the tubing.<br>• Check for leaks and excoriation around the urethral meatus.<br>• Tape the drainage tube securely on the thigh to prevent movement and tension on the catheter.<br>• Watch for signs and symptoms of urinary tract infection, such as hematuria, pyuria, fever, and chills.<br>• Keep the collection bag below the patient's bladder, but not touching the floor.<br>• Drain the bag at least once every 8 hours. Instill 10% povidone-iodine into the drain spout, according to your hospital's protocols.<br>• Wash his perineal area with soap and water several times a day.<br>• Change a latex catheter every 2 to 4 weeks; change a silicone catheter every 6 to 8 weeks.<br>• If catheter drainage decreases, irrigate with 50 ml of sterile normal saline solution, as ordered. |

• an abdominal or flank mass, or both
• vomiting
• paralytic ileus
• decreased urine output
• a ureterovaginal fistula.

An I.V. catheter was inserted for fluid and medication access. Tetanus prophylaxis was given if indicated. An indwelling (Foley) catheter was inserted, and urine was obtained for urinalysis. An IVP and a retrograde pyeloureterogram were taken to detect the location and extent of ureteral injury.

### Priorities

Your first priority is to prepare your patient for surgery as soon as possible, so his ureteral injury can be repaired before his kidney function's affected.

If radiographic studies revealed a partial ureteral tear, the doctor will attempt cystoscopy and insertion of a ureteral splinting catheter. If the patient's ureter continuity is completely

# EVALUATING URINE SPECIMENS

Before sending your patient's urine specimen to the laboratory for complete analysis, make your own minievaluation. As you know, urine is a prime indicator of a patient's genitourinary (GU) status, and any abnormality should alert you to the possibility of GU disease or injury.

Normal urine is, of course, golden yellow and relatively clear. When you check a patient's urine for color and clarity, you shouldn't see any blood or sediment. When you use a urine testing strip for analysis,

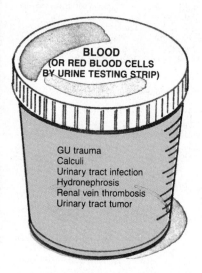

**BLOOD**
**(OR RED BLOOD CELLS BY URINE TESTING STRIP)**

GU trauma
Calculi
Urinary tract infection
Hydronephrosis
Renal vein thrombosis
Urinary tract tumor

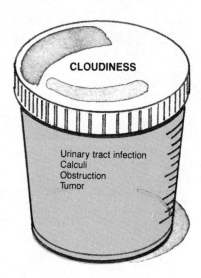

**CLOUDINESS**

Urinary tract infection
Calculi
Obstruction
Tumor

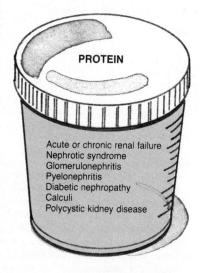

**PROTEIN**

Acute or chronic renal failure
Nephrotic syndrome
Glomerulonephritis
Pyelonephritis
Diabetic nephropathy
Calculi
Polycystic kidney disease

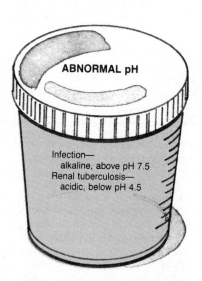

**ABNORMAL pH**

Infection—
   alkaline, above pH 7.5
Renal tuberculosis—
   acidic, below pH 4.5

the urine's pH should be between 4.5 and 8.0. Check its specific gravity, too: normal is 1.005 to 1.030.

If you notice any abnormal urine characteristics (see chart), your patient may have one of the GU disorders listed.

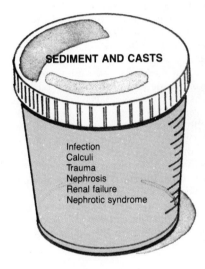

**SEDIMENT AND CASTS**

Infection
Calculi
Trauma
Nephrosis
Renal failure
Nephrotic syndrome

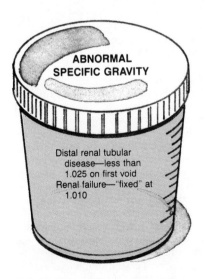

**ABNORMAL SPECIFIC GRAVITY**

Distal renal tubular disease—less than 1.025 on first void
Renal failure—"fixed" at 1.010

broken, the doctor will anastomose the severed parts. In either situation, a nephrostomy tube will probably be inserted to temporarily divert urine from flowing through the healing ureter.

### Continuing assessment and intervention

As soon as your patient returns from surgery, take his baseline vital signs rapidly to assess his hemodynamic status. Perform a complete assessment to discover if he has any trauma-related injuries. Because ureteral injuries are often iatrogenic, be sure to find out if your patient had previous (and recent) abdominal surgery.

Make sure your patient's nephrostomy tube is sutured and taped securely in place: it will be sutured to his skin at the insertion site and reinforced with tape. Instruct him to move slowly and carefully to avoid dislodging the tube. Assess the tube frequently for patency, and notify the doctor *immediately* if it's obstructed. If the doctor asks you to clear the obstruction by irrigating the tube, use 10 ml of normal saline solution, and be sure to introduce the solution slowly; then let it drain out by gravity. To avoid dislodging the tube or traumatizing the patient's delicate tissue, *don't* aspirate the irrigation solution.

To help prevent infection from urine reflux, keep the drainage bag below the level of your patient's bladder and keep the drainage tubing unkinked. Change the dressings around the tube insertion site whenever they become moist, to prevent skin breakdown. Document the number of dressing changes and estimate the amount of drainage (slight, moderate, large, or sufficient to saturate the dressings). Check the patient's tube insertion site for signs of infection, such as redness or purulent drainage. If you note infection, inform the doctor, culture the infection site, and expect to administer antibiotics, as ordered.

Continue to check your patient's vital signs every 15 minutes and to monitor his intake and output every hour. When you document his urine output, include the amount, color, and character of the urine. Be alert for fever, chills, flank pain, decreased output, and cloudy or foul-smelling urine, indicating UTI. If you note these signs and symptoms, obtain a urine culture and expect to administer antibiotics and fluids as ordered. If your patient's blood pressure decreases and his pulse rate become increasingly faint and rapid, he may be going into shock from poor kidney perfusion or rebleeding. Anticipate administering fluids, as ordered, to perfuse his kidneys. The doctor may intervene surgically to control rebleeding.

### Therapeutic care
Infuse supplemental fluids, as ordered, until your patient's able to tolerate clear liquids and an advanced diet. At that time, encourage him to drink lots of fluids. This will flush his kidneys to help prevent urine stasis and infection while his ureteral injury's healing. Expect to continue administering analgesics, to relieve pain, and antibiotics to prevent or treat postoperative infection.

# Urethral Trauma

### Prediagnosis summary
The patient had a history of straddle injury, penile trauma, penetrating trauma, or pelvic fracture. On initial assessment, he also had some combination of the following:
• suprapubic, perineal, or lower abdominal pain
• bleeding from the urethral meatus or associated injuries, or both
• signs of shock, such as tachycardia and hypotension
• a perineal hematoma or urinoma, or both
• penile and scrotal discoloration
• edema of the abdomen, perineum, penis, or scrotum
• urinary urgency, retention, and/or hesitancy
• slight hematuria
• distended bladder
• prostate displacement.

A large-bore I.V. catheter was inserted to replace fluid and to administer medication. Blood was drawn for typing and cross matching and for a CBC. If the patient showed signs of shock from blood loss—such as cool, clammy skin, diaphoresis, hypotension, and tachycardia—fluid replacement was started immediately with crystalloids, colloids, and blood, as needed. If indicated, tetanus prophylaxis was given. Analgesics and antibiotics were also administered. To avoid urine extravasation, the patient was asked not to void. Pelvic X-rays and a retrograde urethrogram were taken with portable equipment to determine the extent and location of the patient's urethral injury. An IVP may also have been taken, to assess the integrity of his renal system. If the patient sustained a pelvic fracture, a KUB X-ray was taken, and a MAST suit may have been applied to stabilize his hemodynamic status. (See *What Happens in Pelvic Fractures*, page 379.)

### Priorities
Your first priority is preparing your patient for emergency surgery to repair his damaged urethra and to divert his urine flow. The specific type of surgery he'll need depends on the nature and location of his injury. For example, if his urethra was injured above his urogenital diaphragm, the doctor will probably perform a suprapubic cystostomy. Then he may manipulate the urethra and bladder over interlocking sounds. As an alternative procedure, he may dissect the severed urethral ends and join them together by end-to-end anastomosis. He'll insert a urethral catheter to act as a stent.

He'll also insert a stenting catheter if the urethra was injured below the urogenital diaphragm. In addition, he may perform a suprapubic cystostomy or a nephrostomy if the catheter doesn't provide adequate urine drainage.

If your patient has accompanying pelvic fracture or penile trauma, the doctor will also attempt to stabilize any associated injuries. (See *What Happens in Pelvic Fractures,* page 379, and the "Avulsion or Amputation of the Penis or Scrotum" entry in this chapter.)

### Continuing assessment and intervention

After your patient returns from surgery, your nursing assessment will focus on preventing postoperative complications.

First, perform a thorough baseline assessment. As you know, a patient may not be aware he has a urethral trauma until several months after the initial injury, when stricture formation obstructs urine flow. Ask if he's been injured recently and, if so, find out when and how the accident happened.

Check your patient's urinary drainage tube for proper placement—it should be taped securely to his abdomen to reduce the risk of increased stricture formation. Check the tube's patency frequently, too, and be careful not to let it become kinked. (This is especially important if the doctor performed a nephrectomy: the resulting buildup of urine in the remaining renal pelvis can damage the renal parenchyma.) Assess your patient for increased perineal swelling and abdominal distention—signs that the tube's obstructed. If it becomes obstructed, notify the doctor and be prepared to irrigate it, if ordered.

Monitor your patient's intake and output closely, and notify the doctor *immediately* about any decrease in output. As you know, this may indicate renal insufficiency or possible extravasation of urine out of the bladder and into the pelvis.

Watch for signs of infection at incisions and catheter insertion sites. If you suspect infection, obtain blood for a CBC and culture. Also culture the patient's urine and wound drainage.

You'll be able to assess the infection's severity on the basis of your patient's signs and symptoms and laboratory results. If the infection's progressed to abscess formation, anticipate insertion of a drain. The doctor will order radiographic studies to pinpoint the site to be drained. Assist as needed, and expect to adjust your patient's antibiotic therapy, as ordered.

Check for gross hematuria, ecchymoses, and hematomas, indicating rebleeding. Also assess your patient frequently for signs of hypovolemic shock. If you suspect rebleeding or shock, notify the doctor *immediately* and anticipate replacing fluids, as ordered.

### Therapeutic care

The goal of therapy is to restore normal urine flow through the healed urethra. Your therapeutic care will focus on preventing infection and stricture formation during the healing process.

Keep your patient on bed rest and, if he doesn't have an accompanying pelvic fracture, turn him every 2 hours to prevent respiratory infection. Encourage him to breathe deeply and to cough frequently, too. To prevent UTI, have him drink lots of fluids. And to prevent skin breakdown, change the dressings applied to the catheter and/or the drain insertion sites as they become moist.

Your patient will continue to wear a catheter to offset stricture formation and to ensure urethral patency while his urethra's healing. Use strict sterile technique when caring for the catheter, and continue administering antibiotics and analgesics, as ordered.

# Renal Calculi

Initially, the patient had some or all of these signs and symptoms:
- excruciating pain in his flank, abdomen, or groin

- abdominal distention
- nausea and vomiting
- fever and chills
- hematuria
- sudden interruption of his urine stream
- urinary frequency and urgency.

A urine sample was obtained for urinalysis to test the patient's urine pH and to detect hematuria, pyuria, crystals, and casts. A KUB X-ray and an IVP were taken to determine the size and location of the patient's renal calculi. Blood was drawn for a CBC and calcium, phosphorus, BUN, creatinine, glucose, uric acid, and electrolyte levels.

## Priorities

Your first priority is to assist with efforts to eradicate the calculi. Expect to insert a large-bore I.V. catheter immediately and to begin infusing large amounts of fluids (2,000 to 3,000 ml). This will increase the patient's urine output, dilute his urine, and possibly flush out the calculi so they can pass through his GU tract. Expect to give a narcotic analgesic, such as Demerol (meperidine) or morphine, to relieve your patient's pain. If urinalysis revealed an accompanying UTI, expect to give broad-spectrum antibiotics, too. (See the "Urinary Tract Infection" entry in this chapter.) You may also need to prepare your patient for emergency surgery to drain accumulated urine, preventing hydronephrosis. (See *Danger: Hydronephrosis,* page 599).

## Continuing assessment and intervention

Perform a thorough baseline examination, including a detailed patient history. Because renal calculi tend to recur and can stem from congenital defects, ask your patient whether he or anyone in his family has a history of kidney stone formation. Find out about your patient's general medical history, too. Certain metabolic factors, such as hyperparathyroidism and renal tubular acidosis, can also predispose your patient to renal calculi; a history of dehydration or infection could mean that calculus-forming substances have concentrated and proliferated. Find out what medications your patient's been taking. Some drugs, including certain vitamin supplements, contain large amounts of calcium. These drugs, along with excessive intake of vitamin D or dietary calcium, for example, have been linked to calculus formation.

If your patient complains of pain that seems to fluctuate throughout his abdomen, calculi may be scraping against the lining of the renal pelvis or ureter as they travel through the urinary tract. Try to locate the painful site—this will help you track the spontaneous passage of the calculi. To make the passage easier, encourage your patient to walk, if possible.

To assess your patient's fluid status and renal function, carefully monitor his intake and output and his daily weight. Keep a 24- to 48-hour record of his urine pH. Strain the urine and reserve any solid material for analysis. Knowing what material the calculi are composed of will help the doctor pinpoint what's causing them to form. Encourage your patient to drink sufficient fluids to attain a daily urine output of 3 to 4 liters. If he can't drink that amount, infuse supplemental fluids, I.V., as ordered.

If your patient has a urinary drainage tube, check its patency frequently. (See *Caring for Urinary Drainage Tubes,* pages 586 to 589.) Change the dressings around the insertion site when they become moist, and weigh them to monitor the amount and rate of drainage accurately. Be alert for bloody or purulent drainage, which may indicate hemorrhage from too-rapid drainage or infection from reflux. If you see bloody drainage, check your patient's vital signs for falling blood pressure and rising pulse rate. If you suspect that he's losing blood, notify the doctor *immediately.* If you see purulent drainage and your patient has fever and chills, suspect that he has an

# HIGHLIGHTING CALCIBIND AND LITHOSTAT

Some hospital staffs are combating renal calculi in patients with histories of previous calculi by using two drugs that prevent stone formation. Here's how these drugs work.

**Sodium cellulose phosphate** (Calcibind) prevents calculi from forming when the patient has hypercalciuria due to excess absorption of dietary calcium. This drug works by binding calcium to its ion exchange resin, preventing the calcium from being absorbed. A patient takes it by mouth, three times a day, with meals.

However, controlling the effects of Calcibind at therapeutic levels may be difficult—the drug can absorb *too* much calcium. So if your patient's taking Calcibind, assess him for these possible complications:

• *Hypocalcemia.* Monitor his serum calcium levels and assess him regularly for signs and symptoms such as muscle cramps, abdominal cramps, cardiac dysrhythmias, tingling at the ends of his fingers, and tetany (manifested by sharp flexion of wrist and ankle joints, carpopedal spasms, muscle twitches, cramps, convulsions, and sometimes stridor). Make sure your patient eats a moderately restricted calcium and oxalate diet and avoids dairy products, spinach, rhubarb, chocolate, and tea. He should also drink at least 2 liters of fluid a day.

• *Osteoporosis.* Your patient may develop lower back pain, reduction in height, and bones that fracture easily. Tell him to take extra precautions against trauma.

**Acetohydroxamic acid** (Lithostat) prevents the formation of struvite or magnesium ammonium phosphate calculi. Usually these occur in patients with recurrent urinary tract infections and form when certain bacteria produce a urea-splitting enzyme called urease. Urease increases the urine's ammonia content and alkalinity. Then the urine becomes supersaturated with magnesium ammonium phosphate; from this, crystals form, accumulate, and result in calculi. Lithostat breaks this chain of events by blocking bacterial production of urease and by lowering urinary pH.

The patient takes Lithostat by mouth three or four times a day, at 6- to 8-hour intervals, when his stomach is empty. If your patient is taking Lithostat, warn him of these possible complications:

• *Hemolytic anemia.* Monitor his complete blood count with a reticulocyte count. Emphasize the importance of continued follow-up care to monitor these blood counts periodically.

• *Rash on the arms and face.* This is especially likely to occur when alcohol is used during the patient's drug therapy. Remind him not to drink alcoholic beverages while taking the drug.

• *Nausea, vomiting, and headaches.*

• *Poor Lithostat absorption.* Iron supplements reduce Lithostat absorption, so tell the patient to consult his doctor before taking any over-the-counter medications.

---

infection and notify the doctor. Expect to administer antibiotics, as ordered.

## Therapeutic care

If the KUB and IVP revealed calculi larger than 6 mm, they may be too large to pass through the patient's ureter, so he'll probably require surgery to remove them. The doctor probably won't attempt surgery, however, until your patient's acid-base, fluid, and electrolyte balances are within normal ranges. Closely monitor serial urinalysis and blood test results to gauge your patient's progress. You should see improvement within 24 hours of initial hydration.

If the calculi are lodged in the ureter, the doctor may use retrieval instruments through a cystoscope to remove them. Calculi are usually removed from other areas, such as the renal calyces or the renal pelvis, through an incision in the patient's flank or lower abdomen. If calculi are embedded in one of the renal calyces (staghorn calculi), the patient may need a nephrectomy.

After the calculus is removed, watch your patient closely for postobstruction

# WHAT HAPPENS IN RENAL CALCULI

Renal calculi, or kidney stones, can form anywhere in the urinary tract, but they most commonly develop in the renal pelvis and calyces. Calculi may stay in the renal pelvis or move through the urinary tract, causing excruciating pain along the way. More common in men than in women, calculi form when substances that are normally dissolved in the urine (calcium oxalate, calcium phosphate, magnesium ammonium phosphate, urate, or cystine) precipitate instead. The following conditions promote urinary precipitation and the development of renal calculi:

• *Dehydration.* When urine production decreases, the calculus-forming substances become concentrated and precipitate out of the urine.

• *Infection.* Chronic urinary tract infections from bacteria that produce urease, a urea-splitting enzyme, increase the urine's ammonia content and alkalinity. The urine becomes supersaturated with magnesium ammonium phosphate and precipitates (struvite calculi).

• *Obstruction.* Urinary stasis allows calculus-forming substances to collect and adhere to one another. It also promotes

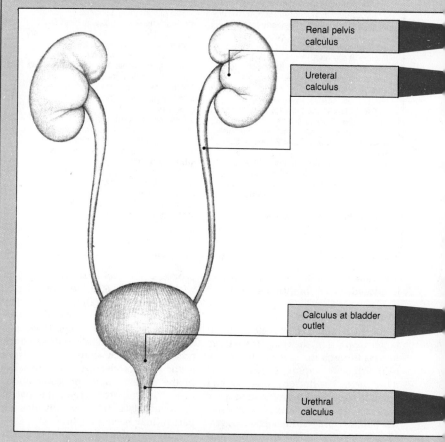

Renal pelvis calculus

Ureteral calculus

Calculus at bladder outlet

Urethral calculus

infection.

- *Hypercalciuria.* A diet high in calcium-rich foods (such as milk and cheese), bone disease, hyperparathyroidism, or prolonged immobilization can cause hypercalciuria. Excess calcium then precipitates to form a calculus.
- *Hyperoxaluria.* Causes of hyperoxaluria, in which excess oxalate may precipitate to form a calculus, include a diet high in oxalate-rich foods (such as fresh vegetables), small-bowel disease, ethylene glycol poisoning, and vitamin $B_6$ deficiency.
- *Hyperuricemia.* Highly concentrated uric acid can precipitate from the urine and form a calculus. Hyperuricemia occurs in people who have gout or renal failure or who use thiazide diuretics and alkylating agents.

No matter how it forms, a renal calculus causes a urinary tract obstruction that damages the area above it. Without treatment, the damage becomes progressively worse. The result? Acute renal failure. This chart shows you how a renal calculus can create problems that may escalate quickly into a life-threatening situation.

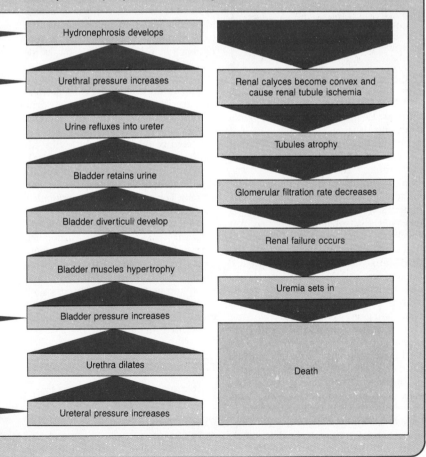

## WHEN YOU SEE RED

When your patient voids red or orange urine, you should tell his doctor you suspect hematuria and possible genitourinary problems, right? Not necessarily. Certain foods, drugs, and diseases can cause psuedohematuria, which looks like hematuria but is simply reddish urine with no detectable hemoglobin or blood cells. So your first move should be to check your patient's chart for pseudohematuria-inducing drugs he may be taking. (Examples include phenazopyridine, phenolphthalein, phenolsulfonphthalein dye, senna, or cascara sagrada.) Then ask him what he's been eating lately—any beets, rhubarb, or blackberries? (Vegetable dyes used to color food also cause pseudohematuria.) Does he have a history of porphyria, which can also redden his urine?

*Now* you're ready to call the doctor and report your findings. If he's able to rule out hematuria, you'll have saved everyone involved needless concern.

diuresis. He may lose massive amounts of water, salt, urea, and electrolytes that were building up during the period of obstruction. This can lead to such complications as hypovolemia, hypotension, hypoglycemia, and electrolyte imbalance. Continue to monitor your patient's fluid balance carefully, and note his electrolyte levels when you check his serial blood tests. Expect to replace fluid and electrolytes until his fluid status and electrolyte balance are maintained and his renal tubules regain their ability to concentrate urine.

Your patient will probably return from surgery with an indwelling (Foley) catheter in place. Unless a nephrectomy was performed, expect to see bloody drainage from the catheter. Check the flank dressing for excessive drainage by turning your patient on his side. Also check his pulse and blood pressure frequently for such changes as tachycardia or hypotension, which may indicate hemorrhage. If you detect such signs, call the doctor *immediately*.

Also continue to watch for signs of infection and to give antibiotics, as ordered. To help prevent respiratory infection, reposition your patient periodically and have him perform deep-breathing and coughing exercises frequently. After he becomes ambulatory, encourage him to walk often.

Depending on what material your patient's renal calculus is composed of, maintain your patient's urine pH at the proper level to erradiate the calculus. For example, if your patient's calculus is composed of phosphate, oxalate, or carbonate, expect to *acidify* his urine. If his calculus is composed of uric acid, cystine, or urate, expect to *alkalinize* his urine. You'll probably administer either ascorbic acid (it can be added to the I.V. or given orally), to acidify his urine, or sodium bicarbonate (I.V.), to alkalinize it. Continue to gauge your patient's acid-base balance by testing his urine pH with Nitrazine paper.

If your patient's calculus was an indicator of an underlying disorder, expect to administer the appropriate drug therapy for that disorder. For example, if your patient had gout, his increased uric acid could be reduced by the administration of allopurinol (Zyloprim).

In addition, consult your hospital's dietitian about the proper diet for your patient. For example, if hypercalciuria caused his calculus, he'll need a diet that's low in calcium and phosphorus. This may mean avoiding carbonated soft drinks, cocoa, cheeses, organ meats, breads prepared from self-rising flour, and other calcium- and phosphorous-rich foods. Discuss with your patient (and whoever prepares his food) the importance of following his prescribed diet and drug therapy.

# Urinary Tract Infection

## Prediagnosis summary

At initial assessment, the patient had some of the following signs and symp-

toms suggesting urinary tract infection (UTI):
- suprapubic pain
- dysuria
- urinary frequency
- urinary urgency
- hematuria
- flank pain
- fever
- chills
- nausea and vomiting.

Urine was obtained for analysis and culture, and blood was drawn for a CBC and for BUN, electrolyte, and creatinine testing.

## Priorities

Your first priority is to begin broad-spectrum antibiotic therapy, as ordered, to prevent the patient's UTI from leading to such serious complications as renal failure and septic shock. (See the "Acute Renal Failure" entry in this chapter and the "Septic Shock" entry in Chapter 14.)

If your patient's infection is in his lower urinary tract, expect to administer oral antibiotics. If his infection includes the upper urinary tract, expect to insert a large-bore I.V. catheter and to start parenteral antibiotic therapy. (This will allow the antibiotic to be absorbed faster and more directly.)

## Continuing assessment and intervention

Check your patient's vital signs and mental status often for trends indicating septic shock. If his body temperature and pulse rate increase, his blood pressure decreases, and his level of consciousness deteriorates, call the

---

WARNING

# DANGER: HYDRONEPHROSIS

If your patient's urinary flow is obstructed, be alert for hydronephrosis, which is a dangerous complication of severe urinary tract infections, renal calculi, and other renal problems. Untreated, hydronephrosis will gradually impair kidney function by distending the renal pelvis and calyces, destroying kidney tissue, and causing renal failure. You can help prevent this by learning to recognize the signs and symptoms of hydronephrosis, so your patient receives prompt treatment.

### Signs and symptoms
The onset of hydronephrosis is usually insidious and asymptomatic. As it progresses, however, the patient may experience the following signs and symptoms:
- severe, colicky flank pain or dull flank pain with backache
- urinary frequency and urgency
- nausea and vomiting
- fever, chills, and pyuria
- hematuria.

### Diagnosis
Expect to see ultrasound studies done along with a complete set of X-rays (intravenous pyelography, cystourethrography, cystoscopy, and retrograde pyelography), to confirm the diagnosis.

### Treatment
Once hydronephrosis is diagnosed, intensive treatment begins. The patient may undergo surgery to remove the obstruction, or the doctor may insert a nephrostomy tube temporarily. Expect to administer antimicrobials for aggressive treatment of the infection.

### Nursing considerations
While caring for your patient with hydronephrosis, you may be responsible for:
- assisting with a nephrostomy and caring for the patient's nephrostomy tube and drainage system
- assisting with ureteral catheter placement and caring for the patient's catheter and drainage system
- giving medication for infection, as ordered
- preparing the patient for surgery to remove the obstruction
- watching for signs and symptoms of renal failure, such as uremia, oliguria, anuria, and circulatory overload.

doctor *immediately*. Anticipate inserting a CVP line for massive hydration to restore your patient's blood volume and to improve his cardiac output, thus increasing his kidney perfusion. You'll also need to insert an indwelling (Foley) catheter and to start monitoring his intake and output closely for signs of renal insufficiency. Expect to administer antibiotics, as ordered.

Perform a thorough nursing assessment to help detect the infection's cause. First, find out whether your patient's had recurrent UTIs. If so, how frequently have they occurred, and how have they been treated? Keep in mind that nephrotoxic antibiotics—often the drugs of choice for treating patients with recurrent UTIs—may have predisposed him to renal complications. (See *Nephrotoxin Alert*, page 572.) Keep in mind, too, that recurrent UTIs can be complications of certain renal disorders, such as renal calculi or urethral trauma. Ask if your patient has a history of renal problems or if he's recently had abdominal trauma or surgery. Also ask whether he has any preexisting chronic conditions—such as arteriosclerosis or diabetes—that affect kidney perfusion. If he does, the accompanying decreased urine output may have triggered his UTI.

Encourage your patient to void every 2 to 3 hours to prevent bladder reinfection from bacteria and urine stasis. Check his intake and output, document his voiding pattern (frequency, amount of urine passed at each voiding, dysuria), and test his urine pH frequently. If he's receiving methenamine mandelate (Mandelamine), encourage him to drink juices that are high in ascorbic acid (such as cranberry or orange juice). Why? Because this will help acidify his urine and increase the antibiotic's effectiveness.

If he's receiving a sulfonamide, such as sulfamethoxazole (Gantanol), administer sodium bicarbonate, as ordered, to help alkalinize his urine. This will aid in preventing associated crystalluria by increasing the sulfona-mide's excretion rate. Because these antibiotics sometimes have a nephrotoxic effect, monitor your patient carefully for renal complications. If his BUN and creatinine levels become elevated and his urine output decreases to less than 30 ml/hour, notify the doctor *immediately*. He'll reevaluate your patient's status, and he may adjust the drug therapy if he suspects renal insufficiency.

### Therapeutic care

Administer antipyretics to reduce your patient's fever, phenazopyridine (Pyridium) to relieve his dysuria, and other analgesics to relieve his pain, as ordered.

If your patient has a history of recurrent UTIs, prepare him for radiologic evaluation studies to determine whether his infection's secondary to a functional or a structural abnormality. If he does have such an abnormality, it will have to be corrected to prevent future UTIs. For example, the doctor may resect your patient's prostate if it's obstructing his urine flow and causing reflux. Hydration or surgery, or both, may be needed to eradicate renal calculi. (See the "Renal Calculi" entry in this chapter.) Or, if your patient has a history of urethral trauma, he may need to have a urethral stent inserted to reduce stricture formation, a common complication. (See the "Urethral Trauma" entry in this chapter.)

If your patient has a first-time lower UTI, he'll be able to go home immediately after the doctor prescribes antibiotic therapy. Make sure that he understands the importance of completing the prescribed therapy and of returning for follow-up urinalysis and culture 2 weeks later. Advise him to drink lots of fluids, to void frequently, and to practice good perineal hygiene to prevent a recurrence. Also instruct him to seek medical attention immediately if he develops fever, fatigue, and loss of appetite. These signs and symptoms may mean he's going into septic shock.

# Avulsion or Amputation of the Penis or Scrotum

## Prediagnosis summary

The patient had a history of trauma to the penis or scrotum. Initially, he may also have had:

- total or partial loss of penile or scrotal skin and tissue
- massive bleeding
- extreme pain
- pallor
- signs and symptoms of shock.

A large-bore I.V. catheter was inserted to administer fluid and medication. Rapid fluid replacement was started to prevent shock. Blood was drawn for typing and cross matching, and the patient received blood transfusions. Tetanus prophylaxis was started, if indicated, and analgesics were administered to relieve the patient's pain. A urethrogram was taken to detect accompanying urethral injury. If available, the avulsed or amputated part was wrapped in dressings soaked with Ringer's lactate containing penicillin and streptomycin and then placed on ice. The injured area was covered with a sterile saline–soaked pressure dressing, and ice was applied to reduce pain, swelling, and bleeding.

## Priorities

Your first priority is to prepare your patient for surgery. Bleeding will be surgically controlled, and the avulsed or amputated part—if available and in good condition—will be replanted. If replantation isn't possible, the wound will be debrided and closed with a skin graft. If your patient's lost extensive amounts of penile or scrotal skin, the injured area will be covered with a split-thickness skin graft and stented with glyceryl-soaked cotton. If the blood supply to your patient's testes is marginal, his testes will be surgically

> ## MANAGING ZIPPER INJURIES
>
> Zipper injuries are common and painful. A zipper injury occurs when the skin of the patient's penis gets caught in his trousers' zipper—and stays caught.
>
> Obviously, this is an injury that's both extremely painful *and* embarrassing. Your first priority is to lessen your patient's anxiety: telling him exactly what the doctor's going to do to help him.
>
> The doctor will begin treatment immediately by applying a topical anesthetic, such as lidocaine—for example, Xylocaine 2% jelly. (Depending on the patient's age, cooperativeness, and degree of pain, the doctor may also ask you to give him a sedative.) When this has taken effect, the doctor will hold the zipper firmly and ease it down, a notch or two at a time, while gently disentangling the patient's skin. (This is *never* a surgical procedure; cutting the skin free of the zipper would increase the tissue trauma and could result in deformity or erectile dysfunction.)
>
> Before the patient's discharged from the ED, expect to apply an antiseptic ointment and sterile dressing. Then give him (or his parents, if the patient's a child) these instructions for home care:
> - Apply cold compresses for 12 hours to reduce swelling and pain.
> - If the patient's an adult, he should wear a scrotal support to relieve discomfort and to protect delicate tissues.

implanted in his thigh. This will maintain vascularization and preserve the patient's fertility by keeping his testes at a temperature that allows spermatogenesis. If the urethrogram revealed a urethral injury, the doctor will insert a catheter (to immobilize the urethra and allow it to heal) or perform a temporary cystostomy (to permit healing prior to anastomosis). (See the "Urethral Trauma" entry in this chapter.)

## Continuing assessment and intervention

Check the doctor's orders to find out what postoperative fluids and medications your patient's receiving and at what infusion rate. Continue administering fluids and medications as indicated.

Check your patient's vital signs every 15 minutes for decreased blood pressure and an increasingly faint, rapid pulse, possibly indicating shock. If you note these changes, inform the doctor *immediately* and expect to alter your patient's postoperative fluid replacement rate as ordered.

Perform a thorough nursing assessment to help determine what precipitated your patient's injury. Try to find out when and how the accident happened. If the injury was self-inflicted, a psychiatrist will be consulted because of the possibility that your patient may attempt additional self-mutila-

## COPING WITH GENITAL TRAUMA

In an emergency involving genital loss or damage, a man faces an emotional and social crisis that may be so great it exceeds his concern for his own life. In fact, he may feel that his life's not worth living anymore. He may become depressed, hostile, and even suicidal. You already know how to help a patient deal with grief due to loss of a body part, but do you know how to help a patient cope with loss of his sexual identity and regain his sense of being a "real" man? Here are some approaches you can use.

Begin by taking your cues from the patient. If he's dangerously hostile or hysterical, ask the doctor to prescribe a sedative for him—this is no time to talk. If he remains hostile or becomes suicidal, obtain a referral to a psychotherapist.

If your patient's calm enough to talk with you, encourage him to discuss his sexual fears and apprehensions. Don't push him to talk, but let him know that you're willing to listen and to help. If appropriate, emphasize that when he's recovered from the physical trauma, reconstructive surgery is a possibility. (Although a reconstruction can't fully replace his original penis, it will look close to normal and it will function for urination—and for sexual intercourse, if a prosthesis is implanted.) You can also remind him that other parts of his body, and a variety of mechanical devices, can provide sexual stimulation and satisfaction.

Your patient probably won't fully accept his new self-image while he's in the hospital. Obtain a referral to a professional sex counselor, and have the counselor see your patient in the hospital. Even if he isn't interested in seeing a counselor now, make sure he knows that this service will be available when his interest in sexual activity returns.

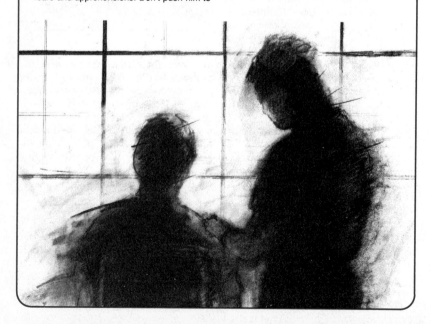

tion. Safeguard your patient by removing environmental hazards, and be prepared to intervene as needed to restrain him. Take your patient's drug history—he may require drug rehabilitation or detoxification.

Your patient will return from surgery with an indwelling (Foley) catheter, perineal urethrostomy, or suprapubic catheter inserted to drain his urine. Check the patency of his urine drainage tube frequently. If it becomes obstructed, notify the doctor *immediately* and be prepared to assist with irrigation. (See *Caring for Urinary Drainage Tubes*, pages 586 to 589.) Monitor your patient's intake and output to assess his fluid status, and take serial urine specimens to note changes in color (indicating increasing or decreasing hematuria) or character (indicating possible infection). Inform the doctor if the patient's urine output drops below 30 ml/hour, or if you suspect increasing hematuria or infection. Expect to adjust your patient's fluid or medication infusion, as ordered.

Check your patient's catheter insertion site, surgical incisions, and graft site for purulent or bloody drainage. Inform the doctor *immediately* if you see copious drainage or if your patient complains of increased pain. (As you know, these signs and symptoms may indicate infection or rebleeding.) Culture the infection site, and expect to change your patient's antibiotic therapy as ordered. If the doctor suspects rebleeding, he'll ask you to apply a pressure dressing to control the bleeding.

A patient who's had skin grafted over his injury will return from surgery wearing a dressing that's thick at the midshaft, to exert pressure on the graft. Check the dressing for proper placement—it should be taped upright on his abdomen to elevate and immobilize the penis so the graft site can heal without contracture. Check the color and temperature of the glans penis frequently to evaluate his circulatory status. Call the doctor *immediately* if the circulation becomes compromised. The

doctor will reassess your patient and loosen the pressure dressing. If the patient's circulation doesn't improve, the doctor may need to amputate your patient's penis, because gangrene can threaten his life.

### Therapeutic care

As with all postoperative patients, maintain pulmonary hygiene by encouraging frequent turning and deep-breathing and coughing exercises. Also continue your patient's antibiotic and analgesic therapy, as ordered.

Your patient will require considerable help to overcome anxiety due to changes in his body image and to actual or potential loss of function. Of course, you'll provide emotional support, but you'll also need to be sensitive to your patient's need for privacy. Be prepared to make arrangements, too, if the doctor feels that your patient requires sexual or psychiatric counseling.

# Testicular Torsion

### Prediagnosis summary

On initial assessment, the patient had some combination of these signs and symptoms:

- sudden onset of testicular pain radiating into his lower abdomen
- a shortened, thickened spermatic cord
- nausea and vomiting
- a testicle riding high in his scrotum
- scrotal edema, tenderness, and firmness
- a scrotal hydrocele
- fever.

Blood was drawn for a CBC, electrolytes, BUN, prothrombin time (PT), and partial thromboplastin time (PTT). A urine specimen was obtained for analysis. Blood flow to the patient's testes was assessed with a Doppler stethoscope and was found to be decreased or absent. The scrotum was transilluminated and may have revealed a hydrocele or a blue-black dot, indicating torsion of the testicular appendage.

## Priorities

Because testicular torsion can quickly result in permanent testicular injury and sterility, your first priority is to prepare your patient for emergency surgery to untwist and permanently stabilize the spermatic cord or to remove the twisted appendage and evacuate the hydrocele, if present. Insert a large-bore I.V. catheter to keep his vein open for fluid and medication administration. While the operating room's being prepared, elevate his testicle on a rolled-up towel—sometimes this will allow the cord to untwist spontaneously. Apply an ice pack on his scrotum to reduce pain and swelling. In addition, the doctor may attempt to untwist the cord manually. First, he'll administer a local anesthetic. Even if either of these preoperative measures is effective, your patient will still need surgery to tack the spermatic cord permanently in place.

## Continuing assessment and intervention

Focus your postoperative assessment on detecting and preventing complications.

Your patient will return from surgery with an I.V. in place. Check the I.V. for the proper postoperative solution and infusion rate, and continue administering fluids and medications as indicated. Expect to administer analgesics, antipyretics (if he has a fever), and prophylactic antibiotics.

Check the dressings for bloody or purulent drainage, and change them when they become moist. If drainage is excessive, notify the doctor. Your patient may also have a Penrose drain inserted to remove accumulated fluid. Whether or not a drain was inserted, he'll be wearing a scrotal support to hold dressings in place.

Monitor your patient's intake and output. Because of postoperative pain at the incision site, he may have difficulty voiding, fearing that this will make his pain worse. If he hasn't voided within 8 hours of surgery, he may have urinary retention. Notify the doctor and expect to insert a straight catheter to drain accumulated urine from the patient's bladder.

### Therapeutic care

Your patient will probably be able to return home 48 hours after surgery. In the meantime, keep him comfortable by

PATHOPHYSIOLOGY

## WHAT HAPPENS IN TESTICULAR TORSION

Testicular torsion—twisting of the spermatic cord and its testicle—usually occurs in boys age 18 and younger. Because of an anatomic abnormality, the patient's epididymis and testicle aren't attached to the scrotal wall. This allows the testicle to dangle in the scrotum so that the cord twists easily. Strenuous activity or an injury may cause a cremaster muscle spasm and torsion, or torsion can happen spontaneously.

Once twisted, the spermatic cord obstructs normal blood flow. This causes swelling and pain and can progress to thrombosis, ischemia, and infarction. If surgical detorsion isn't performed within 6 hours, testicular necrosis and infertility can result.

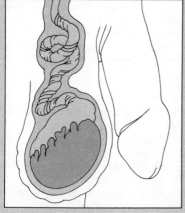

continuing to administer analgesics to relieve his pain. Encourage him to wear his scrotal support both when he's at rest and when he's walking.

To prevent postoperative respiratory infection, have your patient perform deep-breathing and coughing exercises frequently. Also continue to administer antibiotics, as ordered.

The doctor will remove your patient's Penrose drain (if one was inserted) and ask you to discontinue the I.V. infusion. Keep checking his scrotal dressings for drainage. Remind your patient to return for suture removal 7 to 10 days after surgery.

# Priapism

## Prediagnosis summary
Initially, the patient had some combination of the following:
• painful, prolonged erection of the corpora cavernosa
• a flaccid glans penis and corpus spongiosum
• urinary retention
• extreme anxiety
• a history of sickle cell disease, tumor, thrombus, or leukemia.

A large-bore I.V. catheter was inserted for fluid and medication access. Blood was drawn for a CBC and for hemoglobin electrophoresis and sickle cell preparation.

## Priorities
To relieve your patient's pain, apply an ice pack to his penis and administer analgesics, as ordered. Then insert an indwelling (Foley) catheter, as ordered, to relieve urinary retention.

Your next priority is to help evacuate the viscous blood from his corpora cavernosa as quickly as possible. If his priapism's *secondary* to a chronic or malignant condition, your specific intervention will depend on the precipitating cause. For example, if his priapism is a result of sickle cell crisis,

expect to begin massive hydration immediately to break up the sickling cycle, and anticipate administering an exchange blood transfusion. (See the "Sickle Cell Crisis" entry in Chapter 11.) If his priapism's due to a tumor in the corpora cavernosa, prepare your patient for emergency irradiation of the site. Expect to infuse heparin if a thrombus triggered the priapism. And if leukemia's the cause, the doctor may ask you to administer a chemotherapeutic agent, such as cytosine arabinoside, to quickly reduce the number of white blood cells in your patient's circulation. Secondary priapism should disappear once initial treatment of the underlying condition begins.

You may be asked to give your patient an ice water enema or to administer a narcotic, such as Demerol (meperi-

PATHOPHYSIOLOGY

## WHAT HAPPENS IN PRIAPISM

Priapism is continuous and painful penile erection unrelated to sexual stimulation—an emergency that requires swift treatment to prevent irreversible complications. Priapism can be idiopathic or it can be associated with:
• sickle cell anemia or sickle cell trait (found in carriers)
• trauma
• instrumentation
• a tumor within the penis
• acute leukemia
• spinal cord injuries
• side effects of certain drugs (such as trazodone, chlorpromazine, hydralazine, prazosin).

Priapism occurs when nerve damage or a penile or pelvic vascular thrombosis prevents the corpora cavernosa's veins from draining normally. Consequently, the penis becomes engorged and persistently erect.

Unless priapism is treated within a few hours, penile tissue becomes ischemic, the corpora cavernosa becomes fibrotic, and the patient may become impotent. If ischemia persists, penile gangrene may also develop.

dine), to stimulate venous dilation and to help release sequestered blood. If these efforts don't cause the erection to subside, expect to assist the doctor with irrigation of the corpora cavernosa using saline or 10% heparin solution. If this effort also fails, expect to prepare your patient for surgery. He'll receive local caudal or spinal anesthesia, which may cause the penis to become flaccid spontaneously. If it doesn't, the doctor will insert a corpus spongiosum shunt to drain the engorged blood vessels.

### Continuing assessment and intervention

If conservative measures corrected your patient's idiopathic priapism, his presenting signs and symptoms will disappear as soon as his erection subsides, and he'll be released from the hospital. If he required surgery, your assessment will focus on detecting and preventing postoperative complications.

Your patient will return from surgery with a Foley catheter. Check his intake and output for indications of continued urinary retention, and anticipate hydrating him if his output drops below 30 ml/hour.

If your patient's on a postoperative heparin infusion, obtain blood for serial PT and PTT testing. Check your patient's laboratory results, I.V. insertion site, and vital signs frequently for signs of anticoagulant overdose (highly elevated PTT, oozing blood, decreased blood pressure). If you suspect an anticoagulant overdose, *immediately* inform the doctor and stop the heparin infusion. Expect to administer protamine sulfate to neutralize the anticoagulant. (See the "Anticoagulant Overdose" entry in Chapter 11.)

To prevent recurrence of priapism while he's recovering from surgery, your patient's penis will be secured against his perineum with pressure dressings. Make sure the dressings are properly placed, and assess the penis for circulatory compromise. Look for discoloration from poor capillary refill

and for ecchymotic swelling from hematoma formation. Check the penis for warmth, too. If you suspect circulatory compromise, tell the doctor *immediately*. Expect either to flush the corpus spongiosum shunt with heparin solution or to prepare your patient for surgery so the thrombus can be removed.

### Therapeutic care

To prevent postoperative infection and to relieve your patient's pain, continue to administer antibiotics and analgesics, as ordered.

The doctor will ask you to remove your patient's Foley catheter to establish whether he can urinate normally. If he doesn't void within 8 hours, and if efforts to stimulate urination are unsuccessful, inform the doctor and anticipate recatheterizing your patient.

Remember: Priapism can be both frightening and puzzling for your patient. To help relieve his confusion, take the time to explain all the procedures you're doing. He may also need sexual or psychiatric counseling; arrange for consultations with the appropriate hospital staff, if necessary.

## A FINAL WORD

As a nurse, you may know that the signs and symptoms of GU emergencies can be difficult to detect—particularly in patients with other serious illnesses or injuries. For example, if a patient's been hit by a car, you expect to see obvious trauma-related injuries that demand your immediate attention. But equally serious damage to his GU system may not be readily apparent. Why? Because the ribs and other organs protect the GU organs (except for the male genitalia). So be sure to take the time to carefully assess your patient with multiple trauma for GU injuries, especially if he has trauma to his abdomen, back, or genitalia.

Many nontraumatic GU emergencies are also difficult to detect. Yet, if they go unnoticed and untreated, GU conditions such as renal calculi or UTI can become emergencies—fast. For instance, an untreated UTI can lead to sepsis, which has a 50% mortality.

Fortunately, recent advances in managing patients with GU disorders are helping to prevent many of these patients' problems from escalating into emergencies. The incidence of shock, infection, and organ failure associated with GU disorders is decreasing, and new techniques are simplifying therapy. For example, single-dose antimicrobials for UTIs not only combat infection but also can indicate your patient's need for further diagnostic tests. New drugs, such as sodium cellulose phosphate, suppress formation of renal calculi. And new techniques are gradually replacing major surgery for renal calculi. For instance, extracorporeal shock wave lithotripsy uses underwater sound waves to break renal calculi into fine particles that can be excreted painlessly. Another method for removing calculi is percutaneous ultrasound lithotripsy. This technique involves passing an instrument through a nephrostomy tube and shattering the patient's calculi with ultrasound waves. The therapy is low in cost and has few complications and a short recovery period.

And now that clean intermittent self-catheterization is starting to be preferred over long-term catheter drainage, fewer patients will develop cystitis, epididymitis, urethritis, or fistulae.

Providing emotional support for patients with GU emergencies is especially challenging. Why? Because some GU emergencies (penile amputation or avulsion, for example) affect much more than your male patient's physical well-being—such a mutilating injury can confuse his sexual identity, too, and this may ultimately be more debilitating than his physical problem. Fortunately, new advances in reconstructive surgery and penile implants make today's prostheses more lifelike *and* more functional. So a prosthesis can do much to restore your patient's sexual function and his self-esteem. But he'll still need your strong support to complete his recovery.

## Selected References

Harwood, A.L. "Urologic Emergencies," *Emergency Medicine* 15(6): 112-26, March 30, 1983.

Kidd P.S. "Trauma of the Genitourinary System," *Journal of Emergency Nursing* 8(5): 232-38, September/October 1982.

McDougal, W. Scott, and Persky, Lester. *Traumatic Injuries of the Genetourinary System*, Vol. 1. Baltimore: Williams & Wilkins, Co., 1980.

Rosen, Peter, et al. *Emergency Medicine: Concepts and Clinical Practice*, 2 vols. St. Louis: C.V. Mosby Co., 1983.

Smith, Donald R. *General Urology*, 10th ed. Los Altos, Calif.: Lange Medical Pubns., 1981.

# 14

# Shock

## Introduction

At 7:15 one morning, you're getting a report as you start your shift. The night nurse, Mary Carrington, tells you she's concerned about Mrs. Laura Wolther in room 303—in fact, Mary's just called the doctor, and he's on his way. Meanwhile, he's ordered oxygen and asked that Mary and you prepare Mrs. Wolther for transfer to the intensive care unit.

While you begin caring for Mrs. Wolther, Mary summarizes her case, explaining that the 50-year-old woman was admitted 2 days ago because of her stress incontinence and frequent urinary tract infections. Blood work was done on admission; her complete blood count (CBC) showed an elevated white blood cell count. Her chest X-ray was normal. Her admission urine sample was cloudy and dark, with a foul odor; a culture-and-sensitivity test was sent. She had a cystoscopy today, and her vital signs were stable after the procedure (blood pressure 140/80, pulse 74, respiratory rate 22, temperature 99.6° F. [37.6° C.]).

Next, Mary tells you that the evening nurse noticed that Mrs. Wolther's temperature was increased—to 103.2° F. (39.6° C.)—and that her skin was flushed and warm. Her blood pressure and urine output were normal, but she was tachycardic, tachypneic, and slightly confused. The evening nurse gave Mrs. Wolther acetaminophen (Tylenol), believing that her tachypnea, tachycardia, warm skin, and slight confusion were due to her elevated temperature.

Throughout her night shift, Mary checked on Mrs. Wolther regularly. She observed no significant change in her patient's condition until 4 a.m. when Mrs. Wolther's temperature had decreased to 102.2° F. (39° C.). Mary's other findings included:

• normal blood pressure
• cool skin
• thirst
• decreased urine output
• slight ankle edema.

At first, these findings weren't alarming. But by 7:00 a.m., Mrs. Wolther's condition was clearly deteriorating. Now, as you come on your shift, Mrs. Wolther's skin is cold and clammy, her pulse is thready, and her blood pressure is sharply decreased. She's also confused and struggling to breathe. You know the doctor's on his way, but you don't need to wait for his diagnosis to recognize that she's a high-risk patient who probably has septic shock.

Now that Mrs. Wolther's so sick, you realize that her signs and symptoms correspond to the three stages of septic shock: warm (early, or hyperdynamic), cool (intermediate, or normodynamic), and cold (late, or hypodynamic). Why

# MANAGING AN ALLERGIC REACTION TO A BEE STING

As a nurse, you probably know that the incidence of severe allergic reactions to bee stings is very low. But, of course, you also know that when it happens, this type of reaction can be a life-threatening emergency. Are you fully confident that you know how to recognize the signs and symptoms of anaphylactic shock and how to intervene appropriately? What if the victim stopped breathing and didn't respond to your resuscitation efforts—could you perform an emergency cricothyrotomy to open his airway? Here's how to respond *when you're the only one around to help.*

Quickly assess your patient's skin around the sting. If it's red and inflamed, and if hives are forming, he's having an allergic reaction and is in danger of developing anaphylactic shock.

Immediately ask him if he has an anaphylaxis kit (many people with known allergies carry such kits). If he does, help him inject the epinephrine, then massage the injection site vigorously to speed the distribution of epinephrine throughout his body.

The injection should relieve the reaction; but if a kit's not available, the patient's anaphylaxis will worsen rapidly.

Assess his airway, and ask him if he's having trouble breathing or if he feels as though his throat is closing up. Quickly check his pulse—a rapid, thready pulse is an early sign of shock—and inspect the sting site. Remove the stinger if you can do so quickly, to prevent further antigen release. If no stinger's visible and the site's extremely inflamed, you may want to apply a tourniquet (using a scarf or a belt) just above the sting site. But don't dwell on this problem, because your patient's airway may be severely compromised within a very short time.

The patient may become dyspneic as bronchospasm and laryngeal edema develop and compromise his airway and breathing. If he stops breathing, you'll have to open his airway and begin CPR.

Laryngeal edema can progress so that it completely closes the patient's airway, making CPR ineffective. If this happens, and if all your resuscitation efforts fail, prepare to perform a criocothyrotomy.

Place the patient in a supine position, and hyperextend his head slightly while keeping his neck straight. Gently grasp his trachea and slide your fingers downward. You'll feel a large prominence, the thyroid cartilage, and then a smaller prominence directly below, the cricoid cartilage. The cricothyroid membrane lies between the two cartilages.

Cut or stab a small (½″) hole through the cricothyroid membrane into the trachea. Insert something hollow to keep the airway open—a drinking straw or the barrel of a ballpoint pen, for example.

Once the airway's in place and the victim's breathing is restored, get him to a hospital as quickly as possible. He'll need treatment for anaphylactic shock (epinephrine administration and fluid infusion), as well as establishment of a patent airway by intubation or tracheostomy.

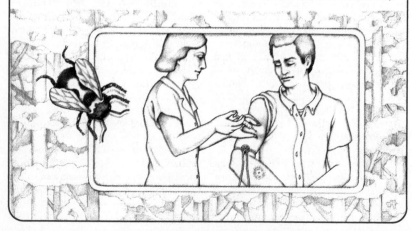

didn't the fact that Mrs. Wolther was going into septic shock become apparent sooner? Because, as you know, *all* types of shock have several stages, some with confusing signs and symptoms that can be very difficult to assess accurately. This is why many patients in shock unfortunately end up like Mrs. Wolther—in situations where even aggressive medical treatment and expert nursing care may come too late to ensure their survival.

Anytime a patient's serious illness or injury includes a disturbance of his circulatory system, he's at risk for going into shock. You may see:

• hypovolemic shock, when a patient's circulating *blood volume* is decreased

• cardiogenic shock, when a patient's *heart* can't pump effectively

• septic shock, neurogenic shock, or anaphylactic shock (collectively called vasogenic shock), when a patient's *vessel tone and size* are altered.

Each of these shock processes leads to inadequate tissue perfusion and, eventually, to inadequate cellular perfusion and deranged microcirculation.

Because all types of shock are complex conditions associated with high mortality, a patient in shock challenges your nursing skills to the limit. But if you can recognize, assess, and care for his shock state promptly, you can improve his chances of overcoming this life-threatening emergency.

## INITIAL CARE

# Prehospital Care: What's Been Done

The insult that precipitated your patient's shock was probably evident: for example, trauma with hemorrhage, suspected myocardial infarction (MI), overwhelming infection, spinal cord injury, or a recent insect sting (in a patient with a history of allergies).

Your patient had signs of shock that probably included a decreased level of consciousness, some degree of hypotension, and alterations in skin color and moisture. If rescue personnel suspected *hypovolemic shock* because of the patient's obvious external bleeding or signs of trauma suggesting internal bleeding, they may have placed the patient supine with his feet elevated 20° to 30°. They attempted to stop external bleeding by applying pressure and, if an extremity was affected, by elevating it. They probably gave him oxygen by nasal cannula or mask and (if qualified) started cardiac monitoring and started an I.V. line with a rapid infusion of Ringer's lactate solution. If the patient was obviously hemorrhaging, they may have applied medical antishock trousers (a MAST suit).

If the patient had signs and symptoms that suggested an MI causing *cardiogenic shock,* they probably gave him oxygen and, if qualified, started cardiac monitoring and started an I.V. at a keep-vein-open rate. They may have given him nitroglycerin sublingually, and they may have given him morphine if his blood pressure was stable. (If it was decreased, they *won't* have given morphine, because this further decreases blood pressure.)

Warm skin, diffuse erythema, or difficulty breathing after recent drug administration or an insect bite or sting alerted rescue personnel to suspect the patient had *anaphylactic shock.* They immediately took steps to protect his airway, if necessary, and—if qualified and equipped to do so—they may have intubated him and administered subcutaneous or possibly I.V. epinephrine. If these steps weren't possible, they provided high-flow oxygen by mask and rushed him directly to the hospital. (The laryngeal edema that accompanies anaphylactic shock may cause airway occlusion quickly, making intubation impossible.) If the patient had signs and symptoms of vascular collapse but hadn't yet developed an airway problem, they placed him supine with his feet elevated 20° to 30°, gave him oxygen, observed his airway closely, and started I.V. fluids.

In caring for a patient with flushed, warm skin and an increased temperature, rescue personnel may have suspected infection and *septic shock.* They probably gave this patient oxygen, started an I.V. at a keep-vein-open rate, and kept him cool.

A patient who suffered spinal cord trauma was first immobilized with a hard collar and then was placed on a backboard. Then, if rescue personnel suspected that the patient might develop *neurogenic shock,* they administered oxygen and started an I.V. at a keep-vein-open rate.

Because shock is so life-threatening, rescue personnel rushed the patient to the hospital with all possible speed.

# What to Do First

As you know, your patient won't just "get" shock—it's a complex syndrome he'll develop as his body responds to a disorder that's causing inadequate circulation or tissue perfusion. Shock's a dynamic process—when your patient's body begins to feel the effects of his compromised circulation, he enters a cycle of compensatory and decompensatory responses that can easily end in death. (See *Shock: Compensation,* pages 620 and 621, and *Shock: Decompensation,* pages 622 and 623.) Once he enters this cycle, his recovery potential depends on what caused his shock, whether his shock is treatable, and how far it's progressed.

With a patient in shock, you won't always be able to anticipate what's going to happen next. But you can count on this: His condition will change rapidly, sometimes from minute to minute. If you intervene rapidly and appropriately, you may help reverse the shock cycle. If you don't, he'll move from compensated shock to decompensated shock—and, he may die.

What does this mean to you when you first assess a patient in shock? Mainly this—that your accurate monitoring of *trends* may be more important than individual assessment observations. Keep this in mind when you perform your initial assessment of your patient's airway, breathing, and circulation. As always, you must be prepared to intervene immediately if you detect any threat to these vital functions. Also remember to start accurate record keeping, because this is the best way to measure changes and uncover trends in your patient's condition.

## Airway

Check the patency of your patient's airway. Look, listen, and feel for air movement, and note any gurgling or gasping. If food, blood, vomitus, or the patient's tongue is obstructing his airway, clear it immediately using the techniques described in the "Life Support" section in Chapter 3. If necessary, insert an oral or nasal airway or assist with endotracheal intubation as required.

If your patient has *anaphylactic shock,* rapid onset of airway-obstructing edema is a life-threatening hazard. He may have laryngeal edema, general airway edema, or edema of his tongue; the edema may have been so severe that rescue personnel were unable to insert an endotracheal tube and could only give him oxygen by mask as they rushed him to the hospital. Expect to assist with emergency cricothyrotomy if the doctor can't intubate the patient once he reaches the hospital. (See the "Life Support" section in Chapter 3.) Expect to give subcutaneous, I.V., or I.M. epinephrine to reduce bronchospasm and edema. You may also give epinephrine directly, through the patient's endotracheal tube (if the doctor's been able to insert one).

## Breathing

Assess the quality of your patient's respirations. His breathing may be compromised by his shock state or by the injury or illness that caused his shock—for example:

• chest trauma (see Chapters 4 and 5)
• central nervous system (CNS) damage resulting from head injury, spinal cord injury, or anesthesia (see Chapter 6)
• pulmonary edema resulting from heart failure (see Chapter 5).

For a patient with compromised breathing, provide oxygen as needed to support his breathing, or begin assisted ventilation if necessary.

If your patient's shock state is compromising his breathing, watch particularly for tachypnea—a valuable warning sign that occurs early in all forms of shock. (The mechanisms that cause shock-related tachypnea may differ—if your patient has hypovolemic shock, for instance, his respirations will increase in an attempt to maximize red blood cell oxygen saturation, whereas in septic shock they'll increase in response to circulating endotoxin.) If your patient has tachypnea, notify the doctor *immediately*. Expect him to order arterial blood gas (ABG) analysis. Provide oxygen by nasal cannula or mask, remembering that the patient will need more oxygen because of the tissue hypoxia that all shock states cause. If your patient continues to have tachypnea, he may tire and need intubation and ventilatory support.

## Circulation

Assess your patient's circulatory status by evaluating his pulse, capillary refill, and blood pressure. Expect some degree of circulatory dysfunction, because shock always causes hemodynamic problems. Hypovolemia, pump failure, and massive vasodilation, in particular, may be immediately life-threatening.

Start by checking your patient's pulse. Palpate for a radial pulse first—if it's present, you know his systolic pressure's 80 mm Hg or greater and

that he has some measure of perfusion. If you don't feel a radial pulse, palpate for a femoral or carotid pulse. If you can palpate his femoral pulse, you know his systolic pressure's 70 mm Hg or greater. If you can palpate his carotid pulse, you know his systolic pressure's 60 mm Hg or greater. Note his

PRIORITIES

## INITIAL ASSESSMENT CHECKLIST

**Assess the ABCs first and intervene appropriately.**

**Check for:**
• altered mental status, indicating decreased cerebral tissue perfusion (early sign)
• tachycardia, indicating decreased cardiac output (early sign)
• tachypnea, indicating poor tissue perfusion (early sign) and acidosis (late sign)
• pale, cool, and clammy skin, indicating compensatory sympathetic response (early sign); or warm, flushed, dry skin, indicating vasodilation (early sign of septic shock).

**Intervene by:**
• positioning the patient properly
• administering supplemental oxygen
• inserting at least one large-bore I.V. and administering fluids
• taking a 12-lead EKG and establishing cardiac monitoring
• administering appropriate medications, such as antibiotics, vasoactive drugs, or corticosteroids.

**Prepare for:**
• blood transfusion, if the patient's hemorrhaging
• central venous pressure line insertion
• Swan-Ganz catheter and arterial line insertion
• medical antishock trousers (MAST suit) application
• autotransfusion
• colloid and crystalloid replacement.

# YOUR ROLE IN AN EMERGENCY

## APPLYING AND REMOVING A M.A.S.T. SUIT

As an early step in treating your patient in hypovolemic shock, expect to apply medical antishock trousers (a MAST suit). The suit has three inflatable chambers—one for the abdomen and one for each leg. Inflating the chambers with a foot-operated air pump exerts external pneumatic pressure on your patient's lower body, much like a large blood pressure cuff. This helps to stem or reverse the hypovolemic shock process by redirecting blood from his legs and pelvis to his central circulation. The result? Restored central blood volume, which increases perfusion to your patient's heart, lungs, and brain and increases blood pressure, stabilizing him while you begin fluid replacement therapy. Caution: Never apply a MAST suit to a patient with pulmonary edema or congestive heart failure. Apply it cautiously to a dyspneic or pregnant patient or to one who's sustained head injuries.

### Applying a MAST suit
• Place your patient in the supine position.

If he's wearing a belt or shoes, remove them.
• If possible, insert a nasogastric tube and an indwelling (Foley) catheter before inflating the suit; otherwise, the increased intraabdominal pressure from the suit can cause the patient to vomit, defecate, or urinate.
• Unfold the MAST suit and lay it flat at your patient's feet.
• Slide the suit under your patient until it reaches the margin of his lowest rib.
• Wrap a leg chamber around each of his legs and secure it with the Velcro strips. Then wrap and secure the abdominal chamber.
• Connect the pressure control unit to the tubing on each chamber; connect the foot pump to the pressure control unit.
• Take your patient's baseline vital signs; leave the blood pressure cuff on his arm for repeat readings as you inflate the suit.
• Starting with his legs, inflate each chamber to an initial pressure of 20 to 30 mm Hg. Always inflate the abdominal

**MAST suit ready to receive patient**

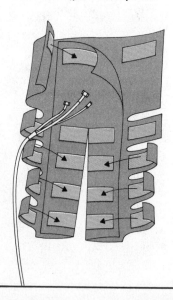

**MAST suit application**

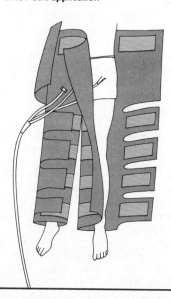

chamber last to prevent blood from pooling in his legs.

• Monitor your patient's blood pressure as you inflate each chamber. Increase the suit pressure in increments of 20 mm Hg until his systolic pressure reaches 100 to 110 mm Hg.

• Once the suit's inflated, monitor your patient's arterial blood gases and tidal volume to detect possible respiratory acidosis.

• Check the pressure of each compartment hourly for any increase or decrease—it should remain stable.

• Check the arterial pulses of your patient's feet to be sure his arterial blood flow isn't obstructed.

**Removing a MAST suit**

• When deflating the suit, always have

blood and I.V. fluid replacements available.

• Deflate the suit one chamber at a time, starting with the abdominal chamber. *Slowly* decrease the pressure over 30 to 60 minutes, in increments of 5 mm Hg, checking your patient's blood pressure each time. (Never deflate the suit suddenly—your patient's blood pressure may fall too quickly, causing irreversible shock.)

• If, during one of the times you're decreasing the suit's pressure, your patient's systolic pressure drops more than 5 mm Hg, stop deflation immediately until his blood pressure stabilizes, or reinflate the suit if necessary.

• Leave the deflated trousers in place for 12 hours before removing them.

**MAST suit fully inflated and connected**

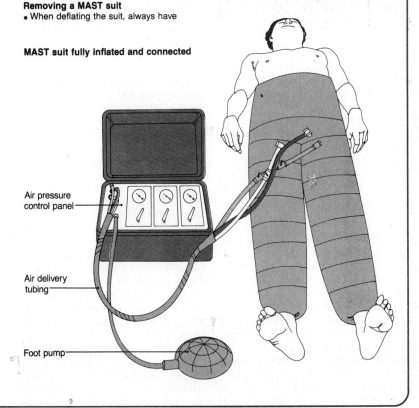

Air pressure control panel

Air delivery tubing

Foot pump

## FINDING A VEIN

As you know, your first priority for a patient in hypovolemic shock is beginning fluid replacement therapy. But when you prepare to do a venipuncture for an I.V., don't be surprised if you can't find a vein. Shock causes your patient's veins to constrict, making them difficult to locate. Here are some tips to help you find a vein when your patient's in shock:

• Drape his arm over the side of his bed so it's below the level of his heart; then apply a soft-rubber tourniquet. This will inhibit venous return and cause the arm veins to fill with blood, bringing them to the surface.

• If you can't locate an arm or hand vein, try to find a vein in your patient's legs or feet.

• If you still can't find a vein, try a blind stick—attempt a venipuncture at a spot where you expect a vein to be, based on your knowledge of vein locations and previous experience.

pulse quality and rate—as you probably know, a weak, thready, rapid pulse is a danger sign indicating decreased volume or decreased tissue perfusion. A slow pulse may indicate your patient's developing cardiogenic shock or neurogenic shock.

Quickly check your patient's capillary refill time by pressing his nail beds or forehead and counting the seconds from the time you release the pressure until color returns. If refill time is greater than 2 seconds, your patient has decreased perfusion and peripheral vasoconstriction.

Auscultate his blood pressure only if the patient's pulse and capillary refill time aren't seriously compromised. Most patients with shock won't develop hypotension until the compensatory mechanisms of tachycardia and vasoconstriction fail and cardiac output begins to drop—in fact, blood pressure in a patient who's in early shock may be normal or even slightly elevated, so it won't tell you much initially. This means you shouldn't rely on hypotension as an indicator of shock; you need to intervene *before* your patient develops this sign.

As shock progresses, your patient's blood pressure will drop, and perfusion to his heart and brain will be compromised if his arterial pressure falls below 70 mm Hg.

If your patient has changes in his pulse rate (rapid or slow) and pulse quality (weak and thready), or delayed capillary refill, assess him quickly for external wounds and for signs or symptoms of internal bleeding. Control any external hemorrhage with direct pressure; place him in the supine position with his feet elevated 20° to 30°; and apply a MAST suit, if ordered, to increase vital organ perfusion and central volume (see *Applying and Removing a M.A.S.T. Suit*, pages 614 and 615). Start several large-bore I.V. lines, and prepare to infuse fluids rapidly (see *Understanding Colloid and Crystalloid Solutions* in the Appendix and *Finding a Vein*). If your patient has no signs of hemorrhage, his shock state may be due to sepsis, cardiac injury, anaphylaxis, or spinal cord injury. Start an I.V. at a keep-vein-open rate to provide access for medications and rapid fluid infusion, if necessary.

Expect to assist the doctor with insertion of an arterial line, a Swan-Ganz catheter, or a central venous pressure (CVP) line. (See *Hemodynamic Monitoring*, pages 636 and 637, and *Monitoring Central Venous Pressure*, pages 642 and 643.) Insert an indwelling (Foley) catheter, if ordered, to measure the patient's urine output. Take a 12-lead EKG and start cardiac monitoring. *Watch closely for dysrhythmias.* All forms of shock (especially cardiogenic and septic shock) predispose your patient to dysrhythmias, which can make his hemodynamic problems even worse (see the "Cardiac Dysrhythmias" entry in Chapter 5).

Draw blood for laboratory studies as ordered and, if your patient's hemorrhaging, draw blood for typing and cross-matching as well.

## General appearance

Check your patient's skin color, temperature, and moisture. If your patient has hypovolemic or cardiogenic shock, he'll probably have cool, pale, clammy skin—a reflection of the peripheral vasoconstriction induced by his decreased perfusion. However, if he's in an early stage of septic, neurogenic, or anaphylactic shock (the vasogenic forms of shock), he'll probably have warm, flushed skin. This is a reflection of the vasodilation that occurs initially. So a patient can be in shock *without* having cool, clammy skin—which *will* develop later if his shock isn't detected early.

## Mental status

Pay close attention to alterations in your patient's mental status. Restlessness, anxiety, and apprehension may, of course, reflect his pain or fears about his emergency illness or injury. But they're also early indicators of decreased cerebral perfusion and hypoxia. (In fact, these may be your earliest indication that your patient's going into shock.) If your patient's confused, stuporous, or comatose, you know that his cerebral perfusion is probably reduced and that he may be in a late stage of shock. (See *Recognizing the Stages of Shock*, page 618.)

## What to Do Next

Begin your secondary assessment only after you've assessed your patient's airway, breathing, and circulation and intervened as necessary. As soon as possible:

• identify the *precipitating factors* that led to your patient's shock state
• identify his *type of shock*.

Caring for a patient in shock is a two-track process that involves correcting the underlying cause *and* reversing the physiologic shock cycle. Your assessment must be rapid, because you need to start intervening immediately. (See the "Definitive Care" section for specific interventions for each type of shock.) But you can't afford to be in such a hurry that you overlook subtle signs and symptoms. These may help you identify the type of shock your patient's developing, so you can provide the best possible care.

Here's a useful approach to determining whether your patient's going into shock.

Remember that shock always develops in response to injury or illness, so identifying your patient's emergency condition may help you quickly determine his risk of going into shock. If your patient's suffered a massive MI, for example, you know he's at risk for *cardiogenic* shock. If he's been in a car accident and has a fractured pelvis, he's at risk for *hypovolemic* shock.

Learn to recognize the early-warning signs common to all types of shock that indicate your patient's entered the shock cycle: alterations in consciousness, tachycardia, and tachypnea.

An *alteration in consciousness* may be your earliest indication that your patient's going into shock, because decreased tissue perfusion and subsequent hypoxia affect the CNS rapidly (see *Recognizing the Stages of Shock*, page 618). Initially, increased epinephrine secretion will cause anxiety and restlessness in your patient; then, as his intravascular volume drops, cerebral hypoprofusion will cause apathy, confusion, and lethargy. Suspect shock whenever your previously alert and oriented patient becomes confused. Report such a change to the doctor *immediately*.

*Tachycardia,* another early-warning sign of shock, results directly from one of the body's first compensatory responses: sympathetic nervous system stimulation aimed at improving cardiac output and tissue perfusion. This is effective for a while. But, as a skilled nurse, you know that this compensa-

# RECOGNIZING THE STAGES OF SHOCK

Because shock is a dynamic process, your patient's stability is difficult to maintain; he may improve or deteriorate rapidly, as the process reverses or progresses. Recognizing the signs and symptoms of each stage of shock will help you classify your patient's condition according to its severity so you can intervene appropriately.

## EARLY OR COMPENSATORY STAGE
- Restlessness, irritability, apprehension
- Slightly increased heart rate
- Normal blood pressure, or slightly elevated systolic pressure or slightly decreased diastolic pressure
- Mild orthostatic blood pressure changes (15 to 25 mm Hg)
- Normal or slightly decreased urine output
- Pale and cool skin in hypovolemic shock; warm and flushed skin in septic, anaphylactic, and neurogenic shock
- Slightly increased respiratory rate
- Slightly decreased body temperature (except fever in septic shock)

## INTERMEDIATE OR PROGRESSIVE STAGE
- Listlessness, apathy, confusion, slowed speech
- Tachycardia
- Weak and thready pulse
- Decreased blood pressure
- Narrowed pulse pressure (except widened in septic shock)
- Moderate to severe orthostatic blood pressure changes (25 to 50 mm Hg)
- Oliguria
- Cold, clammy skin
- Tachypnea
- Decreased body temperature

## LATE OR DECOMPENSATORY STAGE
- Confusion and incoherent, slurred speech; possibly unconsciousness
- Depressed or absent reflexes
- Dilated pupils slow to react
- Slowed, irregular, thready pulse
- Decreased blood pressure with diastolic pressure reaching zero
- Oliguria or anuria
- Cold, clammy, cyanotic skin
- Slow, shallow, irregular respirations
- Severely decreased body temperature

## DEATH

tion will soon fail if you don't correct the underlying cause of the shock and the fluid imbalance that results (see *Shock: Compensation,* pages 620 and 621, and *Shock:Decompensation,* pages 622 and 623). Check your patient's pulse frequently to detect increases or decreases in rate or volume.

*Tachypnea* occurs early, as the result of chemoreceptor stimulation, in all forms of shock. Your patient's increased respiratory rate helps increase red blood cell and tissue oxygenation. But this won't be sufficient if tissue perfusion continues to decrease.

You may have learned that hypotension, oliguria, and cool, clammy skin are the cardinal indicators of shock. But consider this: Hypotension and oliguria occur only *late* in the shock cycle, when your patient's compensatory mechanisms begin to fail. And cool, clammy skin is an early sign only in patients with hypovolemic and cardiogenic shock—in patients with vasogenic forms of shock (septic, neurogenic, or anaphylactic), it's a *late* sign indicating decompensation. So by the time your patient develops hypotension, oliguria, and cool, clammy skin, he may be in a late—possibly irreversible—stage of shock. Obviously, you'll increase your patient's chances of surviving shock if you learn to recognize it early and to intervene appropriately.

As soon as you see signs and symptoms of shock in your patient, concentrate on quickly identifying the type: hypovolemic, cardiogenic, septic, anaphylactic, or neurogenic.

Suspect *hypovolemic shock* in any patient with an illness or injury that predisposes him to decreased intravascular volume, whether volume's lost *from* his body or *into* body tissues. Causes of volume loss include:
- hemorrhage (such as from GI or vaginal bleeding or from surgery)
- trauma (massive injuries causing external or internal bleeding)
- burns
- excessive diarrhea, vomiting, or diuresis or prolonged nasogastric suc-

tioning (causing severe dehydration)
- intestinal obstruction (causing third-space fluid shifts).

Look for these signs and symptoms in a patient who's at risk for hypovolemic shock:
- mottled knees and elbows
- pale, cool, clammy skin
- tachycardia
- weak, thready pulses
- tachypnea
- anxiety and restlessness
- decreased urine output
- flat neck veins
- hypotension and narrowing pulse pressure
- thirst.

Suspect *cardiogenic shock* in any patient with an illness or injury that causes inadequate cardiac pumping. Causes include:
- myocardial infarction (MI), the most common cause
- congestive heart failure
- dysrhythmias
- cardiac tamponade.

These cardiac emergencies, of course, are themselves life-threatening, and you must intervene immediately to correct them (see Chapter 5). But, as you know, a patient may initially survive an acute MI or other cardiac emergency only to fall victim to the life-threatening effects of cardiogenic shock. To help prevent this tragic outcome in your patient with a cardiac emergency, watch for these signs and symptoms of cardiogenic shock:
- pale, cool, clammy skin
- tachycardia (occasionally you may see bradycardia)
- an $S_3$ heart sound
- weak or absent peripheral pulses
- tachypnea
- anxiety and restlessness
- decreased urine output
- distended neck veins
- hypotension and narrowing pulse pressure
- peripheral edema
- pulmonary congestion.

Suspect *septic shock* if your patient's at risk for massive infection due to the

PATHOPHYSIOLOGY

# SHOCK: COMPENSATION

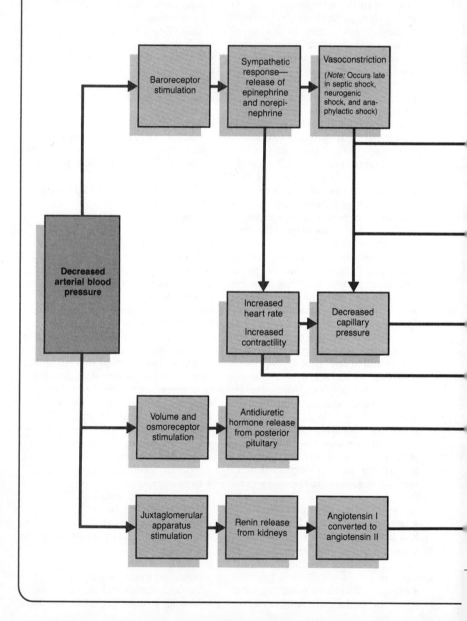

Baroreceptor stimulation

Sympathetic response—release of epinephrine and norepinephrine

Vasoconstriction

(*Note:* Occurs late in septic shock, neurogenic shock, and anaphylactic shock)

Decreased arterial blood pressure

Increased heart rate

Increased contractility

Decreased capillary pressure

Volume and osmoreceptor stimulation

Antidiuretic hormone release from posterior pituitary

Juxtaglomerular apparatus stimulation

Renin release from kidneys

Angiotensin I converted to angiotensin II

No matter what type of shock your patient has, his body will respond initially with the same compensatory mechanisms. His circulatory, neurologic, and endocrine systems will all react in an effort to restore circulating blood volume and to increase tissue perfusion. The flowchart below details how this compensation occurs.

If his shock state's not too severe (or with proper intervention), compensation may successfully reverse the shock process, allowing your patient to recover. However, the compensatory mechanisms are effective for only a short time. If the patient doesn't begin to recover before these mechanisms lose their effectiveness, they actually begin to contribute to the shock process (decompensation), and your patient's condition will deteriorate rapidly (see *Shock: Decompensation,* pages 622 and 623).

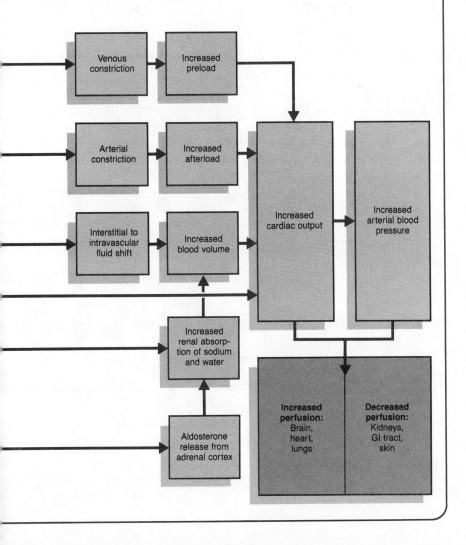

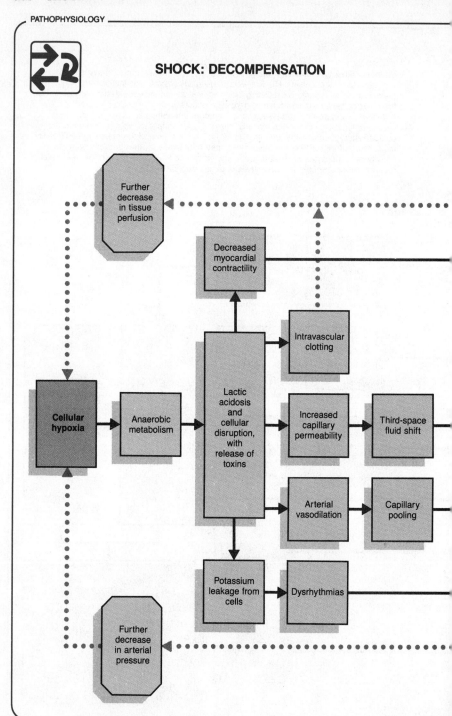

# SHOCK: DECOMPENSATION

When compensation fails, a cycle of decompensation is set in motion that almost invariably results in death. In the flowchart below, the dotted lines show how this cycle develops; note how decreased cardiac output exacerbates the preceding steps of the decompensatory process, until heart failure and brain stem ischemia cause total vasomotor collapse and death.

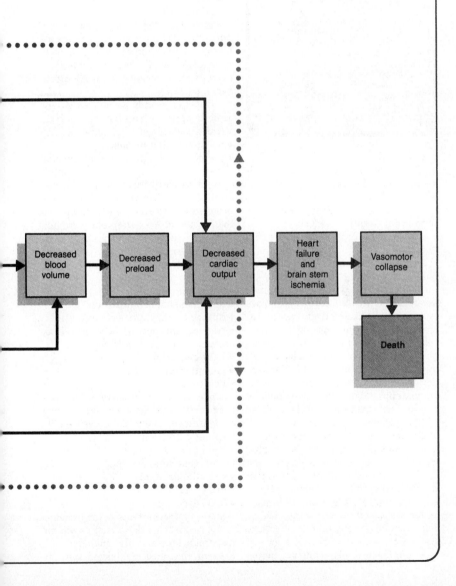

---

## POSITIONING POINTER

When you suspect your patient's developing hypovolemic shock, have someone notify the doctor; then position the patient *flat* on his back with his legs elevated about 20°. This position promotes blood flow to your patient's vital organs by keeping most of his blood in central rather than peripheral circulation. *Don't* place his head, neck, and shoulders lower than his trunk (Trendelenburg's position)—this inhibits venous return to the heart from the upper body and may aggravate cerebral edema. (The increased pressure on his diaphragm may also inhibit breathing.) Elevate his head *slightly* if you suspect brain injury or if he's in respiratory distress.

---

presence of:
- a local infection that's invaded his systemic circulation
- a systemic infection
- a urinary tract infection (especially with gram-negative bacteria)
- a postpartum or postabortal infection.

Remember that invasive procedures (such as inserting an I.V. line or an indwelling [Foley] catheter), immunosuppression, and certain diseases (such as diabetes and liver disease) increase your patient's risk of infection.

Septic shock often occurs in three distinct stages—warm (early, or hyperdynamic), cool (intermediate, or normodynamic), and cold (late, or hypodynamic). Signs and symptoms of cool and cold shock are similar to those of hypovolemic shock, but you'll differentiate these stages from hypovolemic shock by your patient's differing history. By the time he's entered the cool or cold stage of septic shock, you should be aware of his infection. However, the warm stage is more difficult to recognize—it occurs early, before you may be aware of his infection. Watch your patient who's at risk for any infection for these signs and symptoms

of warm septic shock:
- warm, flushed, moist skin; possibly petechiae and ecchymoses
- tachycardia
- full, bounding pulses
- tachypnea
- restlessness and confusion
- normal or slightly increased urinary output
- normal or slightly decreased blood pressure
- chills and fever.

Suspect *anaphylactic shock* in any patient at risk for a severe systemic allergic reaction. Expect your patient to have a history of allergies and to have been exposed recently to an allergenic agent, such as:
- a drug (especially an antibiotic, anesthetic agent, or vaccine)
- transfused blood or plasma
- an insect sting or bite
- an injected diagnostic agent, such as a dye.

Your patient's reaction may be immediate and life-threatening, compromising his airway or breathing (see the "What to Do First" entry in this chapter). To detect the onset of anaphylactic shock, watch your patient for the rapid development of any or all of these signs and symptoms:
- warm, moist skin
- apprehension or uneasiness
- diffuse erythema or urticaria
- edema, especially of the eyelids, lips, tongue, hands, feet, and genitalia
- light-headedness
- paresthesias
- itching.

Suspect *neurogenic shock* in any patient at risk for vasomotor center injury or depression due to the presence of:
- spinal cord trauma
- head trauma
- deep general anesthesia
- spinal anesthesia
- drug overdose
- hypoglycemia.

Signs and symptoms of neurogenic shock result from decreased or absent vasomotor tone and may include:
- warm, dry, possibly flushed skin

- confusion, stupor, or coma
- bradycardia or, possibly, tachycardia
- full, regular pulses
- tachypnea
- decreased urinary output
- hypotension
- nausea and vomiting
- poikilothermy (fluctuating body temperature).

## Special Considerations

### Pediatric
Your infant patient is particularly susceptible to hypovolemic shock—even from a slight hemorrhage or a short period of dehydration. Why? Because his compensatory mechanisms are different from an adult's, and because his obligatory water losses are greater. Watch for these signs and symptoms of hypovolemic shock in a seriously ill or injured infant:
- lethargy
- mottled or gray skin
- tachycardia
- tachypnea.

His blood pressure may remain stable for some time after the shock process begins. This is because infants have an increased vasoconstrictive response.

Watch any infant with signs and symptoms of infection closely: his immature immune system makes him particularly vulnerable to septic shock. But remember—his temperature may rise sharply with even a minor infection, so you can't rely on fever *alone* as a sign of sepsis. Be particularly careful to watch for irritability, lethargy, skin changes, and breathing changes, as well.

### Geriatric
Your elderly, debilitated patient has a weakened immune system, so he's at risk for acquiring almost any infection he's exposed to (for example, from insertion of lines for invasive monitoring). And any infection he acquires can quickly lead to septic shock. If he has underlying cardiovascular disease, this may decrease his cardiac output and his vasoconstrictive response so that he'll move from compensated to decompensated shock more quickly. (See *Shock: Compensation,* pages 620 and 621, and *Shock: Decompensation,* pages 622 and 623.)

When you assess your elderly patient for shock, remember that his baseline mental function may *already* be decreased as a result of cerebral hypoperfusion from atherosclerotic disease. Measure any changes in his level of consciousness against this baseline to determine if shock's present. Remember, too, that he may have weak or absent pulses because of preexisting peripheral vascular disease.

## DEFINITIVE CARE

## Hypovolemic Shock

### Initial care summary
On initial assessment, the patient had a history of trauma, hemorrhage, or another serious condition that decreased his intravascular volume. He also had some combination of these signs and symptoms:
- mottled knees and elbows
- pale, cool, clammy skin
- tachycardia
- weak, thready pulses
- tachypnea
- anxiety and restlessness
- decreased urine output
- flat neck veins
- hypotension and narrowing pulse pressure
- thirst.

The patient was given oxygen by mask or endotracheal tube. A 12-lead EKG and a chest X-ray were taken, and

# WHAT HAPPENS IN HYPOVOLEMIC SHOCK

Vascular fluid volume loss causes the extreme tissue hypoperfusion that characterizes hypovolemic shock. *External fluid loss* results from severe bleeding or from severe diarrhea, diuresis, or vomiting. Causes of *internal fluid loss* include internal hemorrhage (such as GI bleeding) and third-space fluid shifting (such as in diabetic ketoacidosis). Inadequate vascular volume leads to decreased venous return and cardiac output. The resulting drop in arterial blood pressure activates the body's compensatory mechanisms in an attempt to increase vascular volume. If compensation's unsuccessful, decompensation and death may rapidly ensue.

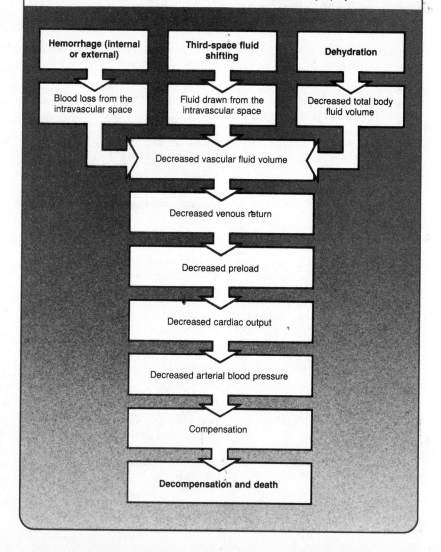

cardiac monitoring was started. Two large-bore I.V. catheters were inserted (one peripherally and one centrally) for rapid fluid administration. An arterial line, an indwelling (Foley) catheter, a CVP line, and a Swan-Ganz catheter were inserted. Initial readings indicated that the patient had decreased CVP, decreased pulmonary artery pressure (PAP), and decreased pulmonary capillary wedge pressure (PCWP). Blood was drawn for ABGs, CBC, electrolytes, blood glucose, prothrombin time/partial thromboplastin time (PT/PTT), platelet count, blood urea nitrogen (BUN), bilirubin, creatinine, serum lactate, serum osmolarity, and typing and cross-matching.

The cause of the patient's blood, fluid, or plasma loss was determined, and, depending on the body system affected, treatment was initiated to correct this. The patient was placed supine, with his feet elevated 20° to 30°, and a MAST suit may have been applied to increase his vital organ perfusion.

**Priorities**

A patient with hypovolemic shock has lost large amounts of blood, plasma, or water and electrolytes, causing decreased perfusion of vital organs. So your initial priority is restoring perfusion to your patient's vital organs to prevent cell damage and death.

Your patient should have at least two large-bore I.V. lines in place—preferably one CVP line and one peripheral line. If a CVP line couldn't be inserted, expect him to have two large-bore peripheral lines or expect the doctor to perform a venous cutdown to insert an appropriate line. Replace fluids by continuous infusion of normal saline or Ringer's lactate solution while you try to estimate the type and amount of fluid your patient's lost. Remember, he may have few or no signs and symptoms of shock until he's lost 15% or more of his intravascular volume. Use these guidelines to assess your patient for the signs and symptoms of hypovolemic shock as

they develop:

• If your patient has mild tachycardia (100 to 120 beats/minute), mild tachypnea (20 to 30 breaths/minute), elevated diastolic blood pressure, decreased pulse pressure, a positive response to a tilt test, anxiety, and normal or slightly increased urinary output, expect that he's lost 20% to 25% (1,000 to 1,250 ml) of his intravascular volume.

• If your patient has moderate tachycardia (over 120 beats/minute), moderate tachypnea (30 to 35 breaths/minute), decreased systolic blood pressure, decreased pulse pressure, anxiety or confusion, decreased capillary refill time, and decreased urinary output, expect that he's lost 30% to 35% (1,500 to 1,750 ml) of his intravascular volume.

• If your patient has severe tachycardia (140 beats/minute or greater), severe tachypnea (35 breaths/minute or greater), severely decreased or no systolic blood pressure, confusion and lethargy, minimal urine output, and cool, pale skin, expect that he's lost 40% to 50% (2,000 to 2,500 ml) of his intravascular volume.

Expect to continue crystalloids (such as normal saline solution or Ringer's lactate), or expect the doctor to order colloids (such as dextran or albumin), plasma, or blood, depending on the amount of intravascular volume your patient's lost and whether the loss is water and electrolytes, plasma, or blood. (See *Understanding Colloid and Crystalloid Solutions* in the Appendix.)

If your patient's lost *water and electrolytes* (for example, from diabetic ketoacidosis, hyperglycemic hyperosmolar nonketotic coma, or prolonged vomiting or diarrhea), expect to continue crystalloid administration—normal saline solution or Ringer's lactate. You'll have to infuse 3 to 4 ml of crystalloid solution for every 1 ml your patient's lost, because the solution moves quickly from the intravascular space to the interstitial spaces.

If your patient's lost *plasma* (for example, from third-space fluid shifts due to burns, bowel obstruction, or severe peritonitis), the doctor may ask you to infuse fresh plasma, fresh-frozen plasma, or plasma protein fraction (Plasmanate), along with crystalloid solutions. (See *Understanding Third-Space Shifting* and Chapter 15, BURNS.)

If your patient's lost *blood* (for example, because of hemorrhage from bleeding disorders, GI bleeding, trauma, or recent surgery), the doctor may ask you to infuse colloids, such as dextran or albumin, while the patient's blood is being cross-matched. Or he may ask you to give type-specific blood. (Crystalloids and colloids won't help your patient if he's lost 40% or more of his circulating blood volume—he won't have enough red blood cells to carry the oxygen his body needs.) You may also give blood if infusion of crystalloids doesn't stabilize your patient's CVP, or if you don't have a MAST suit available. Remember to warm the blood before you give it, to protect your patient's core temperature. If you're infusing large amounts of blood, expect to give plasma (1 unit for every 3 to 4 units of blood) to replace coagulation factors and platelets.

Monitor your patient's vital signs at least every 15 minutes. If he has an arterial line and a Swan-Ganz catheter in place, observe waveforms and pressures frequently. Your priorities are:
• to maintain the patient's systolic blood pressure at 100 mm Hg or higher
• to maintain his mean arterial blood pressure at 80 mm Hg or higher
• to raise his CVP up to 15 cmH$_2$O
• to raise his PCWP up to 18 mm Hg.

You may remove your patient's MAST suit after fluid infusion has started (see *Applying and Removing a M.A.S.T. Suit,* pages 614 and 615).

Your patient may develop an acid-base imbalance before his hypoperfusion is corrected. Expect his ABG values to reflect metabolic acidosis due to anaerobic cellular metabolism. The doctor may ask you to administer an initial dose of sodium bicarbonate to correct this. In addition, he may order subsequent doses based on serial ABG measurements.

If your patient's ventilations are depressed, he may develop respiratory acidosis. Make sure you maintain adequate ventilation—he'll need 1½ to 2 times the amount of oxygen you'd give someone who isn't in shock. If his respiratory acidosis persists, expect the doctor to intubate him and to start him on mechanical ventilation—possibly with positive end-expiratory pressure (PEEP), because this allows you to maintain an increased PO$_2$ without increasing fraction of inspired oxygen (FIO$_2$).

Watch your patient's cardiac monitor for dysrhythmias, which may result from hypoxemia, acidosis, or administration of unwarmed blood. Call the doctor *immediately* if you detect life-threatening dysrhythmias. Check your patient's urine output every 15 minutes. With adequate fluid infusion, you'll see a urine output of 30 ml/hour, or 7 to 8 ml/15 minutes. If not, call the doctor—he'll probably increase the infusion rate or order a fluid challenge.

## Continuing assessment and intervention

Continue to infuse fluids. Your goals are to further improve your patient's perfusion, to restore his intravascular volume to normal, and to protect him from a relapse into shock. Other measures to help improve his perfusion include keeping him quiet (to reduce the work load of his heart), medicating him for pain as ordered (to reduce his anxiety, which reduces his vasoconstriction), and keeping him warm (to promote vasodilation). Don't let him become overheated, though—this increases his cellular oxygen demand, further straining his cardiovascular system.

Your patient's hemodynamic parameters should reach the goals you set earlier:
• systolic blood pressure of 100 mm Hg or higher

## UNDERSTANDING THIRD-SPACE SHIFTING

Edema and hypovolemia—on first thought, these two states seem directly opposed, don't they? And so they are, as clinical entities. But *both* may occur in a patient in shock. Why? Because both result from the same process: a change in the distribution of body fluid caused by a phenomenon known as *third-space shifting.*

What is third-space shifting? To understand it, you need to review some basic facts about body fluid movement. Normally, body fluid moves freely between the body's *interstitial* and *intravascular* spaces to maintain homeostasis. Four basic pressures control fluid movement through the capillary membrane that separates these spaces:
• capillary hydrostatic pressure (the internal fluid pressure on the capillary membrane)

• interstitial fluid pressure (the external fluid pressure on the capillary membrane)
• plasma osmotic pressure (the fluid-attracting pressure from protein concentration within the capillary)
• interstitial osmotic pressure (the fluid-attracting pressure from protein concentration outside the capillary).

Decreased plasma protein levels (such as occur in a patient with peritonitis or one who's had major surgery) or increased capillary permeability (such as occurs in a patient with burns or an allergic reaction) disrupts the relationship between these pressures. The result? Altered fluid movement that traps fluid in the interstitial space and depletes the patient's intravascular volume.

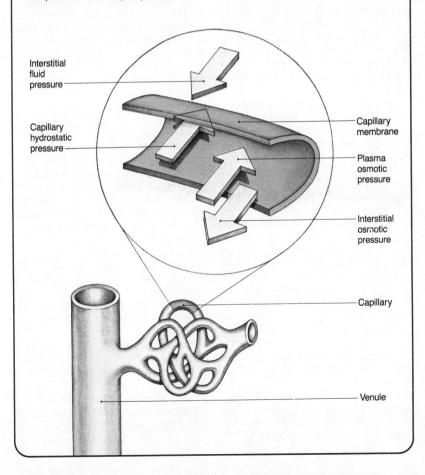

Interstitial fluid pressure

Capillary hydrostatic pressure

Capillary membrane

Plasma osmotic pressure

Interstitial osmotic pressure

Capillary

Venule

- mean arterial pressure of 80 mm Hg or higher
- CVP of up to 15 cmH$_2$O
- PCWP of up to 18 mm Hg.

Check his vital signs, level of consciousness, and urine output every 15 minutes, noting signs of improvement.

Assess your patient's level of consciousness. He should become alert as you restore adequate perfusion.

Check his skin color, turgor, and moisture. Look for a return of normal color and turgor and a decrease in diaphoresis except in his axillae and groin. (Even when his blood volume's adequate, these areas will be damp because of normal sweat gland activity.) Check his capillary refill time by pressing a nail bed and waiting for color to return; refill time should be brisk.

Check your patient's jugular veins. They may have been flat initially; now, with your patient supine, you should see them refill to the level of the anterior border of the sternocleidomastoid muscle.

Your patient's urine output should increase substantially. It may have been as low as a few milliliters per hour before you began fluid therapy. If you've restored adequate perfusion, it may rise to 50 to 100 ml/hour. Make sure it's at least 30 ml/hour; if it isn't, the doctor may ask you to increase the fluid infusion rate.

Your patient's pulse and blood pressure should return to normal. Compare his blood pressure now with his baseline blood pressure (and his normal blood pressure if you know it). Remember that a normal blood pressure for one person may be abnormal for someone who's hypertensive. His pulse should be below 100 beats/minute.

If you don't see these improvements in your patient, notify the doctor and expect that he'll order changes in fluid therapy.

The doctor will order serial hemoglobin and hematocrit tests—check these every 6 hours. If your patient's hemoglobin is in the range of 12.5 to 14 g/dl and his hematocrit is at least 35%, you know you've infused an adequate amount of blood.

### Therapeutic care

Your patient needs constant nursing observation and monitoring even after you've restored adequate perfusion. Why? Because his vital organs were at risk for ischemia and tissue necrosis during the period when he was hypovolemic, and because fluid administration alone may not be enough to restore his normal cellular function. Regularly monitor his cardiac function, kidney function, and mental function to detect developing complications.

The doctor may ask you to administer drugs with vasodilating effects, such as nitroprusside sodium (Nipride) or phentolamine (Regitine), to increase your patient's tissue perfusion and to decrease his tissue hypoxia and acidosis. If you administer these drugs, remember that you must also continue fluid therapy—otherwise, your patient's blood pressure will drop as his peripheral resistance decreases.

If your patient doesn't respond to fluid therapy immediately, expect to administer steroids, such as dexamethasone (Decadron) or methylprednisolone sodium succinate (Solu-Medrol). These drugs improve cellular uptake of oxygen and micronutrients, stabilize lysosomal membranes, increase lactic acid conversion to glycogen, and seem to increase tissue perfusion by increasing capillary vasodilation.

Remember that a patient who's had massive fluid loss and correspondingly large infusions is at risk for fluid overload. If infused fluids (especially crystalloids) move from the intravascular space to the interstitial spaces and become sequestered there, they can cause pulmonary congestion and edema. Assess your patient for rales, dyspnea, a cough with frothy sputum, and jugular venous distention. Check his CVP and PCWP readings—CVP over 15 cmH$_2$O and PCWP over 18 mm Hg are signs that your patient may be developing pulmonary congestion.

If your patient has signs and symptoms of pulmonary congestion, the doctor may ask you to administer albumin, which restores plasma osmotic pressure and draws water from the interstitial spaces back into the intravascular space. As your patient's plasma volume increases, he should excrete the excess water in his urine, increasing his plasma albumin concentration and drawing more water back into the intravascular space for excretion. Check his urine output frequently to see if it's increasing.

If your patient's urine output doesn't increase, the doctor may ask you to administer a diuretic, such as furosemide (Lasix)—but only if your patient has a normal pulse and blood pressure with an increased CVP. He may also ask you to give low-dose dopamine (Intropin), to increase your patient's renal perfusion.

Watch your patient closely for signs and symptoms of cardiac failure—such as dyspnea and rales associated with an S₃ heart sound—or rising CVP and PCWP values *after* fluid therapy. Decreased myocardial oxygenation, decreased coronary blood flow, and increased cardiac pumping from tachycardia may all decrease your patient's myocardial function. If your patient's young and generally healthy, his myocardial function may be fully restored when you correct his volume deficit. But if he's elderly or has cardiac disease, he may need inotropic medications—such as digitalis, isoproterenol (Isuprel), dopamine (Intropin), or dobutamine (Dobutrex)—to improve left ventricular contractility. Administer medications as ordered, and monitor your patient's hemodynamic parameters closely for signs of improved myocardial function.

Provide supportive care as your patient recovers from his shock state. If he's able to eat, give him small, frequent meals high in protein and calories, to replace exhausted carbohydrate and protein reserves. If he can't swallow, expect to provide high-

calorie, high-protein feedings through a gastric feeding tube or by total parenteral nutrition (TPN) through a central venous catheter. (Watch for fluid overload, hyperglycemia, infection, and other complications associated with TPN.)

To prevent your patient from developing a stress ulcer, give I.V. cimetidine (Tagamet), as ordered. The doctor may also ask you to administer an antacid, such as magnesium hydroxide (Maalox). You may give this every hour during the acute phase of shock and then 4 times per day as your patient recovers.

Prevent pulmonary complications by providing respiratory care. Keep the head of your patient's bed elevated, and turn him frequently; provide chest physiotherapy and postural drainage. Encourage your patient to cough and deep-breathe frequently, and give humidified oxygen by mask or endotracheal tube, as ordered.

Don't forget that the patient recovering from hypovolemic shock needs your emotional support. Following initial resuscitation, his stabilization and recovery will be long and complex. Be prepared to answer his questions and to provide concise explanations of the many procedures he must undergo.

---

# Cardiogenic Shock

## Initial care summary

The typical patient with cardiogenic shock has suffered an acute MI that damaged 40% or more of his left ventricle (he may, however, have some other cardiac dysfunction). Your patient had all the signs and symptoms of acute MI (see the "Myocardial Infarction" entry in Chapter 5), if this was the cause of his shock, plus these signs and symptoms:

• pale, cool, clammy skin
• tachycardia or bradycardia
• an S₃ heart sound

PATHOPHYSIOLOGY

# WHAT HAPPENS IN CARDIOGENIC SHOCK

When the myocardium can't contract sufficiently to maintain adequate cardiac output, stroke volume decreases, which means that the heart can't eject an adequate volume of blood with each contraction. Blood backs up behind the weakened left ventricle, increasing preload and causing pulmonary congestion. In addition, to compensate for the drop in stroke volume, the heart rate increases in an attempt to maintain cardiac output.

But, as a result of the diminished stroke volume, coronary artery perfusion and collateral blood flow decrease. All of these mechanisms increase the work load of the heart and enhance left ventricular failure.

The result? Myocardial hypoxia and further decreased cardiac output, which trigger the body's compensatory mechanisms in an attempt to reverse the process and prevent decompensation and death.

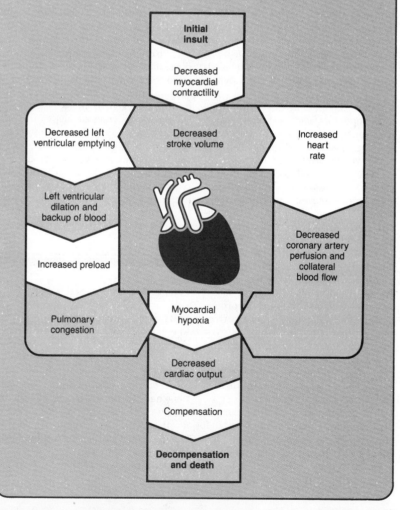

- weak or absent peripheral pulses
- tachypnea
- anxiety and restlessness
- decreased urine output
- distended neck veins
- hypotension and narrowing pulse pressure
- peripheral edema
- pulmonary congestion.

He was given oxygen by mask or endotracheal tube. A 12-lead EKG and a chest X-ray were taken, and he was connected to a cardiac monitor. He was given sublingual nitroglycerin to reduce his chest pain. A large-bore I.V. catheter was inserted for fluid and drug administration, and Ringer's lactate or normal saline solution was started at a keep-vein-open rate. An arterial line was inserted for continuous blood pressure monitoring, and a CVP line and a thermodilution Swan-Ganz catheter with a thermistor port were inserted for hemodynamic monitoring and cardiac output measurements. The patient's initial hemodynamic values indicated:

- increased CVP, unless the patient was hypovolemic
- increased PAP
- increased PCWP
- decreased cardiac output (measured with the thermistor port on the Swan-Ganz catheter, according to your hospital's protocols).

Blood was drawn for ABGs, electrolytes, CBC, blood glucose, BUN, creatinine, PT/PTT, platelet count, and cardiac enzymes (serum glutamic-oxaloacetic transaminase [SGOT], lactate dehydrogenase [LDH], creatine phosphokinase [CPK], and CPK-MB). Appropriate treatment for the patient's MI or other cardiac dysfunction was initiated (see Chapter 5).

### Priorities

Your patient with cardiogenic shock has decreased cardiac output due to his decreased cardiac contractility. As you may know, cardiogenic shock is rapidly fatal in 80% to 90% of patients because of the vicious cycle it initiates: myo-

cardial damage leads to diminished cardiac output, diminished coronary artery perfusion, increased myocardial hypoxia, and further myocardial damage. Once this cycle has begun, only rapid, expert medical and nursing care can help to break it. Your overall priority is to protect your patient's myocardium from further damage by:

- *increasing* his myocardial oxygen supply
- *increasing* his cardiac output
- *decreasing* his left ventricular work load.

Continued hypoxia rapidly increases myocardial damage, so increasing your patient's myocardial oxygen supply is a top priority. Check him for such indications of hypoxemia as restlessness, dyspnea, confusion, and cardiac dysrhythmias. Provide humidified oxygen by nonrebreathing mask, as ordered—a nasal cannula probably won't provide sufficient oxygen. You may give oxygen concentrations ranging from 40% to 100%, depending on the degree of his respiratory distress and the results of his ABG analysis.

If your patient's $PO_2$ is less than 70 mm Hg, his $PCO_2$ is greater than 60 mm Hg, and his pH is less than 7.35 after you initially administer oxygen, expect to assist with endotracheal intubation and to start mechanical ventilation with PEEP (even though decreased cardiac output is associated with PEEP). This increases your patient's $PO_2$ without increasing the $FIO_2$, and using PEEP also avoids increasing the respiratory acidosis that accompanies hypoventilation.

When you give oxygen, help your patient breathe more comfortably by placing him supine with his shoulders and head elevated. This decreases venous return to his heart and so decreases his pulmonary congestion.

If your patient has chest pain, remember that his pain may cause tachycardia, which increases his myocardial oxygen demand. Give medications as ordered—usually *small* doses of morphine sulfate I.V.—to control his pain without decreasing his blood pressure. (You won't give this drug I.M., because his poor peripheral perfusion delays absorption.) Morphine has the additional benefit of causing vasodilation, which reduces your patient's myocardial work load.

Your patient will be anxious and fearful. Of course, you know anxiety increases his sympathetic nervous system response, causing vasoconstriction and hyperventilation—the last things he needs. Watch him for restlessness, irritability, purposelessly repeated movements or comments, and a decreased attention span. If you note any of these signs, check his ABGs and his hemodynamic status to rule out hypoxemia as the cause. If he's simply anxious, take immediate steps to calm him. Stay in the room with him so he knows you're always available. Touch him and maintain eye contact while you provide reassurance, emotional support, and explanations of the procedures you're performing. If you can't control his anxiety with these techniques, notify the doctor *immediately* and obtain an order for a sedative. Otherwise, continued hyperventilation from his anxiety may cause alkalosis, which will decrease his tissue oxygenation.

Remember that your patient may also develop metabolic acidosis because his poor perfusion and subsequent poor tissue oxygenation cause increased anaerobic metabolism and lactic acid production. However, the doctor usually *won't* ask you to give sodium bicarbonate to correct this. Why not? Because sodium bicarbonate administration may lead to sodium and water retention and may also overcorrect his acidosis, leading to metabolic *alkalosis*. Monitor your patient closely, but expect that the acidosis will correct itself as you restore adequate perfusion.

### Continuing assessment and intervention
Your patient will need vigorous medical therapy to control the vicious cycle that occurs in cardiogenic shock. You'll

be responsible for administering medications as ordered, titrating medications to your patient's response, and frequently monitoring his vital signs, ABGs, urine output, and hemodynamic parameters (PAP, PCWP, and cardiac output measurements). If you're not measuring cardiac output, you can assess it by monitoring your patient's urine output, blood pressure, pulse quality, capillary refill, and level of consciousness.

Watch his cardiac monitor for dysrhythmias; if they develop, administer appropriate medications as ordered. (For further information, see the "Cardiac Dysrhythmias" entry in Chapter 5.) If your patient had an acute MI, the doctor may also ask you to administer lidocaine prophylactically to prevent ventricular dysrhythmias from developing. Be particularly alert for changes in your patient's CVP, PCWP, and cardiac output measurements.

If your patient has decreased blood pressure (systolic below 100 mm Hg), narrowed pulse pressure, decreased PCWP (below 12 mm Hg), decreased CVP (below 6 cmH₂O), and decreased cardiac output (below 4 to 8 liters/minute), expect that the continued decrease in his cardiac output may have produced a relative hypovolemia. (Remember that a patient with cardiogenic shock needs a higher filling pressure than normal, so a PCWP within the normal range of 4 to 12 mm Hg won't be adequate.) Expect to administer a fluid challenge of an I.V. crystalloid solution by giving a bolus of fluid over 15 to 30 minutes as ordered, and assess your patient's response. If your patient's CVP, PCWP, blood pressure, cardiac output measurement, and urine output *don't* increase after the initial bolus, repeat the challenge as ordered. The doctor may ask you to give additional boluses of crystalloid solution, or he may ask you to give a colloid, such as 25% albumin. (Albumin produces an osmotic effect: it draws water from the interstitial space and produces proportionately greater intravascular volume expansion than a crystalloid solution does.)

If your patient's CVP and PCWP *do* increase after your fluid challenge, but his blood pressure, urine output, and cardiac output (as measured using the thermistor port in the Swan-Ganz catheter) *don't* increase, stop the fluid challenge and report your findings to the doctor. Increasing CVP and PCWP

## ADMINISTERING NIPRIDE AND DOPAMINE TOGETHER

You may be asked to administer both nitroprusside (Nipride) and dopamine to your patient in cardiogenic shock—despite the two drugs' seemingly opposed effects. To understand why, consider the actions of each drug.

Nipride is a noninotropic (having no effect on cardiac muscle contractility) antihypertensive drug that dilates both arteries and veins. So it's particularly effective in treating cardiogenic shock: its vasodilating action decreases preload and afterload, which results in increased stroke volume, increased cardiac output, and decreased pulmonary congestion. But because Nipride's noninotropic, it enhances cardiac output only slightly. And vasodilation without an adequate increase in cardiac output can cause hypotension and decreased vital organ perfusion.

This is where dopamine comes in. Dopamine, an inotropic adrenergic (sympathomimetic) agent, mimics the effects of natural catecholamines at receptor sites in the sympathetic nervous system. At low to intermediate doses (1 to 10 mcg/kg/minute), it stimulates dopaminergic receptors to preserve renal perfusion and stimulates beta receptors to increase heart rate and contractility.

The resulting increased cardiac output ensures adequate perfusion of vital organs despite the decreased peripheral vascular resistance.

So, by giving your patient both drugs in precisely controlled doses, you can maintain optimum vascular tone. Because both drugs have a quick onset and a short duration, you can titrate them precisely to raise your patient's blood pressure to the desired level. Titrate the Nipride first to reduce preload and afterload; then titrate the dopamine to counteract the Nipride's hypotensive effects and to enhance the patient's cardiac output.

Here are some guidelines to follow when administering Nipride and dopamine together:
• Infuse fluids to correct hypovolemia both before and during the patient's drug therapy; optimum volume status enhances cardiac output.
• Monitor your patient's blood pressure every 5 to 15 minutes during administration; frequently check other signs of blood volume and myocardial function (heart rate, respiratory status, breath sounds, central venous pressure readings, urine output, and Swan-Ganz measurements).
• Mix a 200-mg vial of dopamine in 250 or 500 ml of normal saline solution or dextrose 5% in water ($D_5W$). (Greater concentration may be preferred if fluid restriction is a concern.) Begin the infusion at 2 to 5 mcg/kg/minute, and titrate up to 50 mcg/kg/minute as necessary. Replace the solution every 24 hours.
• Mix the 50 mg of powdered Nipride with 2 to 3 ml $D_5W$, then dilute this in 250 or 500 ml $D_5W$. (The solution is light sensitive, so wrap it in an opaque material, such as aluminum foil.) Begin the infusion at 0.5 mcg/kg/minute, and titrate to 10 mcg/kg/minute if necessary. Replace the solution every 24 hours.
• Use infusion pumps for both medications.
• Use separate I.V.s in large, stable veins. Prevent infiltration, because both drugs can cause ischemic tissue necrosis. Don't piggyback or add any other medications to these lines, to avoid incompatibility and precipitation of the solution.
• With dopamine, if your patient develops oliguria, tachycardia, and dysrhythmias from too much sympathetic stimulation, slow the infusion, notify the doctor, and be prepared to stop the infusion if necessary. Nausea, vomiting, headache, angina, and hypertension may also occur and require that you slow the infusion.
• Prolonged infusion of Nipride may lead to thiocyanate toxicity. Thiocyanate levels should be checked routinely (levels greater than 10 mg/dl indicate toxicity). Watch for weakness, headache, dizziness, restlessness, shallow breathing, nausea, tinnitus, muscle spasms, disorientation, or psychosis; if present, discontinue infusion.

## YOUR ROLE IN AN EMERGENCY

## HEMODYNAMIC MONITORING

Your patient in shock may have an intra-arterial line inserted to provide continuous arterial blood pressure measurement and to allow immediate access to arterial blood for arterial blood gas measurements. This information allows you to monitor your patient's immediate response to treatments, such as volume replacement and administration of vasoactive drugs.

The doctor will insert a catheter into your patient's radial, brachial, or femoral artery. You'll set up the monitoring system, connect it to the catheter with pressurized tubing, and take pressure readings. (The setup is the same for a Swan-Ganz catheter.) Here's how.

### Equipment
- I.V. pole and mount
- Transducer and dome
- Heparinized I.V. solution and administration set
- Pressure bag
- 4' pressure tubing and 6" extension pressure tubing
- Continuous flush device
- Stopcocks (2 three-way and 1 two-way) and caps
- Monitoring equipment

### Equipment setup
- Turn on the monitor to warm it up while you're preparing the equipment.
- Add 500 to 1,000 units of heparin to a 500-ml bag of I.V. solution, and hang the bag.
- Insert a nonvented I.V. administration set with microdrip chamber into the I.V. bag's port; then prime the I.V. tubing. Remember: Make all connections *tightly.*
- Attach a continuous-flush device to the I.V. line.
- Flush air from the continuous-flush device's Luer-Lok port and Luer-Tip port.
- Attach a 4' pressure tubing to the Luer-Lok port; uncap the tubing and flush it.
- Attach a three-way stopcock to the 4' tubing; flush all the stopcock's ports and cap the middle port.
- Connect a 6" pressure tubing to the stopcock's lateral port; flush the tubing and cap it.

- Attach another three-way stopcock to the continuous-flush device's Luer-Tip port; flush all the stopcock's ports and cap the middle port.
- Screw one arm of the transducer dome into the second stopcock's lateral port.
- Attach a two-way stopcock to the transducer dome's other arm; flush all ports and cap the open port.
- Tightly screw the dome onto the transducer and mount the transducer on the I.V. pole.
- Place the I.V. bag inside a pressure bag. Close the flow clamp, and pump up the pressure bag to 300 mm Hg.
- Zero the transducer to atmospheric pressure, and calibrate the monitor to the transducer according to the manufacturer's instructions.
- After the doctor's inserted the arterial catheter, quickly connect the 6" pressure tubing to the catheter's hub. (Note: To prevent blood backflow, *gently* press on your patient's artery while connecting the tubing.)
- Open the flow clamp to start the infusion. Flush the line by manually activating the continuous-flush device to remove any blood. Check the drip chamber: if the heparin solution's flowing steadily, the catheter's patent and properly positioned. (The infusion rate will automatically be 3 to 4 ml/hour.)
- Position the transducer at the level of your patient's right atrium (along the midaxillary line at the fourth intercostal space).

### Monitoring procedure
- Open the stopcocks between your patient and the transducer and begin monitoring your patient's arterial blood pressure.
- Record your patient's systolic, diastolic, and mean pressure readings and obtain strip charts as required.
- Set the monitor alarm limits at 20 mm Hg higher and lower than your patient's normal pressure.
- Observe your patient's pressure waveform on the monitor's screen or the strip charts; if it's not well-defined, take the following steps. First, check his blood pressure with a sphygmomanometer to see if he's

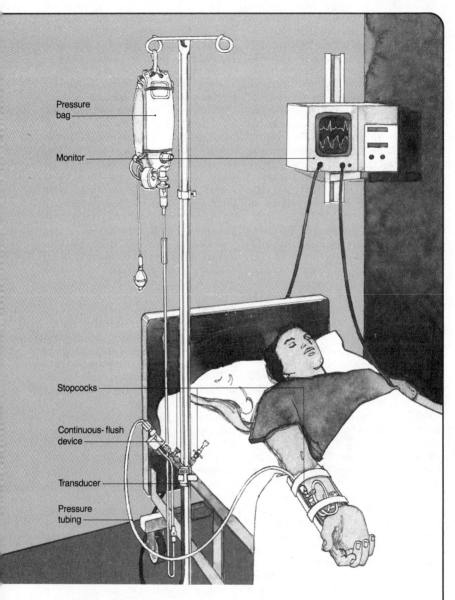

Pressure bag

Monitor

Stopcocks

Continuous-flush device

Transducer

Pressure tubing

hypotensive; if he isn't, then the problem's in the equipment. Flush the line and check whether it's kinked or blocked. If it is, correct the problem. If it isn't, check to see if the stopcocks are open and all connections are tight. Notify the doctor, if necessary.

• Fast-flush the catheter hourly (or accord-ing to your hospital's protocol) to maintain catheter patency.

• Frequently check pulse, color, warmth, sensation, and mobility in your patient's hand (below the insertion site) and his arm (above the insertion site) to ensure ade-quate circulation.

*without a corresponding increase in cardiac output* indicate that your patient's damaged heart can't tolerate additional fluid: continued fluid administration may cause irreversible heart failure or failure of multiple body systems. He may pass from relative hypovolemia to fluid overload almost immediately. To prevent this, assess his pulmonary status when you're checking his hemodynamic parameters, watching for increased dyspnea, frothy sputum, and rales on auscultation. If you note any of these signs, and if your patient's PCWP is greater than 20 mm Hg, expect to administer a diuretic—such as furosemide (Lasix)—to reduce his fluid volume and pulmonary edema.

The doctor may ask you to administer drugs that *increase* cardiac output, either alone or in combination with drugs that *decrease* myocardial work load. Adrenergics with inotropic activity increase the force of left ventricular contraction, thereby increasing your patient's cardiac output. (See *Highlighting Adrenergics*, pages 652 and 653.) The doctor may order dopamine (Intropin), isoproterenol (Isuprel), norepinephrine (Levophed), or metaraminol (Aramine) alone or in combination. He'll choose a drug or combination of drugs based on the patient's condition and his response to therapy; you'll be responsible for titrating doses to the patient's response and monitoring his cardiac output. The doctor will ask you to titrate the dose to keep the patient's vital signs and hemodynamic parameters within certain limits; for example, systolic blood pressure of 100 mm Hg or greater and PCWP of 12 to 14 mm Hg. Administer any of these drugs with an infusion pump so you can control the rate accurately.

The doctor may ask you to administer adrenergics in combination with a vasodilator, such as nitroprusside sodium (Nipride) or nitroglycerin, which increases your patient's stroke volume and cardiac output by decreasing his left ventricular preload and afterload. (See *Administering Nipride and Dopamine Together*, page 635.) Vasodilators also reduce your patient's myocardial oxygen demand. Most often, you'll give nitroglycerin or Nipride by continuous I.V. infusion. Start either of these drugs with a minimum dose, as ordered, then titrate the dose upward to achieve the maximum benefit for your patient. Monitor his PCWP and cardiac output measurement while you're giving these drugs—you want to keep PCWP values in the range of 14 to 18 mm Hg (or within parameters the doctor's ordered) and cardiac output above 4 liters/minute.

Remember this: Whenever you give a vasodilator in combination with an adrenergic, you must use *two* separate infusion pumps and *two* I.V. lines.

## Therapeutic care

Monitor your patient carefully during and after fluid and drug administration. Keep in mind that, although fluids and drugs can improve your patient's condition, they can also cause undesirable effects that strain his weakened heart.

Determine your patient's response to therapy by assessing his clinical condition, hemodynamic parameters, and blood tests. Look for these indications of improvement:

• *clinical condition*—normal pulse rate, decreased diaphoresis, normal skin color and turgor, increased urine output, absent $S_3$ heart sound, clear lungs on auscultation, and improved mental status

• *hemodynamic parameters*—stable PCWP, stable CVP, and stable blood pressure according to the parameters the doctor set, maintained with decreased dependence on vasopressors

• *blood tests*—normal acid-base balance, normal $Po_2$, and normal $Pco_2$.

If your patient's condition doesn't improve with fluid and drug therapy, the doctor may insert an intraaortic balloon pump (see *Understanding How an Intraaortic Balloon Pump Works*, page 181), which augments cardiac output and reduces left ventricular work load. After balloon pump insertion, watch your patient closely for complications due to immobility. You may not be able to turn him or to elevate the head of his bed, but you can help prevent pulmonary complications by encouraging him to cough and deep-breathe. Expect to administer heparin to decrease the risk of thrombus formation. Perform passive range-of-motion exercises on his legs to decrease his risk of venous stasis, and assess pulse strength, sensation, and skin color frequently in all his extremities.

Your patient may need several days of balloon pumping before his condition stabilizes. Then, the doctor may perform coronary artery bypass surgery, if indicated.

As you care for your patient in cardiogenic shock, remember that both he and his family need your emotional support. He's very ill—the odds are against his recovery. And, even if he survives the crisis period, his recovery will be a long and difficult process. He'll need all the support he can get.

# Septic Shock

### Initial care summary
The patient initially had a systemic infection, although this may not have been detected at first. As septic shock developed, his earliest signs and symptoms were probably those of the warm (early, or hyperdynamic) stage of septic shock:
• warm, flushed, moist skin; possibly petechiae and ecchymoses
• tachycardia
• full, bounding pulses
• tachypnea
• restlessness and confusion
• normal or slightly increased urinary output
• normal or slightly decreased blood

pressure
• chills and fever.

These signs and symptoms may have lasted 30 minutes to 16 hours. If his shock wasn't diagnosed and treated at this stage, he developed signs and symptoms of septic shock's cool (intermediate, or normodynamic) stage:
• cool skin
• normal or slightly decreased blood pressure
• decreased urinary output
• tachycardia
• hyperventilation
• peripheral edema
• pulmonary congestion
• thirst.

These signs and symptoms may have lasted only briefly. If his shock continued to progress without diagnosis and treatment—or if treatment was unsuccessful—he developed signs and symptoms of septic shock's cold (late, or hypodynamic) stage:
• cold, clammy skin
• severely decreased blood pressure
• severely decreased urine output
• tachycardia and a thready pulse
• respiratory failure.

Obviously, assessment findings depended on how early in the shock cycle your patient was diagnosed and treated and on whether his signs and symptoms were consistent with his hemodynamic status. (Some patients may have the signs and symptoms of only one stage—for example, warm septic shock—throughout, even though physiologic deterioration continues.)

The patient was given oxygen by nasal cannula or mask. If his respiratory distress was severe, he was intubated and started on mechanical ventilation. A 12-lead EKG was done, and a chest X-ray was taken. Cardiac monitoring was started, and a large-bore I.V. was inserted for fluid and drug administration. An indwelling (Foley) catheter was inserted to measure the patient's urine output. Ringer's lactate or normal saline solution was infused. An arterial line was inserted for continuous blood pressure monitoring, and a CVP line

# WHAT HAPPENS IN SEPTIC SHOCK

Massive infection, most commonly from gram-negative bacteria, is the cause of septic shock. As the body fights the infection, the bacteria die, releasing endotoxins. These endotoxins, through as-yet-unknown mechanisms, impair cell metabolism and damage surrounding tissues. The damaged cells release lysosomal enzymes and histamine. The lysosomal enzymes travel through the bloodstream to other tissues, causing more cell damage. They also trigger the release of bradykinin, a powerful vasoactive substance. Combined with histamine from the damaged cells, bradykinin causes massive peripheral vasodilation and increased capillary permeability (the so-called warm stage of septic shock). This leads to increased third-space fluid shifting and relative hypovolemia. The heart's preload, afterload, and stroke volume all decrease, triggering compensation (the cool stage) in an attempt to stave off decompensation (the cold stage) and death.

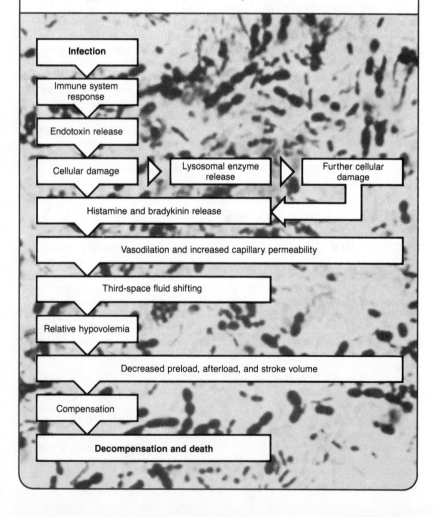

Infection

Immune system response

Endotoxin release

Cellular damage → Lysosomal enzyme release → Further cellular damage

Histamine and bradykinin release

Vasodilation and increased capillary permeability

Third-space fluid shifting

Relative hypovolemia

Decreased preload, afterload, and stroke volume

Compensation

**Decompensation and death**

and a thermodilution Swan-Ganz catheter with a thermistor port were inserted for hemodynamic monitoring and cardiac output measurements. Initial readings revealed:

• increased cardiac output, increased CVP, and increased PCWP if the patient was in the *warm* stage

• decreased cardiac output, decreased CVP, and decreased PCWP if he was in the *cool* stage

• severely decreased cardiac output, decreased CVP, and decreased PCWP if he was in the *cold* stage.

Blood was drawn for a CBC, electrolytes, blood glucose, PT/PTT, platelet count, bleeding time, fibrinogen, fibrin-split products, ABGs, and blood cultures. Urine, sputum, throat, vaginal, and wound drainage or exudate specimens were cultured.

## Priorities

Your first priority is to support your patient's cardiovascular and respiratory function while efforts to identify the organism that caused his shock continue and efforts to eradicate it begin.

Give your patient oxygen—by nonrebreathing mask—up to a 100% concentration, as ordered. If your patient's serial ABG values indicate a progressively decreased $PO_2$ and increased $PCO_2$, the doctor may intubate your patient and start him on mechanical ventilation. Assess his pulmonary status frequently, because patients with septic shock are especially prone to adult respiratory distress syndrome (ARDS). (See the "Adult Respiratory Distress Syndrome [ARDS]" entry in Chapter 4.)

Start fluid replacement, as ordered. Your patient may have relative hypovolemia due to vasodilation and third-space fluid shifts or to fever, diaphoresis, and increased respiration. Monitor your patient's CVP, PCWP, and cardiac output values, and report trends and changes to the doctor. He'll use these to guide your patient's fluid replacement. Depending on your patient's volume status, the doctor may ask you to administer a continuous infusion of normal saline solution or Ringer's lactate with electrolytes (see *Understanding Colloid and Crystalloid Solutions* in the Appendix). Or he may ask you to give your patient a small fluid challenge—for example, 50 to 150 ml of fluid over 15 minutes—and to notify him of the results before repeating it as ordered. This helps reduce the patient's risk of fluid overload and further cardiac decompensation.

As you know, the results of your patient's blood, urine, and other cultures won't be available immediately. Until the infecting organism's identified (and especially if the source of the infection's unknown), expect to administer broad-spectrum antibiotics, such as chloramphenicol, clindamycin, aminoglycosides (gentamicin, tobramycin), penicillins (ticarcillin, carbenicillin), or cephalosporins (cefazolin). If he's *already* on antibiotics for a preexisting infection, expect to continue these or to administer additional broad-spectrum antibiotics. You'll probably give drugs effective against both aerobic and anaerobic organisms.

If you know the source of your patient's infection (for example, if your patient's signs and symptoms indicate a urinary tract infection), the doctor will ask you to give antibiotics specific for the most likely causative organism. Then, as soon as the laboratory identifies the causative organism, he'll ask you to administer specific antibiotics. He'll determine appropriate doses by evaluating blood and urine tests that reflect your patient's renal function (creatinine, creatinine clearance, and urine output) and hepatic function (SGOT, LDH, serum glutamic-pyruvic transaminase [SGPT]). Because these organs metabolize and excrete antibiotics, the doctor will want to evaluate their function before he gives your patient large doses. If renal or hepatic function is impaired, he'll weigh the risks of giving large doses against the risks of uncontrolled septic shock. If only a large dose will reverse the infection, he'll give it even if the patient's renal or hepatic function is impaired, but he'll ask you to monitor the patient very closely and to check laboratory values frequently.

## Continuing assessment and intervention

Check your patient's vital signs and urine output every 15 to 30 minutes.

Apply a hypothermia blanket, if his temperature is increased, to reduce his core temperature and metabolic rate. Monitor his pulmonary function vigilantly, and check his ABG results to detect hypoxemia and acidosis. If he's persistently acidotic after fluid therapy, the doctor may ask you to administer sodium bicarbonate. When you change your patient's position, do so carefully

PROCEDURES

### YOUR ROLE IN AN EMERGENCY

## MONITORING CENTRAL VENOUS PRESSURE

To enable continuous monitoring of your shock patient's fluid status, the doctor may insert a central venous pressure (CVP) line. To do this, he'll thread a catheter through your patient's subclavian or jugular vein (or, less commonly, through the basilic, cephalic, or saphenous vein) until it reaches the right atrium. Once the catheter's in place, you'll connect it to a CVP manometer with a three-way stopcock. Then you'll operate the stopcock to obtain manometer readings. By taking a series of readings and comparing them, you can assess your patient's right heart function and determine his circulating blood volume.

Here's how to take and interpret CVP readings.

**Equipment**
• Disposable CVP manometer set with three-way stopcock, extension tubing, and leveling device
• Container of I.V. solution, as ordered
• I.V. administration set
• Nonallergenic tape or indelible marker

**Before the procedure**
• Set up the I.V. solution, an administration set, and the CVP manometer and its extension tubing; flush the I.V. solution through the tubing.
• Explain the procedure to your patient and assist the doctor with catheter insertion.
• *To prevent formation of an air embolus,* ask your patient to perform the Valsalva's maneuver. As he does so, quickly connect the manometer tubing to the catheter.
• If your patient's unconscious or on mechanical ventilation, lower the head of

his bed, then quickly connect the tubing after a complete inspiration.
• Adjust the administration set's flow clamp to the desired infusion rate.
• Adjust your patient's bed to the horizontal position and place him supine. If he can't tolerate this position, raise the head of the bed slightly. However, make sure you maintain the same position for subsequent CVP readings *to provide an accurate comparison.*
• Adjust the position of the manometer with a leveling rod so that the zero level aligns horizontally with your patient's right atrium. *To find the position of his right atrium,* locate his fourth intercostal space, and measure the depth of his chest from front to back at this level. Divide the depth in half, and mark the site with an indelible marker or a strip of nonallergenic tape. This site becomes the *zero reference point*—the location for all subsequent readings.
• When the manometer's stopcock is level with the right atrium, tape the manometer set to the I.V. pole. Recheck the level before each pressure reading and adjust it, if necessary.
• Check the line's patency by briefly increasing the infusion rate. If the line isn't patent, notify the doctor.

**During the procedure**
• Turn the stopcock to the *I.V. solution-to-manometer* position to *slowly fill the manometer.*
• Turn the stopcock to the *manometer-to-patient* position; the fluid level should slowly fall, with slight fluctuations as your patient breathes.

to decrease the effects of postural hypotension.

Monitor his CVP, PCWP, and cardiac output values, and report any changes to the doctor. With fluid therapy, your patient's condition should improve and you should note:
• increased urinary output
• increased CVP
• increased PCWP

• increased blood pressure
• improved skin turgor
• decreased pulse.

If your patient has edema, assess the degree and kind (pitting or nonpitting) to determine whether it's increasing or decreasing. This will help you estimate your patient's third-space fluid loss (see *Understanding Third-Space Shifting,* page 629).

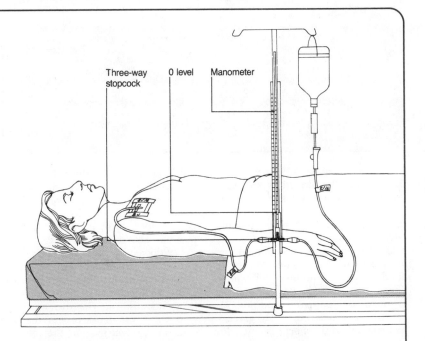

Three-way stopcock    0 level    Manometer

After the fluid column stabilizes (usually between 5 and 15 cmH₂O), tap the manometer lightly to dislodge air bubbles that may distort pressure readings. Take your readings at the *lowest* level the fluid reaches. If the fluid fails to fluctuate during breathing, the end of the catheter may be pressed against the vein wall. Ask your patient to cough to change the catheter's position slightly.

**After the procedure**
• Turn the stopcock to the *I.V. solution–to–patient* position as soon as you take the reading. Then check for blood backflow.
• Readjust the infusion rate, if necessary, and make sure all connections are secure.
• Return your patient to a comfortable position.

**Interpreting CVP readings**
To correctly interpret CVP readings, be aware of the normal range (5 to 15 cmH₂O) and note your patient's previous readings. If your patient's CVP varies from normal range by more than 2 cmH₂O, or if you note a drastic change from the last reading, check the CVP line for patency and repeat the measurement. If you're sure the abnormal reading is accurate, *notify the doctor immediately.* Don't rely on your patient's vital signs as an indicator of his cardiovascular status; CVP measurements can detect disorders before altered vital signs are apparent, which is critical to the early detection of shock. For example, a high CVP reading may signal cardiogenic or warm septic shock; a low reading may signal hypovolemic shock.

## RECOGNIZING TOXIC SHOCK SYNDROME

Toxic shock syndrome (TSS) is an acute form of septic shock caused by infection with *Staphylococcus aureus*—a gram-positive bacterium that may invade any part of your patient's body. Once *S. aureus* has invaded every part of your patient's body, the bacteria secrete enterotoxins that cause TSS.

TSS is most common in menstruating women using tampons, but it strikes patients of either sex and any age. On the average, two new cases are reported each day in the United States, and two deaths occur each month.

TSS is difficult to recognize and diagnose. No positive diagnostic test exists, the onset of TSS is insidious, and its systemic signs and symptoms mimic many other diseases, including viral influenza, food poisoning, scarlet fever, Kawasaki disease, and Rocky Mountain spotted fever.

Remember to consider the possibility of TSS whenever you see a patient with this clinical picture:
- fever above 102° F. (38.9° C.)
- systolic blood pressure below 90 mm Hg
- diffuse rash
- signs and symptoms indicating involvement of at least three body areas (mucous membranes or GI, musculoskeletal, renal, hepatic, hematologic, or central nervous systems)
- negative blood and cerebrospinal fluid culture tests; negative serologic tests for measles, leptospirosis, and Rocky Mountain spotted fever
- positive results of testing for *S. aureus* cultured from the nose, throat, vagina, or any wound
- desquamation (especially of the palms and soles) a week or more after the onset of signs and symptoms.

The doctor may ask you to administer a sympathomimetic (vasopressor) to improve your patient's cardiac output and arterial pressure. Expect to give dopamine (Intropin) or dobutamine (Dobutrex). The doctor may ask you to give either drug with fluid therapy, or he may ask you to give it *after* fluid therapy if fluid therapy alone has failed to produce the desired improvement in your patient's condition. Dopamine is most commonly given to patients in septic shock, because low doses of it increase myocardial contractility and heart rate and selectively dilate renal, mesenteric, and coronary arteries. Administer these drugs with an infusion pump so you can control the rate accurately. The doctor will ask you to start with a small dose initially and then to titrate the dose upward until it reaches the most effective level. Record your patient's cardiac output, arterial pressure, level of consciousness, and ABG results while you're administering these drugs, to monitor their therapeutic effect. Assess his peripheral pulses and urinary output frequently, too, because these drugs may cause arterial shunting, reduced arterial blood supply to the kidneys, and increased tissue ischemia due to vasoconstriction. If your patient develops reduced peripheral pulses or reduced urine output, notify the doctor and expect that he'll adjust the dose.

The doctor may also ask you to administer a vasodilator, such as nitroprusside sodium (Nipride), hydralazine hydrochloride (Apresoline), isosorbide dinitrate (Isordil), or nitroglycerin. These drugs reverse the peripheral vasoconstriction that occurs as a compensatory response in the cold stage of septic shock or as a response to a vasopressor.

If your patient's shock is diagnosed in an early stage, the doctor may order steroids. These drugs seem to block the complement cascade, stabilizing cell membranes, lysosomal membranes, and capillary epithelia and preventing cell lysis and third-space fluid shift. However, this hasn't been proved. In fact, the use of steroids in patients with septic shock is controversial because these drugs are effective only when given within a few hours of onset—after that, their immunosuppressive effects may do more harm than good.

## Therapeutic care

Watch your patient carefully while he's receiving high doses of antibiotics. Make sure blood is drawn at appropriate times to measure peak and trough antibiotic levels—these help determine if his blood levels stay within a therapeutic range without causing toxicity. Your patient may experience ototoxicity or nephrotoxicity—laboratory values can help detect these early so the doctor can reduce drug doses. Assess your patient for nephrotoxicity by monitoring his urine output and by obtaining blood and urine samples for creatinine clearance tests, which reflect kidney function.

Expect to give your patient I.M. vitamin K to promote production of clotting factors. (As you may know, antibiotics can destroy the intestinal flora that normally produce these factors.) And, expect to give him cimetidine (Tagamet) or antacids, as ordered, to help prevent stress ulcers.

Because mortality from septic shock is so high, the doctor will treat it aggressively. If your patient's condition doesn't improve with fluid therapy, antibiotics, or vasopressor or vasodilator therapy, the doctor may try investigational treatment with naloxone (Narcan) or prostaglandin inhibitors, such as indomethacin (Indocin), salicylates, or ibuprofen (Motrin).

Observe your patient closely for signs of disseminated intravascular coagulation (DIC) and ARDS—serious complications that are common in patients with septic shock.

If your patient's developing DIC, he'll have:
• bleeding from mucous membranes, I.V. insertion sites, and injection sites
• prolonged coagulation time
• decreased platelet count
• positive fibrin-split products.

Expect to give this patient plasma, whole blood or packed red blood cells, platelets, and—possibly—heparin. Monitor his laboratory studies carefully, and avoid excessive injections and suctioning. (See the "Disseminated Intravascular Coagulation" entry in Chapter 11).

If your patient's developing ARDS, you'll note:
• decreasing $PO_2$ (despite oxygen administration)
• increasing $PCO_2$
• evidence of consolidation on chest X-ray
• rales and dyspnea.

Notify the doctor *immediately,* and expect to restrict fluids, to provide oxygen, and to administer appropriate treatment as necessary (see the "Adult Respiratory Distress Syndrome [ARDS]" entry in Chapter 4).

Provide emotional support, which includes preparing his family for the possibility that he'll die in spite of aggressive medical treatment and conscientious nursing care. If he does recover, his progress will be slow and difficult, and he'll need constant reassurance and support.

# Anaphylactic Shock

## Initial care summary

The patient had a severe allergic reaction after he was exposed to an antigen. His initial signs and symptoms included rapid onset of:
• warm, moist skin
• apprehension or uneasiness
• diffuse erythema or urticaria
• edema, especially of the eyelids, lips, tongue, hands, feet, and genitalia
• itching
• light-headedness
• paresthesias.

If he wasn't treated immediately, he developed further signs and symptoms, including:
• abdominal cramps
• vomiting and diarrhea
• urinary incontinence
• vaginal bleeding (if female)
• wheezing and stridor
• dyspnea
• air hunger

PATHOPHYSIOLOGY

# WHAT HAPPENS IN ANAPHYLACTIC SHOCK

Anaphylactic shock is a violent systemic allergic reaction to a sensitizing substance (antigen), causing respiratory distress and vascular collapse.

In response to the first exposure to a sensitizing antigen, antibodies form on mast cells (pericapillary cells) and basophils (a type of white blood cell), but no reaction occurs. On subsequent exposure, these antigens and antibodies combine, forming an antigen-antibody complex on the cells' surfaces. This causes cell breakdown

(degranulation) and the release of histamine, the histamine-like substance SRS-A (slow-reactive substance of anaphylaxis), and chemical mediators that eventually cause the release of bradykinin and serotonin. All these vasoactive substances rapidly produce respiratory distress and decreased cardiac output, which activate the body's compensatory mechanisms. If these mechanisms (or treatment) don't reverse the shock process, decompensation and death rapidly ensue.

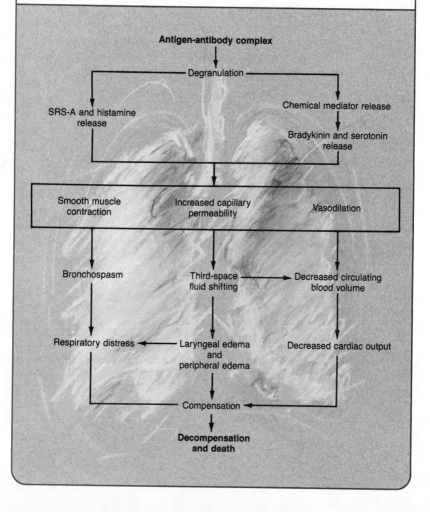

- difficulty speaking
- a barking or high-pitched cough
- laryngeal edema
- hypotension and narrowed pulse pressure
- tachycardia.

His laryngeal edema and respiratory problems may have caused airway obstruction. If so, he was intubated or had an emergency cricothyrotomy. An initial dose of epinephrine was given. An I.V. was started for fluid and drug administration, and he was connected to a cardiac monitor. Blood was drawn for CBC, electrolytes, blood glucose, clotting profile, serum immunoglobulins, BUN, and creatinine. (If his airway was obstructed, these studies were deferred until he was breathing adequately.)

### Priorities

Your initial priorities are to prevent further exposure to the antigen and to restore adequate ventilation. You'll deal with both problems almost simultaneously, because resolving both is critical to your patient's survival.

The antigen that caused your patient's reaction may be immediately apparent—for example, when your patient comes in with a bee stinger still in place or when his reaction starts just after you've given him a drug or a blood transfusion. Quickly determine what antigen your patient's been exposed to. Then prevent further exposure of your patient by:

- stopping any I.V. drug or dye infusion
- stopping a blood transfusion
- removing an insect stinger by scraping it (so additional venom expelled by the venom sac doesn't exacerbate your patient's shock), applying a tourniquet if the stinger can't be removed, elevating the affected part, and applying ice.

If your patient's respiratory status worsens and he hasn't been intubated

---

DRUGS

## HIGHLIGHTING EPINEPHRINE IN ANAPHYLACTIC SHOCK

Although epinephrine is the drug of choice in treating anaphylactic shock, a delicate balance exists between its therapeutic value and its adverse effects. If you give your patient even a slight overdose or infuse the drug too rapidly, he may develop cardiac dysrhythmias and a sudden rise in blood pressure, even a cerebral hemorrhage. So observe the following guidelines when administering epinephrine to your patient:

- Use epinephrine cautiously in patients with angina, dysrhythmias, or hyperthyroid conditions.
- Because an I.V. bolus of epinephrine can cause dysrhythmias, administer epinephrine by subcutaneous (S.C.) injection unless your patient's in profound shock or refractory to S.C. injection. I.V. epinephrine can be given by slow bolus or infusion. I.M. injection is also possible; however, impaired absorption may occur. Endotracheal tube administration is a last resort for a patient in severe shock who doesn't have

an accessible I.V. line.
- Start with a small dose, and repeat it every 10 minutes until your patient stabilizes. The dosage for S.C. or I.M. administration is 0.3 to 0.5 mg (0.3 to 0.5 ml of 1:1,000). I.V. dosage is 0.1 to 0.25 mg (0.1 to 0.25 ml of 1:1,000 or 1 to 2.5 ml of 1:10,000). Dilution of I.V. epinephrine, at least to 1:10,000 concentration, is strongly advised.
- Check your patient's vital signs frequently and, if possible, continuously monitor his cardiac rhythm. If you detect dysrhythmias, immediately stop administering the drug and notify the doctor.
- Keep emergency medications and resuscitation equipment on hand in case cardiac arrest occurs.
- Be alert for other—less serious—side effects, including anxiety, restlessness, headache, tremors, weakness, dizziness, dyspnea, and palpitations. Reassure your patient by explaining that these side effects will subside shortly.

# CASE IN POINT: FAILURE TO RELAY IMPORTANT HISTORY INFORMATION

Mae Pendleton, age 43, was admitted to your unit just before the end of a very busy shift. Your final task: Take Mae's history and prepare her chart. You quickly complete this task, then go off duty. When you return to begin your next shift, you hear more about Mae Pendleton:

A few hours after having a vaginal dilatation and curettage, Mae was feeling better—she was ambulatory and complained of only slight pain. The nurse on duty asked the doctor to order an oral medication for pain. He ordered Percodan. Within a half hour after taking the Percodan, Mae complained of itching and became short of breath. Her blood pressure dropped, too. Recognizing these as signs of a hypersensitivity reaction and possibly of anaphylactic shock, the nurse quickly notified the doctor, then injected epinephrine, as ordered. Fortunately, Mae survived, but she had to remain in the hospital for one more day.

Mae explained to the doctor that she'd informed the nurse who admitted her about her allergy to aspirin. But the doctor didn't find this information on her chart. If he'd known about it, he would've ordered a different medication, because Percodan contains aspirin. Now Mae threatens to sue for negligence.

What would happen if you were really involved in this situation and Mae sued the hospital? Would the court find you negligent?

That's what happened to the nurse named in *Ramsey et al. v. Physicians Memorial Hospital, Inc. et al.* (1977). She failed to inform a doctor of important history related to the illness of two young brothers. The court considered this failure as contributing to one child's death and to the misdiagnosis of his brother's serious illness.

To protect yourself from legal consequences related to communication and documentation errors, follow these guidelines:
• If you're working in the ED, be sure to verbally inform the doctor of any information you've obtained from your nursing assessment and from the patient or a family member—don't wait for a chart to be prepared *after* the patient's received emergency treatment.
• Record information promptly, and be sure to include all the facts—record all your actions and all doctors' orders, especially orders to give or to discontinue medications.
• If you suspect an order was improperly charted, seek clarification from the doctor and correct it if necessary.
• As always, write clearly, use only standard abbreviations, and spell correctly on every patient's chart.

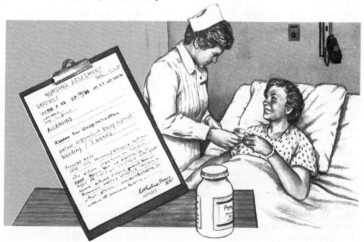

*Ramsey et al. v. Physicians Memorial Hospital, Inc., et al., 373 A. 2d 76 (Md. 1977).*

and hasn't had an emergency cricothyrotomy or tracheotomy, expect to assist with one of these procedures now. (A simple oral airway won't help your patient if his laryngeal edema progresses.) Provide supplemental oxygen by mask or through his endotracheal tube.

As soon as you've provided adequate ventilation and controlled the risk of further exposure of your patient to the antigen, expect to administer medication to block the histamine his body's releasing in response to the antigen. The doctor will probably order epinephrine because it has the additional advantage of counteracting bronchospasm and circulatory failure. Expect to give subcutaneous or I.M. injections of a 1:1,000 dilution, repeated at 10-minute intervals as needed. If the patient doesn't respond, the doctor may ask you to give a slow I.V. push of a 1:10,000 dilution of epinephrine, or he may ask you to give a 1:10,000 dilution through the patient's endotracheal tube (see *Highlighting Epinephrine in Anaphylactic Shock*, page 647).

Watch your patient's cardiac monitor continuously when you administer epinephrine, because he may develop dysrhythmias (particularly tachydysrhythmias). Monitor his blood pressure (with an arterial line if one was inserted), because epinephrine may cause a rapid increase.

Keep your patient supine and begin infusing fluids to replace those lost through third-space fluid shifts from damaged capillary walls. The doctor may insert a central venous line for rapid fluid infusion and CVP measurement. Give normal saline solution, Ringer's lactate, or albumin, as ordered. (Albumin not only replaces lost intravascular volume, it also draws water from interstitial spaces into the intravascular space where it can pass through the kidneys and be excreted.) The amount of fluid your patient needs will vary, but you must give enough to maintain an adequate urine output (30 ml/hour or more). This is particularly important in a patient with anaphylactic shock. Why? Because many antigens are excreted in the urine, so the antigen may not be removed from his body if his urine output is low.

## Continuing assessment and intervention

Observe your patient's blood pressure, pulse, temperature, skin color and turgor, urine output, and respiratory rate, depth, and quality frequently. Signs that his shock is worsening and that he needs more fluid (and possibly more epinephrine) include:

• decreased blood pressure, temperature, and urine output *or*

• increased pulse and respiratory rate, flushing, and edema.

If your patient has a CVP line, monitor his CVP to detect signs of fluid overload. Report increasing CVP to the doctor so he can adjust the amount of fluid if necessary. Remember, however, that you'll have to give enough fluid to maintain an adequate urine output until your patient's completely excreted the antigen that caused his reaction. If you don't, his reaction may recur when the epinephrine wears off.

Fluid administration may not be enough to maintain your patient's blood pressure if he's had a severe reaction. If his blood pressure's still low after fluid therapy, administer a vasopressor, as ordered. The doctor may order dopamine (Intropin) or norepinephrine (Levophed), which have both alpha- and beta-adrenergic effects. Or, if your patient has good cardiac function, the doctor may ask you to give a drug·that has purely alpha-adrenergic effects, such as phenylephrine hydrochloride (Neo-Synephrine) or methoxamine hydrochloride (Vasoxyl). These agents constrict blood vessels without altering cardiac function. Start small doses of these drugs, as ordered, and then titrate them upward.

Administer steroids, such as hydrocortisone sodium succinate (Solu-Cortef) or methylprednisolone sodium succinate (Solu-Medrol), if ordered.

These drugs stabilize your patient's damaged capillary walls and reduce leakage of fluid and plasma protein from the intravascular space. They also stabilize mast cells, preventing further release of chemical mediators.

Expect to give your patient antihistamines and aminophylline, too. An antihistamine, such as diphenhydramine (Benadryl), blocks the effect of histamine on your patient's vasculature and bronchioles. You may give this by I.M. injection or by *slow* I.V. push. (Watch carefully for signs and symptoms of hypotension.) Aminophylline acts as a bronchodilator and prolongs the epinephrine-induced bronchodilation. Give this as an I.V. drip diluted in dextrose 5% in water, at a rate not exceeding 25 mg/minute.

### Therapeutic care
If you've given your patient a vasopressor, begin weaning him from it by reducing the dose gradually, as ordered, and by monitoring his blood pressure at each step until it's stable.

Once your patient's stable, you can take measures to determine the agent that caused his reaction. Of course, if it was something you administered, such as an I.V. drug or a blood transfusion, you identified it early and noted it on the patient's chart. And you noted if the reaction followed a bee sting or ingestion of a food the patient knows he's allergic to. But if the agent hasn't been identified, and the patient hasn't been exposed to a substance he knows he's allergic to, the doctor may perform allergy testing and desensitization after the patient's discharged.

If your patient's hospitalized after his reaction, don't give him a vasodilator or let him take hot baths or showers for at least 24 hours. If he's discharged, remind him to avoid hot baths and showers and alcoholic beverages.

Your patient should wear a Medic Alert bracelet identifying his allergy (or allergies) and carry a list of his allergies in his wallet. Underscore the importance of taking these precautions—

*and* of avoiding exposure to substances he's allergic to. If he's allergic to something he can't avoid (such as bee stings), make sure he plans to carry an anaphylaxis kit and that he and his family understand how to use it.

# Neurogenic Shock

### Initial care summary
The patient developed decreased or absent vasomotor tone in response to general or spinal anesthesia or to such conditions as spinal cord injury or head trauma. Initial assessment findings included:
• warm, dry, possibly flushed skin
• apprehension or restlessness, possibly progressing to drowsiness, stupor, or coma
• bradycardia (or, possibly, tachycardia)
• full, regular pulses
• tachypnea
• decreased urinary output
• hypotension
• nausea and vomiting
• fluctuating body temperature.

If spinal cord trauma caused his neurogenic shock, he may also have had:
• bowel and bladder dysfunction
• flaccid paralysis
• absent reflexes.

He was given oxygen by mask—or, if he had severe respiratory distress, he was intubated and mechanically ventilated. An EKG and chest X-ray were done, and cardiac monitoring was started. Two large-bore I.V. lines were started for fluid and medication administration. Blood was drawn for CBC, electrolytes, blood glucose, and ABGs.

### Priorities
Although neurogenic shock is commonly of short duration and self-limiting, it can affect your patient's car-

# WHAT HAPPENS IN NEUROGENIC SHOCK

In neurogenic shock, the major problem is altered blood vessel capacity. A neurologic insult (from injury, disease, drugs, or anesthesia) disrupts transmission of sympathetic nerve impulses from the brain's vasomotor center, causing unopposed parasympathetic stimulation. This causes a loss of vasomotor tone, resulting in massive vasodilation: the vascular bed increases in size and blood capacity. So, even though the patient's blood volume isn't actually depleted, it's nevertheless inadequate to fill the enlarged vascular bed. The result? Relative hypovolemia, decreased venous return, and decreased cardiac output, which trigger the body's compensatory mechanisms. Usually, these mechanisms are successful—vasoconstriction occurs, reducing the relative hypovolemia and improving vasomotor tone—or the condition spontaneously resolves itself.

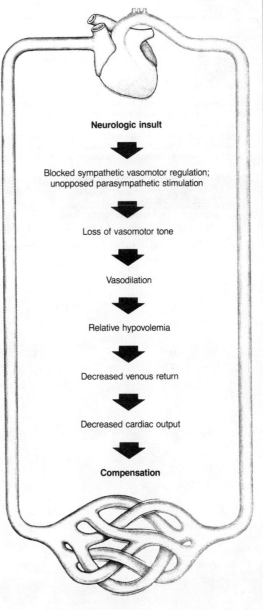

**Neurologic insult**

Blocked sympathetic vasomotor regulation; unopposed parasympathetic stimulation

Loss of vasomotor tone

Vasodilation

Relative hypovolemia

Decreased venous return

Decreased cardiac output

**Compensation**

diovascular and respiratory systems profoundly during its course. So your first priority is to support these systems.

Give your patient supplemental oxygen as needed. If he has a high spinal cord injury, his respiratory muscles will be paralyzed. This means you'll need to assist with endotracheal intubation and mechanical ventilation (see the "Spinal Cord Injury" entry in Chapter 6). If anesthesia caused your pa-

---

DRUGS

## HIGHLIGHTING ADRENERGICS

You'll commonly administer an adrenergic agent I.V. to treat a patient in hypovolemic, cardiogenic, neurogenic, or septic shock. These drugs act on receptors in the patient's cardiovascular system—stimulation of alpha receptors causes vasoconstriction; stimulation of beta receptors increases heart rate and contractility. Although these effects are drug and dosage dependent, the general result is increased blood pressure and cardiac output. Review this chart for important information about adrenergics you may administer to patients in shock.

| DRUG | POSSIBLE ADVERSE EFFECTS | NURSING CONSIDERATIONS |
|---|---|---|
| **dopamine** (Intropin, Dopastat) | Headache, dysrhythmias, anginal pain, palpitations, hypotension, nausea, vomiting, dyspnea, and local necrosis and tissue sloughing with extravasation | • Use a large vein to minimize the risk of extravasation, and watch the infusion site carefully for signs of extravasation. If it does occur, change the infusion site immediately and call the doctor.<br>• During infusion, check the patient's blood pressure, pulse rate, color, and temperature every 15 minutes; check his urinary output every ½ to 1 hour. If the dosage exceeds 50 mcg/kg/minute, check his urinary output more frequently.<br>• Observe the patient closely for adverse side effects. If any develop, notify the doctor, who may adjust or discontinue the dosage.<br>• Slow the infusion rate gradually when discontinuing the drug, and watch the patient closely for a sudden drop in blood pressure.<br>• Don't mix dopamine with alkaline solutions; use dextrose 5% in water for normal saline solution. Mix just before use.<br>• Don't mix other drugs in a bottle containing dopamine; don't give alkaline drugs (sodium bicarbonate, phenytoin sodium) through an I.V. line containing dopamine.<br>• Discard the solution after 24 hours, or earlier if it's discolored. |
| **dobutamine** (Dobutrex) | Headache, nausea, vomiting, chest pain, shortness of breath, premature ventricular beats | • Monitor the patient's EKG, blood pressure, pulmonary capillary wedge pressure, cardiac output, and urinary output while administering the drug. |

tient's neurogenic shock, he may also need ventilatory support because of depressed respirations from the anesthetic itself.

Expect to insert a nasogastric tube if your patient's nauseous or if he has a spinal cord injury that produced a paralytic ileus. The tube will empty your patient's stomach contents and prevent vomiting and aspiration.

Remember to keep your patient supine to prevent orthostatic hypotension

| DRUG | POSSIBLE ADVERSE EFFECTS | NURSING CONSIDERATIONS |
|---|---|---|
| **dobutamine** (Dobutrex) *(continued)* | | • Dobutamine remains stable for 24 hours; oxidation may slightly discolor admixtures but doesn't indicate significant loss of potency.<br>• Don't mix dobutamine with alkaline solutions. |
| **isoproterenol** (Isuprel*) | Headache, weakness, palpitations, dysrhythmias, tremors, anxiety, nausea, vomiting | • Stop the infusion if precordial distress or angina occurs.<br>• Check with the doctor about decreasing the infusion rate or temporarily stopping the infusion if the patient's heart rate exceeds 110 beats/minute (infusion rates that increase the heart rate to 130 beats/minute may induce ventricular dysrhythmias).<br>• Monitor the patient's blood pressure, central venous pressure, EKG, arterial blood gases, and urinary output while administering the drug. |
| **norepinephrine** (Levophed*) | Headache, anxiety, dizziness, hypertension, tachycardia, ventricular fibrillation, metabolic acidosis, decreased urine output | • Discard solutions after 24 hours.<br>• Use a large vein to minimize the risk of extravasation; stop the infusion immediately if extravasation occurs, and notify the doctor.<br>• Keep 5 to 10 mg of phentolamine and 10 to 15 ml of normal saline solution on hand to counteract local irritation occurring with extravasation.<br>• Keep emergency antiarrhythmic drugs on hand.<br>• Check the patient's blood pressure every 5 minutes; check his pulse rate, urinary output, color, and skin temperature frequently during the infusion.<br>• Slow the infusion rate gradually when discontinuing the drug.<br>• Monitor the patient's vital signs even after the drug is stopped—watch particularly for a severe drop in blood pressure. |

*Available in U.S. and Canada. All other products (no symbol) available in U.S. only.

from the relative hypovolemia his increased vascular capacity may cause. Don't allow him to sit upright—if he does, his blood pressure may fall drastically and he may even lose consciousness.

Start I.V. fluids (usually crystalloids), as ordered, to expand your patient's intravascular volume. Give these cautiously, however, because they may cause fluid overload when his vasomotor tone is restored—for example, when his anesthesia wears off or when you give him a vasopressor. Insert an indwelling (Foley) catheter, as ordered, to measure his urine output frequently. A Foley catheter also helps prevent urine retention if your patient has a spinal cord injury that paralyzed his bladder muscles.

### Continuing assessment and intervention

Keep your patient supine, and continue to assess his response to fluid therapy by checking his pulse, blood pressure, and urine output frequently.

If fluid therapy alone doesn't relieve your patient's signs and symptoms, and especially if anesthesia caused his shock, the doctor may ask you to administer an adrenergic. Expect to give an adrenergic that causes alpha-adrenergic stimulation (see *Highlighting Adrenergics,* pages 652 and 653), such as phenylephrine hydrochloride (Neo-Synephrine), I.V. or I.M. (Keep atropine handy when you give your patient this drug, because it may cause bradycardia.) Or you may give methoxamine hydrochloride (Vasoxyl), also I.V. or I.M. If the doctor prefers not to use a vasopressor that's a pure alpha-adrenergic stimulator, he may ask you to give your patient dopamine (Intropin) I.V. Give any of these drugs in small amounts initially, and then titrate the dosage upward as ordered to maintain your patient's blood pressure. You won't typically give these drugs over a long period—this is because some patients develop a tolerance for them, making withdrawal difficult.

Monitor your patient's temperature frequently during his care. His body may lose the ability to control his cutaneous vasodilation, causing his body temperature to fluctuate with the temperature of his environment. If he's *hy*pothermic, keep him warm and cover him with a light blanket; if he's *hy*perthermic, remove his blankets and keep him cool.

### Therapeutic care

The only definitive care for your patient's neurogenic shock is correction of the underlying cause. If anesthesia induced his shock, continue to support his cardiovascular and respiratory function until the anesthesia wears off and his vasomotor tone returns. If spinal cord injury caused his neurogenic shock, his recovery will be influenced by the extent of the injury as well as by the shock state. Vasomotor tone may return when spinal cord edema subsides. Remember, however, that you may need to continue ventilatory support if he has any of certain types of spinal cord injury. (See the "Spinal Cord Injury" entry in Chapter 6.)

## A FINAL WORD

As a nurse, you'll probably agree that shock is an emergency that challenges every aspect of your nursing skill. First, of course, because it's a life-threatening condition that can affect all your patient's body systems, but also because it occurs together with one or more *other* emergency conditions. When you think about shock, you can't help but think about high mortality—cardiogenic shock, for example, has a mortality as high as 80%. And a patient who survives shock will probably confront morbid complications.

Here, at least, help is on the way. Recent advances in the treatment of shock, such as the increasing use of MAST suits and autotransfusions, are helping to reduce shock's adverse consequences. And researchers are always testing new products to treat these patients. One such product still being tested, a blood substitute called Fluosol-DA, can be used at the scene of an emergency or in transport vehicles to help expand blood volume and transport oxygen quickly, so a patient's risk of developing serious complications related to shock is greatly reduced.

Perhaps the most significant advance in treating shock is a clearer understanding of shock's pathophysiology. With this knowledge, you and the rest of the emergency team can take extra precautions to prevent some of shock's devastating effects.

Remember, shock is extremely unpredictable. So, if you think any patient is at risk for shock, you'll have to use preventive techniques whenever possible. Use such techniques as carefully monitoring your patient's intake and output—if you think he's at risk of developing hypovolemic shock—and reporting *any* change. Of course, you know that adhering to sterile techniques is your best way to prevent sepsis and septic shock; and that obtaining an accurate patient history, especially identifying all of your patient's allergies, is your best way to prevent anaphylactic shock.

Of course, despite your preventive efforts, some of your patients with emergencies will develop shock. To care for these patients, you'll need your most accurate assessment skills, because the signs and symptoms of shock may be subtle at first. The early stage of septic shock, for example, may resemble uncomplicated systemic infection; the early stage of hypovolemic shock may cause only mild anxiety and slight changes in respiratory rate and pulse rate. You'll have to act fast to avert such complications as acute respiratory failure, ARDS, DIC, or renal failure. As you know, these are emergencies as serious as the shock itself. So be sure that you're prepared to recognize these complications and to intervene swiftly and appropriately.

Caring for patients in shock not only requires your expert assessment, quick intervention, and up-to-date knowledge of emergency care; it also tests your expertise in providing emotional support. Keep your patient informed about the procedures you and other team members are performing. Keep assuring him that the entire emergency team is doing all it can to help him. And don't forget to keep his family informed—they're just as frightened as the patient. Answer their questions and do what you can to help them make it through the crisis stage. Unfortunately, your role must sometimes be to prepare them for the patient's probable death.

## Selected References

Cohen, Stephen, et al. "Nursing Care of Patients in Shock," Parts 1, 2, 3. *American Journal of Nursing* 82 (June, September, November 1982):943-64, 1401-22, 1723-46.

Crumlish, C.M. "Cardiogenic Shock: Catch it Early," *Nursing81* 11:34-41, August 1981.

Perry, Anne G., and Potter, Patricia A. *Shock: Comprehensive Nursing Management.* St. Louis: C.V. Mosby Co., 1983.

Rice, V. "Shock, A Clinical Syndrome. Definition, Etiology, and Pathophysiology," Part 1. *Critical Care Nurse* 1:44-50, March/April 1981.

Sumner, S.M., et al. "To Defeat Hypovolemic Shock: Anticipate and Act Swiftly," *Nursing81* 11:46-51, October 1981.

# 15

# Burns

## Introduction

You're in the ED getting a history from a patient with an ankle injury when rescue personnel bring in Frank Talarico. "Got a bad flame burn here," one of the paramedics tells you. You promptly send another nurse to call the doctor, and you send an aide for the sterile linen pack. Then you lead the paramedics to the trauma room, where burned patients are cared for. Quickly, you wash your hands and pull on a mask and cap, then a sterile gown and gloves. You know infection control has to start immediately with *any* burned patient.

Helping the rescue personnel transfer Frank to the stretcher, you guess his age as late 20s or early 30s. You see right away that his chest and arms have large areas of burned skin. His respirations are rapid and shallow, and a quick look at his face—the burned-off eyebrows, singed nasal hairs, and blisters forming around his mouth—tells you that, besides his pain and anxiety, an inhalation injury is probably causing his rapid breathing.

While you're making this quick assessment, the paramedics tell you what happened: "He was getting ready to cook hamburgers on a charcoal grill in his yard. His wife said the coals were lit and he was squirting in some charcoal lighter fluid when the fire flamed up. It set his shirt on fire. She forced

him to the ground and rolled him in a blanket to put the fire out. When we got there, we made sure he was breathing and had a pulse; then we got his burned shirt off. We put a clean sheet over him to keep him warm and brought him in. He lives a couple of blocks from here, so we haven't had time to do anything else."

You know, of course, that a burned patient like Frank needs immediate assessment and intervention. Are you sure that you'd know how to assess the seriousness of Frank's condition? Remember, every burned patient—whether he has a thermal burn, chemical burn, or electrical burn—is a high-risk patient. Why? Because the patient may have airway, respiratory, and cardiovascular damage that initially threatens his life more than the burn does.

He may also have multiple trauma—fractures, dislocations, or organ damage. If he does, these injuries will take priority, during emergency assessment and intervention, over his burns—once the burning process has been stopped. (Of course, nothing takes priority over airway, breathing, or circulation problems.)

So the quality of care your patient receives initially can make an important difference in his recovery. This chapter tells you what you need to know—and do—in the first critical minutes *and* during the course of any burned patient's emergency treatment.

# INITIAL CARE

## Prehospital Care: What's Been Done

Prehospital care for a patient who's been seriously burned depends not only on the type and extent of the burn but also on the rescue personnel's training and equipment. In assessing the burned patient, rescue personnel first assessed and stabilized his airway, breathing, and circulation. They then turned their attention to:

• stopping the burning process
• assessing him for signs and symptoms of shock
• stabilizing any fractures or dislocations
• caring for his burns.

If, in assessing your patient's airway, breathing, and circulation, rescue personnel found him apneic and pulseless, they started CPR. (Note: They wouldn't have inserted an esophageal obturator airway in a burned patient with any chance of airway injury, because of the risk of asphyxiation due to airway edema.) If the patient's airway and breathing were stable, rescue personnel nevertheless started humidified oxygen by face mask at 5 to 10 liters/minute. Why? Because of the likelihood that a seriously burned patient will also have inhalation injuries. (See *Understanding Inhalation Injuries*, pages 692 and 693.)

Rescue personnel may have taken several steps to stop the burning process at the scene. If the patient had a *thermal burn*, the rescuers poured wa-

ter or saline solution over the burn area until it was cool to the touch. Then, they removed the patient's clothing and any heat-retaining and constricting items, such as jewelry or a watch.

If he had a *chemical burn*, they removed any clothing that came in contact with the chemical, brushed any dry chemical off his skin with a clean cloth (protecting themselves in the process), and quickly irrigated the burned area with copious amounts of water to dilute the chemical.

To stop a patient's *electrical burn*, of course, rescue personnel removed him from contact with the current's source and began CPR, if necessary. If the patient also had flash burns from the electrical current, rescue personnel assessed and intervened as they would for a thermal burn.

If the patient had a *tar or asphalt burn*, rescue personnel lavaged the area with cold water to cool the tar and stop the burning process. (When tar or asphalt is heated for use, it can reach a temperature of 250° to 850° F. [121.1° to 454.4° C.]—so it can cause a serious burn.) They didn't attempt to remove any of the tar before the patient arrived in the ED.

Burns, as you know, are a kind of trauma, and every patient with burns is treated as if he had a traumatic injury. But if your burned patient also has multiple trauma, then stabilizing those injuries takes priority over caring for his burn wound. So, if your patient was burned in a vehicular accident or other situation that can cause multiple trauma (such as falling from a height or being thrown by the impact of an explosion), rescue personnel carefully assessed his other injuries and intervened appropriately. This may have involved splinting his fractured extremities or stabilizing his cervical spine.

Because fluid loss always follows serious burns, I.V. fluid management may have been necessary to restore sufficient circulating blood volume. Rescue personnel started infusing Ringer's lac-

tate via a large-bore I.V. line if the patient was:
- over age 60 or under age 2
- burned over 20% or more of his body surface area (BSA)
- dehydrated, bleeding heavily, or suffering from trauma
- burned by an electrical source.

Uncomplicated burns (involving less than 20% of the patient's BSA) may not require fluid management by I.V. Oral fluid replacement is usually sufficient.

# What to Do First

Your immediate priority, as always, is to assess your patient's airway, breathing, and circulation and to intervene as necessary. Don't let your patient's burns or other injuries, no matter how serious they are, distract you from this.

### Airway
Start your assessment of the burned patient by making sure his airway is clear and his cervical spine is stabilized. (Remember, electrical current passing through muscle can cause severe tetanic contractions that, in turn, can cause fractures. In any patient with a severe electrical burn, suspect spinal cord injury and keep his cervical spine stabilized until such injury is ruled out.)

Can you feel air over his nose and mouth? If you can't, suspect an upper airway obstruction. This may be caused either by debris (particularly if he was burned in an explosion) or by his tongue or edema. Clear the debris from his airway using finger sweeps, back blows, or suction. If his tongue's obstructing his airway, use the jaw-thrust method—described in the "Life Support" section in Chapter 3—to prevent cervical spine damage. If these procedures don't open the patient's airway, edema may be causing the airway obstruction. The doctor may insert a laryngoscope to visualize the obstruc-

PRIORITIES

## INITIAL ASSESSMENT CHECKLIST

**Assess the ABCs first and intervene appropriately.**

**Check for:**
- stridor, coughing, hoarseness, sooty sputum, and singed nasal hairs, indicating inhalation injury
- decreased blood pressure and increased pulse rate, indicating impending shock
- diminished peripheral pulses, indicating impaired circulation from edema or thrombosis
- fractures, hemorrhage, or other injuries from a fall or tetanic contractions.

**Intervene by:**
- dousing the burn with normal saline solution or water, if the burning process hasn't yet been stopped
- administering supplemental oxygen by face mask
- starting at least two large-bore I.V.s and rapidly infusing fluids
- elevating edematous areas
- covering the patient with a sheet or blanket to prevent hypothermia
- inserting an indwelling (Foley) catheter and a nasogastric tube.

**Prepare for:**
- intubation and mechanical ventilation
- cutdown with central I.V. line insertion
- cleansing and debridement
- bedside X-rays.

tion, or he may intubate the patient.

Edema is likely to occur if your patient inhaled heated air, steam, or chemical fumes. Suspect inhalation injury if he has any of these signs:
- extreme restlessness
- stridor
- singed nasal hairs
- circumoral or pharyngeal burns
- sooty sputum
- hoarseness or voice change
- increased secretions.

WARNING

## AVOIDING DEXTROSE IN EARLY FLUID REPLACEMENT

Don't give dextrose to your burned patient during the first 24 hours of fluid replacement. Why? Because dextrose isn't effective as the primary fluid replacement for this patient. It doesn't remain in the vascular space, where fluid's needed—instead, it passes into the interstitial space. What's more, your patient can't metabolize the dextrose given in massive fluid replacement; he's already overloaded with internal glucose released during his stress response to the burn, and the effectiveness of his insulin is decreased. An isotonic-balanced electrolyte solution, such as Ringer's lactate, is preferred, since it has an electrolyte balance similar to that of blood.

Notify the doctor *immediately* if you see any of these; he'll intubate the patient promptly to prevent developing edema from compromising or completely occluding the patient's airway, and he'll connect the endotracheal tube to a mechanical ventilator or a T-piece. Early intubation is critical for this patient—once his airway becomes completely occluded by edema, the doctor won't be able to intubate him, and he'll have to perform an emergency cricothyrotomy or tracheotomy. Assemble the necessary equipment, and be prepared to ventilate the patient temporarily with an Ambu bag until mechanical ventilation's established. Assist the doctor as necessary—these procedures are difficult to perform, because edema alters landmark structures.

### Breathing

After you've made sure your patient's airway is patent, assess his breathing. If he has cherry red skin or mucous membranes and complains of confusion, headache, and nausea, he may have carbon monoxide poisoning. You may be asked to start 100% oxygen using a tight-fitting mask, or the doctor

may intubate the patient and start him on mechanical ventilation. (See the "Carbon Monoxide Poisoning" entry in Chapter 17.)

If he suffered a severe electrical burn with respiratory arrest, he may already be intubated and oxygenated via an Ambu bag. Expect to connect him to a mechanical ventilator. If he suffered a thermal or chemical burn, he may have dyspnea, tachypnea, wheezing, stridor, or bronchospasm from inhalation of the products of combustion (smoke or chemical fumes), superheated air, or steam.

For a patient with any type of burn, expect to draw blood, to obtain baseline arterial blood gas (ABG) and carboxyhemoglobin levels, and to begin treatment with humidified oxygen by mask. You may also need to give a bronchodilator and to provide ventilatory support—probably with positive end-expiratory pressure (PEEP) if the patient develops respiratory distress or failure.

Trauma to your patient's chest from associated injuries may compromise his breathing. Look for asymmetry and paradoxical breathing, which may indicate a flail chest (see the "Flail Chest" entry in Chapter 4). Note whether he's using accessory muscles to breathe. Listen for stridor, wheezing, rales, rhonchi, or decreased breath sounds, indicating pulmonary complications. Report your findings to the doctor. When you evaluate your patient's breathing, don't rely solely on his respiratory rate to gauge whether his ventilation's adequate. Estimate his tidal volume by observing the depth of his respirations—this is more accurate. Why? Because many noxious gases have a depressant effect on the central nervous system (CNS) that causes the patient's respiration depth to become increasingly shallow—even though *his respiratory rate may not change.*

Pain and anxiety may further compromise your patient's breathing. To relieve his pain and anxiety, expect to give an I.V. narcotic analgesic (for example, morphine sulfate). Don't forget the contribution that your emotional support can make to your patient's comfort.

If your burned patient is hypotensive, you may have to withhold medication for pain because it may decrease his blood pressure further. In this situation, cover the burned area with a sterile sheet. Keeping air off the burn will help ease your patient's pain—and as a bonus, it may reduce his breathing difficulty.

## Circulation

Any patient with a serious burn (over 30% of his BSA burned) will need aggressive intervention to prevent circulatory collapse from *burn shock*—a type of hypovolemic shock that incorporates these factors, as well:
• fluid shifts (as fluid moves from the vascular space into the interstitial space)
• decreased cardiac output (from release of a myocardial depressant factor and decreased circulatory volume)
• neurogenic shock (from the patient's pain and psychological distress)
• adynamic ileus.
Burn shock is one of the most common complications of serious burns, because fluid shifts into the interstitial space in the burned areas result in decreased circulatory volume and cardiac output. This fluid shifting is also the reason why you must give all of a burned patient's medications I.V.—except, of course, tetanus toxoid, which is always given I.M.

If your patient doesn't have an I.V. immediately, expect to start one. If you can't find a peripheral vein in unburned skin, prepare to assist with insertion of a subclavian I.V. or with a cutdown. Number the I.V. bags or bottles infused, to avoid mistakes later when you're totaling the amount of fluid the patient received. Insert an indwelling (Foley) catheter, as ordered, to monitor urine output. Draw blood, as ordered, for necessary laboratory tests.

With any seriously burned patient, the doctor will probably order cardiac enzymes, a 12-lead EKG, and continuous cardiac monitoring. Cardiac dysrhythmias may result from:
• hyperkalemia due to intracellular release of potassium (secondary to cell destruction)
• ventricular irritability due to cardiac effects from an electrical burn
• myocardial tissue hypoxia due to hypoxemia from inhalation injury or shock.
Expect to administer an antiarrhythmic, such as lidocaine I.V., if your patient's dysrhythmia is due to irritability. If it's due to hypoxemia, expect to increase his oxygen percentage and to add PEEP as ordered. Monitor his ABGs frequently. As the hypoxemia is corrected, his dysrhythmias should abate accordingly.

Record your patient's pulse rate, strength, and regularity, using his femoral pulse if edema makes his peripheral pulses difficult to find. (See *Using Doppler Ultrasound,* page 663.) Remember that as edema and eschar (an inelastic, leatherlike necrotic layer) develop in an extremity with circumferential burns, circulatory compromise may result. Notify the doctor and prepare for escharotomy if your patient's peripheral pulses are absent.

Check your patient's blood pressure (on an unburned limb, if possible). Use Doppler ultrasonic flowmeter if necessary. Even if all his extremities are burned, you *can* take his blood pressure. Here's how: Place a 4″ x 4″ sterile gauze pad (or a towel) on the extremity before applying the blood pressure cuff. If you can't assess his blood pressure by any other means, expect to assist with insertion of an arterial line for this purpose. As always, record your findings.

In a patient with severe burns and insufficient fluid replacement, his blood pressure will be low, indicating hypovolemia and, possibly, shock.

You can also assess your patient's circulation by checking his capillary refill time and by frequently reassessing his peripheral pulses.

## General appearance

After providing the necessary care to stabilize your patient's airway, breathing, and circulation, assess the extent of your patient's burn. Use the "rule of nines" or the Lund and Browder chart to estimate the extent of his injury quickly and to form an initial estimate of his fluid needs. (See *Using the "Rule of Nines,"* page 664, and *Using the Lund and Browder Chart,* page 665.) Keep in mind that the "rule of nines" doesn't apply to children, because the percentages are for adult BSA. Use the Lund and Browder chart if your patient's a child.

*Look at all areas of your patient's body.* Expect burned areas to be white, reddened, or darkened and possibly charred or blistered (see *Assessing Burn Depth,* pages 666 and 667).

## Mental status

Most patients with burns are alert, oriented, and very frightened. If your burned patient is drowsy, disoriented, lethargic, or confused, *find out why quickly.* Assess him for carbon monoxide poisoning, hypoxia, hypovolemic shock, head injury, and alcohol or drug abuse. A patient with an electrical burn is more likely to have a decreased level of consciousness from cardiovascular or CNS injury. Start high-flow humidified oxygen, if you haven't already done so; perform a quick neurologic check; and check his blood alcohol and drug levels, as ordered.

# What to Do Next

Now that you've stabilized your patient's airway, breathing, and circulation, you're ready to perform a detailed emergency assessment and to intervene appropriately. While you're performing your assessment, obtain history information from the patient, his family, or rescue personnel. This will help you to identify any associated injuries.

If your patient has a *thermal burn,* determine:
• what caused it—sun; steam; scald; contact with tar, grease, molten metal, or some other superheated substance; direct contact with flames; or an electrical flash
• whether the accident occurred in a closed or open area
• how long the patient was in contact with the heat source
• whether the patient inhaled smoke or chemical fumes
• what type of material was burning
• whether an explosion occurred
• whether the patient was unconscious—and if he was, for how long.

Remember, the longer the period of contact with the heat source, the more the patient's likely to have extensive burns and to need massive fluid replacement. If he suffered a thermal burn in a closed area, be alert for signs of smoke inhalation or carbon monoxide poisoning. Auscultate his lungs, and report any signs of respiratory distress, including *wheezing, rales, rhonchi,* and *increased inspiratory effort.*

With a patient who has an *electrical burn,* you need to know:
• what estimated voltage was involved
• how long the patient was in contact with the current
• whether the current was alternating (the type used in most U.S. homes and industries) or direct (the type used in street car systems and ships, and the type lightning's composed of)
• whether the patient was thrown, or fell from a height, when he contacted the current.

If your patient remained in contact with the electrical current for an extended period of time, he may have massive internal injuries along with serious cardiovascular, renal, and neurologic complications.

If your patient has a *chemical burn* on his skin, remove his clothing and then lavage the burned area with copious amounts of water or saline so-

## USING DOPPLER ULTRASOUND

If your burned patient's peripheral edema or severe hypotension prevents you from palpating his peripheral pulses or auscultating his blood pressure with a stethoscope, try using a Doppler ultrasonic flowmeter. Here's what to do:

Apply coupling gel to the Doppler's probe. Tilt the probe at a 45° angle to your patient's skin, then slowly move it in a circular motion until you hear an optimal arterial or venous flow sound. Count the sounds for 60 seconds to determine your patient's pulse rate. Next, apply a blood pressure cuff and inflate it until the arterial sound disappears. Then slowly deflate the cuff until the sound reappears, and note the systolic pressure reading on the sphygmomanometer.

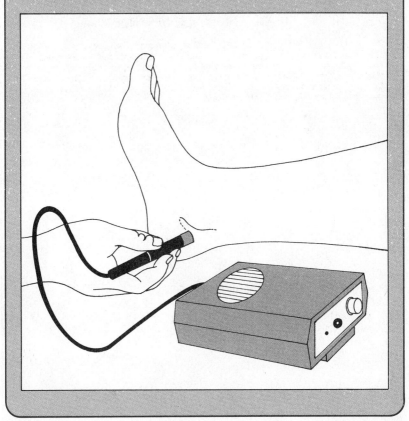

lution *before you do anything else.* Do this by hand or by placing him under the shower. Meanwhile, also try to identify:

- what the chemical is
- what its concentration is
- how long he was exposed to it
- whether noxious fumes accompanied the chemical injury.

If your patient's burn is from *hot tar* or *asphalt,* cool it with cold water and then try peeling the cooled tar away. If it doesn't pull away easily, dissolve it with a petroleum solvent such as Neosporin ointment or mineral oil. Apply the solvent liberally until the tar begins to dissolve, then gently wash the dissolved tar off. Some residual tar may remain in place—this will gradually be removed as dressings are changed.

For all types of burns, you need to estimate what percentage of your patient's BSA is burned. To do this, you may use the "rule of nines" (see *Using the "Rule of Nines"*) or the Lund and Browder chart (see *Using the Lund and Browder Chart*).

Assess your patient for circumferential, full-thickness, or deep partial-thickness burns of the thorax. Assess him, too, for eschar formation—which, by restricting respiratory excursion, may impair his respirations and cause hypoxia.

Find out, too, if your patient suffered associated trauma from an experience such as jumping from a window when he was burned. Palpate his extremities and his head and neck for areas of *tenderness*, and look for *edema*, *ecchy-*

## USING THE "RULE OF NINES"

You can quickly estimate the extent of an adult patient's burn by using the "rule of nines." This method divides an adult's body surface area into percentages that, when totaled, equal 100%. To use this method, mentally transfer your patient's burns to the body chart shown here, then add up the corresponding percentages for each burned body section. The total, a rough estimate of the extent of your patient's burn, enters into the formula to determine his initial fluid replacement needs.

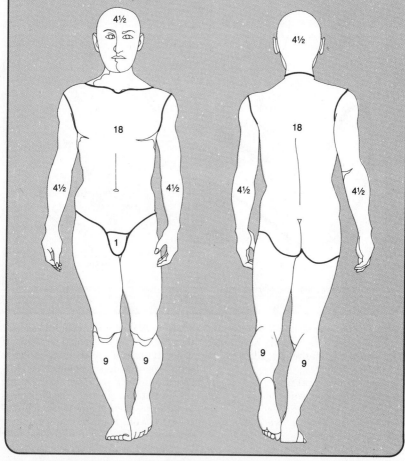

# USING THE LUND AND BROWDER CHART

The "rule of nines" is a quick way to roughly estimate the percentage of your patient's body surface that's been burned. But you can't use it for infants and children. Why? Because their body section percentages differ from those of adults. (For example, an infant's head accounts for about 19% of his total body surface area, compared to 9% for an adult.) To determine the extent of an infant's or child's burns, use the Lund and Browder chart shown here. This chart, unlike the "rule of nines," takes proportional age-size differences into account.

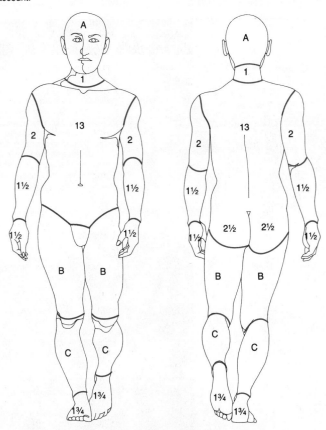

### Relative percentages of areas affected by growth

|                  | At birth | 1 yr   | 5 yr   | 10 yr  | 15 yr  | Adult  |
|------------------|----------|--------|--------|--------|--------|--------|
| A: Half of head  | 9½%      | 8½%    | 6½%    | 5½%    | 4½%    | 3½%    |
| B: Half of thigh | 2¾%      | 3¼%    | 4%     | 4¼%    | 4½%    | 4¾%    |
| C: Half of leg   | 2½%      | 2½%    | 2¾%    | 3%     | 3¼%    | 3½%    |

# ASSESSING BURN DEPTH

A moderate-to-severe skin burn may be classified as either superficial or deep *partial-thickness* (also known as a second-degree burn) or *full-thickness* (also known as a third- or fourth-degree burn), based on its depth and on the postburn presence or absence of deep epithelializing elements—hair follicles and sweat glands. Less severe (first-degree) burns damage only the epidermis, producing tender, reddened skin as in common sunburn; they're not considered at length here.

Burn depth depends on how hot the burn-causing element was and how long the

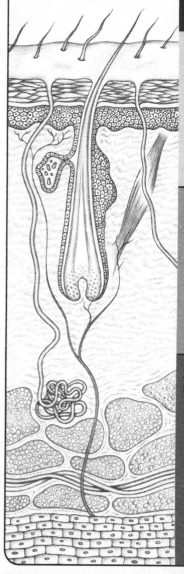

## DESCRIPTION AND EFFECT ON HEALING

**Superficial partial-thickness burn**

- The epidermis and portions of the dermis are damaged or destroyed.
- The burn can become a deep partial-thickness or a full-thickness injury without proper treatment or if infection occurs.
- Epithelialization usually occurs within 2 weeks, because hair follicles and sweat glands that lie in the deep dermis and subcutaneous tissue remain.
- Healing usually occurs with normal hair regrowth and return of skin texture. However, discoloration and scarring may occur.

**Deep partial-thickness burn**

- The epidermis and up to ⅞ of the dermis are damaged or destroyed.
- Slow epithelialization (more than 2 weeks postburn) may occur if hair follicles and sweat glands that lie in the subcutaneous tissue remain.
- If the burn's allowed to heal spontaneously, the skin may be thin, poorly pigmented, and hairless, possibly with hypertrophic scarring.
- Skin grafts are usually necessary for the best cosmetic appearance and skin quality. They also help prevent infection.

**Full-thickness burn**

- The epidermis, dermis, and portions of subcutaneous tissue (and possibly muscle or bone) are destroyed.
- Epithelial elements are destroyed, so healing occurs only at the wound edges.
- Thrombosis of blood vessels causes ischemia, necrosis, and eschar formation.
- Skin grafts are required to replace destroyed tissue.
- Even with grafting, hypertrophic scarring will occur without additional therapy (for example, massage and pressure garments).
- No hair regrowth will occur.

patient's body was exposed to it. To assess the depth of your patient's burns, use the chart below, which describes the three classifications of moderate-to-severe burns and their characteristic assessment findings.

## COMMON ASSESSMENT FINDINGS

- Erythema with blanching due to vasodilation
- Blisters, swelling, and moist surface due to fluid shifts into the burned area
- Pain with possible hyperalgesia due to exposure of nerve endings

- Clinically indistinct differentiation from a full-thickness burn
- Hypo- to hyperalgesia, depending on burn depth, due to damaged nerve endings
- Generally dry surface with a thin layer of eschar, but blisters and blanching may be present

- White, reddened, darkened, or charred skin
- Eschar due to tissue dehydration and loss of elasticity; no blanching, due to destruction of blood vessels
- Blisters (rare)
- Loss of pain sensation and temperature differentiation due to destruction of nerve endings

moses, and any obvious *deformity,* indicating a possible fracture or dislocation.

Auscultate his heart sounds: if you hear an $S_3$ or $S_4$ *gallop* or *murmur,* he may have myocardial injury or decompensation. The doctor will probably order an EKG. (Myocardial injuries frequently accompany high-voltage electrical burns.)

Begin your neurologic assessment by checking your patient's level of consciousness and his pupil symmetry and reactivity. Test his motor strength and reflexes, too.

If your patient has *minor superficial partial-thickness burns* with no other injuries, the doctor will probably release him. (The exception to this rule is a patient with electrical burn injuries. The doctor will probably admit this patient for 24 hours to monitor his cardiac status.) Remind a discharged patient to return to the ED or clinic within 24 hours for follow-up care. Clinic staff will reevaluate the extent and depth of his injury and check for any indications of infection or neurovascular compromise.

All burned patients need tetanus prophylaxis (see *Guidelines for Tetanus Prophylaxis,* pages 66 and 67). Even if your patient's already been immunized, the doctor will order a booster of tetanus toxoid 0.5 ml. If the patient's immunization history is uncertain or the burn is more than 24 hours old, the doctor will order 250 units of I.M. tetanus immune globulin. This is the *only* medication you'll give I.M. to your patient who has burns over 20% or more of his BSA (see *Tetanus Toxoid: An Exception to the "I.V.-Only Rule,"* page 671).

Inspect your patient's abdomen, looking for *distention, rigidity,* or *guarding.* Palpate for *areas of tenderness.* Listen for *bowel sounds;* if they're absent, he has an ileus—which almost always accompanies a burn over 25% of the patient's BSA. Serious burns cause ileus because blood is shunted away from the patient's GI tract to com-

# GUIDELINES FOR FLUID REPLACEMENT

While fluids are being replaced, assess your patient's response and use it to titrate the rate of fluid replacement. But use caution in giving massive fluid replacement to elderly and pediatric patients and to anyone with a history of heart failure. Osmotic diuretics or low-dose dopamine infusion may be necessary to maintain adequate urine output and to prevent fluid overload in these patients, or to aid myoglobin clearance in patients with deep-muscle damage.

| ASSESSMENT FACTORS | NURSING CONSIDERATIONS |
|---|---|
| Intake and output (hourly) | Maintain minimum urine output at 30 to 50 ml/hr in an adult, 0.5 to 1 ml/kg/hr in a child, or 70 to 100 ml/hr in a patient with a deep burn injury affecting muscle tissue, to prevent renal failure from myoglobinuria. |
| Vital signs (every 15 minutes to hourly) | Maintain the patient's blood pressure above 90/60. Increase the fluid infusion rate and notify the doctor if the patient's blood pressure drops more than 20 mm Hg below baseline or if his pulse rises above 110 beats/minute. |
| Mental status (continuously) | Note changes such as restlessness, confusion, or agitation in a previously quiet patient, indicating poor cerebral perfusion. |
| Body weight (same time daily) | Expect the patient to gain weight during the first 48 to 72 hours, due to third-space fluid shifting. Thereafter, expect the patient's weight to slowly decrease toward normal dry weight. |
| Respiratory status (hourly) | Check the patient's breath sounds for rales and note dyspnea, which may indicate fluid overload. If rales or dyspnea is present, decrease the fluid administration rate and notify the doctor. |
| Cardiac status (frequently) | Monitor the EKG continuously with an elderly patient or a patient with a history of heart failure, and auscultate heart sounds at least hourly; notify the doctor if rales, dysrhythmias, or abnormal heart sounds—which may indicate fluid overload—develop. |
| Blood tests (at least daily)<br>• hematocrit<br>• sodium | Notify the doctor if the patient's values are elevated (possibly indicating underhydration) or decreased (possibly indicating overhydration). He may change the infusion rate and the type of fluid administered, and may order a blood transfusion. (Note: Expect an initial rise in hematocrit values.) |
| Urine specific gravity (every 4 hours) | If elevated, expect to increase the infusion rate; or if decreased, to decrease the infusion rate. |

Your patient with serious burns needs massive fluid replacement—especially for the first several days postburn. Expect to give a combination of crystalloids (such as dextrose in water) or colloids to meet your patient's fluid needs. Your hospital may use one of the following formulas to calculate your patient's initial fluid requirements, depending on his age, his ability to tolerate fluids, and the preferred formula.

| FORMULA | ELECTROLYTE-CONTAINING SOLUTION | COLLOIDS | DEXTROSE |
|---|---|---|---|
| **FIRST 24 HOURS POSTBURN** | | | |
| Baxter (Parkland) | Ringer's lactate—4 ml/kg/% burn | Not used | Not used |
| Hypertonic sodium solution | Volume of fluid containing 250 mEq of sodium per liter to maintain hourly urinary output of 30 ml | Not used | Not used |
| Modified Brooke | Ringer's lactate—2 ml/kg/% burn | Not used | Not used |
| Burn budget of F.D. Moore | Ringer's lactate—1,000 to 4,000 ml; 0.5 normal saline—1,200 ml | 7.5% of body weight | 1,500 to 5,000 ml |
| Evans | Normal saline—1 ml/kg/% burn | 1 ml/kg/% burn | 2,000 ml |
| Brooke | Ringer's lactate—1.5 ml/kg/% burn | 0.5 ml/kg/% burn | 2,000 ml |
| **SECOND 24 HOURS POSTBURN** | | | |
| Burn budget of F.D. Moore | Ringer's lactate—1,000 to 4,000 ml; 0.5 normal saline—1,200 ml | 2.5% of body weight | 1,500 to 5,000 ml |
| Evans | ½ of first 24-hour requirement | ½ of first 24-hour requirement | 2,000 ml |
| Brooke | ½ to ¾ of first 24-hour requirement | ½ to ¾ of first 24-hour requirement | 2,000 ml |
| Parkland | Not used | 20% to 60% of calculated plasma volume (within 24 to 32 hours) | As necessary to maintain urinary output |
| Hypertonic sodium solution | ⅓ isotonic salt solution orally, up to 3,500-ml limit | Not used | Not used |
| Modified Brooke | Not used | 0.3 to 0.5 ml/kg/% burn | As necessary to maintain urinary output |

pensate for developing hypovolemia. Expect to withhold all food and fluids, and insert a nasogastric (NG) tube to maintain gastric decompression and to prevent distention and vomiting. Connect the NG tube to low intermittent suction. After emptying the patient's stomach, test the pH of the gastric aspirate with Nitrazine paper. This will give you a baseline figure. (Never allow your patient's pH to fall below 5, because this will increase his risk of ulcer formation.) Begin antacid therapy (probably with Maalox or Amphojel) every 1 to 2 hours. Instill 30 ml into the NG tube, then clamp the tube. After 30 minutes, restart the suction and retest his pH. If it falls below 5, notify the doctor. He may want you to increase the antacid therapy. Send a urine sample for urinalysis and osmolarity, electrolyte, protein, and myoglobin testing; and begin recording intake and output hourly. Don't forget to include your pa-

tient's gastric aspirate in your output record.

If your patient has an electrical burn, try to identify the path the current took through his body. You probably can only approximate this. Why? Because although entry and exit wounds provide clues, they can't help you predict the current's path, which is simply that of least resistance. This means that the current's path can't be predicted by any rule or formula; only the patient's signs and symptoms can guide you. If current passed through an extremity, assess it hourly for increased swelling, vascular compromise, decreased capillary refill time, diminished or absent pulses, and increased pain on motion (see *Understanding Compartment Syndrome,* pages 370 and 371).

The doctor will order a chest X-ray to be done using portable equipment. Although evidence of inhalation injuries won't show up on chest X-rays for

---

## ENCOURAGING YOUR PATIENT'S COOPERATION

When your patient with serious burns realizes the difficult, painful, and frustrating obstacles he faces during treatment and rehabilitation, he'll probably feel completely overwhelmed. Unfortunately, his despair may translate into refusal to cooperate in his treatment.

To encourage his cooperation, try establishing a contract with him each time you begin a difficult procedure.

Why a contract? Because, if your patient has a part in planning his care, he'll begin regaining some sense of control over his life. And, besides reminding him of his responsibility for keeping up his end of the agreement, a contract lets the patient know he can count on *you* to maintain *your* part of the agreement. A contract also gives both of you a chance to recognize each milestone of his progress and to feel a sense of accomplishment when difficult procedures are finished. Of course, day-to-day, informal, verbal contracts will do. Here are some guidelines:
• First, identify a short-term achievable goal. For example, you might tell your patient, "I'm going to remove the wet-to-dry dressings I applied this morning."
• Next, explain to the patient why the goal

is important. For example: "When the dressings come off, they take the burn drainage and dead tissue with them, so your wound will begin to heal with less risk of infection."
• Then explain what you expect from your patient: "This procedure may be quite uncomfortable for you. If you feel like crying or shouting, go ahead. But I need you to hold still; try not to squirm around or fight me." Offer choices—but only if they really exist. (For example, don't ask your patient if he'd like to put off the dressing change for an hour, if you know you have to change it now.) Choices give your patient some control over the procedure. Here's a choice you can give your patient: "If you need me to stop, just tell me and I will for a moment. Then, after you've taken a couple of deep breaths, I'll continue."
• Finally, be sure to explain what your patient can expect from *you.* For example, you might tell him you'll give him an analgesic before you begin (if appropriate). And explain that you'll be as gentle as possible. Tell him, too, that you'll be finished within a specific amount of time—for example, "no more than 15 minutes."

at least 24 hours postburn, this first X-ray will serve as a baseline and, of course, will indicate whether the patient had preexisting pulmonary disease. If a central venous pressure (CVP) line is inserted, wait until this procedure is complete before permitting the X-ray to be taken. Then the X-ray can help confirm—or rule out—correct placement of the CVP line.

Weigh your patient as soon after admission as possible, to provide baseline information for gauging his nutritional status and fluid balance. If you can't weigh him, ask his family to provide you with his approximate weight.

## TETANUS TOXOID: AN EXCEPTION TO THE "I.V.-ONLY RULE"

As a nurse, you know that patients with burns receive virtually all their medications I.V. Why? Because in these patients, widespread shifts in body fluids make absorption by the subcutaneous and I.M. routes erratic.

But one exception exists. It's tetanus toxoid, which is always given I.M. to burned patients—in fact, to *all* patients. So don't be surprised when your burned patient's medication order reads: "Tetanus toxoid I.M." It's the exception to the "I.V.-only" rule.

## Special Considerations

### Pediatric

Pediatric patients who've been burned require specialized care. One reason for this: a child's extremely large BSA in proportion to his weight causes him to lose more fluid and body heat than an adult. And the child's poor antibody response and decreased immunoglobulin levels make him more susceptible to infection and sepsis. Because of these increased dangers, some doctors recommend hospitalizing any burned child under age 2.

To classify a child's burn, use the same indications for burn depth that you'd use for an adult. (See *Assessing Burn Depth*, pages 666 and 667.) But to evaluate the percentage of BSA burned, use the Lund and Browder chart (see *Using the Lund and Browder Chart*, page 665). Fluid replacement is critical because of the pediatric patient's fragile balance between underhydration and overhydration. You may need to assist the doctor in performing a cutdown to obtain access to a vein for I.V. fluid replacement. Use a volume-control chamber (Solu-set) or infusion pump to precisely measure the fluids the patient receives. Keep accurate intake and output records. Weigh the child in the ED and then daily, and reassess him frequently for signs of fluid overload—such as rales and edema.

Remember that your pediatric patient's metabolic rate is higher than an adult's because he's still growing, making his protein and calorie needs proportionally higher. This patient's healing process is accelerated, too—both helping and hindering his recovery. The rapid process speeds recovery, but it can also increase the problems of scarring and contractures. The burn-care team must maintain constant vigilance to prevent these complications.

Unfortunately, you always need to consider whether a pediatric patient's burns may be due to child abuse. The distribution of the burns may provide a clue: for example, clearly demarcated circumferential burns of the hands may indicate that the child's hands were held in scalding water. Make sure you ask the patient privately for details about his burns and any bruises or other associated injuries. Record all your findings, including indications of poor nutritional status and how the child's family reacted to the burn incident. Don't forget: You have an obligation to report any suspected incident

DRUGS

# HIGHLIGHTING TOPICAL AGENTS USED IN BURN MANAGEMENT

You may apply a variety of topical agents on large burns that develop infections or fail to heal. This chart compares the method of application and the effects of some of the most common agents.

| AGENT | APPLICATION METHOD | NURSING CONSIDERATIONS |
|---|---|---|
| **0.5% silver nitrate solution** | Soak a 1″ (2.5-cm) thick gauze dressing with the solution every 2 hours. Change the dressing every 12 to 24 hours, using sterile technique. | This solution doesn't penetrate eschar, so watch the wound carefully for possible infection under the eschar. Keep the entire dressing wet at all times, using a catheter as necessary to moisten the inner layer of thick dressings. Be sure to watch laboratory values closely and report electrolyte abnormalities, such as hyponatremia, hypokalemia, and hypocalcemia. This ointment may blacken unburned skin and clothing, so apply it carefully. |
| **10% mafenide acetate cream (Sulfamylon)** | Remove the ointment from the wounds every 8 to 12 hours, and reapply a ¹⁄₁₆″ thick (1.6-mm) layer, using sterile technique. No dressing is necessary. Generally, limit use to patients with no more than 20% of body surface area burned. | Check arterial blood gas values, as ordered, if your patient has any respiratory problems. Metabolic acidosis and sensitivity reactions can develop. Give your patient an analgesic before every application, to reduce the possibly severe pain from the ointment. Prolonged pain may indicate allergy. Use cautiously if the patient has a history of sensitivity to sulfonamides. |
| **1% silver sulfadiazine cream (Silvadene)** | Remove the ointment from the wounds every 12 hours, and reapply a ¹⁄₁₆″ (1.6-mm) thick layer; replenish as needed. Cover with a dressing of fine mesh gauze, or leave open, as ordered. Use sterile technique. | This ointment doesn't penetrate eschar well, so watch the wound carefully for possible infection under the eschar. Check the complete blood count as ordered, and report any depression of the white blood cell count, because neutropenia may occur in the first week. Report any sensitivity reactions such as a skin rash or itching in unburned areas— the doctor will reevaluate use of the ointment. Use cautiously if the patient has a history of sensitivity to sulfonamides. |

of child abuse. (See the "When to Make a Report" entry in Chapter 2).

**Geriatric**
Geriatric patients with burns are likely to have preexisting diseases that can complicate their burn care. Underlying cardiac disease, for example, complicates fluid replacement because of the patient's decreased myocardial reserve, so you need to monitor his CVP or pulmonary artery pressure (PAP) as well as his blood pressure. If his blood pressure is low and his CVP or PAP is high, expect to decrease his infusion rate. Keep in mind that diabetes increases the geriatric patient's susceptibility to infection and slows wound healing. Degenerative diseases, such as arthritis, also affect this patient's ability to make a complete recovery.

Your elderly patient will probably have poor skin integrity. This prolongs the healing process and makes grafting procedures more difficult. He's also likely to be undernourished, complicating your nutritional management.

# CARE AFTER DIAGNOSIS

# Thermal Burns

### Initial care summary
The patient was burned in an incident involving exposure to flames, splashed hot tar or asphalt, scalding liquid, excessive amounts of ultraviolet rays (from the sun or a sunlamp), or an electrical flash.

Depending on the severity and extent of his burns, the patient had some or all of the following signs and symptoms on initial assessment:
• red, white, blistered, or charred skin (see *Assessing Burn Depth,* pages 666 and 667)

• hypotension
• tachycardia
• respiratory distress, particularly dyspnea, with a sooty tongue or pharynx and singed nostrils
• pain.

Depending on his respiratory status, the patient was either given humidified oxygen by mask or intubated and connected to a mechanical ventilator. An I.V. infusion of Ringer's lactate was started to replace depleted intravascular fluid and to prevent shock, with the infusion rate based on the percent of BSA burned and on the patient's body weight. Blood was drawn and sent to the laboratory for clotting studies, complete blood count (CBC), electrolytes, bilirubin, phosphorus, alkaline phosphatase, blood urea nitrogen (BUN), blood glucose, total serum protein, creatinine, albumin, globulin, calcium, phosphate, and typing and cross matching. (Arterial blood was drawn for ABG analysis, including arterial carboxyhemoglobin.) Chest X-rays were taken with a portable unit to provide a baseline and to verify correct CVP line and endotracheal tube placement. (Note: X-rays won't show changes due to smoke inhalation for at least 24 hours.) An indwelling (Foley) catheter was inserted to monitor the patient's urine output, and urine was sent for analysis. If he had decreased or absent bowel sounds, an NG tube was inserted and attached to intermittent low suction to maintain gastric decompression. The patient received:
• medication to relieve pain (typically morphine sulfate 0.1 mg/kg I.V.), after his vital signs were stabilized
• prophylactic antibiotics I.V. (Note: The benefits of this procedure aren't fully proven.)
• tetanus prophylaxis I.M.

### Priorities
You have five priorities in caring for a patient with a serious thermal burn:
• to maintain cardiorespiratory support
• to restore adequate fluid and electro-

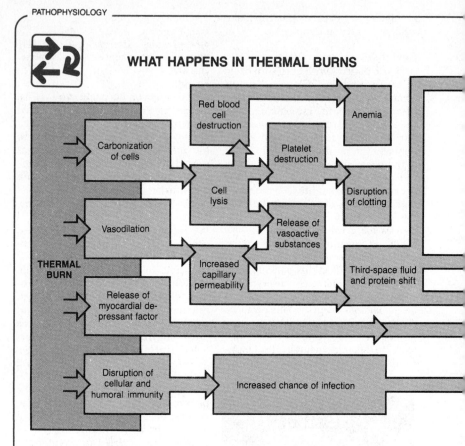

## WHAT HAPPENS IN THERMAL BURNS

A serious thermal burn not only produces traumatic skin wounds but also sets in motion many processes that ultimately disrupt the patient's metabolic state, affecting virtually every body system. Basically, this is what happens.

Initially, heat damages local tissues by denaturing cellular proteins and interfering with heat-labile enzyme systems. Besides skin cells, red blood cells and platelets in the skin's blood vessels are destroyed, which can lead to disruption of clotting. If exposure to intense heat is prolonged, muscle, tendons, nerves, and even bone may be destroyed, as well.

Because of cell membrane destruction, potassium (the chief intracellular cation) escapes into the vascular and interstitial fluid. This causes initial serum hyperkalemia, with a severe intracellular potassium deficit. Serum hypokalemia subsequently results from:

• shifting of body fluids from the interstitial

back into the intravascular space
• fluid loss through burn wound exudate
• (later) renal tubular excretion.

But the main feature of thermal burn injury is *increased capillary permeability.* Water, electrolytes (sodium), and plasma proteins (chiefly albumin) pass from the intravascular space into the interstitial compartment. This massive third-space fluid shifting results in edema and leads to hypovolemia ("burn shock") as circulating blood volume decreases.

Also contributing to hypovolemia is the evaporative fluid loss from the burn wound. As a result of fluid shifts, evaporation loss, and red blood cell destruction, hemoconcentration occurs; this may lead to sludging in the microcirculation. This sluggish microcirculation can cause formation of thrombi and emboli, which contribute to inadequate tissue perfusion.

The release of a myocardial depressant factor has been identified in patients

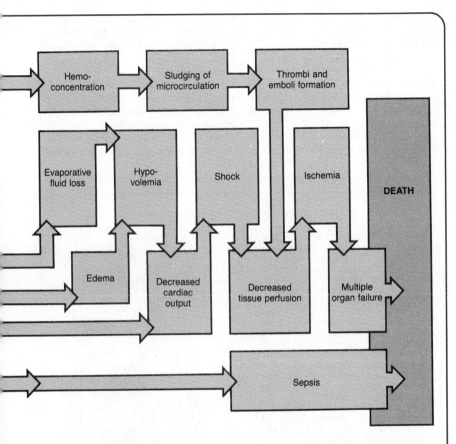

with extensive burn injuries. This depressant factor, along with hypovolemia, decreases cardiac output. The result? Further decreased tissue perfusion, multiple organ failure, and possibly death.

During this process, however, the body's neuroendocrine stress response to the burn injury triggers several compensatory mechanisms. Vasoconstriction occurs as a result of sympathetic nervous system stimulation, maintaining perfusion of vital organs at the expense of peripheral organ perfusion. The kidneys, as well as the GI system, may be affected, with resulting paralytic ileus and, possibly, Curling's ulcers. The release of antidiuretic hormone from the posterior pituitary and aldosterone from the adrenal cortex causes compensatory sodium and water retention—to counteract the fluid and electrolyte losses. Catecholamine release from the adrenal medulla results from sympathetic stimulation, causing the hypermetabolism charac-

teristic of patients with burns. Glucose metabolism, oxygen consumption, and catabolism are all increased. Catabolism, coupled with the protein loss from the burn wound exudate, eventually leads to a state of negative nitrogen balance. If the burned patient's increased nutritional needs aren't met, he may suffer complications of malnutrition, such as poor wound healing and over-whelming infection.

Additional insults to the burned patient involve the kidneys, immune system, and respiratory tract. Renal failure may develop from severe shock or from the kidneys' inability to filter the large amounts of hemoglobin and myoglobin released from damaged muscle and red blood cells.

Researchers don't yet understand why thermal burns reduce immunocompetence, limiting the burned patient's ability to fight infection and predisposing him to sepsis.

lyte balance
- to prevent infection
- to relieve his pain
- to provide psychological support.

After you secure your patient's airway, breathing, and circulation, continue to assess his ABGs, neurologic status, and respiratory rate for signs and symptoms of hypoxemia.

Calculate his fluid needs. His need for massive fluid replacement is greatest during the first 8 hours after the burn occurs. Why? Because circulating burn toxins alter capillary permeability, resulting in fluid shifts. Electrolytes, protein, and water extravasate from the capillary bed, decreasing the patient's circulating blood volume and leading to hypovolemia. (If the patient's burn covers more than 30% of his BSA, capillary permeability will increase throughout his body.) Capillary permeability begins to reverse itself after 8 to 12 hours and is usually restored within 24 hours.

To decrease the patient's hypovole-

## UNDERSTANDING ESCHAROTOMY

A patient with a full-thickness burn develops eschar—a thick layer of devitalized, inelastic tissue. In a circumferential burn of an extremity or the thorax, edema forming below the eschar causes increased tissue pressure, sometimes to the point of impairing blood flow to the extremity or restricting respiratory movement. If this occurs in your burned patient, the doctor may have to perform a bedside escharotomy to relieve the pressure.

As a nurse, you'll probably be the first to see the signs and symptoms indicating that your burned patient needs an escharotomy. In *any* patient with a circumferential full-thickness burn, watch for:
- loss of distal pulses (measured by a Doppler ultrasonic flowmeter, if possible)
- cyanosis and impaired capillary filling
- progressive paresthesia
- unrelenting deep-tissue and muscle pain
- respiratory impairment.

If you note any of these signs and symptoms, notify the doctor *immediately*—prompt surgical intervention is necessary. Using a scalpel, the doctor will make an incision along the entire burned area, penetrating the eschar to the depth of the superficial fascia (see the illustration). This will let the underlying tissues spread as edema increases—relieving tissue pressure, permitting full lung expansion (if it's a thoracic escharotomy), and preventing necrosis and ischemia in uninjured tissue.

After the escharotomy, control your patient's bleeding with pressure dressings or by assisting the doctor with electrocoagulation. Then apply an antimicrobial agent and resume burn care as indicated. Continue to monitor your patient's respiratory and circulatory status to assess the procedure's effectiveness.

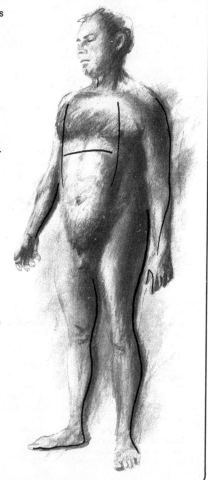

mia and to prevent burn shock, the doctor will order half the calculated 24-hour fluid replacement quantity infused during the first 8 hours. Expect to give Ringer's lactate for the first 24 hours. A simple formula for calculating how much Ringer's lactate the patient should receive in the first 24 hours is the Baxter (Parkland) formula: 4 ml Ringer's lactate/kg body weight/% BSA. Here's an example:

$$\begin{array}{r} 50\% \text{ BSA} \\ \times \quad 70 \text{ kg} \\ \hline 3,500 \\ \times \quad 4 \text{ ml Ringer's lactate} \\ \hline 14,000 \text{ ml Ringer's lactate} \end{array}$$

Using this example, you'd administer:
• 7,000 ml over the first 8 hours
• 3,500 ml over the second 8 hours
• 3,500 ml over the third 8 hours.

Other formulas call for giving the patient colloids together with crystalloids, or hypertonic saline solution. (See *Guidelines for Fluid Replacement*, pages 668 and 669, and *Understanding Colloids and Crystalloids* in the Appendix.)

Take steps to prevent infection from the moment your patient comes to the hospital—this is a top priority. Follow these steps:
• Use sterile linen, if possible.
• Use sterile technique when performing wound care or invasive procedures.
• Keep your patient in isolation, or limit visitors, as ordered.
• Insist that everyone who comes in contact with a patient who has a moderate-to-severe burn wear a mask, cap, and sterile gown and gloves—especially if the burn wounds are exposed.
• You may be asked to administer prophylactic I.V. antibiotics and to apply topical antimicrobial cream to the burn wound to decrease the likelihood of infection.

Signs of infection, if it occurs, won't appear until at least 48 hours postburn.

Administer I.V. analgesic medications, as prescribed, and monitor your patient's response. After each dose, check and record his vital signs and responses.

## Continuing assessment and therapeutic care

Continue to monitor and reassess your patient frequently. Keep in mind that signs and symptoms of respiratory complications, shock, hypothermia, cardiac dysrhythmias, and peripheral vascular compromise may not develop for several hours or days, so your close monitoring is critically important.

Your patient's need for massive fluid replacement (probably with Ringer's lactate) will continue for the first 24 hours after he's burned. Then the patient will begin to receive colloids, dextrose 5% in water, and electrolyte replacement. Remember to keep an accurate intake and output record to monitor his fluid balance closely.

Monitor his vital signs, urine output, and mental status frequently to help determine whether his fluid replacement's adequate. Your patient's baseline pulse rate will probably be rapid (about 100 to 120 beats/minute) because of his body's compensatory response to a major burn. His blood pressure should remain normal. (If he becomes hypotensive, this may indicate that he's going into hypovolemic shock from failure to respond to massive fluid replacement.) Expect to administer a fluid challenge or colloids if your patient's vital signs still don't improve. As a last alternative, the doctor may order a vasopressor, such as dopamine.

You may assist the doctor with insertion of an arterial catheter for frequent monitoring of the patient's ABGs and continuous monitoring of his blood pressure. Remember, never rely solely on arterial line pressure measurements. Continue to check his blood pressure manually and to assess circulation in his burned extremities frequently for circulatory compromise. Use a Doppler ultrasonic flowmeter if his blood pressure is too weak for you to hear with a stethoscope. (See *Using Doppler Ultrasound*, page 663.) This may occur because of increasing edema or because your patient's burn shock is causing poor cardiac output.

To assess the adequacy of fluid replacement, follow these guidelines:

• *Urine output*—Monitor your patient's urine output closely; it's the most reliable indicator of adequate tissue perfusion. Assess his output every 15 minutes until his hydration's adequate—then hourly. (See *Guidelines for Fluid Replacement*, pages 668 and 669.) When his hydration's adequate, his urine output should increase and his urine specific gravity should return to normal.

• *Urine color*—While monitoring your patient's urine output, note the urine's color, as well. As you know, a deep burn destroys red blood cells and muscle tissue, releasing free hemoglobin and myoglobin into the patient's bloodstream. This may cause hemoglobinuria or myoglobinuria, resulting in dark red or brown urine. Free myoglobin may pass through the kidneys—but it also may plug renal tubules, decrease renal perfusion, and cause acute renal failure from acute tubular necrosis (see the "Acute Renal Failure" entry in Chapter 13).

• *Vital signs*—Maintain the patient's blood pressure above 90/60. If it falls more than 20 mm Hg below his normal blood pressure or if his pulse rate increases to above 120 beats/minute, notify the doctor *immediately*—these changes may indicate burn shock.

• *Mental status*—In a previously quiet patient, changes such as restlessness, confusion, or agitation may indicate poor cerebral perfusion, hypoxemia, or insufficient hydration.

• *Body weight*—Expect that your burned patient will *gain* weight during the first 48 to 72 hours postburn because of third-space fluid shifting. After the 3rd day, expect that he will *lose* weight as fluid shifts to the vascular compartment and diuresis occurs. Consider a loss of 1 lb (0.45 kg) per day for about 10 days acceptable. Your goal is to provide sufficient nutritional

therapy to maintain his preburn weight.

• *Respiratory status*—Auscultate your patient's breath sounds for rales, and note any dyspnea, especially if your patient's elderly or has a history of heart failure. In such a patient, dyspnea may indicate fluid overload. If you note rales or dyspnea, auscultate his heart sounds. You may hear an $S_3$ heart sound, another indicator of congestive heart failure (CHF). If you note any of these signs, call the doctor *immediately*.

• *Serial laboratory values*—After the first 24 hours, monitor his laboratory test results. An increased hematocrit level may indicate hemoconcentration. A hematocrit level below 35% may indicate hemodilution or a need for blood replacement. Monitor your patient's electrolyte levels, too. If his sodium level is greater than 145 mEq/liter (indicating hyperosmolarity), notify the doctor and adjust the patient's infusion rate as ordered. If his sodium is less than 130 mEq/liter (indicating water intoxication), you should also notify the doctor.

Assess your patient's body temperature frequently. Be careful to maintain his core body temperature by covering him with a sterile blanket and exposing only small areas of his body at a time. (The rapid fluid loss that accompanies a burn causes corresponding heat loss of about 540 calories/liter.) If he starts to shiver or his temperature drops below 96° F. (35.5° C.), close the treatment room doors (to decrease air currents) and place blankets, a heat lamp, or (if available) a heated bed shield over the patient. A drop in core temperature places him at risk for hypothermia, shock, ventricular fibrillation, and cardiopulmonary arrest.

Monitor your patient's respirations frequently, especially during the first 72 hours postburn (when inhalation injury is most likely to develop). Watch for any change in the character or rate of his respirations—do you note dyspnea or stridor? Anxiety, restlessness,

## CARING FOR TEMPORARY SKIN GRAFTS

A patient with deep partial-thickness or full-thickness burns needs skin grafts to prevent infection and to promote healing of the wounds. These grafts may be applied as soon as eschar is removed. Extremely serious burns may require temporary grafts, to provide early wound closure until autografting (permanent grafting of skin taken from the patient's own body) can be done. These grafts, also called biological dressings, prevent the loss of large amounts of fluid and protein from the wounds and protect the wounds from infection. They also protect exposed structures such as nerves, blood vessels, and tendons.

Types of temporary grafts include:
• allografts (homografts) consisting of human skin from a cadaver (usually obtained from a skin bank)
• xenografts (heterografts) consisting of animal skin (commonly pigskin)
• biosynthetic grafts consisting of a combination of collagen and synthetics.

Whatever type of temporary graft your burned patient receives, he'll need constant care to ensure that his burns heal properly and are protected from infection. So be sure to follow these guidelines when caring for a patient with a temporary graft:
• Keep the graft exposed to air, or dress it as ordered, and protect it from pressure and friction.
• Inspect the burn site frequently. The temporary graft "takes" by adhering to the wound tightly. If separation or sloughing occurs, notify the doctor—he may have to replace the graft.
• Assist the doctor in changing the temporary graft if rejection occurs.
• Watch for signs and symptoms of systemic infection and infection at the graft site. Infection may necessitate removal of the graft; if this occurs, expect to treat the burn site with antimicrobial ointment and the patient with systemic antibiotics.
• You may use a synthetic material, such as Opsite, to temporarily cover superficial partial-thickness burns.

---

or alteration in consciousness may indicate poor ventilation and hypoxemia from edema or inhalation injury. (See *Understanding Inhalation Injuries,* pages 692 and 693.) Anticipate frequent ABG analyses and chest X-rays to monitor your patient's respiratory status. At the first sign of respiratory difficulty, provide humidified oxygen by mask (if he's not already receiving it) and call the doctor *immediately.*

Pain control will become increasingly difficult as your patient's burn heals, because his pain will intensify as healing progresses and as his nerves regenerate. Give an analgesic such as morphine sulfate, as ordered, *at least 20 minutes before dressing changes and other painful procedures.* Consider making short-term verbal contracts with your patient when you need his cooperation to complete difficult or painful procedures. (See *Encouraging Your Patient's Cooperation,* page 670.)

Clean and debride your patient's burns, as ordered. The doctor may ask you to use a combination of procedures and dressings, including (unless you are using a biologic or synthetic dressing) a topical antimicrobial for local care of the patient's burn wound. The following are some of the most frequently used techniques:
• *Exposure*—The burn wound is left exposed to the air, with the patient kept in isolation and the ambient temperature maintained at 82° to 84° F. (27.8° to 28.9° C.). Antimicrobial cream is applied to the wound at specified intervals. As the eschar begins to separate, the necrotic material is carefully trimmed away. This technique minimizes bacterial growth by decreasing moisture on the wound surface.
• *Occlusive dry dressings*—This technique involves applying a multilayered set of dressings. The *innermost layer,* of fine mesh gauze, helps entrap necrotic tissue. If the dressing is being applied over a new or healing graft site, this innermost layer consists of a fine mesh gauze or nonadherent sheeting lightly lubricated with a water-soluble antibiotic or petrolatum. The *middle layer* must be bulky enough to allow absorption of wound exudate from the

## YOUR ROLE IN AN EMERGENCY

## DEBRIDEMENT AND HYDROTHERAPY

As you know, your patient's severe burns need daily cleansing and debridement to prevent infection, to aid the healing process, and to prepare the burn site for skin grafts. You may be asked to do this either at your patient's bedside or in a hydrotherapy tub (Hubbard tank). The following guidelines will help you perform bedside and hydrotherapy debridement safely.

### Bedside debridement
*Procedure*
• If this is your patient's first bedside debridement, explain the procedure to him to encourage his cooperation. Limit the number of people in his room to prevent bacterial contamination of the exposed wound.
• Administer an analgesic 20 minutes before starting debridement, as ordered.
• Wash your hands and put on a sterile cap, mask, gown or apron, and gloves.
• Remove any existing burn dressings, then gently cleanse the wound with povidone-iodine (Betadine) or another appropriate cleansing agent.
• Shave all hair 2″ (5 cm) out from the wound site.
• Change to a fresh sterile gown or apron and gloves.
• Pick up loosened edges of the eschar with sterile forceps. Then, with the blunt edge of sterile scissors or another forceps, probe the eschar and cut the dead tissue away from the wound with the scissors. Leave a ¼″ (6.4-mm) edge of remaining eschar, to avoid cutting into viable tissue. *Don't* debride closed blisters.
• Because debridement removes only dead tissue, bleeding should be minimal. If significant bleeding occurs, apply gentle pressure on the wound with 4″ × 4″ dry, sterile gauze sponges or apply a hemostatic agent, such as a silver nitrate stick. If the bleeding persists, notify the doctor and maintain pressure on the wound until he can control the bleeding with sutures or electrocauterization.
• Rinse the wound surface with saline-saturated lap sponges, then place a sterile burn pad under the cleansed body part. Obtain wound cultures, as ordered.

• Remove the contaminated gown and change to sterile gloves.
• Replace dressings or antimicrobial ointment, as ordered.
*Special considerations*
• To prevent chilling and fluid loss from evaporation, keep your patient warm and avoid exposing large areas of his body. Don't debride more than a 4-in² (10.2-cm²) area per procedure.
• As you know, debridement can be extremely painful. Try to complete the procedure quickly to spare your patient unnecessary pain. If possible, ask another nurse to assist you, and limit the entire procedure to no more than 20 minutes.

### Hydrotherapy debridement
*Procedure*
• To prevent cross-contamination, make sure the tub, all equipment, and the tub room are thoroughly cleaned and disinfected before beginning hydrotherapy. You may line the tub with a sterile plastic liner for extra protection against infection.
• Fill the tub with water warmed to 98° to 104° F. (36.7° to 40° C.), turn on the agitator (if appropriate), and add electrolyte solutions and germicidal solutions, as ordered. Make sure the air temperature is 80° to 85° F. (26.7° to 29.4° C.) or heat lamps are in place, so your patient won't be chilled when he enters or exits the tub.
• If this is the patient's first tub debridement, explain the procedure to him.
• Administer an analgesic 20 minutes before beginning the procedure, as ordered.
• Wash your hands and put on a sterile gown, shoe covers, mask, surgical cap, and axilla-length sterile gloves.
• Place your patient on the plinth, then lower him into the tank so the headrest supports his head. Allow him to soak for 3 to 5 minutes.
• Cleanse all unburned areas (encourage your patient to do this himself, if he can). Wash the unburned skin (shave the hair near the wound), shampoo his scalp, and give mouth care. Provide perineal care (often done before tubbing, too), and clean inside your patient's nose and the folds of his ears and eyes with cotton-tipped applicators.

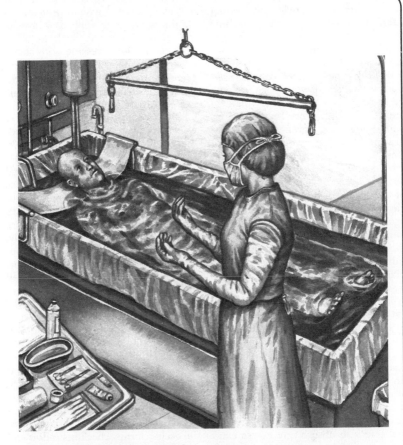

• Change into a fresh, sterile gown and gloves, and gently wash burned areas with gauze pads or sponges to remove topical agents, exudate, necrotic tissue, and other debris.
• Turn off the agitator and use sterile forceps and scissors to debride, as needed.
• When debridement's complete, spray-rinse the patient's entire body to remove all debris.
• Transfer the patient to a stretcher covered with a sterile sheet and bath blanket; then cover him with a warm, sterile sheet (a blanket may be added for warmth), and pat unburned areas dry.
• Replace dressings or antimicrobial ointment, as ordered, before returning the patient to his room.
*Special considerations*
• Remain with the patient at all times during the procedure, to prevent him from injuring himself in the tub.

• Limit hydrotherapy to 30 minutes, to avoid electrolyte loss.
• During the procedure, watch your patient for signs of chilling or fatigue, for altered vital signs, and for unusual pain. Inspect the burn site and surrounding tissues carefully for signs of infection.
• Hydrotherapy's contraindicated if your patient has an electrolyte or fluid imbalance, a body temperature over 103° F. (39.4° C.), or a sudden increase or decrease in respiration, pulse, or blood pressure. It's also contraindicated for a patient who has a mending fracture, an endotracheal tube, or a tracheostomy, or who otherwise needs respiratory assistance.
• In some centers, hydrotherapy has been discontinued in favor of suspending the patient over a tank and spray-rinsing him. This is done to prevent cross-contamination and sepsis.

wound's surface. The *outer layer* is a stretch bandage that holds the dressing firmly in place. Properly applied, this type of dressing can increase the patient's comfort and help prevent contractures.

• *Wet dressings*—These can be used during all stages of wound healing. The *inner layer* is a single layer of gauze and is helpful in debriding the wound and in preparing a granulation bed for grafting. (If the dressing is covering a fresh graft, this layer needn't be removed at each dressing change.) The *outer layer* consists of multiple layers of 24-ply gauze pads; these are sufficiently bulky so that they hold fluid against the wound surface with minimal rewetting. Solutions used to wet this type of dressing range from normal saline solution to complex antimicrobial solutions.

• *Single-layer gauze dressings*—This type of dressing is used over an application of antimicrobial topical cream, to keep the medication against the wound surface. That way, the patient's body motions can't dislodge it, and he has maximum range of motion. This dressing is applied using a single layer of stretch gauze or a net tube dressing. If you use this type of dressing, place absorbent wound underpads over the bed linens to absorb any excess exudate.

• *Subeschar injection*—This technique is only used as ordered for an infected burn wound. The burn wound is exposed during this procedure, and antimicrobial solution is injected beneath the eschar via hypodermoclysis. Following this therapy, appropriate dressings are reapplied to affected areas.

• *Hydrotherapy*—The patient is immersed in a tub for a short period (no longer than 30 minutes) while his wound is thoroughly cleansed. Tubbing also facilitates removal of dressings and loosening of slough, eschar, exudate, and topical medications.

• *Enzymatic debridement*—A proteolytic enzyme, such as sutilains (Travase) ointment, is applied directly to the burn wound, where it liquefies and degrades necrotic wound protein. After the ointment is applied, a layer of topical antimicrobial, such as Silvadene, and a wet dressing with sterile water or normal saline solution is kept over the ointment film. When this technique is used, the treated area shouldn't exceed 15% of the BSA.

• *Antimicrobial agents*—A variety of agents are used to treat burns, including povidone-iodine (Betadine), 1% silver sulfadiazine (Silvadene), 10% mafenide acetate (Sulfamylon), and 0.5% silver nitrate solution. Each has its particular advantages and disadvantages—for example, if your patient's receiving silver nitrate solution, be sure to monitor his electrolyte levels closely. This is because hypocalcemia, hyponatremia, or hypokalemia may occur. (See *Highlighting Topical Agents Used in Burn Management,* pages 672 and 673.)

If tar or asphalt caused your patient's burn, change his burn dressing and reapply a silver sulfadiazine cream or Neosporin ointment every 12 hours until the tar is dissolved completely and removed.

If the patient has burns on any extremity, keep it elevated to decrease edema. If full-thickness circumferential eschar forms, check his radial and pedal pulses and capillary refill time hourly. At the first sign of decreased circulation to his extremities (blanching, tingling, decreased pulses, cyanosis, or increased pain on motion), notify the doctor *immediately* and prepare for escharotomy to relieve the compression (see *Understanding Escharotomy,* page 676). If eschar forms on the patient's neck, chest, or abdomen, be alert for signs of respiratory compromise, such as dyspnea and hypoventilation, and for signs and symptoms of hypoxemia, such as confusion and lethargy. Emergency excisional or enzymatic escharotomy may be necessary to relieve the pressure that burn edema causes.

Assess your patient's burn wounds

## MEETING YOUR BURNED PATIENT'S NUTRITIONAL NEEDS

Your burned patient's nutritional needs will be greatly increased until his wounds heal. He'll need a diet formula high in potassium, protein, vitamins, fats, nitrogen, and calories to keep his weight as close to his preburn weight as possible.

A common formula used to calculate adult calorie needs is 25 kcal/kg + 40 kcal/% body surface area (BSA) burned; for children, 60 kcal/kg + 35 kcal/% BSA burned. Use the following guidelines to ensure that your patient's fluid, calorie, and protein needs are met:
• If your patient's had a paralytic ileus and has burns over more than 20% of his BSA, begin feedings through a nasogastric (NG) tube, using a small and flexible catheter, as soon as his bowel sounds return (typically within 48 hours). Raise the head of his bed 30° to prevent aspiration during feedings. Leave the tube in place and begin a slow, continuous infusion; check every 4 hours for any undigested feedings.
• Also begin oral feedings, and increase as tolerated, except when the patient has facial burns with edema or his level of consciousness is decreased.
• You may begin antacid therapy such as aluminum hydroxide (Maalox) every 2 hours to help prevent Curling's ulcer.
• Help assess your patient's tolerance for the feedings by reporting any nausea, vomiting, or diarrhea.
• If your patient has a prolonged ileus or a large burn, or he can't absorb enough calories through oral feedings and an NG tube, you may give some or all of his nutrients by total parenteral nutrition (TPN). (Remember, however, that TPN increases your patient's chance of infection.)
• Collect 24-hour urine specimens to measure your patient's urea nitrogen level and to evaluate his nitrogen balance. Also monitor his serum protein, glucose, and electrolyte levels. Expect the doctor to adjust the formula, as necessary.
• Keep daily intake and output records and daily calorie and protein counts, and weigh your patient at the same time each day to determine whether his metabolic needs are being met.

---

frequently for signs of infection. Depending on your hospital's policy, obtain wound cultures three times per week until eschar has separated. Report any signs of infection:
• *localized*—Signs include erythema, pain, edema, or induration around the wound and purulent drainage or darkening of the wound eschar.
• *systemic*—Signs include confusion, ileus, hypo- or hyperthermia, hypotension, tachycardia, and decreased urine output. (See the "Septic Shock" entry in Chapter 14.)

After you've assessed your patient's condition and recorded baseline values, obtain a complete medical history—he may have a chronic illness that could complicate his recovery. Here are some examples:
• If your patient has *sickle cell disease*, he may have a sickle cell crisis triggered by the hypovolemia that immediately followed the burn.
• If he has a *cardiovascular disease*, he's vulnerable to developing CHF or pulmonary edema if his fluid replacement is too aggressive.
• If he has *chronic obstructive pulmonary disease*, assess him for complications from obstructed airflow and excessive secretions. Use low-flow oxygen (2 liters/minute) to avoid carbon dioxide retention.
• If the laboratory reported a *high blood alcohol or drug level*, assess any changes in mental status carefully. They could be early withdrawal signs.
• If your patient has a history of abusing alcohol, the doctor will check for *hepatic disease*. If your patient has severe hepatic disease, multiple serious complications may occur. Why? Because of fluid excess, ascites, impaired skin integrity, electrolyte imbalance, vitamin deficiency, and decreased ability to fight infection.
• If your patient has *diabetes*, monitor his fluid replacement and blood glucose tests very carefully until the burn wound is closed. Expect your diabetic patient to have nutritional deficits, slow

wound healing, and altered demand for insulin.

• If your patient has a history of mental illness, consider the possibility that his burns were self-inflicted. If a suicide attempt is suspected, observe precautions according to your hospital's policy.

After your patient's stabilized, one of your most important roles is to provide a therapeutic diet.

The burned patient's increased metabolic needs and his decreased appetite provide one of your biggest challenges. (See *Meeting Your Burned Patient's Nutritional Needs,* page 683.) Expect to try many approaches to meet your patient's nutritional needs during his recovery period. Several formulas have been developed for estimating a burned patient's caloric needs. One is the Curreri formula:

• *For an adult patient:*
(25 kcal × kg of body weight) +
(40 kcal × % BSA burned)

• *For a child:*
(60 kcal × kg of body weight) +
(35 kcal × % BSA burned).

Record all the food and liquid the patient ingests on a calorie count chart. This allows the dietitian to calculate the patient's total calorie and protein intake for each day. Give supplemental feedings between meals, as prescribed, to meet the patient's caloric needs.

If your patient can't eat enough to meet his nutritional needs, start tube feedings. Expect to insert an NG tube or a small-bore feeding tube to administer continual tube feedings. Remember to check for residual contents by aspirating back the patient's gastric contents every 4 hours. If the contents' volume is greater than 100 ml, notify the doctor; he may ask you to slow the rate of infusion until absorption occurs.

If the tube feedings still don't meet your patient's nutritional needs, the doctor may choose total parenteral nu-

trition (TPN) as a final alternative. Because the formula used has a high dextrose content, be extremely careful to maintain sterility at the insertion site—infection often accompanies this form of nutritional therapy. Monitor his blood glucose levels and urine sugar and acetone levels every 6 hours, because he may have difficulty metabolizing the excess glucose load.

Skin care remains a priority until your patient's discharged. To maintain the integrity of his unburned skin and to control edema, change his position often. Position his joints in extension (most contractures occur in the position of flexion). Examples of proper positioning are:

• *shoulder*—Position at a 90° angle abducted from the body's midline (you can use an elbow splint to maintain this position).

• *hips, knees, elbows*—Position all in extension.

Along with proper positioning, exercise—both passive and active—is essential to maintain your patient's full range of motion. As ordered, begin exercise for your patient on the day of admission, starting with simple range-of-motion (ROM) exercises that the patient can do himself. Be sure you don't exceed the point of resistance when you help your patient perform ROM exercises, because this may cause an increase in his inflammatory response that results in calcium deposits and loss of function.

A physical therapist or occupational therapist will initiate your patient's exercise program. Ask him to post a list of recommended exercises in the patient's room, and encourage the patient to perform these. His participation gives him a sense of control and contributes to the speed of his recovery. Remember, inactivity may result in contractures or permanent loss of function. Encourage early ambulation; if your patient has leg burns, apply elastic bandages on his legs whenever they're dependent. This will decrease edema.

Continue giving wound care to burn

and graft sites. The patient with extensive burns will require multiple grafting procedures, and his progress will be slow because of the insufficiency of donor sites. Expect the doctor to use a temporary graft—such as an *allograft* (obtained from the body of another person), a *xenograft* (obtained from an animal), or a *synthetic* or *biosynthetic graft*—until a granulation bed has formed at the burn site. Then he may apply a permanent graft. The principal functions of a temporary graft are to prevent water loss from evaporation and to decrease the risk of infection. This type of graft also allows the patient to move about more easily and covers his exposed nerve endings, making him more comfortable. (See *Caring for Temporary Skin Grafts,* page 679.)

A permanent graft, using the patient's own skin taken from an unburned part of his body, is applied once the wound is free of eschar and infection. These grafts are possible because the blood supply is rapidly reestablished. Until capillaries generate into the grafted tissue, the graft is nourished by an osmotic interchange with the intercellular fluid of the recipient bed. The two types of permanent grafts are:
• *split-thickness,* including the epidermis and part of the dermal layer
• *full-thickness,* including the epidermis and the full dermal layer.
Full-thickness skin grafts are used for cosmetic reconstruction. (Remember, harvesting of a full-thickness graft requires placement of a split-thickness skin graft to heal the donor site.)

Focus your care on watching your patient for signs of infection at both the burn site and donor site. Prevent the graft from slipping out of place, making sure you keep all pressure off the graft to facilitate tissue growth. Use a CircOlectric bed or a low-pressure (Clinatron) bed to help reduce pressure on the area.

Gradually increase his participation in activities of daily living—to increase his strength and to encourage his psychological independence. Encourage his family to take part in counseling sessions, and teach them the importance of having the patient take care of himself as much as possible—despite his pain. Remind them that this is the way he will regain as much function as possible. Arrange for counseling to help him develop strategies for coping with his altered appearance and with functional problems.

Expect him to progress through stages of grieving, depression, anger, and frustration—all are common reactions in patients with serious burns.

# Electrical Burns

### Initial care summary
Initial assessment of your patient with an electrical current burn and related injuries revealed some or all of the following signs and symptoms:
• pain
• skin surface injury, which may have been extensive. He may have had an entry wound that was ischemic, charred, depressed, whitish yellow, and surrounded by blisters. The exit wound may have been small, similar in appearance to the entry site, or larger—possibly even an explosive amputation. If he was struck by lightning, the skin around the entrance wound may have been edematous, charred, or reddened in a burn pattern shaped like tree branches—the so-called arborescent pattern.
• cardiac complications, possibly mild dysrhythmias but also possibly ventricular fibrillation and cardiac standstill
• respiratory complications, possibly tachypnea, apnea, or even respiratory muscle paralysis
• circulatory signs and symptoms, possibly as mild as rapid pulse and decreased blood pressure or as severe as burn shock from fluid shifts associated

# WHAT HAPPENS IN ELECTRICAL BURNS

Electric current, either man-made or natural (lightning), can cause a wide range of injuries, from minor burns to multiple trauma and death. When electric current contacts tissue, three types of injury can occur:
• thermal surface burns from heat and flames that accompany electric current
• arc or flash burns from current that doesn't pass through the body
• so-called true electrical injury from current that does pass through the body.

True electrical injury is more like a crush injury than a burn. Why? Because thermal burns usually destroy only the skin and subcutaneous tissue, whereas electrical injury goes deeper, often destroying muscle tissue and affecting internal organs.

The severity of electrical burns and related injuries depends on these variables:
• the type and the intensity of the current
• the duration of the current's contact with tissue
• the resistance of the tissue the current passes through.

In general, the greater the current's voltage and amperage, and the lower the tissue resistance, the greater the damage to body tissues. However, a low-voltage burn with little resistance (such as when the victim's skin is wet) may produce the same amperage, and thus similar damage, as a high-voltage burn in the presence of higher resistance. This explains why a typical bathtub incident, involving a low-voltage appliance dropped into the water, often causes death.

Electric current is either alternating or direct. Lightning is high-voltage (measured in millions of volts), high-amperage (estimated at between 12,000 and 200,000 amperes) *direct* current. A lightning strike produces both thermal surface burns and true electrical injury as the current flows through the victim's body and into the ground.

Common household electricity is 110-volt or 220-volt *alternating* current. Unlike direct current, alternating current produces tetanic muscular contractions that can cause muscle injury, tendon ruptures, joint dislocations, or bone fractures. These contractions can also prevent the victim from freeing himself from the source of the current (for example, if he grasped a live wire), increasing the damage.

The pathophysiology of electrical burns and related injuries is complex. The current typically produces well-defined, ischemic, painless entrance and exit wounds of varying size, depending on the severity of the injury. As electricity converts to thermal energy in the body, heat coagulates cell proteins, destroying or seriously damaging cells. Electric current generally passes through the body along the path of least resistance—through tissue fluids, blood vessels, and nerves. The resulting degeneration of blood vessel walls and formation of thrombi cause tissue ischemia and necrosis along the current's path.

Muscle damage occurs initially from the current's direct effects and later from disruption of the blood supply. As muscle tissue swells in its fascia, compartment pressures rise, causing more damage as the blood supply to distal parts is cut off.

The most serious injuries occur from electric current passing through vital organs. Ventricular fibrillation or other dysrhythmias can alter heart function, possibly causing cardiac arrest. Neurologic deficits (for example, seizures, coma, and respiratory arrest) may occur if the central nervous system is affected by vascular disruption or demyelinization. Peripheral nerve deficits, from local nerve involvement, may also occur. Compression fractures of the vertebrae or disruption of the spinal cord's blood supply may lead to transient or permanent spinal cord lesions and motor deficits ranging from simple paresis to quadriplegia. Lung and GI organ tissues may also be affected.

Massive ischemic and coagulation necrosis of muscles causes release of great quantities of the proteins hemoglobin and myoglobin. These proteins precipitate in the renal tubules, causing renal tubular necrosis and, possibly, renal failure. In addition, increased anaerobic metabolism occurring in large areas of ischemic muscle injury leads to lactic acidosis. This further decreases myoglobin clearance and accelerates the patient's progress toward renal failure.

Late effects of electrical burns and related injuries may include delayed hemorrhage, cholelithiasis, and cataracts.

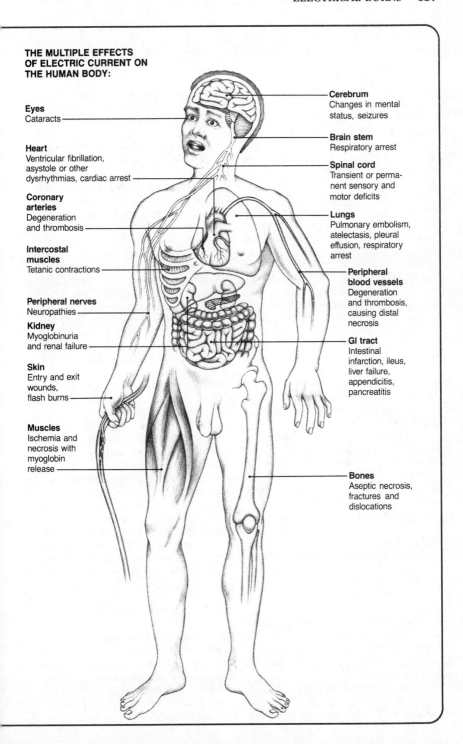

**THE MULTIPLE EFFECTS OF ELECTRIC CURRENT ON THE HUMAN BODY:**

**Eyes**
Cataracts

**Heart**
Ventricular fibrillation, asystole or other dysrhythmias, cardiac arrest

**Coronary arteries**
Degeneration and thrombosis

**Intercostal muscles**
Tetanic contractions

**Peripheral nerves**
Neuropathies

**Kidney**
Myoglobinuria and renal failure

**Skin**
Entry and exit wounds, flash burns

**Muscles**
Ischemia and necrosis with myoglobin release

**Cerebrum**
Changes in mental status, seizures

**Brain stem**
Respiratory arrest

**Spinal cord**
Transient or permanent sensory and motor deficits

**Lungs**
Pulmonary embolism, atelectasis, pleural effusion, respiratory arrest

**Peripheral blood vessels**
Degeneration and thrombosis, causing distal necrosis

**GI tract**
Intestinal infarction, ileus, liver failure, appendicitis, pancreatitis

**Bones**
Aseptic necrosis, fractures and dislocations

with muscle tissue injury
• musculoskeletal complications, possibly including fractures or dislocations, tendon contractures or ruptures, flaccid paralysis due to spinal cord injury, or violent muscle contractures and uncoordinated tremors
• CNS complications, possibly including paresthesias, paraplegia, or convulsions
• decreased level of consciousness, as mild as lethargy or possibly as severe as coma.

Most electrical burns occur in healthy young persons—the majority are men—who have a good chance of being resuscitated after aggressive (and possibly prolonged) CPR. Your patient's cardiac function may have been reestablished with CPR and defibrillations. His airway was checked, and an oral airway was inserted—or the patient was intubated. He was given high-flow oxygen by mask, T-piece, or ventilator. Ringer's lactate I.V. was started to replace fluids, and an indwelling (Foley) catheter was inserted to monitor his urine output. Arterial blood was drawn for ABGs to assess for hypoxemia. Venous blood was drawn for clotting studies and bilirubin, phosphorus, alkaline phosphatase, CBC, electrolyte, BUN, blood glucose, total protein, and creatinine levels. X-rays (including a chest X-ray, a spine series, and long-bone X-rays) and an EKG were taken, and the patient was placed on a cardiac monitor.

## Priorities

Your first priority in caring for a patient who's survived a severe electrical burn involves monitoring his cardiac rate and rhythm. This is important because serious dysrhythmias—such as ventricular fibrillation and cardiac standstill—may occur *after* your patient's cardiac status appears stable. Be prepared to start CPR and to intervene appropriately.

Your next priority is to continue fluid replacement. Expect to infuse Ringer's lactate rapidly for the first 24 hours postburn. Because evaluating the full extent of an electrical burn is difficult, the Baxter formula or any other formula for massive fluid replacement can only serve as a baseline; your patient's urine output is the most accurate gauge of his fluid replacement need. Maintain a minimum output of 70 to 100 ml/hour by titrating the patient's I.V. fluids. If you can't maintain this hourly output with I.V. fluids, expect to give mannitol, as ordered, which increases his fluid output. This in turn increases both his glomerular filtration rate and myoglobin excretion, preventing renal tubule damage.

Check your patient's skin for entrance and exit wounds. As you're aware, electrical current may produce a whitish yellow entrance wound that's ischemic, charred, and depressed, and blisters may form after water vaporizes from the tissues. Remember, however, that major tissue damage usually occurs in deep muscle or subcutaneously (along nerves and vascular pathways), so surface damage may not reveal the full extent of burn-related injuries. The exit wound may look like an explosive injury, with a black and depressed center surrounded by gray-white tissues, extensive skin discoloration, edema, charring, and complete tissue loss that exposes charred bones.

Keep in mind that a patient who sustains an electrical burn may also have a flame burn if the current's heat ignited his clothing. Or, if the flash of electrical energy released intense heat, it may have caused surface burns. Be prepared to assist with emergency escharotomy or fasciotomy if your patient has vascular compromise, from a circumferential burn, or deep muscle injury underlying nonburned areas.

## Continuing assessment and therapeutic care

Your patient with an electrical burn may have serious internal injuries even if he has minimal external burns. And—because the current's pathway will penetrate some tissues and spare

# DANGER: SEPSIS

Sepsis—a potentially life-threatening systemic infection—usually results from the release of gram-negative bacteria and their toxins into the patient's bloodstream. If not recognized early and treated promptly, sepsis can rapidly lead to shock.

Not all infections result in sepsis, of course, but your seriously burned patient is especially at risk because his skin's destroyed, his wounds are moist and seeping, his immune system's impaired, and his injuries require immobilization, and his nutritional needs aren't being adequately met.

When you're caring for a patient who's seriously burned, be alert for these signs and symptoms:
- mental depression
- tachycardia
- restlessness and confusion
- loss of appetite
- decreased bowel sounds
- increased temperature, with or without chills, or decreased temperature
- decreased blood pressure.

If you note any of these in your patient, notify the doctor, who'll order:
- a complete blood count with differential
- a blood culture to isolate the infecting organism
- urine, sputum, and throat cultures and cultures of the arterial and central venous pressure lines and wound drainages
- a chest X-ray.

**Nursing interventions**
Expect to administer broad-spectrum antibiotics until you know the results of your patient's cultures. Once the causative organism's been discovered, start specific antibiotic therapy, as ordered. Change the I.V. site every 48 to 72 hours, and give meticulous catheter care. Keep the urinary drainage system and the I.V. system closed, and remove the indwelling (Foley) catheter and I.V. lines as soon as possible. Continue debriding and cleaning all wounds with careful aseptic technique, to prevent wound colonization from becoming systemic. Apply topical antimicrobials, as ordered. Get your patient out of bed as soon as his condition permits, and encourage ambulation to prevent respiratory infection.

---

others—deep-tissue injury can underlie unburned surface tissues and escape detection on initial assessment.

Monitor your patient's intake and output carefully. Expect to titrate the I.V. infusion to maintain his urine output at 100 ml/hour.

For another estimation of the extent of his internal injuries, expect to send a urine specimen to the laboratory every day for analysis of myoglobin and hemochromogen content, urine sodium, and osmolarity. Tea-colored or brown urine indicates myoglobinuria. Dark red or burgundy-colored urine indicates the release of hemochromogens from muscle—another sign that your patient has significant muscle injury. Myoglobinuria (an excessive concentration of myoglobin in the urine) occurs in patients who have severe and extensive muscle injury. If your patient

has myoglobinuria, expect to continue administering an osmotic diuretic, such as mannitol (Osmitrol), and, possibly, to start low-dose dopamine I.V. for renal perfusion. All these steps ensure adequate renal filtration and increase myoglobin clearance, and they may prevent acute tubular necrosis. The doctor may also order sodium bicarbonate I.V. to prevent precipitation of myoglobin in the patient's renal tubules. Monitor your patient's serial BUN and creatinine levels. If both levels increase, this may indicate your patient has acute renal failure (see the "Acute Renal Failure" entry in Chapter 13).

If the current passed through one or more of your patient's extremities, keep each affected extremity elevated to prevent or decrease edema. Assess him for neurovascular compression from

PATHOPHYSIOLOGY

## WHAT HAPPENS IN CHEMICAL BURNS

The mechanism and severity of a partial- or full-thickness chemical burn depend on the action and penetrability of the chemical and on the duration of the chemical's contact with tissue.

Mechanisms of injury in chemical burns include:
• heat release from acidic or alkaline substances, causing tissue damage
• cell dehydration due to biochemical reaction
• protoplasmic poisoning due to biochemical reaction
• protein coagulation or dissolution of cellular contents from direct biochemical

reaction between the chemical and skin.

These mechanisms damage and destroy the skin and continue to penetrate deeper tissues, causing cell death, until the chemical is completely neutralized. Most chemical burns, like other burns, cause initial vasodilation and hyperemia—involving superficial vessels first, then deeper subcutaneous vessels. Next, as the damage increases, tissue congestion and an inflammatory reaction result from fluid and white blood cell infiltration in the injured tissue. Finally, in severe chemical burns, actual tissue necrosis and dissolution may occur.

---

subfascial muscle edema:
• Tell him to report any numbness, tingling, or pain in his extremities.
• Check him frequently for slow or absent capillary refill.
• Check his peripheral pulses every 15 to 30 minutes.

Pressures usually continue to rise for 48 to 72 hours after the initial burn. At the first sign of neurovascular compromise, contact the doctor *immediately*. He will test, or ask you to test, tissue pressure in the patient's affected extremity. (See *Measuring Compartment Pressure,* page 368.) Pressures that exceed 30 mm Hg will require emergency fasciotomy to allow expansion of the edematous tissue. This will decrease compression on the patient's vascular system and allow perfusion to return. If, however, the electrical current coagulated and thrombosed the vessels, the tissue's perfusion can't be restored. This means that tissue hypoxia, necrosis, and gangrene are inevitable, requiring early and frequent debridement of necrotic tissue. Amputation may be necessary. The total extent of this type of damage may not be apparent for 7 to 10 days postburn.

Evaluate the presence of bowel sounds—if they're absent, your patient

has a paralytic ileus. Expect to insert an NG tube as ordered. Connect it to low suction, and withhold food and oral fluids from your patient. Continue to assess your patient's bowel sounds frequently. When they return, expect to begin oral or NG tube feedings to meet his high caloric nutritional needs. Weigh your patient daily to evaluate whether his nutritional needs are being met.

Perform frequent neurologic assessments, evaluating your patient's level of consciousness, pupil reaction and size, orientation, and ability to conduct a logical conversation. Remember this: If his electrical burn caused CNS injury, he may develop neurologic complications long after you consider him stable. Be alert for secondary effects of CNS damage, such as convulsions, decreased level of consciousness, paresthesias, and respiratory depression and failure.

Burn wound care for your patient is likely to include not only cleansing and debriding but also frequent grafting procedures. Remember, all these procedures are painful; give I.V. analgesics, as ordered.

Assess your patient for signs of wound infection. Culture any drainage and, if he has a wound infection, administer systemic antibiotics, as ordered, and a topical antibiotic, such as mafenide acetate (Sulfamylon), which can penetrate into deep tissue.

Continue to monitor his vital signs frequently. Watch for signs and symptoms of fluid imbalance: hypovolemia due to fluid shifting or fluid overload due to overaggressive fluid replacement. Signs of fluid overload include:
• increased blood pressure
• increased pulse
• rales
• $S_3$ heart sound.

Signs of hypovolemic shock include:
• increased pulse rate
• decreased blood pressure
• orthostatic hypotension.

Auscultate your patient's lungs for wheezing, rales, and rhonchi, indicating such respiratory complications as airway edema or fluid overload. If you hear any of these breath sounds, notify the doctor *immediately*. Expect to obtain stat ABGs and a chest X-ray and to begin (or increase) supplemental oxygen therapy by nasal cannula, face mask, or endotracheal tube. If these tests confirm fluid overload, expect to give aminophylline and diuretics. Encourage your patient to cough, turn, and deep-breathe frequently.

# Chemical Burns

## Initial care summary
The patient had a history of exposure to one of the strong alkalis or acids commonly used in cleaning products or industrial extraction processes. In an industrial accident, for example, he may have been burned by sulfuric, formic, acetic, or trichloroacetic acid; in a household accident, by a cleaning product such as hydrofluoric acid.

If rescue personnel brought the patient to the ED, they intervened by removing clothing from the affected area and brushing off any dry chemical substance remaining on his skin. Then they lavaged the entire burned area with copious amounts of water.

Initial assessment of the patient revealed some or all of the following signs and symptoms:
• erythematous, discolored, raw, white, soft, mushy, or excoriated skin
• edema in the tissues under the burn
• pain or paresthesias
• respiratory distress.

If the patient had respiratory difficulty (such as dyspnea and tachypnea) from inhaling chemical fumes, an airway was probably inserted, and humidified oxygen was started by mask. If his signs and symptoms were severe, an endotracheal tube may have been inserted, and he may have been placed on mechanical ventilation.

The extent of his burns was estimated, using the "rule of nines" or the Lund and Browder chart, and other injuries associated with the burn were assessed. (See *Using the "Rule of Nines,"* page 664, and *Using the Lund and Browder Chart,* page 665.)

If he had an extensive skin burn, an I.V. of Ringer's lactate was started to replace fluid lost because of shifts out of the intravascular bed and into the interstitial space. Blood was drawn for clotting studies, liver function studies, typing and cross matching, CBC, and electrolyte, alkaline phosphatase, BUN, blood glucose, total serum protein, creatinine, albumin, globulin, and calcium phosphatase levels. An indwelling (Foley) catheter was inserted for close monitoring of his output, and a urine specimen was sent for analysis.

Medications he received included tetanus toxoid and analgesics.

## Priorities
The first priority involved in caring for your patient with a chemical burn is to stop the burning process. If his skin or eyes are burned, continue copious lavage of the burn until the skin's pH returns to normal. Neutralization of alkalis and acids by using their respec-

# UNDERSTANDING INHALATION INJURIES

Respiratory tract injury can result when a person inhales steam, superheated air, or a toxic product of combustion, such as smoke from a house fire or fumes from burning chemicals or synthetic materials. Another toxic product of combustion, carbon monoxide, won't injure the respiratory tract directly but will make respiration less efficient by decreasing the blood's ability to carry oxygen. The patient may sustain a thermal injury to his upper respiratory tract, from excessive heat or steam, and/or damage to his lower respiratory tract from inhaling a toxic product of combustion. The effects of these injuries include the following:

• In a patient with a thermal inhalation injury, *laryngeal edema*—from increased capillary permeability in injured mucosal tissue—may rapidly cause airway obstruction.

• In a patient with *tracheobronchitis* from smoke or fume inhalation, airway occlusion may be progressive. This happens because of bronchospasm, laryngeal edema, mucosal sloughing, and hypoxia. Chemical irritants also disrupt the membrane between the alveoli and the pulmonary capillaries in the patient's lungs, allowing fluids and protein to accumulate and, possibly, to cause noncardiogenic pulmonary edema or adult respiratory distress syndrome.

• In a patient who's inhaled carbon monoxide, *hypoxemia* and *hypoxia* occur because carbon monoxide prevents oxygen from combining with hemoglobin. Without intensive oxygen therapy, this inhalation injury can lead to cardiopulmonary failure and death.

## Signs and symptoms
Because an inhalation injury victim can deteriorate rapidly, early recognition and intervention are critically important. Signs and symptoms include:
• singed nasal hairs
• orofacial burns
• soot-stained sputum
• coughing or hoarseness
• rales, rhonchi, or wheezes
• respiratory distress
• additional signs and symptoms related to the source of his injury.

Remember, however, that signs and symptoms of inhalation injuries may not be apparent for up to 48 hours after exposure. Delaying treatment for such a period could have serious consequences—so be sure to *suspect* inhalation injury in any burned patient who:
• lost consciousness at any time
• was exposed to burning agents in an enclosed space.

This patient should be admitted for observation and diagnostic tests—such as bronchoscopy, xenon lung scan, and arterial blood gas analysis—even if he has no initial signs and symptoms.

## Nursing interventions
Your priorities for this patient are to provide adequate oxygenation and to prevent progression to respiratory failure by:
• administering humidified oxygen to your patient immediately
• preparing for (and assisting with) endotracheal tube insertion and placing the patient on mechanical ventilation before airway obstruction can occur
• assessing the patient's breath sounds frequently for wheezes, rales, and rhonchi and suctioning him carefully so as not to further damage the trachea
• taking a sputum culture as soon as possible after intubation
• anticipating pulmonary therapies such as intermittent positive-pressure breathing (IPPB), nebulizer treatments with bronchodilators, coughing and deep breathing, and chest physiotherapy. (These procedures mobilize the thick secretions in the bronchial tree.)
• watching your patient for signs of pneumonia (fever, increased and purulent secretions, and respiratory distress) and culturing as necessary
• watching your patient for complications from therapy, such as rib fracture, wound injury, pneumothorax, and gastric distention.

Expect to administer antibiotics after culture-and-sensitivity tests determine which drugs will be most effective. Anticipate using bronchodilators to control bronchospasm and to lessen the patient's risk of airway obstruction. Steroids have been used, in patients with inhalation injuries, to decrease the inflammatory response and to stop fluid leakage out of capillaries and into the lungs. But steroids aren't generally recommended for long-term use in patients with burns, because of increased risk of infection.

This chart shows you the signs and symptoms of inhalation injury from different products of combustion. It can help you recognize an inhalation injury early and help you prevent additional complications.

| TOXIC PRODUCT OF COMBUSTION | SOURCES | SIGNS AND SYMPTOMS |
|---|---|---|
| **Hydrochloric acid** | Burning products made of polyvinyl chloride, such as unbreakable bottles, electrical insulation, wall coverings, and car interiors | • Dyspnea |
| **Hydrocyanic acid** | Burning products made of polyurethane or nylon, such as thermal insulation, wall coverings, seat cushions, carpeting, and mattress materials | • Light-headedness<br>• Nausea<br>• Dyspnea<br>• Chest pain<br>• Syncope |
| **Styrene** | Burning products made of styrene, such as piping, wall coverings, luggage, appliances, and plastic food and drink containers | • Conjunctivitis<br>• Rhinorrhea<br>• Burning pain in mucous membranes |
| **Acrolein** | Burning products made of acrylics, such as textiles, wood finishes, wall coverings, furniture, and piping | • Burning pain in mucous membranes<br>• Light-headedness<br>• Dyspnea |
| **Ammonia** | Burning products made of nylon, such as carpeting, clothing, and upholstery | • Conjunctivitis<br>• Burning pain in mucous membranes<br>• Laryngeal and pulmonary edema |
| **Carbon monoxide** | Burning of almost all things | • Headache<br>• Light-headedness<br>• Nausea and vomiting<br>• Dyspnea<br>• Visual disturbances<br>• Seizures<br>• Coma |

tive neutralizing agents (a weak acid or a weak base) was once the method of choice but is no longer advocated. Why? Because this method sets up an exothermic reaction between the original chemical and the neutralizing base or acid, and this reaction actually gives off heat in addition to the original chemical's burning effect. The result is increased tissue damage.

A burn from a weak alkali or acid (for example, a household detergent or floor wax remover) will probably require 30 to 60 minutes' lavage before the patient's skin pH returns to normal. But copious lavage doesn't act this quickly in stopping the burning process from a *strong alkali,* such as ammonium hydroxide, which may require up to 24 hours' continuous lavage before the patient's skin pH returns to normal. A burn from a *strong acid,* such as hydrofluoric acid, may require lavaging for 12 hours. For such prolonged lavage, expect to place the patient in a shower on a chair or to use a shower trolley or a hydrotherapy tub.

Here's an important point to keep in mind: Most noninhalation chemical injuries occur on the patient's head, neck, or extremities, because these are the most commonly exposed areas of the body. Any person who sustains a chemical burn to the head or neck should have, in addition to skin lavage, extensive lavage of his eyes plus a follow-up examination by an ophthalmologist. This is because corneal ulcerations and eye infections commonly follow chemical burns to the eyes. (For more information, see the "Chemical Burns of the Eye" and "Eye Infections" entries in Chapter 9.)

Once the burning process has been stopped, you must simultaneously manage several equally important priorities for your patient:
• anticipating respiratory complications
• stabilizing fluid and electrolytes
• relieving his pain
• preventing infection.
Assess your patient's respiratory sta-

tus, keeping in mind that inhalation of certain chemical fumes can cause irritation of the tracheobronchial tree. (See *Understanding Inhalation Injuries,* pages 692 and 693.) This can result in copious bronchial secretions, which in turn can cause plugs in small bronchi and collapse of the distal alveoli, leading to atelectasis. Adult respiratory distress syndrome (ARDS) may also follow inhalation of toxic fumes. In a patient with ARDS, damage occurs at the alveolocapillary membrane. (See the "Adult Respiratory Distress Syndrome [ARDS]" entry in Chapter 4.)

Continue to auscultate your patient's lungs for rales, rhonchi, and wheezes and to assess his breathing for rate, depth, and pattern. Stridor, dyspnea, or tachypnea indicates probable respiratory complications. (You may note tachypnea even before your patient complains of being short of breath.)

Continue fluid replacement as ordered. Keep in mind that underestimation of fluid needs can easily occur, because:
• The total BSA of most chemical burns is relatively small—but such a burn may be deep, requiring split-thickness skin grafting.
• If chemical penetration isn't halted, the damage continues to increase for up to 72 hours after the injury.
• Respiratory difficulty from inhaling toxic fumes may not develop until hours after the initial injury. When it does develop, your patient's need for fluids will increase.

Many strong chemicals can cause both full-thickness and partial-thickness burns that are extremely painful. So expect to give a narcotic analgesic I.V. as soon as the patient's stable.

As with any burn, infection control is a priority from the moment your patient enters the hospital. Begin your efforts to prevent infection as soon as you begin caring for him. Give systemic antibiotics and apply topical antibiotic cream, as ordered.

# DRESSING FOR SUCCESS

As a nurse, you know that infection control is essential for any burn site. But do you know that some areas of the body are more susceptible to infection and scarring than others? The following guidelines will help you give special care to patients with burns over these sensitive areas.

• **Face:** Generally use open-wound treatment for all patients with facial burns. Clean the burns every 4 hours with sterile saline–soaked gauze pads or sterile water. Then rinse the burns with sterile saline and gently apply a thin layer of antibiotic ointment. Debride with sterile scissors and forceps, as necessary. If applicable, shave the patient's beard daily, and clean his face every 8 hours.

• **Eyes:** Administer ointment or eyedrops, if ordered. Remove built-up ointment and secretions every 4 hours. The patient's eyelids may swell shut—don't force them open.

• **Ears:** Shave all hair within 2″ (5 cm) of a patient's ear burn and apply a topical antimicrobial. Remove the pillow from the patient's bed so it won't put pressure on his ears.

• **Nose:** When caring for a patient with nose burns, use the open-wound treatment and clean the area with sterile saline–soaked gauze pads every 4 hours. Clean his nostrils frequently, using cotton-tipped applicators. If the patient's had a nasogastric tube inserted, be sure to check his nostrils periodically for signs of pressure necrosis.

• **Mouth:** Apply antimicrobial ointment to the patient's burned lips. Have him gargle often with diluted hydrogen peroxide or mouthwash and brush his teeth.

• **Hands:** Wash the burned area with a mild cleansing solution, such as povidone-iodine (Betadine), then rinse it with sterile saline. Next, apply an antimicrobial ointment and wrap the burn with a fine mesh gauze. If your patient is alert and cooperative, encourage him to use his hands as much as possible. If he can't use his hands, wrap gauze between each finger to maintain separation. Next, splint his wrist, fingers, and entire hand so they're in functional positions, with his thumb abducted. (If his palm's burned, splint his hand in the extended position.) After splinting, wrap gauze around his entire hand. (See the illustration.) Remove the splint at regular intervals to encourage the patient to exercise his hand.

• **Perineum:** Never cover your patient's perineal area with gauze—this locks in moisture and can cause infection. Instead, clean the area with sterile saline, apply antimicrobial cream, and place sterile towels around his upper thighs. After each voiding and bowel movement, cleanse the area and reapply antimicrobial cream.

• **Feet:** To prevent loss of function in your patient's burned foot, apply an antimicrobial ointment and wrap the foot in a dorsiflexed position. When wrapping his toes, make sure you place gauze between them to maintain separation and to prevent webbing.

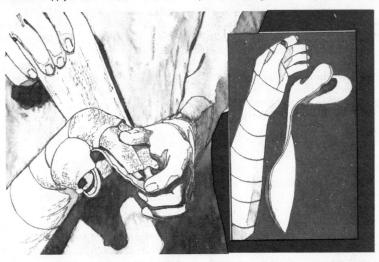

## Continuing assessment and therapeutic care

With your patient's airway, breathing, and circulation stabilized—at least temporarily—you're ready to perform a complete assessment and to intervene as necessary for additional problems he may have.

If he's having respiratory difficulty or possible pulmonary complications, monitor his ABGs closely. And be alert for signs and symptoms of hypoxemia such as restlessness, lethargy, and confusion. (These may not develop until 4 to 72 hours postburn.) If you note any of these signs or symptoms in your patient, expect to give supplemental oxygen by face mask or—if hypoxemia persists—by intubation and mechanical ventilation or by T-piece.

The doctor will probably perform fiber-optic bronchoscopy to inspect this patient's bronchial tree for damage. If your patient's airways are inflamed and edematous, expect to assist the doctor with intubation. He may ask you to give aminophylline to reduce small-airway constriction.

Obtain a complete medical history from your patient. Be particularly alert for indications that he has a preexisting respiratory or cardiac disease. If he has a chronic metabolic or endocrine disease (such as diabetes) or a nutritional deficiency, expect delayed healing and increased susceptibility to infection.

After the initial stage of caring for the patient's burn by continuous lavage is completed, treatment is similar to what you'd do for a thermally burned patient. But keep in mind that many chemicals cause both topical and systemic effects because they're readily absorbed into the systemic circulation. For example, chromic acid, formic acid, phosphorus, and tannic acid can cause nephrotoxicity and hepatic necrosis, whereas creosol causes methemoglobinemia and hemolysis. Phenol may cause cardiovascular collapse even if absorbed through only a small area. So you can understand why you need to identify all the properties of the chemical that burned your patient. Your regional poison control center is an excellent source of current information.

Once the chemical's systemic effects on your patient are identified, monitor his serial laboratory studies carefully for indications that he's developing complications. Be particularly careful to study his BUN and creatinine results if he was exposed to a nephrotoxic chemical, his liver function tests if he was exposed to a hepatotoxic chemical. Urinalysis will help detect possible myoglobinuria—be alert for port–wine colored urine, another indicator of this complication. If your patient does develop myoglobinuria, expect to give increased amounts of fluid to maintain his urine output at 100 ml/hour. This will keep his kidneys patent and flush the myoglobin out.

To prevent underestimating your patient's need for fluid replacement, watch for changes in the size and appearance of his chemical burn and tell the doctor *immediately* when any change occurs. Monitor his fluid replacement closely, and watch for signs of hypovolemia (such as decreased urine output) and for changes in his vital signs (such as increased pulse rate and decreased blood pressure). Keep accurate intake and output records (see *Guidelines for Fluid Replacement,* pages 668 and 669). Expect to adjust the I.V. rate to maintain a 50 ml/hour output.

Before dressing changes (and any other painful procedures), give your patient an analgesic, as ordered. Remember, the degree of pain relief he experiences is a clue to the success of his treatment. Monitor his reactions to each dose. If he tells you he isn't getting as much relief from pain as the same dose of analgesic gave him earlier, he may have:

• increased tolerance for the drug
• increased pain, possibly indicating a new complication, such as compartment syndrome or infection.

Perform a thorough assessment, and notify the doctor so he can reevaluate the patient.

# CASE IN POINT: WHEN A PATIENT REFUSES TREATMENT

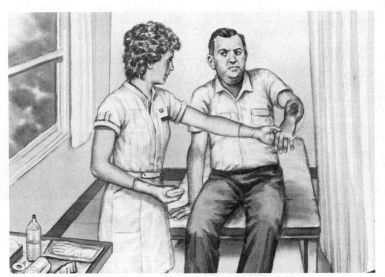

Kent Parker, age 54, has arrived in the ED with a serious thermal burn on his left arm. Unfortunately, before bringing him to the ED, a co-worker applied an ointment to the burn. Now, looking at Kent's arm, you realize that you'll have to remove the ointment before you or the doctor can treat the burn. You explain this to Kent and he agrees to the treatment. So you administer a fast-acting pain medication, as ordered, and begin scrubbing. After only a few seconds, Kent withdraws his arm and begs you to stop because of the pain.

You reach for Kent's arm, explaining that the medication will take effect soon and that you'll be more gentle. Then you try to continue scrubbing. But Kent just says, "Forget it!"—and abruptly leaves the hospital. Then, several weeks later, you receive notice that he's suing you for assault and battery. Would the courts allow such a suit? Would you be liable?

In the case of *Winters v. Miller* (1971), a woman who'd been involuntarily admitted to a state psychiatric hospital sued the hospital after she was discharged. She claimed that, while hospitalized, she received medication and treatment that she didn't agree to. An appeals court ruled that

because a patient has the right to refuse treatment, the plaintiff had the right to sue for assault and battery.

To avoid a similar legal problem, remember that a person may refuse even emergency treatment. If a competent adult refuses any treatment, under any circumstances, don't treat him or assist in treating him. Instead, determine his reason for refusing and report the incident to your supervisor and to the doctor (who may, if the patient's condition threatens his life, limb, or organ functions, request that the hospital's attorney obtain a court order). Have the patient sign a refusal-of-treatment form. If he won't sign it, be sure to document his refusal. If no grounds exist for obtaining a court order, you must defend his right to refuse treatment.

But if a patient refuses treatment in an *irrational* way, with disjointed statements or inappropriate gestures, he may be incapable of a valid refusal. You still have a duty to provide treatment; in fact, you and the doctor could be liable for *not* treating him. You also have a responsibility to continue to inform a competent patient about treatment he's refused, because he may change his mind.

*Winters v. Miller*, 446 F. 2d 65 (1971)

Use strict aseptic technique when you care for your patient's burn wound. Debridement may be necessary to remove necrotic or sloughed tissue. If the patient has a partial-thickness or full-thickness burn, he may need a partial-thickness or full-thickness skin graft. Assess the graft and donor sites for increased swelling, drainage, a "soupy-looking" graft, or pain. This may indicate that the wound is infected. Culture an open wound, as ordered, and report any indications of local or systemic infection *immediately*. (See *Danger: Sepsis,* page 689.) Expect to administer antibiotics I.V. and topically, as ordered.

As a nurse, you know that meeting a burn patient's nutritional needs can be a formidable challenge. (See *Meeting Your Burned Patient's Nutritional Needs,* page 683.) A patient with a serious chemical burn is no exception. He's probably psychologically depressed, so you shouldn't be surprised if his appetite's depressed, too. And he may become uncooperative with the people caring for him—even refuse to eat. To help him, be flexible in your approach:

• Provide small, frequent meals.

• Try making contracts with your patient to get him to eat (see *Encouraging Your Patient's Cooperation,* page 670).

• Ask family members to bring in his favorite foods.

• Avoid performing painful procedures just before he has his meals.

Expect that, despite these efforts, you may have to give some of his feedings by NG tube or by TPN.

Weigh your patient daily—at the same time each day, with the same scale—to keep an accurate record of his weight gain or loss and to gauge the success of his nutritional support.

Helping your patient regain his independence psychologically—as well as physically— is an important part of your nursing care. As soon as his condition permits, give him increasing responsibility for his activities of daily living. Encourage him to exercise. Help his family understand the need to encourage his independence, even when self-care is painful for him.

Encourage the family's participation in other ways, too. For example, include them in as many of your patient's activities as possible during his long hospitalization. Extend your psychological support to the family as well as to the patient, and arrange for counseling if they request your help. As for any burned patient, assess the need for a work or school reentry program.

## A FINAL WORD

More than 2 million people require medical treatment for burn injuries each year. Of these, over 70,000 require hospitalization; many of these patients are children under age 6.

Fortunately, most of these burn victims will survive. And thanks to recent advances in all aspects of burn care—infection control, wound management, treatment of burn shock, and scar management—their chances for complete recovery are improving.

But one aspect of a burn patient's care is little changed: The road to both physical and psychological recovery from serious burns is long and painful. Besides the pain he must endure while his burns are healing, your patient must suffer painful debriding and grafting procedures. And he must undergo these ordeals while isolated from his family and in anticipation of an altered appearance that may devastate him—and his family—psychologically. Of course, complications and discouraging setbacks in his recovery are also likely.

To you, as a nurse and as a caring person, this means that your seriously burned patient needs an unusual degree of emotional support. For him, each day's successes or setbacks can have long-term effects, so your support is a strong factor in building and maintaining his momentum toward recovery. Along with making sure your assessment and intervention skills are up to date, be prepared to give generous emotional support and encour-agement to your patient. Whenever you can, applaud and reinforce his successes as he copes with self-care, with painful therapy procedures, and with depression and despair. Together, you and your burn patient can keep his road to recovery open.

## Selected References

Artz, Curtis P., et al. *Burns–A Team Approach.* Philadelphia: W.B. Saunders Co., 1979.

Brunner, Lillian, and Suddarth, Doris. *Textbook of Medical-Surgical Nursing,* 5th ed. Philadelphia: J.B. Lippincott Co., 1984.

Budassi, Susan A., and Barber, Janet M. *Emergency Nursing: Principles and Practice.* St. Louis: C.V. Mosby Co., 1981.

*Critical Care Quarterly* Issue on Burn Management. 1(3): December 1978.

*Diseases.* Nurse's Reference Library. Springhouse, Pa.: Springhouse Corp., 1981.

Sabiston, David C., ed. *Davis/Christopher Textbook of Surgery,* 2 vols. Philadelphia: W.B. Saunders Co., 1981.

Salisbury, Roger E., and Newman, Nancy. *Manual of Burn Therapeutics.* Boston: Little, Brown & Co., 1983.

Wachtel, Tom, et al. *Current Topics in Burn Care.* Rockville, Md.: Aspen Systems Corp., 1983.

Wagner, Mary M., ed. *Care of the Burn-Injured Patient: A Multidisciplinary Involvement.* Littleton, Mass.: John Wright/PSG Publishing Co., 1981.

Wilkins, Earle W., Jr. *MGH Textbook of Emergency Medicine,* 2nd ed. Baltimore: Williams & Wilkins Co., 1983.

# 16

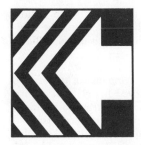

# Environmental Emergencies

## Introduction

You're working in the ED one hot, humid August afternoon. From the athletic field nearby, you hear the shouts of the high school's football team. They've been out practicing all afternoon, running and doing drills; you wonder how they stand the heat. A wave of hot air pushes into the ED whenever the doors open, and you're glad to be inside, with air conditioning.

At 4:00, a car pulls up in front of the ED. The football coach and a player still in uniform pull another uniformed player from the back of the team station wagon and half-carry him toward the ED door. You rush to meet them with a stretcher.

The coach tells you that the player is Neil Simmons, age 17. You see immediately that he's unconscious, flushed, and drenched in sweat. "What happened?" you ask.

"He collapsed doing laps," the coach says.

You touch Neil's face—it's burning hot. Quickly, you call for help and begin to remove his uniform, while Neil's coach and teammate fill you in on the rest of what happened.

"He was acting real weird during exercises," his teammate tells you. "He threw up after drinking a lot of water, and then he started acting silly. I asked him a couple of times if he felt okay, and he said he was fine. But when we

were doing laps his legs gave out and he collapsed."

When you question the coach, he tells you that a few other players threw up during practice, but that nobody seemed too sick. "It always happens on days like this," he says. "The kids drink too much water no matter what I tell them." You ask him if he ever gives them balanced salt solutions instead, but he tells you he doesn't believe in "fancy drinks."

"Besides," he says, "I keep a close eye on them. They were all sweating hard—and everyone knows you can't get heat stroke if you're still sweating."

Unfortunately for Neil, his coach is wrong this time. Exertional heat stroke *does* occur in people who are still sweating profusely. And—when you assess Neil's condition and find he has a rectal temperature of 106° F. (41° C.), hypotension, tachypnea, and signs of dehydration—you're pretty sure heat stroke is what's wrong with him.

As soon as you've removed Neil's uniform, you place him on a hypothermia blanket, apply ice packs to his axillae and groin, and start sponging him down with cool water. You can only hope that your prompt cooling measures will reduce Neil's temperature quickly enough to prevent permanent organ damage.

Heat stroke, of course, is only one of

the many and varied environmental emergencies you'll encounter. This is because everybody—from healthy young adults who enjoy a variety of outdoor activities to elderly persons who only go out for evening walks or shopping—is exposed to a number of environmental insults every day. In addition to heat stroke (and heat exhaustion), you may also see hypothermia, frostbite, near-drowning, altitude-related illness, and bites and stings—depending on the geography and climate where you live.

So count on it—you'll have many opportunities to help patients with environmental emergencies *and* to prevent these types of emergencies. This chapter will tell you how to recognize them and intervene appropriately.

# INITIAL CARE

# Prehospital Care: What's Been Done

Prehospital care for your patient depended on the type of environmental insult he was exposed to and on the extent and severity of his signs and symptoms.

If the patient was exposed to cold and had signs and symptoms of *hypothermia,* rescuers immediately moved him to a warm, protected area, removed any wet clothes, and covered him with blankets. If his respirations were depressed, they gave him 100% oxygen by mask or ventilated him with an Ambu bag at half the normal rate. They started an I.V. at a keep-vein-open rate, and they initiated cardiac monitoring. If they were sure that the patient had no pulse, they started CPR on the way to the hospital. If the patient had areas

of *frostbite,* a rescuer began rapidly rewarming the affected area by holding it or by cradling it in his axilla or groin.

If the patient was exposed to heat and had signs and symptoms of *heat stroke,* rescuers removed his clothes, opened the windows in the transport vehicle, sponged him down with alcohol or cold water, and applied cold packs to his axillae and groin. They started an I.V. and cardiac monitoring, and they may have inserted an esophageal obturator airway or an endotracheal tube to protect his airway if he developed seizures or started vomiting.

If the patient was recovered from the water after a *near-drowning* accident, rescuers started CPR immediately if he was pulseless, taking steps to protect his cervical spine. If the patient was conscious and breathing, they gave him 100% oxygen by nonrebreathing mask, started an I.V., and began cardiac monitoring.

If the patient was evacuated from the mountains after an episode of *altitude-related illness,* rescuers gave him supplemental oxygen and watched him closely for signs of developing cerebral or pulmonary edema.

If the patient suffered a serious or venomous *bite or sting,* rescuers provided care specific to the animal, insect, spider, or aquatic organism involved. If the patient had a large animal or human bite that caused substantial bleeding, rescue personnel applied direct pressure, or pressure at pressure points, and elevated the part (if possible). If it was a dog bite, they may have attempted to recover the animal so it could be observed for rabies. If a snake or aquatic organism bit the patient, rescuers may have been able to recover it so hospital personnel could identify it, provide appropriate care, and—if the animal was venomous—administer appropriate antivenin. While keeping the patient quiet and monitoring his breathing and circulation, rescuers rushed the patient to the hospital for further care.

Make sure you get a full report from rescue personnel about the incident, the patient's other injuries, and the interventions the rescuers provided.

# What to Do First

Environmental emergencies can cause a variety of different insults to your patient's body—insults that can affect multiple body systems. His signs and symptoms, of course, will vary depending on whether he's been exposed to:

- heat or cold
- water
- high altitude
- a venomous insect, spider, snake, or aquatic organism.

You'll need an accurate history to determine the cause of his emergency and to provide definitive care—a patient suffering from exposure to cold, for example, will need very different care than a patient bitten by a snake.

Remember, no matter what's caused your patient's environmental emergency, your first priority is still to stabilize your patient's airway, breathing, and circulation.

### Airway

Quickly assess the patency of your patient's airway, listening for wheezing or stridor. If his airway's obstructed, clear it immediately using the techniques described in the "Life Support" section in Chapter 3. (Observe cervical spine precautions if you have any reason to suspect cervical spine injury, especially if you see an indication of trauma above his shoulders.)

Wheezing indicates small-airway obstruction, such as may occur when your patient aspirates vomitus. This is particularly likely to occur if your patient's experienced hypothermia or near-drowning. If he's aspirated vomitus, clear his oral cavity and suction him, then turn him on his side to pre-

---

PRIORITIES

## INITIAL ASSESSMENT CHECKLIST

**Assess the ABCs first and intervene appropriately.**

**Check for:**
- wheezing or stridor, indicating laryngeal edema from anaphylaxis (due to bites or stings) or aspiration from near-drowning
- hypotension, indicating shock from hypothermia, hyperthermia, or a bite or sting
- increasing dyspnea, cough, stertorous respirations, and hemoptysis, indicating high-altitude pulmonary edema
- increasing headache, weakness, and altered level of consciousness, indicating high-altitude cerebral edema
- cyanosis, indicating hypoxemia in altitude-related illness, hypothermia, or near-drowning
- altered behavior and consciousness, indicating altitude-related illness, hypothermia, or hyperthermia
- dysrhythmias, indicating hyperkalemia, hypokalemia, or acidosis.

**Intervene by:**
- administering 100% oxygen by face mask (warmed, if the patient's hypothermic)
- inserting a nasogastric or endotracheal tube (*except* in a patient with hypothermia, because vagal stimulation could cause ventricular fibrillation)
- starting an I.V. and administering fluids
- applying warm blankets or ice packs, as indicated.

**Prepare for:**
- applying hypo- or hyperthermia blankets
- beginning internal rewarming procedures, such as heated peritoneal, bladder, or gastric lavage
- administering antivenin, sodium bicarbonate, antiarrhythmics, or diuretics, as ordered.
- taking a chest X-ray.

vent further aspiration. Insert a naso-gastric (NG) tube, as ordered, to suction his stomach contents and to prevent further aspiration.

If your patient's unconscious, the doctor may ask you to assist with en-dotracheal intubation to provide a se-cure airway. (He may ask you to assist with nasal intubation if he suspects a neck injury.) However, he'll probably avoid intubation if the patient's hy-pothermic. Why? Because hypothermic patients are particularly at risk for ven-tricular fibrillation, and intubation causes vagal stimulation that may trig-ger this dysrhythmia. Position this pa-tient's head carefully, to prevent his tongue from falling back and occluding his airway, and watch him closely.

Stridor may be due to laryngeal edema resulting from an anaphylactic response to a toxic bite or sting. Call the doctor *immediately* if you suspect this, and prepare for emergency cri-cothyrotomy, if necessary (see the "An-aphylactic Shock" entry in Chapter 14).

### Breathing

Assess the quality of your patient's res-pirations, noting rate and depth. Note any nasal flaring, retractions, or ac-cessory muscle use. Respirations may be extremely depressed if your patient's hypothermic—as low as a few per min-ute. Count his respirations for a minute or longer, and remember that a slow respiratory rate in this patient may be acceptable as long as his pulse is also slow. If he's in respiratory arrest, pro-vide ventilation with an Ambu bag at half the normal rate.

If your patient's hyperthermic, his respiratory rate may increase to 60 breaths/minute or more. Provide sup-plemental oxygen by mask or endotra-cheal tube, to support his increased need for oxygen. Also provide supple-mental oxygen if your patient has dys-pnea or such other signs of respiratory distress as may occur with altitude-related illness or in response to certain venomous bites and stings.

If your patient's had a near-drowning

accident, he may not be breathing at all. Start CPR, if necessary (see the "Life Support" section in Chapter 3). Even if he's conscious and breathing, he'll be severely hypoxemic; so provide 100% oxygen by nonrebreathing mask or as-sist with endotracheal intubation, as ordered. (A cross-table lateral X-ray of the patient's cervical spine will be done first to evaluate him for cervical spine injury.) The doctor may ask you to start mechanical ventilation with positive end-expiratory pressure (PEEP) or continuous positive airway pressure (CPAP).

### Circulation

Assess your patient's circulation by taking his pulse and blood pressure. His pulse may be extremely slow, as in hypothermia, or extremely fast, as in hyperthermia. Remember that a hy-pothermic patient's pulse may be very slow or even undetectable. Look for other signs that he's still alive, such as slight body movements. You probably won't start CPR in a hypothermic pa-tient unless you're *sure* he has no pulse, because starting chest compressions before you've rewarmed him may pre-cipitate ventricular fibrillation and death. If you do start chest compres-sions, give them at half the normal rate until the patient's completely re-warmed. If he has no pulse after near-drowning, start CPR *immediately* at the normal rate.

Your patient may have some degree of hypotension from hypothermia, hy-perthermia, or venom (particularly snake venom). Insert an I.V. line for fluid and medication administration, and expect to infuse fluids if he shows signs of volume depletion. If ordered, insert an indwelling (Foley) catheter to measure his urine output.

Obtain a 12-lead EKG tracing to ob-serve for dysrhythmias, and initiate cardiac monitoring. If your patient's condition permits, draw blood for lab-oratory tests. A patient who's experi-enced near-drowning, altitude-related illness, or hypothermia will be hypoxemic to some degree, so make sure his arterial blood gases (ABGs) are tested. (Note: If your patient's hypothermic, make sure you record his body temperature at the time blood was drawn—otherwise his blood will be analyzed incorrectly and his $PO_2$ and $PCO_2$ values will be falsely elevated; his pH falsely depressed.) If your patient has an immediately life-threatening condition such as severe heat stroke or an anaphylactic reaction, you'll have to defer drawing blood until you've started definitive care.

### General appearance

Quickly assess your patient's general appearance. Keep in mind that his environmental emergency may be associated with trauma—as when near-drowning occurs after the patient strikes his head. Other environmental emergencies, such as altitude-related illness and hypothermia, may cause severe confusion and disorientation that impair your patient's judgment and may cause him to injure himself further. Look for signs of external or internal bleeding and for bruises or contusions that may indicate associated injuries. Check for abnormal breath odor, especially alcohol, acetone, or gasoline odor, because this may provide you with a clue to the underlying condition—such as diabetic ketoacidosis—that may have contributed to or caused his environmental emergency.

Keep in mind, too, that environmental injuries may occur in combinations. Examples include:
• hypothermia and frostbite
• altitude-related illness and hypothermia
• near-drowning and hypothermia or stings or bites from aquatic organisms.

### Mental status

When you check your patient's mental status, look for alterations in consciousness ranging from irritability and anxiety (as in mild heat exhaustion or altitude-related illness) to confusion,

stupor, or coma (as in hypothermia, heat stroke, or near-drowning). Record your initial findings as baseline data. Consistent monitoring of your patient's level of consciousness will help you detect subtle changes that may signal impending problems.

# What to Do Next

After you've assessed your patient's airway, breathing, and circulation and intervened as necessary to stabilize them, determine the type and extent of his environmental injury. You need to find out where the patient was and what he was doing when his signs and symptoms developed. Was he:
• exposed to *cold?*
• exposed to *heat?*
• submerged in *water?*
• at *high altitude?*
• *bitten* or *stung?*

Many times, you'll be able to determine this information almost instantly from your patient's complaints, from his appearance, and from local environmental conditions (for example, if it's a hot summer day or a cold, windy day). If your patient's condition per-

---

## WHAT BIT HIM?

Unfortunately, your patient may not be able to name what bit (or stung) him. But if he saw the organism, and if you've previously prepared aids to help him identify it, you'll be able to provide the specific treatment he needs.

First, develop a list of biting and stinging organisms that are common to your geographic region. Then obtain full-color pictures of them or actual specimens of the smaller ones (such as insects), mounted or in jars. With these aids, your patient can *show* you what bit or stung him, instead of providing a possibly misleading description.

mits, take a quick history to identify chronic and current illnesses, allergies, and medications, including over-the-counter drugs, he may be taking.

If the nature of his environmental injury isn't immediately obvious, ask the patient or his family to tell you what happened. This information will identify signs and symptoms to assess for. Then you can proceed to determine their extent and seriousness and intervene as necessary.

### Exposure to cold

If your patient was exposed to cold or to cool, wet, windy conditions and appears weak, apathetic, confused, or unconscious, suspect that he has some degree of *hypothermia*. Take his rectal temperature immediately, using a rectal probe or a thermometer that registers at least as low as 75° F. (23.9° C.)—core temperature below 94° F. (34.4° C.) indicates hypothermia. If he has *mild* hypothermia (core temperature of 90° to 94° F. or 32.2° to 34.4° C.), he's probably conscious (although somewhat lethargic) and shivering, with cold, pale skin and diminished respiratory rate and blood pressure. He probably also has trouble walking and performing purposeful movements. His speech may be slurred as well.

If your patient has *severe* hypothermia (core temperature less than 90° F. or 32.2° C.), his signs and symptoms are more pronounced. He may be unconscious, with some muscular rigidity. Or, if his core temperature's extremely low, he may be completely comatose and rigid. When you assess this patient's pulse and respiratory rate, they're very slow—he may breathe only three or four times per minute. His blood pressure's decreased, and he may develop severe hypotension if his temperature continues to drop.

Cover the patient with blankets and monitor his temperature with a rectal probe—or use a rectal thermometer every 5 to 10 minutes. Watch his cardiac monitor closely: if he has severe hypothermia, he also has sinus bradycardia and possibly supraventricular dysrhythmias such as atrial fibrillation. Increased myocardial irritability means he's at risk for ventricular fibrillation as well, so handle him very carefully, avoiding any sudden movements that may precipitate this dysrhythmia. (See *Danger: Cold Blood*, page 711.)

If your patient complains of a cold, numb extremity or body part after exposure to cold, he may have *frostbite*. Check his body temperature quickly, because hypothermia—which often accompanies frostbite—must be treated first. If he's not hypothermic, or after you've taken measures to control his hypothermia, assess the frostbitten area. Look at the skin color, and palpate the area gently with your fingers. If the skin is whitish but blanches when you press it, he doesn't have true frostbite. But, if it *doesn't* blanch and the patient reports sharp, aching pain or some loss of feeling or sensitivity to cold, he may have *superficial* frostbite. If the affected area is white and waxy and doesn't blanch, and the patient reports numbness, heaviness, or complete loss of sensation, he probably has *deep* frostbite. Degrees of frostbite are difficult to differentiate on initial assessment, but another clue is the way the tissue feels to your touch. If the tissue below the skin is soft and resilient, the frostbite may be superficial, involving only the skin and subcutaneous tissue. If the tissue beneath the skin is hard and solid, he probably has deep frostbite involving the skin, subcutaneous tissue, muscles, tendons, nerves, and vessels.

If you suspect any degree of frostbite, elevate the affected area and place sterile cotton balls between digits. Then, begin rapid rewarming.

### Exposure to heat

If your patient collapsed or felt ill after he was exposed to high temperature and humidity, or after he exercised vigorously in warm weather, he may have a heat-related illness. Quickly take his rectal temperature and assess his signs and symptoms. If your patient has a minor form of heat illness *(heat edema, heat tetany, heat syncope, anhidrotic heat exhaustion,* or *heat cramps)*, his life isn't in danger and you can intervene for his signs and symptoms (see *Understanding Minor Heat-Related Illnesses,* page 725). However, if he has signs and symptoms of *heat exhaustion* or *heat stroke,* he'll need further care. Do you know how to identify these two serious—and similar—conditions? Heat stroke is more serious than heat exhaustion: the differences are in body temperature, the severity of signs and symptoms, and the presence or absence of central nervous system (CNS) disturbances. Here's a summary of clues to differentiating these two conditions:

• body temperature typically 100° F. (37.8° C.) or less in heat exhaustion; typically above 105° F. (40.5° C.) in heat stroke

• headache, dizziness, or syncope in heat exhaustion; confusion, stupor, delirium, seizures, or coma in heat stroke

• orthostatic hypotension in heat exhaustion; frank hypotension in heat stroke

• hot, flushed, and diaphoretic skin with heat exhaustion; hot, flushed, and possibly anhidrotic skin with heat stroke.

If the patient appears to have heat exhaustion, keep him quiet and in a cool environment. Moisten his skin, and use a fan to direct cool air on his body. Check his pulse and blood pressure, and draw blood for blood urea nitrogen (BUN), hematocrit, and serum sodium levels, to determine how severely he's dehydrated. If your patient's mildly dehydrated, the doctor may ask you to give him an oral electrolyte solution. For severe dehydration, expect to give normal saline (NS), sodium chloride 0.45% (½NS), or dextrose 5% in sodium chloride 0.45% (D₅½NS) I.V.

If your patient's temperature is above 100° F. (37.8° C.) and you suspect heat stroke, start more aggressive cooling measures immediately. Don't wait to draw blood or to assess him further, because *heat stroke may be rapidly fatal.* Remove his clothes and pack him in ice, soak him in ice water, or wet him down with a slurry of ice chips and water. Place sheets over the patient's body and soak them, to keep the water and ice in close contact with his skin. Use a fan to speed evaporation and cooling. Monitor his temperature constantly with a rectal probe, or take his temperature every 10 to 15 minutes with a rectal thermometer. Provide I.V. fluids, as ordered, to replace lost fluid volume.

## Near-drowning

If your patient was submerged in water and had a *near-drowning accident,* he may have a wide variety of clinical problems ranging from mild respiratory distress to severe respiratory distress, hypothermia, and cardiac arrest. He may also be lethargic, combative, confused, disoriented, or semicomatose, depending on his degree of hypoxemia. Continue supplemental oxygen and ventilatory assistance, and observe him closely for developing pulmonary problems. Ask the patient's family or rescue personnel how long the victim was under water, how cold the water was, and how quickly resuscitation was begun, because these factors will influence your patient's recovery. The doctor will order a chest X-ray to detect pulmonary complications.

## Altitude-related illnesses

If your patient's recently been at a high altitude (and wasn't acclimated to it) and now has respiratory signs and symptoms and alterations in his level of consciousness, he may have an altitude-related illness. Ask him how high he ascended, how quickly he ascended, and when his signs and symptoms first appeared. Then ask him to describe how he feels. If he reports headache, malaise, nausea, loss of appetite, problems sleeping, confusion, and dyspnea on exertion, he probably

## GUIDELINES FOR RABIES PROPHYLAXIS

When caring for a victim of an animal bite, don't forget to assess his need for rabies prophylaxis. As you know, untreated rabies is invariably fatal—so take every precaution to protect your patient. This chart contains the information you'll need.

If rabies prophylaxis is indicated, give your patient both rabies immune globulin (RIG) and human diploid cell rabies vaccine (HDCV) *immediately,* as ordered. If RIG isn't available, expect to administer antirabies serum, equine.

| ANIMAL | CONDITION OF ANIMAL AT TIME OF ATTACK | RABIES PROPHYLAXIS |
|---|---|---|
| **Domestic** (dog, cat) | Healthy and available for 10 days of observation | None, unless animal develops rabies during observation* |
| | Rabid or suspected rabid | RIG and HDCV |
| | Unknown (escaped) | Consult public health officials; if treatment's indicated, give RIG and HDCV |
| **Wild** (raccoon, skunk, bat, fox, and other carnivores) | *Consider all rabid* unless proven negative by laboratory tests on captured animals** | RIG and HDCV |
| **Others** (livestock, rodents, and rabbits) | Consider individually; consult public health officials. Rodent and rabbit bites rarely cause rabies in humans. | Consult public health officials |

*During the 10-day holding period, begin treating your patient with RIG and HDCV at the first sign of rabies in the animal, when the animal should be killed and tested immediately.
**The animal should be killed and tested as soon as possible; holding it for observation delays your patient's treatment (if needed).

Adapted from "Rabies Prevention," *Morbidity, Mortality Weekly Report,* 29:279, 1980.

has *acute mountain sickness (AMS),* a self-limiting syndrome that will resolve itself in 1 to 5 days. However, you must be alert for the more serious forms of altitude-related illness: *high-altitude pulmonary edema (HAPE)* and *high-altitude cerebral edema (HACE).*

Signs and symptoms of HAPE include:
• increasingly severe dyspnea on exertion
• tachycardia
• persistent cough (dry or producing frothy sputum)
• noisy, gurgling respirations
• weakness
• orthopnea

• hemoptysis
• rales and rhonchi.

Signs and symptoms of HACE include:
• increasingly severe headache
• confusion, possibly progressing to stupor or coma
• emotional lability
• hallucinations
• ataxia
• motor weakness.

Continue to provide oxygen and observe for improvement. He started improving when he descended below 8,000 to 10,000 feet, where you're presumably seeing him. If you work in a high-altitude area, the doctor may ask you to arrange for the patient's transport to a facility at a lower altitude.

### Bites and stings

If your patient's been bitten or stung, try to determine what bit or stung him so you can intervene appropriately and administer antivenin if necessary (and as ordered). This will be obvious if the animal was a pet, such as a dog or cat, or a farm animal. If it was a wild animal, however, or a snake, insect, or aquatic organism, the patient may not know its specific type. Ask him to describe it and, if you have books, charts, or specimens available, show these to the patient and see if he can identify it. Watch the patient closely for a developing anaphylactic reaction (see the "Anaphylactic Shock" entry in Chapter 14).

## Special Considerations

### Pediatric

An infant or neonate is particularly at risk for hypothermia, because his large surface-to-mass ratio and his lack of subcutaneous tissue allow him to lose heat rapidly. And because a neonate's thermoregulatory center isn't fully developed, he's unable to generate heat by shivering.

Because young children typically aren't strong swimmers (or can't swim at all), they're more likely than adults to experience near-drowning. They're also more likely to sustain serious bites to the face, head, and neck from playing at close quarters with household pets.

### Geriatric

Your elderly patient's also at particular risk for hypothermia—in fact, he may even be chronically hypothermic because of his decreased basal metabolic rate, appetite, physical activity, vasoconstrictive response, and subcutaneous fat layer. This means he may become severely hypothermic when exposed to a moderately cold environment, such as an apartment with the heat turned down, that wouldn't affect a younger, more active person. And as you probably know, arteriosclerosis and other disorders of peripheral circulation increase an elderly patient's risk of frostbite.

Age also increases the risk of heat stroke, which is especially dangerous in an elderly patient. Why? Because an elderly patient who develops heat stroke is more likely to develop severe cardiovascular and respiratory problems along with it—particularly if he has underlying heart disease.

## DEFINITIVE CARE

## Hypothermia

### Initial care summary

Initial assessment findings varied, depending on the degree of the patient's hypothermia. If he had *mild hypothermia* (core temperature of 90° to 94° F. or 32.2° to 34.4° C.), he had some combination of these findings:
- shivering
- fatigue, weakness, lethargy, or apathy
- slurred speech
- ataxia
- muscle stiffness
- tachycardia (and possibly tachydysrhythmias)
- hyperactive deep-tendon reflexes
- diuresis
- decreased respiratory rate and blood pressure
- cold, pale skin.

If he had *severe* hypothermia (core temperature less than 90° F. or 32.2° C.), his signs and symptoms were more pronounced and included some combination of the following:

- cold, pale skin
- confusion, stupor, unconsciousness, or profound coma
- muscle rigidity
- hyporeflexia or areflexia
- bradycardia (and possibly bradydys-rhythmias and conduction distur-bances)
- J waves on EKG
- hypotension
- severely decreased respirations
- oliguria.

He was given supplemental oxygen or, if necessary, ventilation was as-sisted with an Ambu bag at half the normal rate. A large-bore I.V. was in-serted for fluid and medication admin-istration. If the patient was pulseless and apneic, CPR was started, and he was intubated despite the risk of ven-tricular fibrillation.

A 12-lead EKG and a chest X-ray were taken. Continuous cardiac monitoring was initiated, and blood was drawn for a complete blood count (CBC), platelet count, electrolytes, blood glu-cose, ABGs, BUN, creatinine, lactate

### DETECTING HYPOTHERMIA

As you know, a patient's hypo-thermia may be very subtle; you may detect it only after tak-ing his temperature. But if you always use a standard clinical thermometer, you still run the risk of overlooking hypothermia and of under-estimating its severity. Why? Because most standard thermometers only register low temperatures to 94° F. (34.4° C.).

So, if you suspect that your patient has hypothermia (based on his history of exposure or immersion), be sure to take his temperature with a low-reading thermometer. Use a continuous-monitoring rectal probe, if possible. It has two important advantages: Rectal temperature most closely reflects core temperature, and you won't have to move your patient every 10 to 15 minutes to take manual rectal tempera-ture readings.

dehydrogenase (LDH), serum glutamic-oxaloacetic transaminase (SGOT), serum glutamic-pyruvic transaminase (SGPT), fibrinogen, fibrin-split products, prothrombin time (PT), partial thromboplastin time (PTT), serum calcium, and serum magnesium.

### Priorities

Before you begin any interventions, re-member that you must handle the hy-pothermic patient *gently,* because any excessive handling or mechanical stim-ulation before he's rewarmed may pre-cipitate ventricular fibrillation. (See *Danger: Cold Blood.*)

With this in mind, your two initial priorities are fluid replacement and re-warming. Insert a metal thermistor probe into his rectum, so you can mon-itor his temperature constantly. (See *Detecting Hypothermia.*) Expect to start fluid administration *before* you begin rewarming; this is because I.V. fluids decrease blood viscosity and pe-ripheral vasoconstriction and increase blood flow to the heart, reducing the risk of dysrhythmias.

Begin a rapid infusion of dextrose 5% in water (D$_5$W) or D$_5$½NS, as or-dered. The doctor probably *won't* order Ringer's lactate, because your patient's hypothermic liver can't metabolize lac-tate properly. If possible, warm I.V. fluids before you give them—heated fluids don't contribute much to active rewarming of your patient, but they at least prevent further heat loss. Insert an indwelling (Foley) catheter to mon-itor his urine output. The doctor may insert a central venous pressure (CVP) line to monitor the patient's fluid status more accurately.

After you've started fluids, begin re-warming your patient. Depending on your patient's degree of hypothermia, the doctor may order passive external rewarming, active external rewarm-ing, or active core rewarming; he'll take your patient's age and general health into account when deciding which method or combination of methods will be most effective.

Expect to start *passive external rewarming* if your patient's young and healthy and has mild hypothermia due to exposure or if he's elderly and has mild hypothermia that developed gradually. Place the patient in a warm room, and cover him with blankets or a similar insulating material. This minimizes the heat your patient loses by evaporation, convection, and radiation, and allows him to generate enough heat for spontaneous rewarming. Passive rewarming has the advantage of maintaining peripheral vasoconstriction, which minimizes the risk of vascular collapse during rewarming.

If your patient's hypothermia is more severe, or if passive external rewarming doesn't raise the patient's core temperature at least 1.8° F./hour (1° C./hour), the doctor may order active external rewarming, active core rewarming, or a combination of the two. Provide *active external rewarming* by applying an electric blanket, warmed blankets, a heating pad, a hyperthermia blanket, or hot water bottles to your patient's thorax, or by immersing him in warm water (105° to 110° F. or 40.6° to 43.3° C.) in a tub or Hubbard tank as ordered. If possible, avoid warming his extremities during active external rewarming, so he can maintain some degree of peripheral vasoconstriction. Why? Because rapid peripheral vasodilation may precipitate cardiovascular collapse as his vascular capacity increases. Furthermore, as vasodilation allows cold blood to rush from your patient's periphery to his core, his core temperature may actually *drop* (a phenomenon known as *core temperature afterdrop*).

*Active core rewarming,* alone or in combination with active external rewarming, minimizes the patient's risk of cardiovascular collapse and core temperature afterdrop. The doctor may ask you to give additional heated I.V. fluids and to give heated, humidified oxygen by mask, endotracheal tube, or intermittent positive-pressure breath-

ing device. He may also start heated peritoneal dialysis, with an isotonic dialysate of dextrose 1.5% heated to 110° F. (43.3° C.), or he may start heated gastric or bladder lavage. Assist him as necessary with these procedures.

If your patient's hypothermia is extremely severe, and the active-core-rewarming methods described don't elevate his temperature rapidly, the doctor may insert a chest tube or perform a thoracotomy and start a mediastinal lavage with heated NS or Ringer's lactate. He may also initiate extracorporeal blood rewarming, which will elevate the patient's temperature even if he's in cardiac arrest. Assist with chest tube insertion or prepare the patient for surgery, as ordered.

If your patient's in cardiac arrest, expect to continue CPR for hours, if necessary, until his pulse and respirations return or until he's completely re-

# WHAT HAPPENS IN HYPOTHERMIA

Hypothermia occurs when the body's core temperature drops below 94° F. (34.4° C.). The cause is prolonged exposure to cold temperatures or to a cool, wet environment, but many clinical conditions that upset the body's thermoregulatory center in the hypothalamus can also predispose a patient to hypothermia. These include malnutrition, hypopituitarism, myxedema, hypoglycemia, diabetes, alcoholism, trauma to the head or spinal cord, myocardial infarction, and shock. Because the body's biochemical functioning is

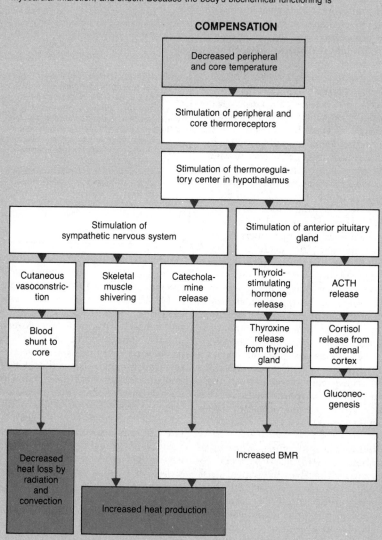

**COMPENSATION**

Decreased peripheral and core temperature

Stimulation of peripheral and core thermoreceptors

Stimulation of thermoregulatory center in hypothalamus

Stimulation of sympathetic nervous system

Stimulation of anterior pituitary gland

Cutaneous vasoconstriction

Skeletal muscle shivering

Catecholamine release

Thyroid-stimulating hormone release

ACTH release

Blood shunt to core

Thyroxine release from thyroid gland

Cortisol release from adrenal cortex

Gluconeogenesis

Decreased heat loss by radiation and convection

Increased BMR

Increased heat production

temperature-dependent, reduced core temperature slows the basal metabolic rate (BMR) and all cellular activity. When the core temperature remains above 90° F. (32° C.), *compensation* is usually effective in reducing heat loss, generating heat, and increasing the BMR. However, below 90° F., compensation isn't sufficient to offset heat loss. Continued core temperature drop triggers hypothermic *decompensation*, which eventually leads to death if the process isn't reversed. These flowcharts show how hypothermic compensation and decompensation occur.

## DECOMPENSATION

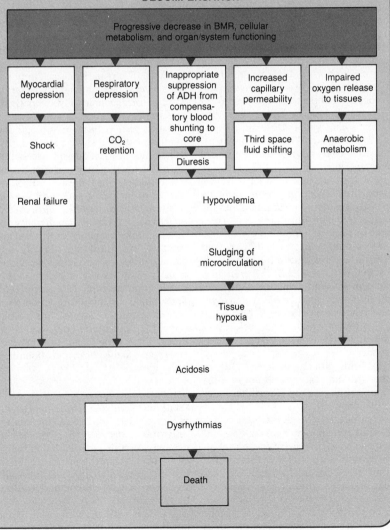

warmed. Remember, full recovery is possible even after a long period of cardiac arrest when the patient's severely hypothermic. The doctor won't declare him dead unless he still has no heartbeat or respirations after he's rewarmed to at least 89.6° F. (32° C.).

## Continuing assessment and intervention

After you've begun rewarming your patient, perform a complete assessment to provide baseline information. Monitor his vital signs every few minutes throughout the rewarming period, and keep accurate records of the changes in his temperature. Keep alert for core temperature afterdrop, and watch for a return to normal body temperature. If you're using active core rewarming, the doctor will probably ask you to discontinue dialysis or lavage when the patient's core temperature approaches 96° F. (35.6° C.). Why? To avoid "temperature overshoot"—unintentional hyperthermia.

Watch his cardiac monitor closely— atrial fibrillation, premature ventricular contractions, conduction blocks, and ventricular fibrillation are common in patients whose core temperature is below 86° F. (30° C.), and difficult to reverse until temperature is restored to 90° F. (32.2° C.) or higher. (Remember, antiarrhythmics and defibrillation *may not be effective* in a patient whose temperature is below 90° F. Continue to handle your patient very carefully, and avoid any vagal stimulation.

Examine him closely for frostbite or other trauma that may accompany his hypothermia (see the "Frostbite" entry in this chapter).

Continue to give fluids as ordered. Monitor your patient's intake and output, and watch his CVP values closely— the vasodilation and hyperemia that occur with rewarming may increase your patient's fluid needs. However, he's also susceptible to fluid overload, so be sure to watch for jugular venous distention and to auscultate his lungs

for rales and other signs of pulmonary edema.

Check your patient's initial blood tests. Typically, they'll reflect dehydration, electrolyte abnormalities, and acidosis. Draw blood for additional tests as your patient rewarms, being particularly careful to check his ABG and electrolyte levels. (When you send ABG results to the laboratory, make sure you record your patient's body temperature at the time the blood was drawn—otherwise, the results will be interpreted incorrectly.) As your patient rewarms, his electrolyte abnormalities and metabolic acidosis should correct spontaneously. If they don't, the doctor may ask you to administer potassium, if your patient's serum potassium level is less than 3.0 mEq/liter, or sodium bicarbonate if your patient's acidosis is severe.

Assess your patient's neurologic status frequently—it should also improve as he rewarms. If it doesn't, assess him for problems that may underlie his hypothermia or may have predisposed him to it, including such problems as trauma, sepsis, hypothyroidism, hypoglycemia, adrenal insufficiency, or uremia. Take a history from your patient or his family to identify any chronic diseases or signs and symptoms he may have had before he became hypothermic. If appropriate, draw blood for thyroid function tests, serum cortisol levels, toxicology screening, and blood cultures, as ordered. Expect the doctor to order cervical spine, skull, chest, and abdominal X-ray films.

## Therapeutic care

Continue to monitor your patient's temperature closely for 24 to 48 hours after rewarming, because some rewarmed posthypothermic patients fail to maintain a normal body temperature. Monitor his cardiac rhythm continuously, and keep a defibrillator and sodium bicarbonate on hand. Why? Because your patient's still at risk for ventricular fibrillation for 2 to 24 hours after rewarming, depending on how fast he was warmed.

Watch for these complications of hypothermia:

• *pneumonia,* the principal complication of hypothermia. Check your patient's breath sounds frequently, and watch for fever, purulent sputum production, and other signs of infection. The doctor may ask you to give antibiotics prophylactically.

• *thromboembolism* secondary to an increase in blood viscosity. Watch your patient for calf pain and redness (possibly indicating phlebitis) and for chest pain and dyspnea (possibly indicating pulmonary embolus). Report these findings to the doctor *immediately.*

• *a syndrome resembling disseminated intravascular coagulation* (DIC) from increased viscosity and intravascular stasis. Watch your patient for bleeding from the gums, nose, and I.V. sites. (See the "Disseminated Intravascular Coagulation" entry in Chapter 11.)

• *acute renal failure.* Hypothermia may precipitate rhabdomyolysis, which can cause acute renal failure. (See the "Acute Renal Failure" entry in Chapter 13.)

---

# Frostbite

## Initial care summary

The patient was exposed to cold and complained of a cold, numb extremity or body part. Initial assessment findings depended on the degree of injury (which can be difficult to determine initially).

If he had *superficial* frostbite, his signs and symptoms probably included:

• sharp, aching pain, or a loss of feeling and sensitivity to cold in the affected area

• white, waxy skin that doesn't blanch when pressed but feels soft and resilient.

If he had *deep* frostbite, his signs and symptoms probably included:

• complete loss of sensation plus numbness and a feeling of heaviness in the affected area

• white, waxy skin that doesn't blanch when pressed and feels hard and solid.

The patient was assessed for hypothermia, which may have accompanied the frostbite—if present, this was treated first (see the "Hypothermia" entry in this chapter). Blood was drawn for a CBC and electrolyte, blood sugar, BUN, and creatinine levels and a clotting profile. X-rays of the injured area were also taken. An I.V. was started at a keep-vein-open rate for fluid and medication administration.

## Priorities

Begin thawing the patient's frostbitten area *immediately* and *rapidly*— most cellular damage occurs during the freezing and thawing processes, so you want to avoid slow thawing.

Immerse the frostbitten part in a warm water bath (100° to 108° F., or 37.8° to 42.2° C.), preferably with a whirlpool. (If your patient's face or ears are affected, pour warm water over the area or apply warm, moist soaks. Change soaks frequently to maintain the desired temperature.) Handle the affected part gently, and protect it from friction and pressure. *Don't massage it*—this can cause tissue damage. If clothes are frozen to the area, don't try to remove them until after the area's thawed.

Your patient will experience considerable pain as the affected area thaws. Expect to administer an analgesic and a sedative such as I.M. or I.V. morphine or meperidine (Demerol), as ordered.

As the area thaws, a pink flush will appear and (on an extremity) will progress distally until the area's flushed to the tip. Keep the area immersed until it's completely flushed, is warm to your touch, blanches when you press it, and stays flushed when you remove it from the water bath. Don't apply any dressings to the area. If the patient's fingers or toes are affected, place sterile cotton

# WHAT HAPPENS IN FROSTBITE

The body's response to extremely cold temperatures is vasoconstriction. This decreases blood flow and oxygen supply to peripheral tissues as blood is shunted to the core. Thus deprived of oxygen, the peripheral tissues are especially susceptible to damage from cold.

Frostbite occurs when tissue temperature drops below its freezing point of −2° F. (−18.9° C.). Extremities and exposed areas—especially the hands, feet, ears, and face—are most susceptible. The extent of tissue damage depends on the degree of cold and the duration of exposure. The diagram below shows how frostbite develops.

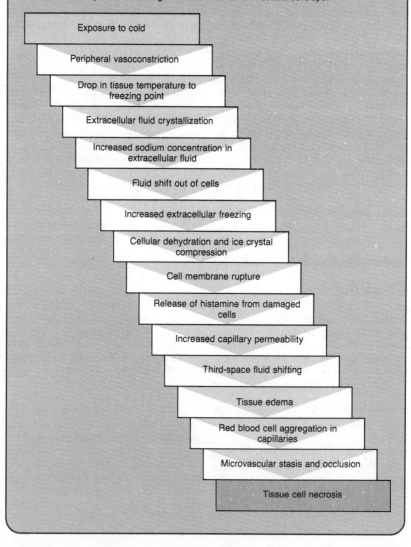

Exposure to cold

Peripheral vasoconstriction

Drop in tissue temperature to freezing point

Extracellular fluid crystallization

Increased sodium concentration in extracellular fluid

Fluid shift out of cells

Increased extracellular freezing

Cellular dehydration and ice crystal compression

Cell membrane rupture

Release of histamine from damaged cells

Increased capillary permeability

Third-space fluid shifting

Tissue edema

Red blood cell aggregation in capillaries

Microvascular stasis and occlusion

Tissue cell necrosis

between the digits to minimize friction. Check the color of the flush after you rewarm the area, because it may help indicate the severity of the injury: it may be mottled blue or purple if your patient has *superficial* frostbite, and blue, violet, or gray if he has *deep* frostbite. If his frostbite is extremely severe, the affected area may remain gray and cold even after it's completely thawed. If so, it won't regain function.

Check your patient's neurovascular status as soon as the affected area's completely thawed. The area may appear transiently cyanotic, but this should disappear unless the patient has an underlying injury such as a fracture or sprain. You should be able to feel pulses in the affected area—if they're weak or absent, this may indicate thrombus formation. Report your findings to the doctor *immediately*—he may ask you to give I.V. low-molecular-weight dextran to reverse intravascular red blood cell aggregation and to improve microcirculation.

Expect to give tetanus prophylaxis, as ordered. (See *Guidelines for Tetanus Prophylaxis*, pages 66 and 67.)

## Continuing assessment and intervention

After you've rewarmed the frostbitten area, the doctor will order protective (reverse) isolation for your patient, to minimize the chances of infection. Use sterile sheets, and protect the affected area from pressure and friction—use a bed cradle, for example, if his legs are affected. Keep the patient on bed rest, and keep the affected area elevated.

When your patient's stable, perform a thorough assessment and take a complete history to provide baseline information. Pay particular attention to the preinjury state of the affected part, because any neurovascular dysfunction will affect his recovery. Take his vital signs every 4 hours after rewarming, and perform frequent assessments. Watch for:

• persistent cyanosis or ischemia of the affected area
• persistent, increasing pain
• edema
• weak or absent pulses.

These signs and symptoms may indicate that your patient's developing compartment syndrome (see *Understanding Compartment Syndrome*, pages 370 and 371, and *Measuring Compartment Pressure*, page 368). Don't overlook the significance of these signs and symptoms—they may mimic the signs and symptoms you expect your patient to have immediately after rewarming, but if they're *persistent*, something's wrong. Be sure to keep careful track of them and to report them to the doctor.

The doctor may order pain medication, such as propoxyphene (Darvon) or acetaminophen with codeine (Tylenol with codeine). He may also order phenoxybenzamine hydrochloride (Dibenzyline) orally. An alpha-adrenergic blocking agent, Dibenzyline decreases vasospasm and also causes vasodilation. When you give this drug, watch for orthostatic blood pressure changes and provide plenty of fluids, because vasodilation makes your patient subject to relative hypovolemia.

The doctor may administer reserpine or tolazoline hydrochloride intraarterially—vasodilators that cause a temporary medical sympathectomy that decreases pain, edema, and vasospasm and increases blood flow to the area, improving the probability of survival of marginal tissue.

Inspect the affected area frequently. Blebs will begin to form 12 to 24 hours after the injury and are a positive prognostic sign. (If your patient develops few or no blebs, this may indicate that circulation isn't returning to the area.) Don't rupture the blebs—they're sterile and help protect the underlying tissue.

Start whirlpool treatments of the patient's affected area, as ordered, to clean and debride the area. The doctor will probably ask you to provide baths twice daily for 20 minutes each, using water heated to 90° to 98° F. (32.2° to

## EXERCISE THERAPY FOR FROSTBITE VICTIMS

A patient with frostbitten hands or feet must regularly exercise the affected parts to prevent muscle atrophy and to improve circulation. Teach your patient the exercises shown below, and explain their importance to him. Make sure he does at least four 20-minute sets each day.

### HAND EXERCISES

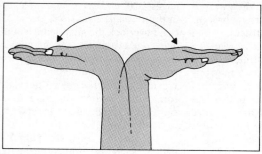

Flex and extend the wrist.

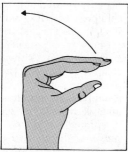

Bend and straighten each finger at the metacarpal-phalangeal joints; keep other fingers straight.

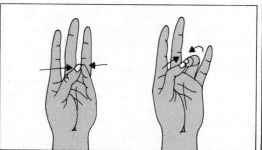

Touch the tip of the thumb with each finger.

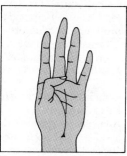

Touch the thumb to the base of each finger.

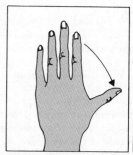

Spread the web space of the thumb widely.

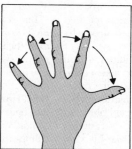

Spread the fingers.

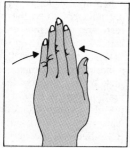

Squeeze the fingers together; then repeat the sequence twice.

## BERGER'S (LEG) EXERCISES

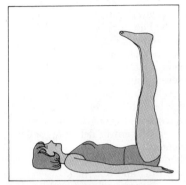

Raise the legs overhead for 2 minutes.

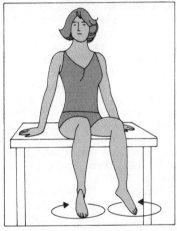

Dangle the legs over the bedside and swirl them in circles for 2 minutes.

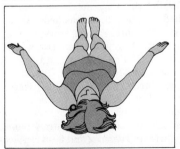

Lie flat for 2 minutes, and then repeat the sequence twice.

36.7° C.) and pHisoHex or another mild disinfectant soap. Encourage the patient to move the area actively during whirlpool treatments. After each whirlpool treatment, allow the area to air dry, and place sterile cotton between affected digits and other affected areas that touch. Don't dress the area.

Start him on a regular exercise program to increase blood flow to the area, to prevent stiffness, and to prevent formation of a tight eschar. (See *Exercise Therapy for Frostbite Victims.*)

If your patient's frostbite was severe and he continues to have significant edema and pain, the doctor may perform a surgical sympathectomy. This procedure has several beneficial effects: it reduces edema rapidly, decreases pain, speeds demarcation of viable from nonviable tissue, stops vasospasm, and promotes healing.

### Therapeutic care

Your patient's blebs will rupture spontaneously 3 to 7 days after he was rewarmed. *Don't* remove the flaps of skin that remain—they'll provide some coverage and help reduce his pain. Instead, continue the whirlpool treatments, which will debride the bleb flaps slowly and naturally.

Watch for infection after the blebs rupture. (You know, of course, that open, wet areas increase the risk of infection.) Culture any purulent drainage, and expect to administer antibiotics as ordered once the culture results return from the laboratory. Continue protective isolation of your patient, and keep the affected area dry, protected, and on sterile sheets. Remind the patient to perform his exercises frequently, and check his neurovascular status regularly.

After they rupture, your patient's blebs will dry into a hard, dark eschar. The doctor won't debride this unless it's infected. If it becomes tight and stiff and restricts movement of the area, the doctor may split the eschar gently along its dorsal surface (if a digit is involved) or along its lateral borders. Don't remove the eschar—as with ruptured blebs, allow the eschar to slough off naturally during whirlpool treatments.

The full extent of your patient's injury may not be apparent for several weeks. Watch for demarcation between viable and nonviable areas—where tissue has been completely destroyed, soft tissue will spontaneously mummify and slough off, causing a spontaneous amputation. The doctor may inject technetium 99 (a radioactive isotope) intraarterially, to determine the extent of the patient's microcirculatory damage and to help predict what areas will ultimately be nonviable. After the process of spontaneous amputation is complete (usually 3 to 4 weeks), the doctor will perform surgery to remove any remaining nonviable tissue and to create a clean stump.

Be prepared to help the patient cope with the emotional stress of his frostbite injury. He needs your emotional support because he's sure to be discouraged and depressed. Explain to him that as the healing process continues, his injury will temporarily look worse rather than better. If tissue starts to mummify and slough off, he'll wonder what's going to be left! Reassure him that he's making progress, but don't minimize the fact that the healing process will be lengthy or that he may need surgery and may lose some function permanently.

# Heat Stroke and Heat Exhaustion

## Initial care summary

The patient was exposed to some form of heat stress and developed signs and symptoms of severe heat-related illness: either heat exhaustion or heat stroke. If he had *heat exhaustion*, initial assessment findings may have included:
• malaise, irritability, and anxiety
• tachycardia

• tachypnea
• orthostatic hypotension
• moderately increased temperature (usually not above 100° F. or 37.8° C.)
• headache, dizziness, or syncope
• hot, flushed, diaphoretic skin.

If he had *heat stroke*, initial assessment findings may have included:
• severe tachycardia
• severe tachypnea
• severe frank hypotension
• severely increased temperature (usually above 105° F. or 40.5° C.)
• alterations in consciousness, ranging from confusion to delirium, seizures, or coma
• hot, flushed, possibly anhidrotic skin
• vomiting and diarrhea.

The patient was intubated if he was comatose or had severe respiratory distress or seizures. Supplementary oxygen was provided, and he may have been given an oral electrolyte solution. An I.V line was started with NS, ½NS, or D₅½NS, and an EKG was taken. His clothing was removed, and cooling measures were started immediately. Cardiac monitoring was initiated. If the patient's condition permitted, blood was drawn for a CBC, platelet count, PT, PTT, fibrin-split products, blood sugar, creatinine, electrolytes, BUN, serum protein, serum lactate, calcium, ABGs, SGOT, LDH, and creatine phosphokinase (CPK). If the patient's condition was poor, these studies were postponed until cooling was underway.

## Priorities

Initially, you may not be able to tell whether your patient has heat exhaustion or heat stroke: signs and symptoms often overlap, and sometimes only frank CNS disturbances and grossly elevated SGOT, LDH, and CPK values in heat stroke distinguish the two disorders. But you won't have the results of laboratory tests immediately, and you may not even have time to draw blood. So start rapid cooling and fluid replacement if you have any reason to suspect heat stroke.

Insert a rectal thermistor probe to

monitor your patient's temperature (glass thermometers are dangerous if your patient develops seizures, and they're not usually adequate for measuring extremely elevated temperatures.) If a thermometer's all you have, measure the patient's rectal temperature every 5 to 10 minutes.

Continue surface cooling measures, as ordered:

• You may cover the naked patient with sheets or towels wetted with a slurry of ice chips and water—change them frequently to maintain the cooling effect.

• You may apply ice packs to areas of maximum heat transfer (axillae and inguinal area) or you may apply a hypothermia blanket to his thorax. These provide some cooling while avoiding cutaneous vasoconstriction.

• You may spray the patient's body with warm water and then direct *dry* air over him with a fan, which maximizes evaporative cooling. (If air in the treatment area is humid, this method won't work as well.) If you use this method, make sure you provide a *rapid* air flow.

While you provide surface cooling measures, massage your patient as necessary to reduce the cutaneous vasocontriction that may occur if his skin temperature drops below 82.4° F. or 28° C. (Keep in mind that maximum vaporization depends on a high skin-to-air temperature gradient as well as an adequate cutaneous blood flow.)

In addition to these surface cooling measures, the doctor may also ask you to give cold I.V. fluids and cold enemas, and he may start a cold gastric or peritoneal lavage. These methods provide only a small fraction of the cooling necessary, but they may be useful if your patient's temperature is extremely elevated and he doesn't respond quickly to surface cooling measures.

Your patient may start shivering violently after you initiate cooling measures. Take steps to control this (as ordered), because shivering increases your patient's metabolic rate and heat production. Watch his cardiac monitor to detect shivering artifacts—an early sign. If he starts to shiver, anticipate giving chlorpromazine (Thorazine) I.V., which decreases shivering and metabolic oxygen consumption and dilates cutaneous blood vessels. (Use chlorpromazine with caution and monitor your patient's blood pressure carefully, because chlorpromazine may cause a marked decrease in your patient's blood pressure.) Or the doctor may ask you to give barbiturates. These drugs have effects similar to chlorpromazine's, but keep in mind that they may mask your patient's neurologic status. If the patient's shivering is very severe, the doctor may give him sodium thiopental.

Your patient's uncontrolled shivering may progress to frank seizures. If this occurs, expect to administer I.V. diazepam (Valium) or phenobarbital. Although you might expect the doctor to order phenytoin sodium (Dilantin) because it's commonly used to control seizures, in this situation he probably won't. Why? Because it's been reported to be ineffective in patients with heat-related illnesses.

Check your patient's fluid status once cooling's underway. If you haven't already done so, draw blood for laboratory tests to determine the degree of his dehydration. His BUN, hematocrit, serum sodium, and serum protein levels will probably be elevated. The doctor will probably insert a CVP line to assess the patient's hydration and heart function and to allow rapid fluid administration. (If the patient's severely hypotensive, the doctor may insert a Swan-Ganz catheter instead.) Expect to insert an indwelling (Foley) catheter and to administer I.V. fluids rapidly. The doctor will probably order NS, ½NS, or D₅½NS—depending on the results of your patient's laboratory tests.

## Continuing assessment and intervention

Stop cooling your patient when his temperature reaches 102° F. (39° C.). This way, you'll avoid *overshoot hypother-*

# WHAT HAPPENS IN HEAT STROKE

Normally, the body's thermoregulatory center—located in the hypothalamus—maintains body temperature. Two mechanisms help dissipate excess heat and maintain the core temperature: diaphoresis and cutaneous vasodilation. These mechanisms release body heat through radiation, convection, and most importantly, evaporation.

Overexposure to high environmental temperatures (especially when combined with high humidity and low wind conditions, which interfere with normal body surface cooling) impairs the release of body heat, leading to heat storage and an abnormal rise in body temperature. In addition, a number of other factors predispose a person to heat stroke:
• age (the elderly are particularly susceptible)

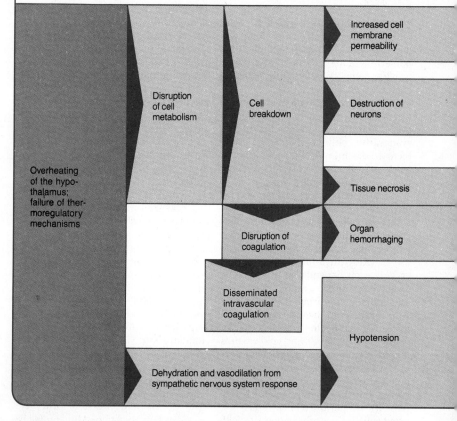

mia from overcooling your patient. Check his vital signs and neurologic status frequently.

Perform a thorough assessment to provide baseline information. Take a history, including whether he has pre-existing cardiac or endocrine disease. Also note if he's taking any medications that may precipitate heat-related illness. These include:
• thyroid extracts and amphetamines, which increase heat production
• haloperidol (Haldol), which decreases thirst

- obesity
- fever
- dehydration
- strenuous exercise
- chronic cardiovascular illness
- alcohol consumption
- use of diuretics, thyroid hormones, amphetamines, anticholinergics, phenothiazines, or tricyclic antidepressants.

Heat stroke occurs when the hypothalamus becomes overheated—generally when body temperature rises above 105° F. (40.5° C.). Thermoregulation fails, cellular metabolism is disrupted, and then—as internal temperature rises—cell breakdown begins. Heat stroke affects virtually every body system, as shown in the flowchart.

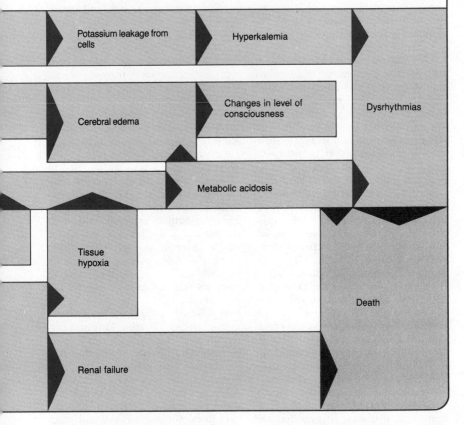

- antihistamines, anticholinergics, phenothiazines, and beta-adrenergic blockers, which decrease diaphoresis. Report your findings to the doctor.

Continue to give fluids as ordered, and expect to draw blood for serial assessments of BUN, hematocrit, serum protein, and serum sodium, to determine the degree of your patient's dehydration and his response to fluid replacement. Monitor his fluid status carefully by checking his CVP values, urine output, urine osmolarity, blood pressure, and pulse. Remember that he's susceptible to fluid overload: as his body temperature drops, cutaneous vasoconstriction will push a large volume of plasma into his central circulation and may cause pulmonary edema. This is especially likely to happen if renal hypoperfusion secondary to hypotension is compromising his renal function. Watch for signs of pulmonary edema, such as a frothy cough, distended neck veins, rales, and elevated CVP. Report these to the doctor; he may ask you to administer a diuretic. Also report oliguria that continues after you've given fluids, because it may indicate developing renal failure. The doctor may order mannitol, to increase your patient's urine output.

Your patient may be hypotensive as the result of high-output heart failure that develops when blood is shunted through his dilated vessels. With treatment, as his body temperature decreases and his vessels constrict, his blood pressure should increase. However, if his hypotension persists after he's cooled a few degrees, the doctor may ask you to give an I.V. fluid challenge of 200 to 500 ml of NS over several minutes. Monitor the patient's blood pressure and CVP readings as you do this—if they increase, expect to administer more fluid until his blood pressure reaches 90/60 mm Hg or until his CVP is greater than 12 cmH₂O. If he doesn't respond to the fluid challenge, or if his CVP is already elevated, the doctor may ask you to give an adrenergic agent such as isoproterenol (Isuprel), dopamine hydrochloride (Intropin), or dobutamine (Dobutrex).

Continue to monitor your patient's temperature or to take it regularly if you're using a thermometer. Remember, he may develop rebound hyperthermia up to 6 hours after cooling, and he'll have thermoregulatory instability for days or weeks. Keep him on bed rest, as ordered, to avoid heat production caused by activity and to decrease his tissue oxygen demands. Continue to provide supplementary oxygen even if his ABGs are satisfactory, because he

may still have tissue hypoxia and increased tissue oxygen demands.

Your patient may be acidotic, especially if he has exertional heat stroke. Expect to give sodium bicarbonate if his pH is below 7.2. If his serum potassium is also low, expect to give I.V. potassium. However, if his serum potassium is low but he's *not* acidotic, this will correct itself after cooling; he won't need to receive potassium.

## Therapeutic care

Continue to monitor your patient's temperature, vital signs, and fluid status. If he had *heat exhaustion*, he'll probably recover fully within 12 hours— but if he's elderly or has cardiovascular disease, he'll need more cautious fluid replacement and more frequent assessments, so expect to care for him longer in the hospital.

If your patient had *heat stroke*, he probably has serious tissue damage. He'll be vulnerable to renal insufficiency and renal failure (due to hypotension and hypoperfusion), myoglobinuria, acute tubular necrosis, and rhabdomyolysis (see the "Acute Renal Failure" entry in Chapter 13). Check his urine output frequently, and check the results of his laboratory tests for BUN, creatinine, and serum potassium levels. If he develops renal insufficiency or renal failure, expect the doctor to start dialysis and to treat him for hyperkalemia.

Watch for bleeding from the patient's gums, nose, or I.V. sites. This may signal DIC resulting from the small vessel thrombi and platelet destruction that accompany heat stroke (see the "Disseminated Intravascular Coagulation" entry in Chapter 11). Report any unusual bleeding to the doctor, and expect to administer heparin and other therapy as ordered.

Perform passive range-of-motion exercises on your patient, and encourage him to do active range-of-motion exercises. This will stimulate his circulation and help prevent thrombosis.

Continue to check your patient's

# UNDERSTANDING MINOR HEAT-RELATED ILLNESSES

Except for heat stroke and heat exhaustion, heat-related illnesses generally aren't life-threatening. This chart will help you recognize and treat patients with these less serious disorders.

## HEAT EDEMA

Signs and symptoms include mild swelling and a feeling of tightness in the hands and feet. Heat edema occurs in unacclimated persons—especially those who are elderly—during the first few days of heat exposure.

**Treatment**
- Elevate the patient's extremities.
- Apply support hose, if necessary.
- No additional treatment's necessary; the edema is self-limiting and should resolve with acclimation.

## HEAT TETANY

Carpopedal spasms (due to rapid changes in pH from hyperventilation) occur during overexposure to heat (heat tetany often accompanies heat exhaustion or heat stroke). Although a positive Chvostek's sign may be present, the patient's serum calcium is normal.

**Treatment**
- Move the patient to a cool environment.
- Heat tetany is self-limiting—it should resolve without treatment.

## HEAT SYNCOPE

Signs and symptoms include brief lapses of consciousness from postural hypotension due to shunting of blood to dilated peripheral vessels. Water and salt depletion occur rarely.

**Treatment**
- Place the patient supine and elevate his legs.
- Hydrate him with oral fluids, if necessary.
- To prevent a recurrence, tell the patient to avoid sudden or prolonged standing in a hot environment.

## HEAT CRAMPS

Painful cramps occur in the most strenuously used muscles (such as the thighs and shoulders) due to a decrease in extracellular sodium through sweating, dilution with free water, or both. Besides cramping, the patient may have nausea, cool and pallid skin, or diaphoresis.

**Treatment**
- To replace fluid and electrolytes, give the patient a balanced electrolyte drink, such as Gatorade.
- Loosen the patient's clothing, and have him lie down in a cool place.
- Massage his muscles. If his muscle cramps are severe, start an I.V. infusion with normal saline solution.

## ANHIDROTIC HEAT EXHAUSTION

A poorly understood syndrome of weakness, polyuria, and failure of normal sweating, this syndrome often occurs after several months of heat acclimation and is usually preceded by prickly heat. Other signs and symptoms include tachycardia, tachypnea, and fever. Anhidrotic heat exhaustion predisposes the patient to heat stroke.

**Treatment**
- Move the patient to a cool environment.
- Place him supine and let him rest.
- Give him potassium supplements to replace the potassium lost through polyuria.
- Tell him to avoid strenuous physical activity until his condition improves.

serum enzyme levels. If he had heat stroke, his CPK, SGOT, SGPT, and LDH levels may remain very high for 7 to 14 days, even with prompt cooling. Assess his neurologic status frequently—permanent CNS damage is probable if he was in a prolonged coma. His prognosis is poor if:

• his temperature remained high despite cooling.
• he was in a coma for a prolonged time despite cooling.
• he developed severe renal insufficiency or failure.
• his SGOT levels were severely elevated during the first 24 hours.

# Near-Drowning

## Initial care summary

The patient was rescued after submersion in water; he may or may not have aspirated water. If he was in cardiac arrest, cardiopulmonary resuscitation was started as soon as he was removed from the water, and continued. (See *Understanding the Mammalian Diving Reflex,* page 728.)

On initial assessment, his signs and symptoms varied depending on how long he was submerged and the water temperature. His age and physical condition were additional factors. He may have had no signs and symptoms, or he may have had some combination of the following:

• dyspnea
• wheezing
• rales and rhonchi
• coughing (possibly producing pink, frothy sputum)
• tachycardia
• cyanosis
• elevated temperature (unless he's also hypothermic)
• vomiting and abdominal distention
• chest pain
• altered mental status—confusion, irritability, restlessness, lethargy, seizures, or coma

• increased muscle tone
• shallow or gasping respirations
• cardiopulmonary arrest.

If he had respiratory insufficiency, severe respiratory distress, or cardiopulmonary arrest, he was given 100% oxygen by intubation; otherwise, by mask. His cervical spine was immobilized if any trauma was suspected, and a cross-table lateral X-ray of his cervical spine was done. If he was hypothermic, rewarming measures were started (see the "Hypothermia" entry in this chapter). An I.V. line was inserted for fluid and medication administration, and an NG tube was inserted if he was vomiting—to protect his airway and to decrease gastric distention. An EKG and a chest X-ray were taken; the chest X-ray may have been normal or may have shown perihilar or generalized pulmonary edema. Cardiac monitoring was started. Urine was obtained for urinalysis, and blood was drawn for a CBC, PT, PTT, and BUN, creatinine, serum calcium, serum magnesium, electrolyte, ABG, and blood glucose levels.

## Priorities

Submersion for any length of time causes hypoxemia, which in turn may cause cerebral, cardiac, and renal hypoxia. So your priorities for a near-drowning victim are to ensure a patent airway, to support adequate ventilation, and to improve gas exchange.

Provide aggressive pulmonary therapy *even if your patient has no signs or symptoms.* Why? Because pulmonary edema or aspiration pneumonia may occur minutes to days after submersion. If the patient hasn't been intubated yet, you may have to assist with intubation if:

• he produces copious secretions.
• he goes into coma or can't clear secretions from his airway.
• his ABG levels indicate a $PCO_2$ greater than 45 mm Hg and a $PO_2$ less than 80 to 90 mm Hg, even after he's given 40% oxygen by mask.

If he's intubated, expect to provide

# WHAT HAPPENS IN DROWNING AND NEAR-DROWNING

Drowning and near-drowning most commonly occur when a submerged person aspirates enough water to cause asphyxia. (However, 10% to 20% of drowning victims die of laryngospasm and asphyxiation *without* aspirating water.) Asphyxia results in hypoxemia and hypercapnia, causing tissue hypoxia, anaerobic metabolism, metabolic and respiratory acidosis, unconsciousness, convulsions, and dysrhythmias that lead to cardiac arrest and death, unless the victim is successfully resuscitated.

The brain responds to hypoxemia by shifting water and sodium from surrounding blood vessels into brain cells. The resulting cerebral edema and increased intracranial pressure can lead to permanent brain damage in a resuscitated victim. In addition, renal failure may result from acute tubular necrosis due to prolonged hypoxia and hypotension, and disseminated intravascular coagulation may occur from the release of certain activators of the extrinsic clotting and fibrinolytic systems from the victim's damaged lungs.

Research shows that fresh water and salt water have different damaging effects on the body's fluid volume and electrolyte balance (although drowning and near-drowning victims seldom aspirate enough water for these differences to be clinically significant).

*Fresh water* is hypotonic compared to body fluid, so it's rapidly absorbed from the alveoli into pulmonary circulation, causing hypervolemia, hemodilution, and hemolysis. All serum electrolytes except potassium decrease, and circulatory overload occurs. Destruction of pulmonary surfactant results in atelectasis.

*Salt water* is hypertonic and irritating to the alveoli, so it pulls fluid and plasma proteins from the pulmonary circulation into the alveoli. The result? Hypovolemia and hemoconcentration. All serum electrolyte levels are elevated, and hypotension may develop. With pulmonary edema adding to the aspirated fluid volume, these nonventilated, fluid-filled alveoli produce a right-to-left intrapulmonary shunt and further hypoxemia.

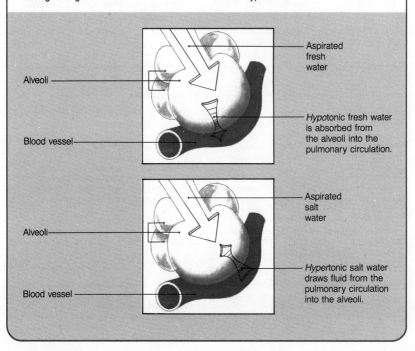

Alveoli

Blood vessel

Aspirated fresh water

*Hypo*tonic fresh water is absorbed from the alveoli into the pulmonary circulation.

Alveoli

Blood vessel

Aspirated salt water

*Hyper*tonic salt water draws fluid from the pulmonary circulation into the alveoli.

mechanical ventilation with PEEP or intermittent mandatory ventilation with CPAP. If your patient doesn't require intubation and mechanical ventilation, use a tight-fitting mask to provide oxygen with CPAP. The doctor will adjust the oxygen concentration and the degree of PEEP or CPAP to achieve an adequate $PO_2$, based on your patient's ABG results. If not contraindicated, elevate the head of the patient's bed slightly.

Expect to give I.V. aminophylline to improve your patient's gas exchange through bronchodilation. The doctor may also ask you to give inhaled or I.V. beta-adrenergic agents, such as epinephrine and isoproterenol hydrochloride (Isuprel), to treat bronchospasms. Suction the patient as needed to remove secretions—you may have to do this frequently.

If the doctor suspects that your patient aspirated water during submersion, he may perform a bronchoscopy. Assist him as necessary with this procedure.

Your patient may have combined respiratory and metabolic acidosis as a result of asphyxia. If he's unconscious, and if his ABGs reveal acidosis, the doctor may ask you to administer I.V. sodium bicarbonate (0.5 mEq/kg of body weight) to help restore a normal pH.

## Continuing assessment and intervention

Monitor your patient's vital signs, and insert a Foley catheter for accurate measurement of his urinary output. The doctor may insert a CVP line or a Swan-Ganz catheter to assess the patient's fluid balance and heart function. Notify the doctor if the patient's hemodynamic measurements indicate hypo- or hypervolemia, or if his urine output drops—he may develop renal failure from acute tubular necrosis due to renal hypoxia and hypotension.

Give I.V. fluids as ordered. If your patient was submerged in fresh water, the doctor may order $D_5W$. If the patient was submerged in salt water, the doctor may order Ringer's lactate or normal saline, and possibly albumin.

Perform a thorough assessment to detect associated injuries and to uncover any conditions that may have caused the accident. Be alert, in particular, for signs and symptoms of intracranial hemorrhage and of head, neck, or back

---

## UNDERSTANDING THE MAMMALIAN DIVING REFLEX

A drowning victim is rushed into the ED. Despite the CPR done at the scene and during transport, he has no detectable pulse, heartbeat, or breathing, he's cyanotic, and his pupils are fully dilated. He's dead. Or is he?

Don't give up your resuscitation efforts yet—he may still be alive. Why? Because, in a small percentage of apparently drowned persons, a protective mechanism—known as the *mammalian diving reflex*—is triggered. People submerged as long as 38 minutes have been resuscitated with little or no brain damage because of this reflex.

As you know, aquatic mammals such as whales and seals can remain underwater for long periods. They can do this because, when they submerge, blood is diverted from their extremities and concentrated in

circulation to their heart, lungs, and brain. Their heart rate and brain metabolism also slow considerably, reducing these animals' need for oxygen and protecting their vital organs.

The same reflex can operate in humans. It doesn't occur in all drowning victims, however, because several factors must operate simultaneously to trigger it. These are:

• *water temperature*—the water must be 70° F. (21.1° C.) or colder; the colder the water, the more pronounced the reflex.

• *age*—young victims have a more easily stimulated diving reflex.

• *facial immersion*—the mechanism of the diving reflex is vagal stimulation with peripheral vasoconstriction, so the victim's face must be suddenly submerged in cold water to trigger the reflex.

injuries. Was the patient affected by drugs or alcohol at the time of the accident? Does he have preexisting heart disease (which may have caused a myocardial infarction), diabetes (which may have caused a hypoglycemic episode), or epilepsy (which may have caused a seizure)? Don't forget to consider that a near-drowning accident may also represent a suicide attempt or child abuse.

Check your patient's neurologic status frequently. If he's had a period of cardiac arrest, the hypoxemia he experienced will lead to cerebral hypoxia and brain tissue acidosis. And cerebral edema may develop even *after* you've restored his circulation. So he'll need rapid and extensive cerebral resuscitation to prevent permanent neurologic damage. Expect the doctor to insert an intracranial pressure (ICP) monitor; he may also insert an arterial line for continuous blood pressure monitoring, so you can calculate your patient's cerebral perfusion pressure (see the "Increased Intracranial Pressure" entry in Chapter 6). Monitor your patient's ICP, blood pressure, and urinary output closely.

To decrease your patient's metabolic rate, cerebral edema, and oxygen requirement, the doctor may ask you to provide several interventions:
• controlled hyperventilation with a mechanical ventilator (this reduces blood $CO_2$ levels, constricting cerebral blood vessels and reducing cerebral blood flow)
• high doses of a corticosteroid, such as dexamethasone (Decadron), which may reduce cerebral edema
• a diuretic, such as mannitol or furosemide (Lasix), which will decrease fluid volume and cerebral edema
• a neuromuscular blocking agent, such as pancuronium (Pavulon)—but only if your patient's on a ventilator, because this drug will completely paralyze his respiratory muscles
• a barbiturate, such as pentobarbital
• controlled hypothermia.
These interventions increase the like-lihood that your patient will survive with unimpaired cerebral function.

Check your patient's ABG levels and assess his pulmonary function frequently to determine how he's responding to pulmonary therapy. Perform chest physiotherapy as ordered, to help loosen secretions, and suction him as necessary afterwards.

### Therapeutic care

Continue to watch for secondary drowning, even if your patient's signs and symptoms improve and he seems to be getting better: he can still develop pulmonary edema or aspiration pneumonia (from secondary infection) even after successful resuscitation and treatment. Be particularly alert for confusion, substernal chest pain, adventitious breath sounds (rales and wheezes), and signs of infection (increased white blood cell count, purulent sputum, and fever). Notify the doctor if infection seems to be developing, and expect to start or continue aggressive pulmonary therapy. If your patient develops pneumonia or sepsis, give antibiotics specific to the causative organism, as ordered.

If your patient required mechanical ventilation, his pulmonary problems may make weaning difficult, so he may be in the hospital for some time. Encourage active range-of-motion exercises if he's conscious, and perform passive range-of-motion exercises if he isn't; exercise helps prevent venous stasis and thrombosis. If ordered, apply antiembolism stockings, such as TEDS. Turn him frequently to prevent pressure sores from developing.

# Altitude-Related Illnesses

### Initial care summary
The patient with some form of altitude-related illness typically ascended rap-

# CASE IN POINT: FAILURE TO FOLLOW HOSPITAL POLICY

Suzie Karton, age 16, is a patient on your unit recovering from a near-drowning accident. Suzie was slightly acidotic when she arrived at the ED, so the doctor gave her sodium bicarbonate. Now, she's receiving supplemental oxygen, I.V. fluids, and nasogastric decompression, and you're monitoring her frequently. When you notice slight bradycardia and widened pulse pressure—possible signs of increased intracranial pressure—you notify the doctor and document your findings. He's not alarmed—but you plan to watch Suzie closely, assessing her every 15 minutes.

After two such assessments, Suzie hasn't improved; so you notify the doctor again. He tells you firmly that he doesn't see the need to reexamine her. Now you're at a crossroads: Your nursing manual requires you to report a doctor's failure to attend to a patient, but the doctor seems so sure his decision's correct... you decide not to report the incident.

When you assess Suzie's condition the next time, she's stuporous, her temperature is elevated, and her respirations are irregular—possibly Cheyne-Stokes respirations. Now you're sure the doctor's needed—but suddenly, Suzie goes into respiratory arrest. Despite all efforts to save her, she dies. Later, after reviewing the record of their daughter's hospitalization, her parents sue for negligence leading to her daughter's death. Are you liable in any way?

In *Utter v. United Health Center* (1977), a nurse documented and reported her findings of a patient's deteriorating condition. But when the doctor didn't attend to his patient, the nurse failed in her duty to report the incident, as her hospital nursing manual required. The court considered this failure as contributing to the patient's further injuries, and found the nurse negligent.

To protect yourself from liability in situations like this, keep these points in mind:

● Always follow the procedures called for in your hospital's nursing manual.
● If any policy of your hospital seems to conflict with your state nurse practice act, don't follow it until you've checked with your supervisor. Remember, your nurse practice act is the law—if you violate it, your license may be suspended or revoked.
● If your hospital lacks clearly written nursing policies, request them. If any of its policies seem questionable, request changes.

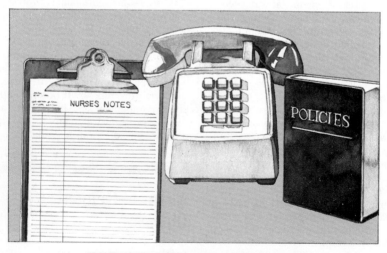

*Utter v. United Health Center*, 236 S.E. 2d 213 (W. Va. 1977)

idly from near sea level to an altitude of at least 8,000 to 9,000 feet, and he probably slept there for at least one night. (He may have been climbing for recreation, or he may have traveled to a city considerably above the altitude he's used to.) He may have engaged in strenuous physical activity immediately after his ascent. His signs and symptoms developed 1 to 4 days after the ascent and were severe enough that he sought medical attention.

Initial assessment findings varied with the type and severity of his altitude-related illness. If he had *acute mountain sickness* (AMS), he had some combination of the following:
• headache and confusion
• exertional dyspnea
• nausea, vomiting, and diarrhea
• malaise
• a decreased appetite
• difficulty sleeping.

If he had *high-altitude pulmonary edema* (HAPE), he had some combination of the following:
• increasingly severe dyspnea on exertion
• orthopnea
• noisy, gurgling respirations
• weakness
• rales and rhonchi
• tachycardia
• persistent cough (dry or with frothy sputum); possibly hemoptysis.

If he had *high-altitude cerebral edema* (HACE), he had some combination of the following:
• increasingly severe headache
• emotional lability
• hallucinations
• motor weakness and ataxia
• confusion, possibly progressing to stupor or coma.

The patient was given supplemental oxygen by mask. A chest X-ray and a 12-lead EKG were taken, and blood was drawn for a CBC and for ABGs.

## Priorities
Your priorities are the same for all three forms of altitude-related illness:
• Remove the patient from the high al-

DRUGS

## HIGHLIGHTING ACETAZOLAMIDE

You know how to recognize the signs and symptoms of altitude-related illness, and you're alert for them in any patient who's recently been exposed to a high altitude. But what would you think if, in addition to (or instead of) the usual signs and symptoms, the patient complained of:
• urinary frequency
• alterations in taste
• tingling of his fingertips and lips
• sudden, transient myopia?
Think acetazolamide (Diamox). Why? Because these signs and symptoms are side effects of acetazolamide—a drug prescribed (among other uses) to counter the effects of acute mountain sickness in persons who frequently climb to high altitudes. If your patient's a "climber," his doctor may have prescribed acetazolamide (a carbonic anhydrase inhibitor) to prevent or lessen his signs and symptoms.

When taken on the day of ascent and continued for 3 to 5 days, acetazolamide causes increased bicarbonate diuresis. This compensates for the respiratory alkalosis your patient experiences at high altitudes and may improve his ventilation, decreasing his signs and symptoms of acute mountain sickness. Side effects are common, however, especially if the drug's used for more than 5 days.

So when your patient's a "climber," consider whether acetazolamide, rather than a systemic illness, may be causing his signs and symptoms.

titude, if he hasn't already descended.
• Provide supplemental oxygen.

Your specific interventions, of course, will depend on how severe your patient's signs and symptoms are and where you see him. If you practice in an area *below* 7,000 feet and your patient comes to you *after* he's descended (or has been evacuated) from the mountain, your most important priority's already been achieved. If he has HAPE or HACE, give him supplemental oxygen by mask before you assess him further. If he has AMS, his condition will improve spontaneously with de-

PATHOPHYSIOLOGY

## WHAT HAPPENS IN ALTITUDE-RELATED ILLNESS

As an unacclimated person ascends to high altitudes, his arterial oxygen saturation decreases in response to the lack of environmental oxygen. If allowed to persist, this lack of oxygen leads to hypoxemia and any of these altitude-related physiologic reactions to hypoxemia:
• acute mountain sickness (AMS)
• high-altitude pulmonary edema (HAPE)
• high-altitude cerebral edema (HACE).

Compensatory mechanisms to offset hypoxemia begin at once. These include:
• *hyperventilation,* in an attempt to increase blood oxygenation
• *tachycardia,* to increase pumping of oxygenated blood to hypoxic tissues
• *stimulation of the kidneys to secrete erythropoietin,* to increase the blood's oxygen-carrying capacity.

In an unacclimated person, however, these mechanisms may be insufficient to relieve hypoxemia, because the environmental oxygen supply is simply too low. AMS then develops, as hyperventilation gives way to respiratory alkalosis and respiratory depression.

AMS typically lasts for only a few days,

and recovery is spontaneous as the person becomes acclimated or is brought to a lower altitude. Within 24 to 36 hours after the onset of AMS, his renal system responds with bicarbonate diuresis—the excretion of bicarbonate ions to correct respiratory alkalosis. As a result, the person's respirations increase, his hypoxemia decreases, and he recovers. (Note: The diuresis may cause dehydration that must be treated.)

If the person's kidneys don't secrete sufficient bicarbonate ions for diuresis, however, his condition will worsen, and HAPE or HACE may ensue. The exact pathophysiologic processes of these potentially fatal disorders aren't known. HAPE probably results from uneven constriction of the pulmonary vascular bed: some parts of the bed are hyperperfused, causing fluid movement out of the capillaries and into the alveoli and interstitial compartments in the lung tissue. A possible explanation for HACE is that cerebral hypoxia damages the brain cell membranes so that they allow fluid to shift into the cells, causing them to swell.

scent, and the doctor will ask you to discharge him after making sure he understands what happened to him.

If you practice in an area *above* 7,000 feet, and if your patient's signs and symptoms indicate severe HAPE or HACE, the doctor may order the patient to be evacuated to a facility at a lower altitude. Give oxygen by mask, and arrange for his transport. If the patient's signs and symptoms suggest only AMS, you can advise him that he'll feel better if he descends but that if he chooses not to, he'll acclimate and begin to feel better within 1 to 3 days. The doctor may ask you to administer analgesics or antiemetics for symptomatic treatment of your patient's headache, nausea, and vomiting. Then he may ask you to discharge the patient with instructions to rest, to avoid alcohol and tobacco, to avoid strenuous exercise,

and to drink plenty of fluids. Although the patient may have difficulty sleeping, the doctor usually *won't* prescribe a hypnotic drug—the patient's already hypoxemic during sleep and a hypnotic will depress his ventilations further, possibly leading to severe hypoxemia.

Check your patient for other problems that may be associated with his altitude-related illness. For example, because of confusion and impaired mental acuity, your patient may have made errors in judgment that exposed him to hypothermia or frostbite (see the "Hypothermia" and "Frostbite" entries in this chapter).

## Continuing assessment and intervention

Most patients with AMS will be discharged or transported to lower altitudes; those admitted will need only bed rest and observation. So your continuing assessment and care will be limited to the patient with HAPE or HACE.

If your patient has *HAPE*, his condition should begin to improve once he's descended to a lower altitude. Provide oxygen by mask at 4 to 6 liters/minute, and check his ABGs frequently. Initially, he may have a low $PO_2$, a low or normal $PCO_2$, and a high pH; these values will improve as you correct his hypoxemia. Keep the patient on bed rest, as ordered.

Expect the doctor to order repeated chest X-rays and EKGs to assess the patient's progress. His initial chest X-ray probably showed a patchy, fluffy infiltrate in one or both lungs; this should clear slowly as his clinical condition improves. His initial EKG probably showed evidence of right atrial and right ventricular overload; this should improve rapidly. (Both these improvements should occur with descent, oxygen, and bed rest.)

The doctor generally *won't* order furosemide (Lasix), as he might to treat pulmonary edema from non-HAPE causes. Furosemide doesn't seem to help patients with HAPE, and it will further reduce your patient's already low circulating volume—with a corresponding effect on his cardiac output.

Auscultate your patient's lungs frequently, and listen for a decrease in rales and rhonchi.

Assess your patient's fluid status frequently. Remember, he's likely to be dehydrated if he's been in the mountains for several days, because of the spontaneous bicarbonate diuresis that occurs as a compensatory response to respiratory alkalosis. Assess him for such signs of dehydration as poor skin turgor and thirst.

If your patient has *HACE*, his condition should also begin to improve once he's descended. Provide high-flow oxygen by mask, and place him on complete bed rest, as ordered. Assess his neurologic status frequently—he

may have neurologic deficits ranging from memory loss and decreased mental acuity to paralysis, psychotic behavior, and coma. If these don't improve with descent, oxygen therapy, and bed rest, the doctor may ask you to administer a corticosteroid for cerebral edema. If the doctor does choose to give a corticosteroid, he'll probably order I.M. dexamethasone (Decadron). Expect to give a diuretic, such as mannitol or urea, if your patient's condition is very poor. Watch your patient on diuretic therapy for signs of dehydration.

### Therapeutic care

Your patient with HAPE or HACE should recover without further intervention after he's been given oxygen and placed on bed rest—or, if he has severe HACE, after treatment with corticosteroids and diuretics. Problems usually arise only when these conditions are misdiagnosed (HAPE, for example, may be confused with asthma or pneumonia) or overtreated.

Continue frequent pulmonary assessments if your patient has HAPE, and frequent neurologic assessments if your patient has HACE, throughout his hospital stay. Check his calves for redness, tenderness, or swelling, which may indicate thrombophlebitis. (Your patient has an increased risk of developing this just after exposure to high-altitude conditions, which increase blood coagulability and viscosity.) Perform passive range-of-motion exercises on your patient's legs to minimize venous stasis. If your patient's elderly and has a history of thromboembolism, the doctor may ask you to apply antiembolism stockings such as TEDS.

# Bites and Stings

As you know, a wide variety of organisms—including insects, spiders, aquatic organisms, snakes, other animals, and even humans—can cause bite or sting injuries. Consult the charts that follow for detailed information on how to identify what bit or stung your patient, what specific signs and symptoms to assess for, and how to intervene appropriately. Remember to obtain a thorough history—not only to record details of your patient's bite or sting incident but also to identify his chronic diseases or allergies and any medications that he's currently taking.

Keep in mind that most patients who've been bitten or stung will require tetanus prophylaxis, and that some may require prophylactic antibiotics and rabies prophylaxis as well. (See *Guidelines for Tetanus Prophylaxis*, pages 66 and 67, and *Guidelines for Rabies Prophylaxis*, page 708.) Be sure you're prepared to intervene for an anaphylactic reaction, too. Keep oxygen, emergency respiratory equipment, epinephrine, and other emergency drugs on hand, and be prepared to use them.

## NURSE'S GUIDE TO BITES AND STINGS

### SNAKEBITES

**All poisonous snakes inject venom through their fangs.**

#### Pit viper
*(Crotalidae)*
(rattlesnakes, water moccasins, copperheads, cottonmouths)

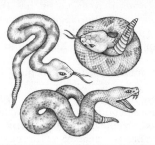

**Clinical features**
• Immediate pain in the bite area
• Edema (begins early and may involve the entire extremity)
• Petechiae and ecchymoses
• Possible systemic signs and symptoms: weakness, fever, nausea, vomiting, circumoral tingling and numbness, metallic taste in the mouth, and muscle fasciculations
• Possible hypotension, widespread hemorrhage, shock, and pulmonary edema

#### Coral snake
*(Elapidae)*

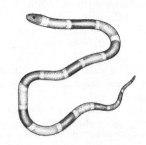

**General information**
• Most common venomous snakes in United States; found in every state except Maine, Alaska, and Hawaii
• Distinguishing characteristics include:
—a flattened, triangular head
—a depression (the pit) midway between the eye and nostril on both sides of the head
—vertically elliptical pupils
—rattle (in rattlesnakes) made by a series of rings on the end of the tail
—large, retractable, anterior maxillary fangs
—single row of subcaudal plates
• Venom primarily hematotoxic

**General information**
• Eastern coral snake prevalent in North and South Carolina, Florida, Louisiana, Mississippi, Georgia, and Texas; western coral snake prevalent in Arizona and New Mexico
• Distinguishing characteristics include:
—a black head
—red, black, and yellow bands *with red bands always bordered with yellow* (Note: Some nonpoisonous snakes have colored

## NURSE'S GUIDE TO BITES AND STINGS *(continued)*

bands, but red bands are bordered with black)
—round pupils
—small, fixed maxillary teeth
• Venom primarily neurotoxic

**Clinical features**
• No local signs or symptoms; systemic signs and symptoms possibly greatly delayed even with severe poisoning
• Possible systemic signs and symptoms (appear after several hours): apprehension, giddiness, dyspnea, nausea, increased salivation, vomiting, and weakness
• Bulbar palsy (appears in 4 to 7 hours)
• Diffuse paralysis (follows in 1 to 2 hours)
• Signs and symptoms progress rapidly; may result in respiratory arrest

**Nursing interventions**
*For all snakebites:*
• Assess the patient's cardiovascular, respiratory, and neurologic status frequently; monitor his vital signs every 15 minutes.
• Measure the wound circumference periodically, to detect increasing edema.
• Obtain a pulse in all edematous extremities with Doppler ultrasound.
• Start an I.V., draw blood for laboratory tests, and obtain an EKG, as ordered.
• Cleanse the wound.
• Give medications as ordered (possibly including analgesics, antibiotics, tetanus prophylaxis, and antivenin). Perform a skin test before you give antivenin. If the patient is sensitive, dilute the antivenin and give it by very slow I.V. dripping, as ordered.
• Watch for an anaphylactic reaction to the antivenin; keep epinephrine, oxygen, vasopressors, and emergency resuscitation equipment on hand.
• Administer packed cells, whole blood, I.V. fluids, and fresh plasma or platelets, as ordered.

### AQUATIC ORGANISMS WOUNDS

**Organisms with nematocysts (tentacles)**
(Coelenterates, including hydroids, jellyfish, corals, anemones, Portuguese man-of-war)

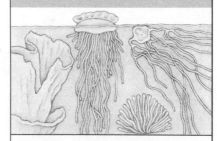

**General information**
• Venom mechanisms in tentacles evert on chemical or mechanical stimulation, penetrating the skin and injecting venom.
• May inject venom on contact or later; tentacles may still discharge venom when the animal is dead or when broken off from the animal

**Clinical features**
• Severe burning pain
• Red, weltlike lesions
• Possible systemic signs and symptoms (depending on species and number of tentacles involved): headache, nausea, vomiting, muscle cramps, diarrhea, convulsions, angioedema, dyspnea, and respiratory arrest

**Nursing interventions**
*For all tentacle wounds:*
• Pour alcohol over the wound to inactivate the tentacles.
• Apply an alkaline solution such as sodium bicarbonate, to neutralize the acid venom.
• Apply a steroid cream and a topical anesthetic to the wound, as ordered.
• Give medications as ordered (possibly including antihistamines, antibiotics, analgesics, and tetanus prophylaxis).
• Watch for signs of a systemic reaction. If it occurs, give I.V. diazepam or calcium gluconate for muscle cramps, or systemic corticosteroids, epinephrine, and antihistamines for an allergic reaction, as ordered.

*(continued)*

## NURSE'S GUIDE TO BITES AND STINGS *(continued)*

### Organisms with spines
(Catfish, stingray, sea urchin, scorpion fish)

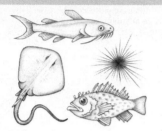

### General information
• Catfish: venomous spines on dorsal and pectoral fins inflict severe, often contaminated injuries.
• Stingray: sharp spine on tail (covered with integumentary sheath) carries venom into skin and can produce extensive lacerations.
• Sea urchin: spines and pedicellaries (tiny, fanglike organs) inject venom.
• Scorpion fish (including California sculpin, stonefish, and lionfish): venomous spines on fins inject venom that may be lethal.

### Clinical features
• Catfish: instant stinging, throbbing pain; infection common
• Stingray: immediate intense, sharp pain; possible systemic signs and symptoms including: nausea, vomiting, diarrhea, syncope, muscle cramps, dysrhythmias, convulsions, and respiratory distress
• Sea urchin: immediate pain; redness, swelling, and numbness; possible paralysis; possible acute respiratory distress
• Scorpion fish: intense pain and swelling, quickly involving entire extremity; possible systemic signs and symptoms including: syncope, shock, dysrhythmias, and respiratory distress; possible cardiopulmonary arrest

### Nursing interventions
*For all spine-inflicted wounds:*
• Irrigate the wound thoroughly with normal saline solution.
• Soak the affected area in hot water (122° F., or 50° C.) for 30 to 90 minutes, to neutralize heat-labile venom.
• Prepare the patient for X-rays, to visualize any imbedded spines and sheaths.
• Assist with removal of spines and sheaths, or prepare the patient for surgery, if necessary.
• Assist with cleansing and possible

debridement of the wound, which may require surgical closure.
• Give medications as ordered. (These may include antibiotics, antihistamines, analgesics, corticosteroid creams, antivenin, and tetanus prophylaxis.)
• Monitor the patient closely for cardiopulmonary signs and symptoms; keep emergency resuscitation equipment available.

### INSECT AND SPIDER BITES AND STINGS

### Tick
*(Dermacentor andersoni and variabilis)*

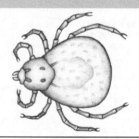

### General information
• Flat, brown-speckled body; 8 legs
• Common in woods and fields throughout the United States
• Attaches to host (usually at head, neck, or groin) by burrowing its head into the host's skin; feeds on blood
• May inject a neurotoxin that can cause acute paralysis
• May transmit diseases such as tularemia and Rocky Mountain spotted fever

### Clinical features
• Painless bite
• Pruritus
• Local irritation (if head remains after removal)
*If tick paralysis develops:*
• Paresthesia
• Lower extremity pain
• Possible respiratory failure from bulbar paralysis

### Nursing interventions
• Remove the tick by covering it with a tissue or gauze pad saturated with alcohol or mineral oil, which blocks the tick's breathing pores and causes it to withdraw from the skin.

## NURSE'S GUIDE TO BITES AND STINGS *(continued)*

• If the tick doesn't withdraw after the pad's been in place for a half hour, remove the tick with tweezers (make sure you get all the parts).
• Wash the area with soap and water and apply an antiseptic.
• If the patient develops respiratory failure, assist with mechanical ventilation as ordered.

### Brown recluse spider
### *(Loxosceles reclusa)*

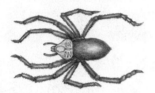

**General information**
• Light brown, small (1 to 1.5 cm long; 0.5 to 1 cm wide); characteristic dark brown violin mark on back
• Most common in south-central United States; usually found in closets, woodsheds, and other dark areas
• Injects a coagulotoxic venom by biting

**Clinical features**
• Mild or no pain with bite; pain increases with time
• Local reaction 2 to 8 hours after bite: small, red puncture wound forms a bleb and becomes ischemic; center becomes dark and hard 3 to 4 days later; ulcer develops in 2 to 3 weeks
• Possible systemic symptoms: fever, chills, nausea, vomiting, malaise, arthralgia, and petechiae
• Hemolytic anemia and thrombocytopenia (rare)

**Nursing interventions**
• Cleanse the lesion with a 1:20 Burow's aluminum acetate solution, and apply an antibiotic ointment as ordered.
• Give medications as ordered (possibly including corticosteroids, antihistamines, antibiotics, tetanus prophylaxis, and I.V. fluids).
• Monitor the patient's vital signs and general appearance; watch for changes at the bite site.

• If necessary, assist with lesion excision and skin grafting.

### Black widow spider
### *(Latrodectus mactans)*

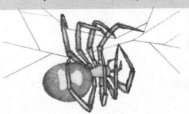

**General information**
• Coal black, with a characteristic red or orange hourglass mark on the ventral side of the female (the male doesn't bite)
• Common throughout the U.S.; usually found in outdoor buildings, such as barns and garages, or under rocks
• Injects a neurotoxic venom by biting; venom affects neuromuscular junctions

**Clinical features**
• Immediate sharp, stinging pain with bite, then dull, numbing pain
• Local edema; tiny red bite marks without necrosis
• Stomach muscle rigidity and severe abdominal pain 10 to 40 minutes after bite; both subside within 48 hours
• Muscle spasms in extremities
• Possible systemic signs and symptoms: extreme restlessness, vertigo, diaphoresis chills, pallor, convulsions (especially in children), hyperactive reflexes, hypertension, nausea, vomiting, headache, ptosis, eyelid edema, urticaria, pruritus, and fever
• Possible shock and respiratory depression

**Nursing interventions**
• Keep the patient warm and quiet; immobilize the affected part.
• Clean the bite site with antiseptic; apply ice to relieve pain and swelling and to slow circulation.
• Give medications as ordered (possibly including I.V. calcium gluconate, muscle relaxants, narcotics, tetanus prophylaxis, and antivenin). Monitor your patient's respiratory status closely if you give narcotics. Perform a skin test before you give antivenin, and desensitize the patient as

*(continued)*

## NURSE'S GUIDE TO BITES AND STINGS *(continued)*

ordered if the test shows a sensitivity to horse serum.
• Watch for an anaphylactic reaction to the antivenin; keep epinephrine and emergency resuscitation equipment on hand.
• Check the patient's vital signs frequently, and report changes to the doctor. Signs and symptoms usually subside 1 to 3 hours after antivenin administration.

### Scorpion
*(Vejovis spinigerus*—nonlethal; *Centruroides sculpturatus*—lethal)

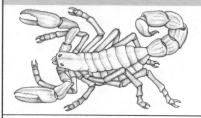

### General information
• Curled tail with stinger on end; 8 legs; 3″ long (7.6 cm)
• Common throughout the southwestern United States; one species (found in Arizona) has potentially lethal neurotoxic venom
• Injects venom by stinging
• Usually stings in the evening, when the temperature cools

### Clinical features
*Nonlethal reaction:*
• Local swelling and tenderness; sharp, burning sensation
• Skin discoloration
• Paresthesia
• Lymphangiitis with regional gland swelling
*Lethal reaction (neurotoxic):*
• Immediate sharp pain without visible local reaction
• Systemic signs and symptoms (usually appear in 1 to 3 hours): itching of eyes, mouth, and throat; impaired speech; hypersensitivity to stimuli; drowsiness; generalized muscle spasms; convulsions; extreme restlessness; nausea; vomiting; and incontinence
• Possible respiratory or cardiovascular failure
• Signs and symptoms last 24 to 78 hours; prognosis is poor if they progress rapidly during first few hours

### Nursing interventions
• Immobilize the patient.
• Apply a tourniquet proximal to the sting.
• Pack the sting area in ice; if possible, immerse the patient in ice water to above the sting area.
• Give medications as ordered (possibly including I.V. calcium gluconate, emetine, and antivenin).
• Monitor his vital signs, watching closely for signs and symptoms of respiratory distress.
• Keep emergency resuscitation equipment on hand.

### Bee, wasp, yellow jacket
*(Hymenoptera)*

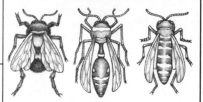

### General information
• Rounded abdomen (honeybee); furry, rounded abdomen (bumblebee); slender body with elongated abdomen (wasp, yellow jacket)
• Common throughout the United States
• Injects venom by stinging (bees leave stingers in their victims; wasps and yellow jackets retain stingers and can sting repeatedly)

### Clinical features
*Local reaction:*
• Painful wound (stinger may protrude)
• Edema
• Pruritus
*Systemic reaction (anaphylaxis):*
• usually occurs within 20 minutes
• weakness
• chest tightness
• dizziness
• nausea and vomiting
• abdominal cramps
• laryngeal edema

### Nursing interventions
• Remove the stinger (if present) by scraping; don't pull it, because this releases more toxin.

## NURSE'S GUIDE TO BITES AND STINGS *(continued)*

● Cleanse the site and apply ice.
● Watch the patient carefully for signs of anaphylaxis; keep emergency resuscitation equipment on hand.
● If anaphylaxis develops, administer oxygen, epinephrine, and other drugs as ordered.

sporins).
● Administer tetanus prophylaxis, as ordered.
● Assist with debridement of infected wounds or devitalized tissue (some doctors routinely debride all hand bites). The doctor probably won't close the wound unless it's on the patient's face.

### HUMAN, DOG AND CAT BITES

#### Human bites

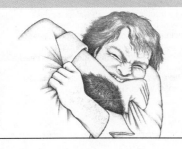

#### Dog bites

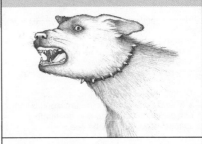

### General information
● Most dangerous of all mammalian bites, due to possible severe complications resulting from infections (common infecting organisms are *Staphylococcus* and *Streptococcus*)
● Most common on the hand (usually associated with fighting), may cause deep lacerations that disrupt fascia, tendons, and joints. If wound occurs when hand is clenched in a fist, the lacerated skin retracts and then returns to its original position, carrying saliva deeper into wound.
● Possible patient delay in seeking treatment, because of embarrassment

### Clinical features
● Laceration with possibly significant amounts of devitalized tissue
● Hematoma formation
● Possible crush injuries
● Possible amputation
● Infection likely; early signs include redness, warmness, tenderness, swelling, and foul-smelling grayish exudate

### Nursing interventions
● Assist with wound exploration, to determine the depth of the injury.
● Cleanse and irrigate the wound.
● Culture the wound site, and start antibiotic therapy, as ordered (usually with cephalo-

### General information
● Most common on extremities, head, and neck
● Most bites from larger breeds, so severe bites common
● Generally associated with a low infection rate

### Clinical features
● Signs and symptoms vary from contusions or superficial abrasions to severe crush injuries, deep puncture wounds, and tissue loss.

### Nursing interventions
● Control bleeding as necessary.
● Support and splint the injured areas.
● For a laceration, assist with local wound care—including thorough cleansing, debridement, and copious irrigation, usually with normal saline solution. The doctor may or may not suture the wound (he'll probably suture a facial wound).
● For a puncture wound, assist with cleansing and excising devitalized tissue; irrigation is not performed. (Alternatively, the entire wound may be excised and closed.)
● Administer tetanus and rabies prophylaxis, as ordered.
● If the dog is a stray, contact the local public health department to determine the need for rabies prophylaxis.

*(continued)*

## NURSE'S GUIDE TO BITES AND STINGS *(continued)*

### Cat bites and scratches

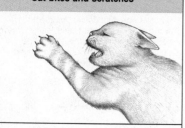

**General information**
• Usually not as serious as dog bites
• 30% chance of infection from both bites and scratches

**Clinical features**
• Typically small, deep puncture wounds that disrupt tendons and may penetrate joint spaces; scratches may be deep

**Nursing interventions**
• Cleanse the wound thoroughly with antimicrobial soap; irrigate it with normal saline solution.
• Assist with debridement of devitalized tissue if needed.
• Obtain a culture and gram stain for grossly infected wounds.
• Administer prophylactic antibiotics for all bites that penetrate the skin, because inoculated bacteria may not be removed by cleansing.
• Administer tetanus and rabies prophylaxis, as ordered.
• Instruct the patient to watch for the development of cat scratch fever. The incubation period is 3 to 10 days; tender papules will develop on the patient's skin, with painful lymphadenopathy, headache, fever, malaise, and erythema. There is no treatment for this, but it will resolve within several months.

# A FINAL WORD

Each year, ED and clinic personnel treat patients with a variety of environmental emergencies; some of these emergencies have high incidences of morbidity and mortality. Environment-related heat stroke, for example, causes over 4,000 deaths yearly in the United States; hypothermia contributes to many fatalities. And besides the injury from the primary emergency, the patient's at risk for developing complications—a life-threatening anaphylactic reaction, for example, can turn even a minor bite or sting into a serious emergency.

Clearly, *any* environmental emergency can be life-threatening. But you can help reduce morbidity and mortality from these emergencies in your patients if you know how to zero in on the most likely causes—*quickly*—and just as quickly select the most appropriate interventions.

To give the best care to patients with environmental emergencies, one very helpful aid is familiarity with your own regional environment. If you live and practice in a region with a temperate climate, for example, you can expect to see a wide variety of environmental emergencies related to the changing seasons and to the many types of animals, insects, and spiders that flourish in such a climate. In contrast, if your region is well above sea level, or predominantly hot or cold all year round, you'll see patients with a narrower spectrum of environmental emergencies—but you'll probably see proportionately more such patients. So a thorough knowledge of your region's climate and indigenous animals, insects, and spiders can provide you with quick clues to what caused a patient's environmental emergency.

The types of recreational activities a region offers provide additional clues. For example, if a nurse lives in a region with many lakes or a seashore, and no high mountains, then she's much more likely to see patients with near-drowning and scuba-diving emergencies than with altitude-related illnesses. You can readily extrapolate from this example to identify the recreation-related environmental emergencies you're most likely to see in *your* patients.

As you probably know, environmental emergencies most often involve young, healthy persons. Why? Because they're very active in outdoor recreational activities and sports. But as you also know, no one's immune from these types of emergencies. Elderly persons, for example—especially those with chronic health problems—are particularly susceptible to hypothermia; they also have low resistance to the effects of other environmental emergencies. And, of course, anyone can suffer an animal, insect, or spider bite.

Once you've successfully cared for a patient with an environmental emergency, don't forget to teach him how to *prevent* such an emergency from recurring. For example, be sure you tell a patient who's recovering from hypothermia that he'll be more sensitive to cold from now on. A patient who suffered a heat-related illness needs to know that he should drink more water than usual, even if he's not thirsty, and acclimate gradually if he's not used to a hot climate. Make sure, too, that climbers, hikers, and swimmers you've cared for understand what caused their emergency problems and how to prevent future ones. When your patients know more about their environment and its potential dangers, they'll be able to avoid many environmental emergencies. And at least some of them will have you to thank.

## Selected References

Alexy, Betty J. "Problems Due to Cold," *Journal of Emergency Nursing* 6(1):22-24, January/February 1980.

Bowman, Warren D., Jr., et al. "Air-related Problems: When Your Patient Treks to High Places," *Patient Care* 16(11):55-83, June 15, 1982.

Boyd, L.T., et al. "Heat and Heat-Related Illnesses," *American Journal of Nursing* 81(7):1298-1302, July 1981.

Budassi, Susan A., and Barber, Janet M. *Emergency Nursing: Principles and Practice.* St. Louis: C.V. Mosby Co., 1981.

Kravis, Thomas C., and Warner, Carmen G. *Emergency Medicine: A Comprehensive Review.* Rockville, Md.: Aspen Systems Corp., 1982.

Rosen, Peter, et al. *Emergency Medicine: Concepts and Clinical Practice,* vol. 1. St. Louis: C.V. Mosby Co., 1983.

Wilkins, Earle W., Jr. *MGH Textbook of Emergency Medicine,* 2nd ed. Baltimore: Williams & Wilkins Co., 1983.

Wingate, Elizabeth. "A Nursing Perspective on Frostbite," *Critical Care Update* 10(1):8-15, January 1983.

Wyngaarden, James B., and Smith, Lloyd H., Jr., eds. *Cecil Textbook of Medicine,* 16th ed. Philadelphia: W.B. Saunders Co., 1982.

Yocum, R.F., and Bohler, S. "Heat Stroke," *Journal of Emergency Nursing* 7:144-47, July/August 1981.

# 17

# Poisoning and Substance Abuse Emergencies

## Introduction

You're working the morning shift in the ED when a distraught young woman rushes in clutching a small boy in her arms. It's Janet McLaughlin and her son, Tim, age 3. Obviously frightened and upset, Mrs. McLaughlin tells you that she walked into her kitchen moments before and found Tim sitting on the counter with an empty vitamin bottle. "I think he must've swallowed the entire bottleful!" she cries. "Now he has diarrhea—and there's blood in it!"

Quickly, you assess the boy's airway, breathing, and circulation and start checking his vital signs. He has a fever of 101° F. (38.3° C.) and he's rubbing his eyes as if he's feeling drowsy.

Speaking in a calm voice, you ask Tim's mother if she's brought the vitamin bottle with her. Nodding anxiously, she pulls a bottle out of her purse and hands it to you. It's a popular brand of children's chewable vitamins—with iron. You ask if she performed any first-aid measures before coming to the ED. "No—I just wanted to get him here as fast as I could," she answers.

You know you'll have to act fast to keep the boy from absorbing a toxic amount of iron into his system—if you don't, he may suffer irreversible liver, heart, or kidney damage; coma; or death.

If you work in an ED, you can expect to see many patients with poisoning or substance abuse emergencies. Are you confident that you'll know how to care for all of them? To do so, you'll need to understand how a wide variety of poisons and other toxic substances exert their effects—*and* how to counteract them.

As a nurse, you probably know that managing a poisoning emergency involves four basic goals:

• supporting the patient's airway, breathing, and circulation
• identifying the poison
• removing as much of it as possible
• arresting its absorption into the patient's system.

For treatment to be effective, you have to achieve all these goals almost simultaneously. This can be a challenge, because some poisons have frighteningly quick effects. (For example, death can occur within 1 to 15 minutes of inhaling or ingesting cyanide.) You need to perform a rapid and accurate initial assessment, followed *immediately* by appropriate interventions. After you've taken the initial steps to remove the poison and to prevent its absorption, you need sharp assessment skills and knowledge of how the poison acts so you can recognize early signs of such complications as organ damage and failure.

Finally, in the midst of all this fast-paced activity, you also have to remember that your patient's family will probably be frightened and concerned. They'll need your reassurance and support.

This chapter will help you recognize the signs and symptoms of poisoning and substance abuse emergencies and will make you familiar with the interventions that must follow.

# INITIAL CARE

## Prehospital Care: What's Been Done

Rescue personnel first assessed the patient's airway, breathing, and circulation, intervening as necessary. (If the patient was exposed to a poisonous gas, such as carbon monoxide, they evacuated him to fresh air first.) They quickly tried to find out what toxic substance the patient took or was exposed to by questioning the patient, his family, or his friends. Depending on the suspected toxic substance, rescue personnel preserved (or attempted to retrieve) a sample of the substance, the poison's container, empty pill bottles, or drug paraphernalia. If a hydrocarbon, carbamate, organophosphate, or caustic substance came into contact with the patient's skin, rescue personnel removed any clothing covering the affected site and washed the area with copious amounts of soap and water. (See the "Chemical Burns" entry in Chapter 15.) If the substance splashed in his eye, they immediately started irrigating the affected eye with normal saline solution. (See the "Chemical Burns of the Eye" entry in Chapter 9.)

Rescue personnel started CPR immediately for a patient who wasn't breathing and had no pulse. If his airway was obstructed, they cleared it with finger sweeps or suction. If he didn't have a gag reflex, they inserted an esophageal obturator airway (EOA) to prevent aspiration. (They used an oral airway instead of an EOA for a patient who ingested a caustic substance, to prevent further damage to his esophagus.) If his respirations were depressed, they gave him oxygen via a nasal cannula or a tight-fitting mask—to prevent hypoxemia.

For a patient who was breathing and had a pulse, but was *unconscious*, rescue personnel started an I.V., administered a bolus of dextrose 50% in water ($D_{50}W$), and gave 50 to 100 mg of thiamine I.M. Why? Because hypoglycemia and acute thiamine deficiency can mimic drug intoxication. Rescue personnel may also have administered naloxone (Narcan) if the patient had a suspected narcotic overdose. As with any unconscious patient, rescue personnel recognized the possibility of accompanying cervical spine injury and stabilized the patient's cervical spine by applying a Philadelphia collar.

With a *conscious* patient, rescue personnel probably started an I.V. and began infusing dextrose 5% in water ($D_5W$) at a keep-vein-open rate. Rescue personnel administered naloxone (Narcan) if the patient had a suspected narcotic overdose or showed signs of central nervous system (CNS) depression (blurred vision, dizziness, disorientation, depressed level of consciousness). If they knew or suspected he'd ingested either an acid or an alkali caustic substance, they gave him up to 4 ounces of milk or water orally, to dilute the poison; they *didn't* induce vomiting. If the patient took any other kind of toxic substance, a paramedic may have induced vomiting by giving him syrup of ipecac—if he was responsive and had a gag reflex.

Rescue personnel next performed a basic neurologic examination. They assessed the patient for decreased level of consciousness and for pupillary changes that might indicate CNS depression from hypoxemia or substance abuse.

When you receive the patient in the ED, remember these important points:
• Find out what (if anything) the patient's been given I.V. and whether he was given any home remedies—such as the so-called universal antidote—which may have wasted precious time by delaying proper treatment. Did anyone perform first aid treatment before calling rescue personnel or bringing the patient to the hospital? If so, what was done?
• Obtain rescue personnel's assessment of the patient's initial neurologic status. You'll need this information as a baseline for evaluating later changes in the patient's condition.
• Get a brief history of the patient's poisoning or drug abuse emergency. Don't attempt to obtain a thorough medical history now—you can do that later, after your patient's stabilized. But as you begin assessing his airway, breathing, and circulation, try to gather pertinent details about the poisoning, toxic exposure, or drug overdose that's causing his signs and symptoms.

# What to Do First

Your first priority is to rapidly assess the patient's airway, breathing, and circulation. If rescue personnel started life-support measures, reassess your patient's status and, if necessary, continue the procedures they initiated. Because the absorption rate of a poison or drug may fluctuate, your patient's status can change quickly and unexpectedly at any time—so you'll need to reassess his airway, breathing, and circulation at frequent intervals. Be prepared to intervene appropriately at a moment's notice.

### Airway
Assess the patency of your patient's airway. If it's obstructed, attempt to clear it using finger sweeps or, if necessary, a large-bore suction catheter or a tonsil-tip (Yankauer) catheter. If he's unconscious, check whether his flaccid tongue has fallen back and occluded his airway, and intervene if necessary by inserting an oral airway. If his gag reflex is absent, accumulated secretions may

PRIORITIES

## INITIAL ASSESSMENT CHECKLIST

**Assess the ABCs first and intervene appropriately.**

**Check for:**
• hypoactivity, decreased level of consciousness, bradycardia, or decreased respiratory rate, suggesting central nervous system (CNS) depression
• hyperactivity, tachycardia, tachypnea, or hyperventilation, suggesting CNS stimulation
• needle tracks, possibly indicating drug injection
• circumoral blisters or crystal residue, possibly indicating corrosive substance ingestion; blisters or erythema on the skin, possibly indicating barbiturate, carbon monoxide, or glutethimide poisoning; or powdered residue on the patient's skin or clothing, possibly from an insecticide.

**Intervene by:**
• inducing vomiting with syrup of ipecac or performing gastric lavage
• starting an I.V. and giving dextrose 50% in water, thiamine, and naloxone (Narcan), as ordered, if the patient's unresponsive
• administering activated charcoal and cathartics, as ordered
• forcing diuresis and altering the patient's urine pH.

**Prepare for:**
• advanced life support
• intubation and mechanically assisted ventilation
• administration of an antidote based on toxicology screening results
• hemodialysis, peritoneal dialysis, or hemoperfusion.

cause aspiration and airway obtruction. To prevent aspiration, place the patient on his side so oral secretions will drain. Be prepared to suction him, if necessary.

If you see blisters or residue in or around your patient's mouth, he may have swallowed an alkaline caustic substance that's causing pharyngeal and esophageal swelling—which can quickly block his airway. The doctor will intubate him nasotracheally (and very gently) to avoid perforating his trachea and damaging the oral mucosa.

If rescue personnel inserted an EOA to prevent aspiration, don't remove it until your patient's level of consciousness improves and his gag reflex returns. At that time, turn the patient on his left side and carefully suction any accumulated secretions from his mouth. Then remove the EOA. Be prepared for large amounts of vomitus once the EOA is removed.

### Breathing

Auscultate your patient's lungs to assess the presence and character of his breathing. Note the pattern, depth, and rate of his respirations. A patient with CNS depression or cardiac dysrhythmias from hydrocarbon poisoning, cyanide poisoning, or a drug overdose may have moist rales, possibly indicating pulmonary edema. If he's suffering from a CNS depressant overdose, his respiratory rate will probably be less than 10 breaths/minute. If he's taken a CNS stimulant, expect his respiratory rate to increase to more than 30 breaths/minute.

If you detect bradypnea and alveolar hypoventilation, administer supplemental oxygen, as necessary, to reduce hypoxemia. Give your patient 100% oxygen if carbon monoxide poisoning's suspected. Notify the doctor *immediately* if your patient develops any respiratory difficulty, and prepare for intubation and mechanical ventilation.

### Circulation

Assess your patient's circulatory status quickly. Start by checking his pulse rate and blood pressure—they may be normal or decreased, if he took a CNS depressant, or elevated if he took an overdose of a CNS stimulant.

If your patient's hypotensive and doesn't already have an I.V., insert one now, using a large-gauge catheter. To increase your patient's perfusion, the doctor may ask you to infuse 200 ml of I.V. fluid—usually normal saline solution or Ringer's lactate—every 5 minutes for the next 15 minutes. Insert an indwelling (Foley) catheter to monitor your patient's urinary output in response to I.V. fluid therapy. Obtain a urine sample, too, for toxicology screening.

Assess the appearance and character of your patient's skin. As you know, skin that's pale, cool, and diaphoretic may indicate shock. To determine whether your patient has adequate circulation, check the color of his arms and legs and assess his nail beds for color and for capillary refill time. Slow capillary refill plus cold, cyanotic nail beds and extremities may signal shock, tissue hypoperfusion, hypoxemia, or all three.

Because your patient's circulatory status can change suddenly as his system absorbs the poison, expect to connect him to a cardiac monitor. His EKGs may reveal dysrhythmias. These can occur as a direct result of ingesting an intoxicant or as an indirect result of hypoxemia and acid-base or electrolyte imbalances. If the poison's impairing his cardiac output and decreasing his tissue perfusion, his EKGs may reveal such dysrhythmias as bradycardia, tachycardia, or premature ventricular contractions (PVCs).

If the patient's condition permits, obtain blood for blood glucose levels to test for hypoglycemia or hyperglycemia, and for a toxicology screen to test for drug toxicity. Draw additional blood for a complete blood count (CBC) and for electrolyte, serum osmolarity, serum creatinine, serum ammonia, blood urea nitrogen (BUN), and arterial blood gas (ABG) levels.

## General appearance

Note whether your patient has any obvious signs of trauma—such as burns, bruises, or lacerations. Also note if he has any blisters or ulcerations in or around his mouth or elsewhere on his skin; these may indicate he's ingested a caustic substance or a barbiturate overdose. Assess the color of his skin, sclera, and mucous membranes, too: a "boiled lobster" (orange-red) appearance may indicate borate poisoning—especially if the patient's a child who may have eaten rat poison or another boric acid derivative. Cherry red skin and mucous membranes are characteristic of carbon monoxide poisoning. Yellowing of the skin or sclera suggests hepatic failure.

If a liquid or gaseous toxic substance has splashed on the patient's skin or clothing, remove his clothing and decontaminate his skin by washing it with copious amounts of soapy water. This will prevent or arrest percutaneous absorption of the poison.

Check his extremities for needle marks; if you find them on his arms, suspect drug abuse. (The patient's probably a diabetic if you find needle marks on his abdomen or thighs.)

Remember to smell the breath of *any* patient with a poisoning emergency, to help determine what poison he may have ingested. Some poisonous substances—ammonia, gasoline, and alcohol, for example—smell the same on a patient's breath as they do in their containers. Other poisonous substances also produce characteristic breath odors:
● Cyanide produces a bitter-almond breath odor.
● Turpentine produces an unmistakable breath odor of violets.
● Organophosphate ingestion produces a garlicky breath odor.
Your patient's breath odor may also provide a clue to a possible underlying condition that will affect the care he needs. For example, a fruity or acetone odor on your patient's breath may indicate diabetic ketoacidosis.

Complete your assessment by observing your patient for signs of seizure activity. Look for generalized tonic and clonic contractions, bowel or bladder incontinence, upward deviation of the eyes, excessive salivation, and oral or lingual lacerations and contusions. If he has a seizure, place him on his side to prevent aspiration of gastric contents, and keep his airway patent. Administer supplemental oxygen through an Ambu bag. Don't forcibly restrain his movements, but guide them to prevent further injury. Administer anticonvulsants, such as diazepam (Valium) or phenytoin (Dilantin) I.V., as ordered.

## Mental status

A patient with an emergency involving poisoning, drug abuse, or exposure to a toxic substance may be conscious or comatose or have an altered level of consciousness, depending on the type and severity of his emergency.

Use the Glasgow Coma Scale to assess his level of consciousness quickly. (See *Assessing Your Patient's Level of Consciousness Using the Glasgow Coma Scale*, page 229.) If he's inattentive, incoherent, or agitated, he may have taken an overdose of a CNS stimulant. If he responds to painful stimuli with decerebrate or decorticate posturing, he may have severe brain damage as a direct result of poisoning or substance abuse.

If he's lethargic, stuporous, or comatose, he may have absorbed a toxic substance systemically. Start an I.V. if the patient doesn't already have one. If rescue personnel didn't administer $D_{50}W$, naloxone (Narcan), and thiamine, the doctor may order these as an I.V. push now.

Checking the patient's pupils for size and reaction to light may help you identify the substance that's causing his emergency. (See *Understanding Pupillary Changes*, page 230, and *Documenting Pupil Size*, page 231.) For example, if both his pupils are dilated and fixed and he shows no reaction to light, he may have an anticholinergic overdose. Test his deep tendon and gag reflexes to further assess the severity of his CNS depression.

# What to Do Next

Now that you've stabilized your patient's airway, breathing, and circulation, obtain a detailed history of his poisoning emergency. Question the patient and anyone who accompanied him to the ED. Ask:

• What poison or drug did the patient take?

• Were empty pill bottles, a poison container, or paraphernalia for abusing drugs found nearby? Did someone bring these items to the ED?

• Where and how was the patient discovered, and what was he doing just prior to the emergency?

But what if your patient's unconscious, uncooperative, or simply unaware of what poison or drug is causing his emergency signs and symptoms? What if no witnesses were present at the time of the emergency? Then you'll need to rely completely on your assessment of the patient's signs and symptoms, being especially alert for clues to his emergency problem.

Perform a quick assessment to help determine:

• the type and extent of his poisoning

• signs and symptoms of other emergency problems, such as accompanying trauma or underlying systemic disease.

While you're performing your assessment, continue to check your patient's airway, breathing, and circulation frequently, and be alert for any change in his condition. Remember, *change may occur suddenly.* Be prepared to stop your assessment and to intervene immediately if his condition deteriorates.

During your initial assessment, you quickly evaluated your patient's level of consciousness. If he's *comatose,* continue your assessment to determine if his coma's the result of poisoning, trauma, or a neurologic or metabolic disorder.

Suspect supratentorial structural lesions if your patient has central neurogenic hyperventilation (sustained rapid breathing), disconjugate gaze, or doll's eye movements. He may be in metabolic coma if he has a persistent pupillary light reflex with severely depressed respirations. (See the "Coma" entry in Chapter 6.)

Assess your patient for any *changes in breathing pattern, depth, or rate* that may provide clues to his emergency problem. Listen to your patient's breath sounds. If you hear rales or rhonchi and he complains of *dyspnea* or *tachypnea,* he may have pulmonary edema—possibly due to poison-induced fluid shifts in his lungs.

Note any decrease in tidal volume; you may see this if your patient has either increased or decreased respirations. When it accompanies compensatory hyperventilation, decreased tidal volume may signal metabolic acidosis. (A number of poisonous substances can cause metabolic acidosis, such as cyanide, carbon monoxide, heavy metals, aspirin, and hydrocarbons.) If your patient's breathing is rapid and deep, with a pattern similar to that of central neurogenic hyperventilation, he may have taken an overdose of salicylate (aspirin). Shallow breathing with a slow respiratory rate may indicate cyanide poisoning. Cheyne-Stokes respirations suggest carbon monoxide poisoning. *If his breathing is completely irregular, be alert for impending respiratory arrest.*

If you note any of these breathing alterations, call the doctor *immediately* and prepare to use life-support techniques, if necessary.

With a patient who complains of *abdominal pain,* find out when he first noticed the pain. Gradual onset may indicate prolonged exposure to a potentially toxic substance—such as lead, organophosphate, carbamate, or salicylate—or an underlying and possibly undiagnosed disorder. Sudden onset of abdominal pain may suggest an acute poisoning emergency. To obtain clues to what's poisoning him, ask your patient to describe the pain:

• Abdominal *cramping* may indicate organophosphate, carbamate, plant, or food poisoning.

• A *burning* sensation may accompany hydrocarbon poisoning or salicylate overdose.

• Intense *colicky* pain suggests heavy metal poisoning.

Inspect your patient's abdomen for further signs of his poisoning emergency and for trauma. Look for distention, possibly indicating ingestion of a caustic substance. Note any petechiae, rashes, or hives—these may indicate salicylate overdose. Listen to his bowel sounds: if he's been exposed to an organophosphate or carbamate, his bowel sounds will be hyperactive. Next, gently palpate his abdomen: lower abdominal tenderness may indicate food poisoning. Right upper quadrant pain or hepatomegaly may signal acetaminophen overdose. If your patient has cyanide poisoning, you may detect a distended bladder from urinary retention.

Patients with poisoning emergencies often complain of *vomiting* or *diarrhea.* If your patient has either of these complaints, explain to him that this is his body's way of expelling the poison, and tell him you'll soon be able to give him some medication to relieve his discomfort. To estimate when the poisoning occurred, ask him when his vomiting or diarrhea began. Obtain a sample of his vomitus for toxicology screening and a stool specimen to check for occult blood.

Your patient may also be *dehydrated* and *thirsty,* either as a direct result of his poisoning or because of poison-induced signs and symptoms such as vomiting, diarrhea, or diaphoresis. Don't give him any oral fluids now—this may trigger spontaneous vomiting,

## WHEN CHARCOAL WORKS TOO WELL

You know that activated charcoal adsorbs, or binds, toxic substances to its surface, so it prevents them from being absorbed by the body and lessens their effects. But do you know that charcoal can do the same thing to *antidotes,* too?

For example, charcoal adsorbs syrup of ipecac. If you give them together, the patient won't vomit the substance he's ingested, and the charcoal won't adsorb it very well, either. So give charcoal only *after* your patient vomits from taking ipecac.

Charcoal can also adsorb acetylcysteine (Mucomyst), acetaminophen's antidote. Before you give oral acetylcysteine to your patient, perform gastric lavage to remove any charcoal.

increasing the risk of aspiration or forcing the poison further down his throat or esophagus.

Now that you've quickly assessed your patient's condition, your next priority is to help remove the poison and to prevent further absorption of it into his system. To do this, you'll either induce vomiting or perform gastric lavage, depending on the substance your patient ingested, his level of consciousness, and whether he has a gag reflex. Keep suction equipment nearby and be prepared to suction his oropharynx to prevent aspiration. Explain to your patient that the procedure selected may be uncomfortable for him, but that it's essential to remove the poison to prevent systemic absorption. This may help you gain his cooperation and reduce struggling, which could provoke aspiration.

If the patient's alert and you don't suspect he has swallowed a caustic substance, induce vomiting by first giving him 8 to 16 ounces of water to drink, followed by 10 to 30 ml of syrup of ipecac orally. Keep him in an upright position to decrease the risk of aspiration, and encourage him to drink plenty of water. He should start vomiting within 10 to 15 minutes; if he doesn't, repeat the dosage—unless his level of consciousness deteriorates during this interval. The danger of aspiration increases greatly if vomiting occurs while a patient's stuporous, so

be ready to perform gastric lavage to remove both the initial dose of ipecac *and* the poison if your patient's level of consciousness deteriorates.

If the patient lacks a gag reflex or has a decreased level of consciousness, expect to perform gastric lavage (see *Performing Gastric Lavage*). If he's

PROCEDURES

## YOUR ROLE IN AN EMERGENCY

### PERFORMING GASTRIC LAVAGE

You'll perform gastric lavage when vomiting's contraindicated or when the patient:
• doesn't vomit after receiving syrup of ipecac.
• is comatose.
• is awake and has ingested a large amount of a highly toxic substance. (Note: *Don't* perform gastric lavage if your patient's ingested a caustic substance; the tube may perforate his esophagus.)
• needs activated charcoal instillation as part of his treatment.
• has central nervous system (CNS) depression with an inadequate gag reflex. (You may also perform gastric lavage for a patient with upper GI bleeding, to remove blood and to promote clotting.)

**Equipment**
• I.V. bottle or bag of warmed normal saline irrigating solution (or tap water, if the patient's an adult)
• Two pieces of connector tubing or (if you're using gravity drainage instead of suction) three large single-lumen rubber tubes, two calibrated containers, and a Y-connector
• Suction machine
• Ewald tube or large-lumen Salem-sump tube
• Hemostat
• Water-soluble lubricant
• Anesthetic jelly
• Stethoscope
• 50-cc syringe

**Before the procedure**
• Explain the procedure to the patient, if possible.
• Hang the irrigating solution and clamp the inflow tubing.
• Assist with endotracheal or nasotracheal

intubation, if needed.
• Position the patient on his left side in a three-quarter prone position, with his feet elevated.
• Anesthetize the back of his throat and lubricate the tube, as ordered.
• Insert the Ewald tube or Salem-sump tube.
• Check tube placement by injecting about 30 cc of air through the tube and listening for air flow in the patient's stomach, using a stethoscope.
• Aspirate the patient's stomach contents with the 50-cc syringe, and send the aspirate sample to the laboratory for analysis.

**During the procedure**
• Connect the Ewald tube to the Y-connector, or connect one port of the Salem-sump tube to the inflow tube and the other port to the outflow (suction) tube.
• Remove the hemostat from the inflow tube, and clamp it on the outflow tube.
• Instill up to 200 ml of solution, as ordered.
• Massage the patient's stomach to mix its contents and to break up any concretions of poisons or drugs.
• Unclamp the outflow tube, and clamp the inflow tube.
• Record the outflow amount—it should equal or exceed the amount instilled. If it doesn't, move the tube by rotating it between your fingers or pulling back on it slightly until enough solution flows back.
• Repeat this inflow-outflow cycle, using 5 to 10 liters of fluid, as ordered.

**Nursing considerations**
• Don't leave the patient alone during the procedure—watch him continuously for

comatose or unresponsive, assist with insertion of an endotracheal tube before performing gastric lavage, to prevent aspiration.

At best, induced vomiting and gastric lavage will remove only 50% to 60% of the patient's gastric contents. For adsorption of the remaining poison, you may be asked to give him a slurry of activated charcoal and water or saline solution. Remember, swallowing large volumes of fluid may force your patient's gastric contents into his duodenum, so administer small amounts of the slurry orally or through a nasogastric (NG) tube, as ordered. If

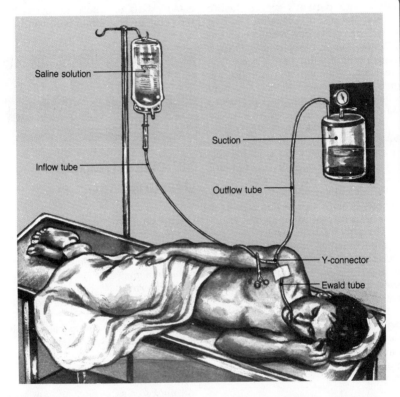

such complications as stomach distention or vomiting and aspiration.
• Monitor his vital signs frequently. Be alert for bradydysrhythmias from vagal stimulation.
• Suction his oral cavity frequently to prevent aspiration and airway obstruction.
• Administer activated charcoal and cathartics, as ordered.
• For GI bleeding, use a disposable irrigation set and a syringe for aspiration. This method is less traumatic than suction.
• Modify the lavage solution according to the patient's need. For example, ice

the saline solution and add a vasoconstrictor, as ordered, for GI bleeding; add calcium for fluoride or oxalate poisoning; add potassium permanganate for cyanide poisoning.
• Document your patient's vital signs, level of consciousness, and intake and output, as well as the date and time of lavage, the size and type of gastric tube used, any drugs given through the tube, the time you removed the tube, the irrigating solution's volume and type, and your observations of the patient's gastric contents.

vomiting was induced, *wait until it's subsided* before administering the charcoal slurry (usually about 15 to 20 minutes). You may also be asked to give your patient a saline or osmotic cathartic to speed the poison's elimination through his GI tract.

Once you've intervened to help remove the poison and to stop its continued absorption, take some time to obtain your patient's general health history. Because a poisoning or drug abuse emergency can readily compromise the patient's respiratory status, a patient with a pulmonary disease is at great risk of developing a complication such as pulmonary edema. A patient with renal disease may have decreased ability to handle the excessive fluids he needs to flush poison from his system. A patient with cardiac disease is at risk for cardiac dysrhythmias from his poisoning and for congestive heart failure from fluid replacement therapy.

For any patient who has a poisoning emergency or a drug overdose, consider the possibility of attempted suicide. Obtain a psychiatric history, and determine whether your patient's been depressed. Find out if he's taking any medications for a known medical problem: he may have taken an unintentional overdose.

Also assemble an occupational history—this is especially important if you suspect the patient may have organophosphate, carbamate, carbon monoxide, or lead poisoning from exposure on the job.

# Special Considerations

## Pediatric

Because of their natural inquisitiveness, children are often victims of accidental poisoning. Chewable vitamins (and other medications), household cleaning products, and poisonous plants are among the leading causes of poisoning in children. Suspect acci-

dental poisoning in any child who has specific *or nonspecific* signs and symptoms. Be sure to ask the child's parents if any possibility exists that *other* children, such as friends or siblings, may also have swallowed the poison.

If your patient's an infant, be alert for signs of hypotonic (floppy) infant syndrome: inability to suck, a weak cry, or floppy head movements. These are classic signs of failure to thrive, but they also suggest infant botulism.

# DEFINITIVE CARE

# Salicylate (Aspirin) Overdose

## Initial care summary

The patient had a history of excessive salicylate (aspirin) ingestion. Initially, he showed a combination of these signs and symptoms:
- hyperthermia
- a burning sensation in his mouth or throat
- altered level of consciousness (lethargy, restlessness, disorientation, or coma)
- petechiae, rashes, or hives.

In addition, if he ingested *less than 150 mg/kg* of salicylate, he may have had:
- deep, rapid respirations
- hyperventilation
- thirst
- nausea and vomiting
- tinnitus
- diaphoresis.

Or, if he ingested *more than 150 mg/kg* of salicylate, he may have had:
- dehydration
- convulsions
- seizures
- hearing loss

- decreased motor ability
- respiratory failure.

The patient's respiratory status was assessed, and supplemental oxygen was provided through a nasal cannula, tight-fitting mask, or mechanical ventilator, as indicated. Blood was drawn for a serum salicylate level, CBC, prothrombin time (PT), partial thromboplastin time (PTT), typing and cross matching, and ABG, electrolyte, blood glucose, and BUN levels. A urine specimen was obtained for analysis to determine acetone and salicylate levels and pH.

Vomiting was induced if the patient was awake and alert; if he wasn't, gastric lavage was performed. Activated charcoal and a saline cathartic were administered, and an I.V. was started with $D_5W$. The patient was connected to a cardiac monitor, and a 12-lead EKG was taken.

## Priorities

Your first priority is to reassess your patient's respiratory status. Why? Because a patient with a salicylate overdose can rapidly develop respiratory distress at any time as a result of his acid-base imbalance. Be prepared to assist with intubation and mechanical ventilation, if necessary.

Begin infusing Ringer's lactate or isotonic sodium chloride at a rapid rate, for fluid replacement and volume expansion. To keep urine alkaline, expect to add sodium bicarbonate to his I.V. fluid or to give tromethamine (THAM) by slow I.V. push. This will help decrease his tubular reabsorption of aspirin and enhance its excretion through his genitourinary (GU) tract.

## Continuing assessment and therapeutic care

Check your patient's vital signs often—especially his blood pressure, pulse rate, and body temperature. If his temperature's higher than 101° F. (38.3° C.), sponge him with tepid water. If this doesn't reduce his fever, you may need to place him on a hypothermia blanket.

Your patient may also have hypotension; to increase his vital organ perfusion, be prepared to elevate his legs and to administer a vasopressor, as ordered. The doctor may also order an increase in your patient's I.V. infusion rate.

Monitor your patient's intake and output carefully to evaluate his fluid status. Auscultate his breath sounds often: rales may indicate fluid overload or pulmonary edema. (If the doctor suspects edema, he'll order a chest X-ray.)

Check the results of your patient's serial blood tests to help gauge the effectiveness of his fluid replacement and alkalinization therapy. His serum salicylate level should steadily decrease as excretion progresses, and his ABGs should show a slightly alkaline blood pH. Remember, your patient's acid-base balance can change rapidly, not only because of his alkalinization therapy but also because of salicylate's toxic acidic effect. If his blood pH drops below 7.15, the doctor will ask you to *immediately* give him an I.V. push of 3 to 5 mEq/kg of sodium bicarbonate, to buffer his acidosis.

When you check your patient's electrolyte balance, be alert for sodium overload and potassium depletion—common side effects of alkalinization therapy. Replenish his potassium stores by adding potassium chloride to his I.V. solution, and expect to change his I.V. solution for one with a lower sodium content. Continue replacing other electrolytes as indicated until his balance is restored.

Continue monitoring your patient's cardiac rhythm and rate. (As you know, acid-base and electrolyte imbalances may cause cardiac dysrhythmias.) If you note frequent PVCs, call the doctor *immediately*. Expect to give your patient lidocaine, as ordered.

Perform hourly neurologic assessments, noting any change in your patient's level of consciousness. Remember—lethargy, confusion, or coma may

PATHOPHYSIOLOGY

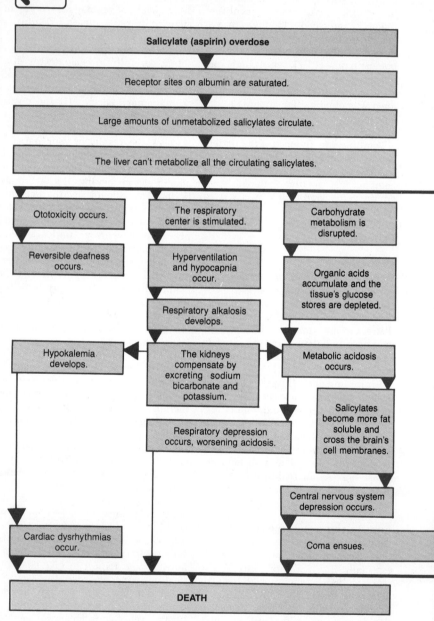

# WHAT HAPPENS IN SALICYLATE (ASPIRIN) OVERDOSE

Salicylate (aspirin) overdose

Receptor sites on albumin are saturated.

Large amounts of unmetabolized salicylates circulate.

The liver can't metabolize all the circulating salicylates.

Ototoxicity occurs.

Reversible deafness occurs.

The respiratory center is stimulated.

Hyperventilation and hypocapnia occur.

Respiratory alkalosis develops.

Carbohydrate metabolism is disrupted.

Organic acids accumulate and the tissue's glucose stores are depleted.

Hypokalemia develops.

The kidneys compensate by excreting sodium bicarbonate and potassium.

Metabolic acidosis occurs.

Respiratory depression occurs, worsening acidosis.

Salicylates become more fat soluble and cross the brain's cell membranes.

Central nervous system depression occurs.

Cardiac dysrhythmias occur.

Coma ensues.

DEATH

A salicylate (aspirin) overdose can occur in any of five different ways. It can be:
• *congenital,* as in a newborn infant whose mother takes a lot of aspirin just before delivery.
• *therapeutic,* as in a child or adult who receives repeated doses of aspirin for fever or pain.
• *accidental,* as in a toddler who eats pills or drinks the brightly colored liquid.
• *nonaccidental,* a form of child abuse, as when a parent deliberately gives too much aspirin to a child.
• *self-induced,* as in depressed teenagers, elderly people, and others who try to commit suicide via aspirin overdose.

Normally, the stomach and small intestine absorb salicylates well. Then most of the salicylates (50% to 80%) bind to the plasma's albumin while the liver metabolizes the unbound salicylates and the kidneys excrete them.

An overdose of salicylates causes the same degree of binding to plasma albumin after absorption—but then many more unbound salicylates remain in circulation. The liver's metabolic pathway quickly becomes saturated with these unbound salicylates. This chart details the serious— even fatal—effects that can result.

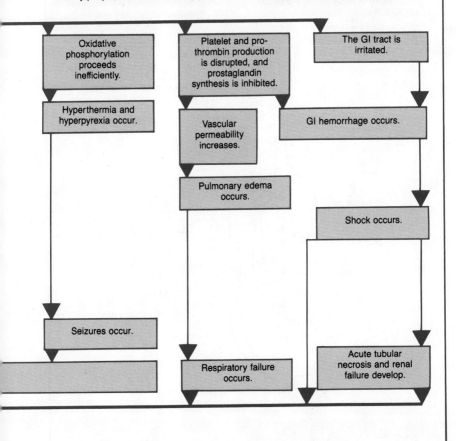

## UNDERSTANDING HEMOPERFUSION

Hemoperfusion removes certain toxins from a patient's system by drawing blood across a bed of activated charcoal, which filters out these poisons. You may expect to see hemoperfusion used for a patient with barbiturate, glutethimide, salicylate (aspirin), methaqualone, meprobamate, or paraquat poisoning—especially if the substance wasn't completely removed from his GI system by emesis, lavage, or activated charcoal given orally.

Before hemoperfusion can begin, your patient needs an arteriovenous shunt or fistula for vascular access. A percutaneous femoral vein catheter can also be used. Then his blood's drawn from an artery into the hemoperfusion circuit, where it's heparinized and monitored for adequate blood pressure. A pump moves the blood at approximately 300 ml/minute from

the arterial drip chamber, then past another pressure monitor, which detects blood clots in the cartridge by calculating the pressure drop across it. Then the blood travels through the charcoal bed in the hemoperfusion cartridge. (Sometimes the charcoal is replaced with a special resin to filter lipid-soluble drugs, such as glutethimide and methaqualone.) The hemoperfusion cartridge traps the poison or drug along with creatinine, uric acid, and middle-weight molecular uremic toxins. A third pressure monitor gauges the patient's venous resistance, and the blood moves through a venous drip chamber and into an air bubble detector before it's pumped back to the patient through a vein.

Hemoperfusion's very effective in treating certain types of poisonings and overdoses. When combined with hemodialysis, it's also a successful treatment for liver failure. Although complications are rare, hemoperfusion can cause thrombocytopenia, transient leukopenia, hemolysis, clotting factor deficiencies, electrolyte imbalances, and hypotension. So, if your patient must have hemoperfusion, be prepared to transfuse platelets or fresh-frozen plasma with clotting factors, to give I.V. fluids, and to administer a pressor agent, as ordered.

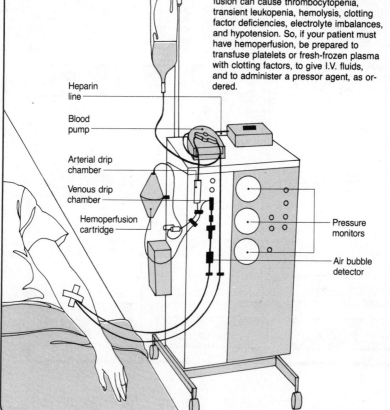

Heparin line

Blood pump

Arterial drip chamber

Venous drip chamber

Hemoperfusion cartridge

Pressure monitors

Air bubble detector

signal that a toxic level of salicylate is causing hypoglycemia or hypoxemia. Inform the doctor, and expect to obtain blood for *immediate* laboratory testing to measure glucose and ABG levels. He may ask you to correct your patient's hypoglycemia by increasing his dextrose infusion. Or, if the patient's hypoxemic, the doctor may order supplemental oxygen.

Each time you assess your patient, be alert for possible indications of internal hemorrhage—especially if his hematocrit and hemoglobin levels start to fall. Check his stools and vomitus for frank or occult blood, which may indicate lower GI bleeding. (Anticipate performing gastric lavage with iced saline solution.) If he has hematuria, he may be bleeding somewhere along his GU tract. A patient with unequal pupil size and changes in his level of consciousness may have an intracerebral hemorrhage. Notify the doctor if you detect *any* of these signs and symptoms. Expect to give your patient vitamin K to stimulate his clotting mechanism, and prepare to transfuse blood, as ordered (see *Administering Blood Transfusions,* page 493).

# Acetaminophen Overdose

## Initial care summary

The patient had a history of ingesting acetaminophen. Initial assessment revealed that he had some combination of the following signs and symptoms:
- anorexia
- nausea and vomiting
- diaphoresis
- dehydration
- an altered level of consciousness
- hypotension
- right upper quadrant pain
- liver tenderness
- jaundice.

Blood was drawn for a plasma acet-

PATHOPHYSIOLOGY

## WHAT HAPPENS IN ACETAMINOPHEN OVERDOSE

Even in normal doses, acetaminophen's a drug that liver cell enzymes convert into toxic metabolites. Fortunately, normal stores of glutathione detoxify these metabolites, which are then excreted in the urine.

But in an acetaminophen overdose, liver cell enzymes form so many toxic metabolites that they overwhelm the liver, deplete glutathione stores, and defy detoxification. The metabolites then bind to cellular proteins, killing liver cells and causing liver failure. The result? Hypoglycemia, encephalopathy, bleeding, shock, coma. Death will ensue if the overdose isn't recognized and treated promptly.

aminophen level, liver function studies (serum glutamic-oxaloacetic transaminase [SGOT], serum glutamic-pyruvic transaminase [SGPT], and bilirubin levels), and ABG, electrolyte, creatinine, serum glucose, and BUN levels. Samples of urine, blood, and gastric contents were obtained for toxicology screening. Vomiting was induced if the patient was awake and alert; if he wasn't, gastric lavage was performed. An I.V. was started to replace fluids and to give medications.

## Priorities

Because large amounts of acetaminophen have accumulated in your patient's liver, he risks developing hepatic necrosis that may quickly lead to hepatic failure and death. Your first priority, then, is to administer acetylcysteine (Mucomyst) to inactivate acetaminophen's toxic metabolites and to help prevent hepatic injury. (See *Highlighting Acetylcysteine,* page 758.) Expect to give a loading dose of the antidote orally; if your patient can't tolerate oral medications, insert an NG tube to administer the antidote. (If your hospital's protocol permits, you may be asked to give the antidote I.V.)

Remember, a patient with an acet-

DRUGS

## HIGHLIGHTING ACETYLCYSTEINE

You may have used acetylcysteine (Mucomyst) before as a mucolytic for patients with respiratory problems. But did you know that this sulfhydryl compound is also the antidote for acetaminophen overdose? Here's why:

Acetylcysteine replenishes the patient's glutathione stores and restarts the acetaminophen detoxification process. It's very effective and well tolerated, with minimal side effects (nausea and vomiting).

Expect to give acetylcysteine orally within 24 hours of acetaminophen ingestion. (Some centers give it I.V. instead.) First, empty the patient's stomach by gastric lavage or by induced vomiting. Then prepare a 5% acetylcysteine solution by diluting it with cola, fruit juice, or water. After the loading dose, give smaller doses every 4 hours, as ordered, until laboratory results show that your patient's plasma level of acetaminophen is low enough that it won't cause liver damage.

---

tylcysteine therapy. Your patient's plasma acetaminophen level should steadily decrease, and his SGOT, SGPT, and bilirubin levels should return to normal. If these improvements don't occur, expect to adjust his dosage of the antidote. If his PT remains prolonged, expect to give vitamin K to stimulate his clotting mechanism. Continue replacing fluids and electrolytes, as indicated, to correct his dehydration and electrolyte imbalance.

Your patient may develop acute renal failure because of acetaminophen's antidiuretic effect. To keep alert for this, monitor his intake and output hourly. If his output drops below 30 ml/hour, call the doctor *immediately*. He'll order immediate BUN and creatinine blood tests and ask you to administer a diuretic. If your patient's output still doesn't increase and his BUN and creatinine levels are elevated, expect to assist with peritoneal dialysis. (See *Assisting with Peritoneal Dialysis,* pages 576 and 577, and the "Acute Renal Failure" entry in Chapter 13.)

---

aminophen overdose shouldn't be given activated charcoal, because this will absorb the acetylcysteine. If your patient received activated charcoal because he ingested several different drugs, expect to perform gastric lavage to remove the charcoal before administering the antidote. (See *Performing Gastric Lavage,* pages 750 and 751.)

### Continuing assessment and therapeutic care
Start performing a complete assessment by checking your patient's vital signs. Tachycardia, hypotension, and a weak pulse may indicate impending shock, possibly from circulatory collapse. Expect to increase your patient's I.V. infusion rate and to give a vasopressor, such as norepinephrine I.V., to correct his hypotension.

Continue to give your patient acetylcysteine at 4-hour intervals. Obtain blood for serial laboratory tests, and monitor the results to help determine the proper dosage for continued ace-

# Heavy Metal Poisoning

### Initial care summary
On initial assessment, the patient had a history of ingesting a substance containing a heavy metal (lead, iron, or arsenic). In addition, he had some combination of the following signs and symptoms:
- vomiting and diarrhea
- colicky abdominal pain
- nausea and loss of appetite
- decreased level of consciousness
- tachycardia and hypotension.

If the patient was suspected of ingesting an *arsenic*-containing substance, these were his only presenting signs and symptoms.

If *lead* poisoning was suspected, onset of these signs and symptoms may have occurred gradually, over the course of 3 to 6 months. This patient

may also have experienced gradual onset of the following signs and symptoms:
- irritability
- peripheral nerve weakness
- stupor.

If *iron* poisoning was suspected, the patient may also have had:

- blood-streaked vomitus, diarrhea, or urine
- rose-colored urine
- fever
- lethargy and hypotonia.

To determine whether chelation therapy was necessary, blood was drawn to evaluate serum iron concentration

PATHOPHYSIOLOGY

## WHAT HAPPENS IN HEAVY METAL POISONING

Normal levels of lead, arsenic, and iron in the air, water, and soil usually pose no health problems. But when a person ingests large amounts of these heavy metals, they can cause severe damage by:
- directly contacting vital organs.
- saturating heavy metal binding sites and invading the cells.
- interfering with cellular enzyme action.

Without prompt treatment, death may result from multisystem failure or shock.

The most common sources of heavy metal poisoning are:
- arsenic-containing pesticides and contaminated water
- lead paint chips
- vitamins and other iron preparations.

Although heavy metals are absorbed in different ways, they often have similar effects, as detailed below.

### GASTROINTESTINAL SYSTEM

**Arsenic causes:**
- formation and subsequent rupture of plasma-filled vesicles under the GI mucosa
- plasma coagulation in the intestinal lumen
- increased peristalsis and severe diarrhea
- shock.

**Iron causes:**
- necrosis of the GI tract's mucosal wall
- hemorrhage that may lead to shock.

### LIVER

**Arsenic and iron cause:**
- liver necrosis
- liver failure.

### KIDNEYS

**Arsenic, lead, and iron cause:**
- tubular degeneration and necrosis
- renal failure.

### CENTRAL NERVOUS SYSTEM

**Arsenic and lead cause:**
- central nervous system depression
- peripheral neuropathies
- encephalopathy
- convulsions
- coma.

### BONE MARROW

**Lead causes:**
- inhibition of the heme synthetic pathway
- acute hemolytic crisis, anemia, and hypoxia.

### RESPIRATORY SYSTEM

**Iron causes:**
- vascular congestion of lungs
- pulmonary edema and hemorrhage
- respiratory failure.

and total iron-binding capacity or blood lead level. Blood was also drawn for CBC, electrolyte, ABGs, liver function studies, coagulation testing, BUN, creatinine, and typing and cross matching. If the doctor suspected lead poisoning, additional blood was drawn to evaluate the patient's serum erythrocyte protoporphyrin level. An indwelling (Foley) catheter was inserted. Samples of the patient's urine, vomitus, blood, and stools were obtained for toxicology screening. (If the patient had a history of possible exposure to arsenic, an additional urine specimen was obtained to determine his urinary arsenic level.) He was connected to a cardiac monitor, and a 12-lead EKG was taken. An abdominal X-ray was taken to visualize any undigested tablets. An I.V. was started to replace lost fluid and electrolytes and to administer medication.

If the patient was responsive and had a gag reflex, vomiting was induced with syrup of ipecac. If he was unresponsive or lacked a gag reflex, gastric lavage was performed. Following the lavage, a 5% sodium bicarbonate or sodium phosphate cathartic may have been given.

## Priorities

Because high concentrations of iron, lead, or arsenic can accumulate quickly in your patient's kidneys, liver, or brain tissue, evacuation of gastric contents may remove only a small percentage of the metal he ingested. Your first priority, then, is to help the patient excrete as much of the remaining metal as possible.

To help accomplish this, the doctor will order forced diuresis. Increase the infusion rate, as ordered, to speed the metal's excretion through the patient's GU tract. If his laboratory tests reveal a high concentration of arsenic, lead, or iron, expect to administer a chelating agent. This will bind with the metal and facilitate its elimination.

If urinalysis reveals a toxic level of *arsenic,* expect to give your patient di-

mercaprol (BAL) I.M. For a patient with severe *lead* poisoning (greater than 70 mcg/ml), expect to administer edetate calcium disodium (calcium EDTA) I.M. To increase the EDTA's binding power, the doctor may order a combined initial dosage of EDTA and BAL. If your patient has severe *iron* poisoning (greater than 500 mcg/ml), expect to give him deferoxamine (Desferal) I.M.

## Continuing assessment and therapeutic care

Check your patient's vital signs often, especially his blood pressure and pulse rate, to determine whether fluid replacement and chelation therapy are correcting his hypotension. If they aren't, expect to administer a vasopressor and to increase his I.V. fluids. Closely monitor his intake and output to evaluate his fluid balance, and continue cardiac monitoring to evaluate his heart rhythm and rate. His hemodynamic status should improve as his plasma volume increases.

Obtain urine and blood samples for serial laboratory analyses, and monitor the laboratory results to determine how effectively the metal's being excreted. If your patient has *arsenic* poisoning, his urine arsenic level should steadily decrease. If he has *lead* or *iron* poisoning, you should note a proportionate decrease in his serum lead or iron level as the metal's excreted. Continue to replace electrolytes, as ordered, until your patient's electrolyte balance is restored. When you check his ABGs, be alert for possible metabolic acidosis, especially if he has iron poisoning. Expect to give sodium bicarbonate I.V. to correct acidosis.

Note any decrease in your patient's urine output, particularly if he also has increased BUN and creatinine levels—which may indicate renal failure. (If your patient has lead poisoning and urinalysis reveals proteinuria, glycosuria, or aminoaciduria, this may mean that lead is accumulating in his renal tubules, causing tubular damage.) Inform the doctor of your findings, and be prepared to assist with peritoneal dialysis, as ordered. (See *Assisting with Peritoneal Dialysis,* pages 576 and 577.)

If your patient's receiving BAL, be alert for possible side effects, such as localized abdominal pain, paresthesias, excessive salivation, and vomiting. Notify the doctor if your patient develops any of these signs and symptoms, and expect to administer antihistamines to relieve the severity of his reaction.

Your patient may also develop GI complications—hemorrhage, for example—as a direct result of heavy metal poisoning. Check his stools for frank and occult blood, and monitor his serial CBCs. If his hematocrit and hemoglobin levels start to decrease, this may also indicate GI bleeding. Let the doctor know of your findings, and expect to perform gastric lavage with iced saline solution. Prepare to give your patient a blood transfusion, as ordered (see *Administering Blood Transfusions,* page 493).

Be alert to the possibility of hepatic damage or failure as a direct result of your patient's poisoning, especially if he ingested lead or iron. When you're assessing him, note if his sclera or skin is becoming yellow, and inform the doctor of your results. Expect to obtain blood for coagulation testing. If your patient has hepatic failure, he may develop severe internal hemorrhage with prolonged clotting time or thrombocytopenia. (See the "Hemorrhage Secondary to Thrombocytopenia" entry in Chapter 11.)

Perform frequent neurologic assessments, and assess your patient's mental status often. A depression in his level of consciousness may signal a decrease in cerebral perfusion—or it may indicate that the poisoning's directly affecting his CNS. Administer supplemental oxygen, as needed, and have someone call the doctor. He may order a change in the vasopressor therapy your patient's receiving.

# Hydrocarbon Poisoning

## Initial care summary

On initial assessment, the patient had a history of ingesting or inhaling a hydrocarbon-containing substance (such as gasoline, aerosol spray propellant, or turpentine). He had a combination of these signs and symptoms:
• breath odor of a petroleum distillate or violets
• dyspnea, coughing, or gagging
• a burning sensation in his mouth, esophagus, and stomach
• redness, blisters, or irritation in his nostrils or mouth and pharynx
• palpitations
• tremors and muscle cramps in his arms and legs
• dizziness
• mental deterioration
• cool, clammy skin
• fever
• euphoria
• headache
• cyanosis or pallor.

If the patient inhaled hydrocarbon fumes, he was evacuated to fresh air. If his skin was exposed to a hydrocarbon substance, his clothes were removed and his skin was washed with soapy water. If the substance splashed in his eye, the affected eye was irrigated with water or normal saline solution for at least 30 minutes.

An I.V. was started at a keep-vein-open rate. A 12-lead EKG and a chest X-ray were taken, and the patient was connected to a cardiac monitor. Urine was obtained for analysis, and blood was drawn for CBC, ABGs, blood glucose, BUN, creatinine, electrolytes, liver function studies, and toxicology screening. The doctor may have ordered induced vomiting or gastric lavage—or neither, if he decided that the risk of aspiration outweighed the risk of poison absorption. A saline cathartic was administered to promote elimination of the hydrocarbon.

## Priorities

Your patient with hydrocarbon poisoning risks aspiration of material that will irritate and inflame his lung's mucosal lining, setting up a chemical reaction that can quickly lead to pulmonary edema. Keep in mind that his respiratory status can change abruptly. This means that your first priority is to reassess his respiratory status and help prevent or treat aspiration. To prevent aspiration, position your patient on his side with his feet elevated 20° to 30°. If he's cyanotic or pale and coughing, gagging, or choking, he may already have aspirated hydrocarbon mate-

PATHOPHYSIOLOGY

# WHAT HAPPENS IN HYDROCARBON POISONING

Hydrocarbons are some of the most frequently used substances in our society. These organic compounds, consisting only of carbon and hydrogen molecules, can be grouped into three categories:
• *aliphatic hydrocarbons,* which are commonly derived from petroleum or petroleum processing

• *aromatic hydrocarbons,* which are found in coal products
• *halogenated hydrocarbons,* containing chlorine or fluorine, which are used as aerosol spray propellants, refrigerants, solvents, and vehicles for paints, varnishes, and other coatings.
    Although a patient may inhale hydrocar-

| | |
|---|---|
| | Acute tubular necrosis develops. |
| | Sensitivity to circulating catecholamines increases. |
| Inhalation of hydrocarbon material | The pulmonary mucosal lining is irritated. → Chemical pneumonitis develops. → Pneumonia ensues. |
| | The central nervous system is depressed. |
| | Fatty degeneration and cellular necrosis of the liver begin. |

rial—even if his initial chest X-ray didn't reveal chemical pneumonitis. If you suspect aspiration, call the doctor *immediately*. He may ask you to give the patient supplemental oxygen or, if your patient's respirations are severely depressed, to assist with intubation and mechanical ventilation.

## Continuing assessment and therapeutic care

Because the body's fatty tissues absorb hydrocarbons, routine toxicology screening may not accurately indicate your patient's level of accumulated hydrocarbon. So while you're assessing your patient, remember that even

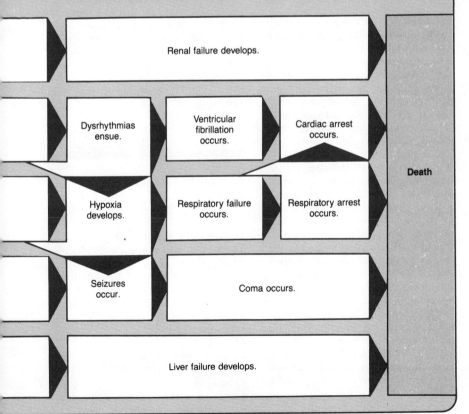

bon material deliberately—glue sniffing's an example of this—accidental poisoning is more common (for example, inhaling aerosol spray). Hydrocarbons are most toxic when they're inhaled or aspirated; ingestion's less likely to cause poisoning because the GI system doesn't absorb hydrocarbons well. Skin contact also produces no serious systemic effects.

A patient with hydrocarbon poisoning can be affected in any or all of the ways shown in this chart. (In addition, exposure to aromatic hydrocarbons over time may cause cancer.) As you can see, death may occur if the patient doesn't receive treatment.

Renal failure develops.

Dysrhythmias ensue.

Ventricular fibrillation occurs.

Cardiac arrest occurs.

Hypoxia develops.

Respiratory failure occurs.

Respiratory arrest occurs.

**Death**

Seizures occur.

Coma occurs.

Liver failure develops.

though he seems stable, his condition can change suddenly as his fatty tissues release stored hydrocarbons.

Check your patient's vital signs often, especially his body temperature. He may have a neurogenic fever as high as 103° F. (39.4° C.) for the first 48 hours after hydrocarbon exposure. Expect to administer antipyretics and to place your patient on a hypothermia mattress, as ordered.

If your patient's fever persists for 48 hours and his blood pressure drops severely, he may have an infection, possibly from aspirating foreign material into his lungs. Culture the patient's sputum, and obtain a chest X-ray. You may be asked to administer a broad-spectrum antibiotic until the infection-causing organism is identified. Then, the doctor will ask you to administer an antibiotic that's specific to the causative organism.

Continue to monitor your patient's respiratory status by checking his serial ABGs and by evaluating his breath sounds frequently. If his ABGs reveal a decreased $PO_2$ or you detect diffuse rales, rhonchi, or decreased breath sounds, call the doctor *immediately*. These signs indicate that your patient may have developed pulmonary complications, such as chemical pneumonitis or pulmonary edema. The doctor will order serial chest X-rays to detect possible infiltrate edema or atelectasis. To prevent cerebral hypoxia, expect to give supplemental oxygen via a mask or mechanical ventilator. To correct noncardiogenic pulmonary edema, expect to give corticosteroids and to place the patient on PEEP. If pneumonitis develops, give a broad-spectrum antibiotic, as ordered.

Continue monitoring your patient's cardiac output. Because hydrocarbons interfere with the heart's conduction system, you may note dysrhythmias, such as ventricular fibrillation, heart block, or asystole. If your patient's heartbeat becomes severely bradycardic, and his blood pressure decreases, expect to give him atropine I.V.

to accelerate his heart rate. Be prepared to defibrillate, too, if your patient develops ventricular fibrillation. (See the "Life Support" section in Chapter 3.)

Perform a neurologic assessment every hour to detect changes in your patient's level of consciousness. If he becomes confused or lethargic, notify the doctor—the fatty tissues in your patient's body may be releasing stored hydrocarbons, or hypoxemia from pulmonary complications may be causing CNS depression.

Check your patient's urine output every hour, as well, and obtain specimens for serial urinalyses. Inform the doctor if you note decreased urine output or hematuria—these may indicate renal damage. (So may a finding of proteinuria on urinalysis.) Be prepared to perform peritoneal dialysis, if ordered (see *Assisting with Peritoneal Dialysis,* pages 576 and 577). Rarely, a patient's signs and symptoms won't abate with peritoneal dialysis. The doctor may then order hemodialysis or hemoperfusion (see *Comparing Hemodialysis and Peritoneal Dialysis,* pages 578 and 579, and *Understanding Hemoperfusion,* page 756).

# Carbon Monoxide Poisoning

### Initial care summary
The patient had a history of inhaling carbon monoxide and, on initial assessment, had some of the following signs and symptoms:
• headache and dizziness
• depressed level of consciousness
• hyperventilation
• Cheyne-Stokes respirations
• cardiac dysrhythmias
• hypotension
• chest pain
• cogwheel rigidity of arms and/or legs
• opisthotonic posturing

# WHAT HAPPENS IN CARBON MONOXIDE POISONING

As you may know, carbon monoxide's a colorless, odorless gas resulting from incomplete burning of organic substances, such as gasoline, coal products, tobacco, and building materials. You'll see carbon monoxide poisoning most often in burn victims with smoke inhalation and in people who've tried to commit suicide by inhaling automobile exhaust fumes. When anyone inhales air that contains a high level of carbon monoxide, he's in serious danger of cardiopulmonary failure and death. Here's why:

Once it's inhaled, carbon monoxide crosses the alveolocapillary membrane, which is the means of gas exchange between alveolar air and capillary blood in the lungs. Because it has a high affinity for hemoglobin (nearly 240 times that of oxygen), carbon monoxide quickly binds to it, forming carboxyhemoglobin. This causes hypoxemia, because the hemoglobin can no longer carry oxygen. Carboxyhemoglobin formation also prevents release of oxygen from unaltered hemoglobin to the tissues. In addition, carbon monoxide binds with the myoglobin in muscle cells and interferes with cellular respiration.

The result? Hypoxia and metabolic acidosis. Because the heart and brain have the most active cellular metabolism, they are the first organs affected:
• Ischemia and dysrhythmias may cause cardiac arrest.
• Cerebral edema can lead to convulsions, coma, Cheyne-Stokes respirations, and respiratory arrest.

Without rapid oxygen therapy, carbon monoxide poisoning is fatal. Here's an illustration to help you understand what happens in carbon monoxide poisoning.

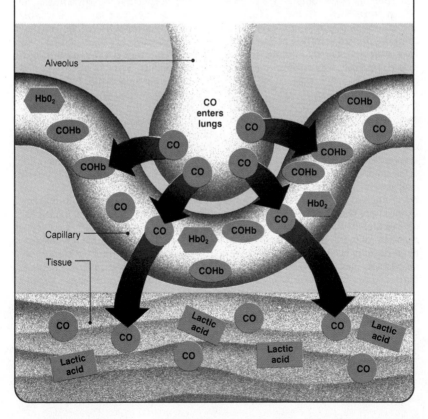

- cherry red mucous membranes
- skin erythema and edema
- blister formation
- impaired hearing or vision.

The patient was evacuated to fresh air, and 100% oxygen was administered through a tight-fitting face mask or an endotracheal tube with mechanical ventilation.

An I.V. was started to administer fluids and medication. If the patient had an altered level of consciousness, a $D_{50}$ bolus and naloxone (Narcan) were administered. A 12-lead EKG and a chest X-ray were taken, and the patient was attached to a cardiac monitor. Blood was drawn for ABGs (including carboxyhemoglobin and creatine phosphokinase), electrolytes, BUN, and creatinine levels. Urine was obtained for myoglobin analysis. Samples of the patient's blood, urine, and gastric contents were obtained for toxicology screening. If the toxicology studies revealed an accompanying drug overdose, forced vomiting or gastric lavage was performed, and the appropriate antidote was administered (if one existed).

## Priorities

Your first priority is to continue administering 100% oxygen to accelerate the patient's elimination of carbon monoxide and to improve his tissue oxygenation. If blood studies reveal that your patient's carboxyhemoglobin level is greater than 40%, expect to administer oxygen (in a hyperbaric chamber, if possible) to speed the separation of carbon monoxide from hemoglobin. If hyperbaric oxygenation isn't available, the doctor may ask you to place the patient on a hypothermia blanket to reduce his metabolic rate and, therefore, his oxygen requirements and to help prevent cardiac and CNS complications.

## Continuing assessment and therapeutic care

Obtain blood for serial ABG levels, and use the blood test results to gauge the effectiveness of your patient's oxygen therapy. Continue to provide supplemental oxygen, as ordered, until his carboxyhemoglobin level falls below 10%. If your patient has acidosis, the doctor will ask you to infuse sodium bicarbonate until your patient's blood pH returns *only* to about 7.2. Why? Because carbon monoxide separates faster from hemoglobin if the patient's blood is slightly acidic.

Keep your patient on strict bed rest to minimize his body's oxygen demand, and continue to monitor his vital signs and cardiac output. Because his blood's delivering less oxygen to myocardial tissue, you may note hypotension and cardiac dysrhythmias—such as tachypnea, atrial flutter, and fibrillation—and PVCs. Expect to give I.V. fluids to increase his circulatory blood volume and to correct hypotension. To prevent ventricular dysrhythmias, the doctor may ask you to give lidocaine through a continuous I.V. drip. You may also be asked to obtain blood for cardiac enzyme and isoenzyme testing if the doctor thinks your patient's at risk for angina or myocardial infarction.

Monitor your patient's fluid balance by checking his urine output every hour. If his urinalysis reveals myoglobinuria, this indicates rhabdomyolysis has occurred as the result of muscle breakdown from prolonged coma. Maintain an hourly output of 50 ml by adjusting your patient's fluid intake as ordered, and monitor BUN and creatinine levels for elevations indicating possible renal failure.

Perform hourly neurologic assessments, notifying the doctor if your patient's level of consciousness changes. (Even if he's had only slight carbon monoxide exposure, he can suffer permanent CNS damage from cerebral edema or ischemia.) If the doctor feels that your patient's intracranial pressure is dangerously increased, he'll order a computerized tomography (CT) scan and ask you to give the patient a corticosteroid and an osmotic diuretic. (See the "Increased Intracranial Pressure" entry in Chapter 6.) If your patient's having seizures, expect to administer diazepam (Valium) I.V., as ordered. Also be sure to protect him from injury by removing potentially hazardous items from his environment.

Watch for and report any changes in your patient's personality or cognition. He may become overly aggressive, euphoric, or hyperactive if he develops encephalopathy involving portions of his frontal and parietal cortex. Because his tissues may not start releasing stored carbon monoxide until 7 to 21 days after exposure, onset of neurologic and psychologic impairment may be correspondingly delayed. Advise the family to be alert for this possibility.

# Organophosphate and Carbamate Poisoning

## Initial care summary

The patient had a history of organophosphate or carbamate poisoning from being exposed to or ingesting a pesticide, insecticide, or herbicide. On initial assessment he revealed some combination of the following signs and symptoms:
• vision disturbances (constricted pupils, blurred vision)
• increased secretions (lacrimation, salivation, pulmonary secretions, or diaphoresis)
• bradycardia
• dyspnea or bradypnea
• nausea or vomiting, or both, accompanied by diarrhea
• increased bowel sounds and abdominal cramping
• involuntary defecation and urination
• pallor or cyanosis
• muscle fasciculations or twitching
• muscle weakness or paralysis
• altered level of consciousness

• seizure activity.

The patient's airway was suctioned to remove secretions. Blood was drawn for a CBC, ABGs, electrolytes, blood glucose, BUN, and creatinine levels. Additional blood was drawn to test cholinesterase activity in the patient's red blood cells and whole blood. Urine was obtained for analysis to detect organophosphate or carbamate metabolites. The patient was attached to a cardiac monitor, and a 12-lead EKG was taken. An I.V. was inserted, and an initial dose of 0.4 to 2.0 mg of atropine was given but failed to elicit an anticholinergic reaction—such as increased pulse rate, dry mouth, flushing, or pupil dilation. (If he was cyanotic, he was given supplemental oxygen first, to correct hypoxemia and to deliver oxygen to the myocardium. This prevents ventricular fibrillation—an adverse reaction to atropine.) The patient's clothing was removed, and his skin was washed with copious amounts of soapy water and alcohol to decontaminate it and to prevent further absorption. If he swallowed the organophosphate or carbamate, vomiting was induced or gastric lavage was performed. Activated charcoal and a saline cathartic were given.

## Priorities

Your first priority is to start your patient on atropine therapy, as ordered. Expect to give him 1 to 2 mg of atropine I.V. or I.M. every 10 to 15 minutes until the parasympathomimetic effects of his poisoning abate. His pupils should become dilated and his heart rate should increase to over 120 beats/minute. This may take 6 to 12 hours if the patient has carbamate poisoning, or up to 24 hours if he has organophosphate poisoning. You'll probably give a total of 25 to 50 mg of atropine—but if your patient's severely poisoned, you may need to give as much as 5 g of atropine before his signs and symptoms are relieved. If he has organophosphate poisoning, you'll also give him pralidoxime chloride (Protopam) to quickly

PATHOPHYSIOLOGY

# WHAT HAPPENS IN ORGANOPHOSPHATE AND CARBAMATE POISONING

Organophosphates and carbamates are widely used insecticides, pesticides, and herbicides that can also poison humans. Both are rapidly absorbed through the skin, eyes, and respiratory and GI systems. Farm workers are most commonly exposed, but children sometimes accidentally ingest these substances (pets' flea and tick poisoning collars and solutions are typical sources). Deliberate ingestion is a rarely employed method of attempting suicide.

Both these substances are powerful cholinesterase inhibitors. As you may recall, the body needs the enzyme acetylcholinesterase to break down acetylcholine (ACh)—the important chemical neurotransmitter at the myoneural junction that controls normal muscle contractions. When an organophosphate or carbamate binds its phosphate radical to acetylcholinesterase, inactivating it, ACh accumulates at the myoneural junction. The overabundance of ACh first enhances, then paralyzes nerve impulse transmissions across the myoneural junctions. Without treatment, this leads to respiratory paralysis, shock, cardiac arrest, and death.

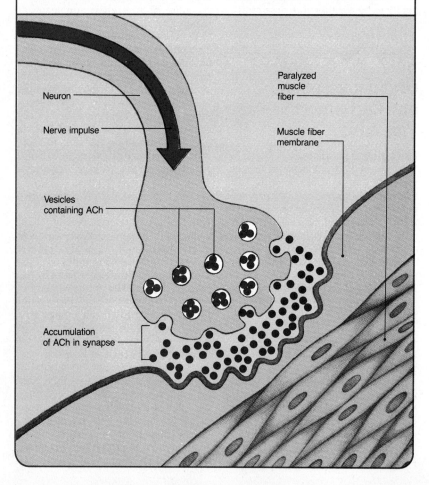

Neuron

Nerve impulse

Vesicles containing ACh

Accumulation of ACh in synapse

Paralyzed muscle fiber

Muscle fiber membrane

reactivate acetylcholinesterase. Expect to give 30 mg/kg by I.V. infusion.

## Continuing assessment and therapeutic care

Check your patient's vital signs frequently, and continue monitoring his heart rate and rhythm. You may note decreasing blood pressure and pulse rate, even heart block, because organophosphates and carbamates slow conduction through the atrioventricular node. Expect to raise your patient's atropine dosage to increase his heart rate. Also expect to begin vasopressor infusion to increase his blood pressure. Place him in a modified Trendelenburg position to increase his vital organ perfusion. If these measures don't increase his heart rate, the doctor may ask you to assist with insertion of a temporary pacemaker. (See *Assisting with Temporary Pacemaker Insertion,* page 191.)

Monitor your patient's acid-base and electrolyte balances by checking his serial ABG and electrolyte levels. Expect to give sodium bicarbonate to correct his acidosis and to replace electrolytes. Check his ABG levels for signs of hypoxemia (decreasing $PO_2$), and give supplemental oxygen, as needed.

You can gauge the success of your patient's atropine therapy by:
• evaluating his salivation response (as the drug takes effect, he should stop salivating excessively)
• observing whether his respirations increase (they should)
• monitoring his heart rate (it should increase to greater than 120 beats/minute)
• checking his pupils (they should become dilated).

As you continue to care for him, be sure to keep his airway patent and to monitor his respiratory status carefully. Auscultate his lungs for rales, and watch for dyspnea, tachypnea, or frothy sputum—possibly indicating pulmonary edema. (If he develops pulmonary edema, expect to give him a diuretic.) Poisoning by organophosphate or carbamate weakens intercostal muscles, so your patient may develop inadequate respirations, even respiratory paralysis. To detect this serious complication as early as possible, measure his tidal volume, vital capacity, and respiratory rate frequently. If atropine therapy doesn't increase his respirations, be prepared to assist with intubation and mechanical ventilation. The doctor may also increase your patient's atropine dosage.

Assess your patient's neurologic status—especially his level of consciousness—hourly. Expect improvement in this area and in his muscle tone; if he isn't improving, the atropine therapy may not be effective. You may see muscle fasciculations and twitching over your patient's cheeks, chest, and upper arms. If these are especially severe, or don't improve with therapy, the doctor may order an EEG to differentiate between fasciculations and possible seizure activity. (If your patient has seizures, expect to give him an anticonvulsant, such as diazepam [Valium] I.V.) The poison may also affect your patient's hypothalamus, causing alterations in his body temperature. The doctor may ask you to place him on a hypo- or hyperthermia blanket to correct his fever or subnormal temperature. Temperature changes may make him more susceptible to bed sores, so reposition him every 1 to 2 hours. Massage his back and pressure points vigorously, using a moisturizing lotion, to stimulate his circulation and to retard skin breakdown.

# Plant Poisoning

## Initial care summary

The patient had a history of ingesting a poisonous plant. Initial assessment findings included some combination of these signs and symptoms:
• severe irritation or a burning sensation in his mouth and throat

## NURSE'S GUIDE TO POISONOUS PLANTS

### PLANT
**Cherry (pits)**

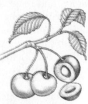

### PLANT
**Dumb cane
(Dieffenbachia)(all parts)**

### PLANT
**English ivy (all parts)**

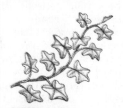

### SIGNS AND SYMPTOMS

- Shortness of breath
- Vocal cord paralysis
- Muscle twitching
- Weakness
- Seizures
- Stupor
- Coma

### SIGNS AND SYMPTOMS

- Tongue and throat swelling, excessive saliva-tion, dysphagia
- Blistering and burning of mucous membranes
- Vocal cord paralysis
- Nausea, vomiting, diarrhea

### SIGNS AND SYMPTOMS

- Nausea, vomiting, diarrhea
- Abdominal pain
- Dyspnea
- Excessive salvation
- Coma
- Skin irritation

### ASSESSMENT AND INTERVENTION

- Maintain an open airway Induce vomiting or per-form gastric lavage, as ordered.
- Watch for signs of cyanide poisoning and use the cyanide antidote kit, if necessary. (This is also true with apricot and peach pits.)
- Give oxygen by nasal cannula or mask.
- Give I.V. fluids and blood transfusions, as ordered, to correct shock.
- Administer phenytoin (Dilantin) and diazepam (Valium), as ordered, to control seizures.

### ASSESSMENT AND INTERVENTION

- Be especially alert for airway obstruction; maintain an open airway.
- Induce vomiting or perform gastric lavage, as ordered, if your patient doesn't have blisters.
- Administer activated charcoal and a cathartic, as ordered.
- Apply cold packs to his lips and mouth to reduce swelling and pain.
- Give a demulcent, such as milk or milk of magne-sia, as ordered, to soothe irritated mucous mem-branes.
- Administer an antihista-mine and epinephrine, as ordered.
- Administer an antiemetic (such as chlorpromazine) and an antidiarrheal, as ordered, if vomiting and diarrhea persist.

### ASSESSMENT AND INTERVENTION

- Perform gastric lavage, as ordered.
- Administer activated charcoal and a cathartic, as ordered.
- Give oxygen by nasal cannula or mask.
- Be prepared to provide artificial respiration, if needed.
- Give an antidiarrheal and an antiemetic, as or-dered, to control persis-tent diarrhea and vomiting.

## PLANT
**Holly (berries and leaves)**

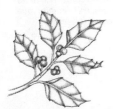

## SIGNS AND SYMPTOMS

• Nausea, vomiting, and diarrhea
• Inflammation and numbing sensation in the mouth
• Stupor
• Convulsions
• Coma

## ASSESSMENT AND INTERVENTION

• Induce vomiting or perform gastric lavage, as ordered.
• Give activated charcoal and a cathartic, as ordered.
• Give oxygen by nasal cannula or mask.
• Give an antiemetic and an antidiarrheal, as ordered, to control persistent vomiting and diarrhea.
• Give an anticonvulsant, as ordered, to control seizures.

## PLANT
**Jimsonweed (thorn apple) (all parts)**

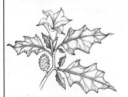

## SIGNS AND SYMPTOMS

• Intense thirst and dry mouth
• Dry, flushed skin
• Dilated pupils
• Headache, hallucinations, delirium, coma
• Convulsions
• Tachycardia
• Hypertension
• Bradypnea
• Fever
• Urinary retention
• Decreased bowel activity

## ASSESSMENT AND INTERVENTION

• Induce vomiting or perform gastric lavage, as ordered.
• Give activated charcoal and a cathartic, as ordered.
• Give oxygen by nasal cannula or face mask.
• Give physostigmine, as ordered, to reverse the symptoms.
• Give an anticonvulsant, such as diazepam or phenytoin, as ordered, to control seizures.
• Give an antipyretic or apply cool, wet packs or a hypothermia blanket, as ordered, to lower the patient's temperature.
• Give pilocarpine eye drops, as ordered, to ease the pupil dilation.
• Place the patient in a quiet room with low lighting, to reduce stimulation.

## PLANT
**Lily of the valley (all parts)**

## SIGNS AND SYMPTOMS

• GI distress
• Dysrhythmias

## ASSESSMENT AND INTERVENTION

• Induce vomiting or perform gastric lavage, as ordered.
• Give activated charcoal and a cathartic, as ordered.
• Give procainamide, quinidine sulfate, or phenytoin, as ordered, to correct dysrhythmias.
• Give atropine, as ordered, to correct severe bradycardia.
• Give sodium polystyrene sulfate (Kayexalate), as ordered, or prepare for hemoperfusion, to correct hyperkalemia.
• If poisoning is severe, anticipate electrical pacing of the heart.

*(continued)*

## NURSE'S GUIDE TO POISONOUS PLANTS *(continued)*

### PLANT

**Mistletoe (berries)**

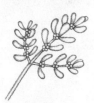

### PLANT

**Mushrooms—Amanita species (*Amanita phalloides*) (all parts)**

### PLANT

**Mushrooms—Amanita species (*Amanita muscaria*) (all parts)**

### SIGNS AND SYMPTOMS

- Severe nausea, vomiting, and diarrhea
- Dyspnea
- Bradycardia
- Cardiovascular collapse
- Delirium, hallucinations
- Coma

### SIGNS AND SYMPTOMS

*6 to 24 hours after ingestion:*
- Sudden onset of severe, colicky, abdominal cramps
- Nausea, vomiting, and bloody diarrhea
- Elevated liver enzymes and bilirubin
- Signs of recovery, followed by hepatic failure, cardiac failure, renal failure, diffuse intravascular coagulation, or convulsions.

### SIGNS AND SYMPTOMS

*2 to 10 hours after ingestion:*
- Stomach cramps
- Vomiting
- Diarrhea
- Dyspnea
- Bradycardia
- Hypotension
- Excessive salivation, tearing, sweating, and pupil contraction
- Hallucinations, delirium, coma

### ASSESSMENT AND INTERVENTION

- Induce vomiting or perform gastric lavage.
- Give activated charcoal and a cathartic.
- Give oxygen by nasal cannula or mask for respiratory distress.
- Give potassium procainamide or quinidine sulfate, as ordered.

### ASSESSMENT AND INTERVENTION

- Induce vomiting with syrup of ipecac; follow with copious amounts of fluid.
- Perform gastric lavage.
- Administer activated charcoal and a saline cathartic, such as sodium sulfate or magnesium sulfate, if needed.
- Give I.V. penicillin, as ordered, to interfere with the toxin's binding to albumin and to enhance renal excretion.
- Give the antidote—thiotic acid I.V.—if available.
- Institute forced diuresis, as ordered, to enhance excretion.
- Prepare for hemodialysis or hemoperfusion, as ordered.

### ASSESSMENT AND INTERVENTION

- Induce vomiting with syrup of ipecac, as ordered.
- Perform gastric lavage, as ordered.
- Administer activated charcoal and a saline cathartic, as ordered.
- Give atropine or physostigmine, as ordered, to reverse the signs and symptoms.

## PLANT

**Potatoes (tubercles)**

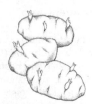

### SIGNS AND SYMPTOMS

- Severe abdominal pain
- Nausea and vomiting
- Diarrhea
- Respiratory depression
- Cold, clammy skin
- Headache
- Progressive weakness
- Paralysis

### ASSESSMENT AND INTERVENTION

- Induce vomiting or perform gastric lavage, as ordered.
- Give activated charcoal and a cathartic, as ordered.
- Give oxygen by nasal cannula or mask for respiratory distress.
- Give an anticonvulsant, such as diazepam or phenytoin, as ordered, to control seizures.
- Perform CPR, if necessary.

## PLANT

**Rhododendron (all parts)**

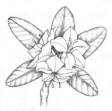

### SIGNS AND SYMPTOMS

- Vomiting
- Increased salivation
- Tearing
- Nasal discharge
- Dyspnea
- Bradycardia
- Hypotension
- Convulsions
- Muscle weakness progressing to paralysis

### ASSESSMENT AND INTERVENTION

- Induce vomiting or perform gastric lavage, as ordered.
- Give activated charcoal and a cathartic, as ordered.
- Give oxygen by nasal cannula or mask.
- Administer atropine, as ordered, to treat bradycardia.
- Administer an anticonvulsant, as ordered, to control seizures.

## PLANT

**Rhubarb (leaves)**

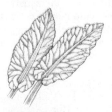

### SIGNS AND SYMPTOMS

- Burning of mouth and throat
- Increased salivation
- Tearing
- Nasal discharge
- Severe intermittent abdominal pain
- Nausea and vomiting
- Dyspnea
- Muscle weakness, cramps, and tetany
- Renal failure, anuria
- Convulsions, coma

### ASSESSMENT AND INTERVENTION

- Induce vomiting with syrup of ipecac or perform gastric lavage, as ordered, with lime water, chalk, or calcium salts to neutralize the toxin.
- Give oxygen by nasal cannula or mask for respiratory distress.
- Administer calcium gluconate, as ordered, to correct hypocalcemia.
- Infuse fluids rapidly, as ordered.

- edema of his mouth and throat
- GI distress
- central and peripheral anticholinergic effects (for example, hallucinations, dilated pupils, hypertension, dry and flushed skin, or urinary retention)
- parasympathomimetic effects (for example, bradycardia, hypotension, constricted pupils, excessive salivation, or involuntary urination or defecation)
- signs of respiratory distress
- signs of CNS depression (for example, decreased level of consciousness) or stimulation (for example, seizure activity).

In addition, the patient may have had signs and symptoms specific to the type of plant he ingested (see *Nurse's Guide to Poisonous Plants,* pages 770 to 773).

A large-bore I.V. catheter was inserted, to replace fluids and electrolytes and to administer medications. If edema was occluding the patient's airway, an artificial airway was inserted. Supplemental oxygen was given if the patient showed signs of respiratory distress. The patient was connected to a cardiac monitor, and a 12-lead EKG was taken. Samples of urine, blood, and vomitus were obtained for toxicology screening to identify the poison contained in the ingested plant. If possible, a sample of the suspected plant was obtained for identification.

Vomiting was induced if the patient was awake and alert; if he wasn't, gastric lavage was performed. (Depending on what plant the patient ingested, a special lavage fluid may have been used. See *Nurse's Guide to Poisonous Plants,* pages 770 to 773.) Activated charcoal and a cathartic were given to help adsorb and eliminate the toxin.

### Priorities
Your first priority is to reassess your patient's airway, breathing, and circulation. Remember, his status can change quickly at any time as his body metabolizes the poison. Keep suction equipment, airway equipment, and oxygen nearby, and be prepared to use them promptly. If he shows signs and symptoms of shock, place him in a modified Trendelenburg position and increase his fluid infusion rate, as ordered. Expect to give a vasopressor for persistent hypotension or shock.

### Continuing assessment and therapeutic care
Gather thorough, accurate information about the poisoning. What plant did the patient ingest? If he isn't sure and hasn't brought a sample with him, ask him to describe how it looked and tasted. How much time has passed since he ingested the plant? When did he first notice his signs and symptoms? Remember, you can call the local Poison Control Center with a description of the suspected plant and the patient's history information. They'll identify the plant over the phone and describe the proper interventions. Does he have any allergies or chronic diseases? Is he taking any medications? Use the answers to these questions to guide your assessments and interventions.

All plant poisonings require symptomatic and supportive treatment, depending on the type of plant ingested and the body systems affected. Perform a general nursing assessment of your patient's condition. Then, use the *Nurse's Guide to Poisonous Plants* on pages 770 to 773 to evaluate your findings. Expect to perform some or all of the interventions described.

# Cyanide Poisoning

### Initial care summary
The patient had a history of cyanide exposure, ingestion, or inhalation and some or all of these signs and symptoms:
- bitter-almond breath odor
- dyspnea
- shallow respirations and slow respiratory rate
- headache
- dizziness

# WHAT HAPPENS IN CYANIDE POISONING

Cyanide's one of the fastest and deadliest poisons known, especially in the form of hydrocyanic acid (hydrogen cyanide) or its potassium and sodium salts. Inhalation of this bitter, almond-scented gas, or ingestion of cyanide pellets, can lead to death within minutes.

In spite of its risks, hydrogen cyanide and its derivatives are commonly used in industry and medicine. Sodium nitroprusside, a cyanide derivative, is used to treat patients with hypertensive crisis and to create a bloodless field for brain surgery. Cyanide's also found in the home in silver polishes, pesticides, almonds, and seeds from apples, peaches, plums, and cherries. It has claimed many lives due to accidental poisonings.

Cyanide prohibits the cells from using oxygen. This causes hypoxia, loss of consciousness, and muscular paralysis, which lead to respiratory and cardiac failure. The patient may die quickly after he's exposed to cyanide, or he may live for several hours if the cyanide's erratically absorbed. But no matter how slowly this poison's absorbed, the patient will die without prompt treatment. You can see what happens in this chart.

**Cyanide's ingested or inhaled.**

Skin, mucous membranes, GI tract, or lungs absorb cyanide rapidly.

Cyanide swiftly penetrates the cells and binds with the iron component of cytochrome oxidase.

Cellular oxygen transport's inhibited.

Cellular respiration's inhibited.

Cellular anoxia occurs.

Tissue hypoxia develops with an inability to regenerate adenosine triphosphate.

Loss of consciousness occurs.

Seizures occur.

Muscular paralysis ensues.

Respiratory failure and arrest develop.

Cardiac arrest occurs.

**DEATH**

- nausea
- bright red venous blood
- decreased level of consciousness
- eye protrusion
- pupil dilation
- seizures
- distended bladder.

Based on the patient's combination of signs and symptoms, the doctor immediately suspected cyanide poisoning. Because death can occur within 1 to 15 minutes of inhaling or ingesting cyanide, the doctor ordered the antidote to be administered immediately.

### Priorities

Administer the antidote, as ordered. If the patient's *receiving supplemental oxygen* through a nasal cannula or mask, remove this device and continue oxygen administration through an Ambu bag to provide access for the antidote. Place the amyl nitrite pearls in a gauze pad, crush them, and hold them over the air inlet of the Ambu bag, without interrupting ventilation. If the patient's *not receiving supplemental oxygen*, hold the crushed amyl nitrite pearls under his nose. As you're doing this, blood will be drawn for a cyanate level, CBC, electrolytes, serum glucose, BUN, and ABGs. Another nurse will start an I.V., draw sodium nitrite into a syringe, and infuse it slowly over the next 2 minutes. The nitrite solution will combine with your patient's hemoglobin to form methemoglobin—a cyanide binder. After the I.V. administration is complete, discontinue the amyl nitrite inhalation and administer sodium thiosulfate I.V. through the same needle and vein. The sodium thiosulfate will break down the methemoglobin-cyanide complex into thiocyanate. As you may know, this cyanate is nontoxic and easily excreted by the kidneys.

If the patient *ingested* the cyanide, the doctor will also order a gastric lavage. Expect to perform gastric lavage with a 1:5,000 solution of potassium permanganate. Then, administer charcoal and a saline cathartic. If his *skin and/or clothing were contaminated* with cyanide, remove his clothing and cleanse his skin with soap and water to arrest percutaneous absorption of the poison.

### Continuing assessment and therapeutic care

After you've administered the cyanide antidotes, monitor your patient's respiratory status closely. *His condition may deteriorate suddenly,* so be prepared to intervene immediately: keep an artificial airway, intubation equipment, an Ambu bag, and suction equipment nearby. Monitor his ABG levels for signs of hypoxia, and provide supplemental oxygen as necessary. Listen to his lungs often; if you hear rales and note dyspnea or tachypnea, your patient may have pulmonary edema. Inform the doctor of your findings. He may order:

- a chest X-ray
- intubation and mechanical ventilation with positive end-expiratory pressure (PEEP).

Insert an indwelling (Foley) catheter, as ordered, to prevent or relieve the urinary retention that often accompanies cyanide poisoning. Monitor your patient's fluid and electrolyte balances by recording his hourly urine output and by checking his serial electrolyte levels. Replace sodium and potassium, as indicated.

Connect your patient to a cardiac monitor and check his vital signs frequently. You may note hypotension, possibly from circulatory collapse. Expect to administer a vasopressor, such as dopamine or dobutamine, and to increase your patient's I.V. fluid infusion rate—as ordered—to stabilize his hemodynamic status. You may also see dysrhythmias, such as PVCs. If PVCs occur frequently, expect to give your patient a bolus of lidocaine followed by a continuous infusion of this drug. The doctor will order *immediate* blood tests to measure the patient's ABG and electrolyte levels; this will help him determine whether the dysrhythmias are due to hypoxia or to an electrolyte imbalance.

Perform a neurologic assessment every hour. Watch your patient closely for these signs and symptoms of cerebral edema:
- severe headache
- disturbances in vision
- widened pulse pressure
- changes in level of consciousness.

If you note any of these signs or symptoms, tell the doctor. He'll order a CT scan and ask you to administer an osmotic diuretic (Mannitol) if your patient isn't already receiving one. If your patient's on a mechanical ventilator, expect to make adjustments to reduce his $PCO_2$. (See the "Increased Intracranial Pressure" entry in Chapter 6.)

Throughout your continuing assessment, keep a fresh cyanide antidote kit nearby. If your patient doesn't improve with the initial dose, or if his vital signs deteriorate, expect to readminister the antidote—giving half the initial dose.

# Caustic Substance Poisoning

## Initial care summary

The patient had a history of ingesting a caustic substance, such as a drain cleaner or a household cleaning agent. Initial assessment revealed some combination of the following signs and symptoms:
- a burning sensation in his oral cavity, pharynx, and esophageal area
- painful swallowing (dysphagia)
- respiratory distress (dyspnea, stridor, tachypnea, and hoarseness)
- soapy-white mucous membranes
- oral ulcerations and/or blisters.

If the suspected caustic substance was a strong *acid*, he may also have had:
- signs of gastric perforation (abdominal pain and rigidity, hypoactive or absent bowel sounds, nausea or vomiting, and hematemesis)
- signs of circulatory collapse (clammy skin, weak but rapid pulse, shallow respirations, and oliguria).

Or, if the suspected caustic substance was a strong *alkali,* he may also have had:
- signs of esophageal perforation (crepitation, from subcutaneous emphysema, and chest pain).

If the patient's a child, he probably showed signs of discomfort, such as pulling at his mouth with his fingers, excessive drooling, crying as if in pain, and refusing to drink or suck.

The patient was given milk to dilute the caustic substance. An I.V. was inserted to administer fluid and medication. If the patient showed signs of circulatory collapse or shock, an indwelling (Foley) catheter was also inserted to monitor his output. Chest X-rays were taken. Blood was drawn for a CBC and for ABG, electrolyte, BUN, creatinine, and blood glucose levels.

If your patient ingested an acid and showed no signs of oral or esophageal erosion, his gastric contents were aspirated through an NG tube; then gastric lavage was performed with large volumes of saline or cold water. (Gastric lavage is *contraindicated* for a patient who's swallowed an alkali.)

## Priorities

Your first priority is to reassess your patient's respiratory status, intervening as necessary. You should be aware that inhalation of *acidic* fumes sets off a chemical reaction in the lungs that can quickly lead to chemical pneumonitis, and ingestion of an *alkali* can severely damage the epiglottis and cause edema that may block the patient's airway. Keep oxygen, emergency airway equipment, and suction devices nearby for immediate use, if needed. If your patient develops severe edema that blocks passage of an endotracheal tube, the doctor may perform a tracheotomy.

Expect to administer broad-spectrum antibiotics, such as ampicillin, to prevent infection of the damaged mucosa. If he swallowed an acid, you'll

PATHOPHYSIOLOGY

# WHAT HAPPENS IN CAUSTIC SUBSTANCE INGESTION

The typical victim of caustic substance ingestion is a child who's accidentally swallowed a household cleanser. But adults attempting suicide also may ingest caustic substances. Both types—acids and alkalis—can cause serious injury, depending on the type, concentration, and quantity ingested. The duration of tissue contact and the individual's tissue resistance also play a part. The chart below shows you the effects of ingesting various caustic substances.

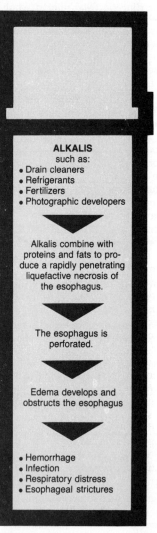

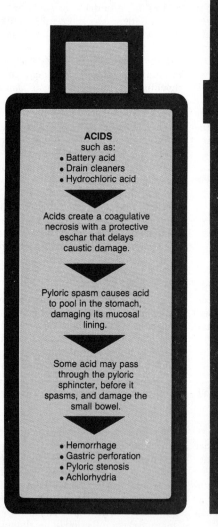

**ACIDS**
such as:
- Battery acid
- Drain cleaners
- Hydrochloric acid

Acids create a coagulative necrosis with a protective eschar that delays caustic damage.

Pyloric spasm causes acid to pool in the stomach, damaging its mucosal lining.

Some acid may pass through the pyloric sphincter, before it spasms, and damage the small bowel.

- Hemorrhage
- Gastric perforation
- Pyloric stenosis
- Achlorhydria

**ALKALIS**
such as:
- Drain cleaners
- Refrigerants
- Fertilizers
- Photographic developers

Alkalis combine with proteins and fats to produce a rapidly penetrating liquefactive necrosis of the esophagus.

The esophagus is perforated.

Edema develops and obstructs the esophagus

- Hemorrhage
- Infection
- Respiratory distress
- Esophageal strictures

also give him an antacid (Maalox, for example, through an NG tube). The antacid will neutralize the acid in his stomach and help prevent erosion of the mucosal lining.

## Continuing assessment and therapeutic care

Continue to give your patient respiratory and circulatory support. Auscultate his lungs frequently, and monitor his ABGs for signs of hypoxemia. Give him oxygen as needed. If he shows signs of circulatory collapse, monitor his vital signs and output often, and be alert for signs of shock. Give him a vasopressor, as ordered, increase his I.V. fluid infusion rate, and monitor his intake and output carefully afterward—to evaluate his fluid balance.

The doctor will perform an endoscopy to reveal the extent of injury. If the patient swallowed an *alkali,* the doctor will perform an esophagoscopy; if the patient swallowed an *acid,* the doctor will perform an esophagogastroscopy.

Prior to endoscopy, give your patient nothing by mouth. After endoscopy, the doctor will order a barium swallow to serve as a baseline and to give further information about the extent and severity of the patient's injury. If the endoscopy or barium swallow reveals necrosis, prepare him for immediate surgery to resect the necrotic segment and to anastomose healthy tissue.

For a patient who swallowed an *alkali,* expect to give corticosteroids to prevent scarring and stricture formation. Assess him for dyspnea, excessive salivation, or decreased respirations; these signs may indicate that stricture's already occurred. If so, the doctor will perform gentle retrograde dilation (bougienage) to maintain patency of the patient's airway so he won't need future resections to correct stricture formation.

If your patient swallowed an *acid,* be alert for signs of metabolic acidosis, especially if he swallowed a formaldehyde acid. Monitor his serial ABGs

and total carbon dioxide content. If he develops acidosis, expect to give him sodium bicarbonate I.V. Monitor his renal function by checking his serial BUN and creatinine results and his intake and output record. An increase in BUN and creatinine levels together with a decrease in output below 30 ml/ hour may indicate acute renal failure. (See the "Acute Renal Failure" entry in Chapter 13.) If your patient has acute renal failure, be sure to monitor his acid-base balance closely: his kidneys won't be able to produce sodium bicarbonate, which could make his metabolic acidosis worse.

Examine your patient's abdomen frequently if he swallowed an *acid,* and be on the alert for abdominal tenderness and rigidity and for hypoactive or absent bowel sounds. If you note any of these signs and your patient complains of nausea or vomiting, he may have developed peritonitis. (See *Danger: Peritonitis,* page 332). Call the doctor *immediately*—peritonitis may signal gastric perforation, and your patient may need emergency surgery.

Give your patient total parenteral nutrition, as ordered, until he's able to tolerate oral liquids. (If he swallowed an *alkali* and has severe stricture formation, you may have to feed him through a gastrostomy tube.) During each assessment, test his ability to swallow; this should improve as his edema decreases.

# Botulism and Salmonellosis

## Initial care summary

The patient, on initial assessment (and depending on the severity of his illness), had some of these signs and symptoms indicating botulism or salmonellosis:

- nausea and vomiting
- diarrhea or constipation

PATHOPHYSIOLOGY

## WHAT HAPPENS IN BOTULISM

Botulism occurs when a spore-forming anaerobic bacillus, called *Clostridium botulinum*, releases one of the world's most potent toxins. The toxins themselves are antigens, but the body develops no immunity to them because the *lethal* dose is *less* than the amount required to produce antibodies. Seven immunologically different types of botulism toxin exist, but three types—A, B, and E—are the most common.

The most common cause of botulism is improperly canned food, especially home-preserved vegetables. Spores are also found in the soil and in certain foods—such as honey. These can cause botulism through deep-wound contamination or through ingestion. (In an infant, this leads to the so-called floppy infant syndrome.) Because botulism's a rare but typically fatal disease, you must report *all* cases to the Centers for Disease Control in Georgia.

After a person ingests *C. botulinum*, this organism releases a toxin that's absorbed by the upper GI tract. The toxin prevents acetylcholine's release at the myoneural junctions, which causes muscular and respiratory paralysis. Without prompt treatment, respiratory arrest and death will follow.

- abdominal cramping and tenderness
- subnormal body temperature
- weakness, lethargy, dizziness
- headache
- blurred vision
- dilated pupils
- a dry, sore throat with hoarseness
- impaired speech
- dyspnea
- muscle paresis or paralysis in arms, legs, or trunk
- progressive muscle palsies

If the patient's an infant, he probably showed signs of hypotonic (floppy) infant syndrome: constipation, depressed gag reflex, inability to suck, and loss of head control.

A history of the patient's food intake during the previous week was obtained, and it revealed ingestion of contaminated water or improperly processed foods. A fresh stool sample, a urine specimen, and, if possible, samples of the suspected food and the patient's gastric contents were obtained for laboratory examination to identify the circulating toxin. Blood was drawn for a toxin assay, ABGs, electrolytes, and osmolarity studies. Culture specimens isolated either the bacterial organism *Salmonella* if the patient had salmonellosis or *Clostridium botulinum* if the patient had botulism. Vomiting was induced if the patient's level of consciousness was adequate and he showed no evidence of seizure activity. Otherwise, gastric lavage was performed. If several hours had elapsed since the patient ate the food that made him ill, a cathartic—such as sodium sulfate or magnesium sulfate—was administered. An I.V. was started to replace lost fluids and to administer medications.

### Priorities

If culture results reveal that your patient has *botulism*, expect to administer equine botulism antitoxin I.V. to neutralize circulating toxin. You may also be asked to give guanidine hydrochloride to bind the toxin and to stop it from being released into the patient's systemic circulation. You'll also need to begin fluid and electrolyte replacements. If your patient has infant botulism or wound botulism, you may give penicillin, as well.

Because the botulism antitoxin is derived from horse serum, be sure to obtain an accurate history of the patient's allergies and to perform a hypersensitivity skin test. (If your patient's allergic to the antitoxin, the doctor may order hydrocortisone to desensitize him.) After administering the antitoxin to your patient, be alert for facial swelling, flushed complexion, rashes, pruritus, stridor, or wheezing: these signs may indicate anaphylaxis, other hypersensitivity, or serum sickness. Keep epinephrine 1:1,000 and emergency airway equipment nearby. If your patient develops a hypersensitivity reaction, inform the doctor *immediately,* and be ready to intervene as needed.

If your patient has *salmonellosis,* your first priority is to begin supportive care. Why? Because salmonellosis is self-limiting. It usually resolves within 2 to 5 days and rarely results in death. Start replacing fluid and electrolytes, as ordered, to correct your patient's dehydration and to restore his electrolyte balance.

After you've stabilized your patient, report the emergency to the Centers for Disease Control.

### Continuing assessment and therapeutic care

Monitor your patient's fluid and electrolyte balances by recording his hourly intake and output and the results of his serial blood tests. Continue to replace fluid and electrolytes as indicated, and check his vital signs frequently to detect whether his body temperature's returning to normal. If your patient has *salmonellosis,* he can return home after his hemodynamic status is stabilized.

You'll continue to assess and care for the patient with *botulism,* however. Because respiratory paralysis poses the greatest threat to your patient's life, assess his respiratory status carefully and often. Turn him every 1 to 2 hours, and encourage deep breathing exercises to prevent atelectasis. If he has difficulty swallowing, continue to suction his oropharyngeal secretions before they can accumulate; this will help to prevent aspiration pneumonia. (If your patient develops pneumonia, culture his sputum and expect to administer antibiotics, as ordered.)

If your patient shows hypoxemia, hypercapnia, or a vital capacity of less than 1,000 ml, provide supplemental oxygen and be prepared to assist with intubation and mechanical ventilation, if necessary. If he continues to have difficulty breathing or swallowing and his serial ABG levels and vital capacity decrease despite ventilatory assistance,

call the doctor *immediately.* He may perform a tracheotomy and start your patient on a volume respirator. However, to evaluate the patient's unassisted respiratory function, the doctor may ask you to check the patient's ABG levels periodically and to measure his vital capacity at regular intervals *off* ventilatory support.

Keeping a close watch on your patient's neurologic status is very important. During frequent neurologic assessments, evaluate his bilateral motor status (reflexes and ability to move his arms and legs) and level of consciousness. If his mental status starts to deteriorate, notify the doctor *immediately.* He may ask you to adjust the patient's fluid replacement. If he foresees that the patient may have seizures, he'll probably order a prophylactic anticonvulsant, such as phenytoin sodium (Dilantin).

You may also be asked to give your patient with botulism diphenoxylate hydrochloride with atropine sulfate to help alleviate his abdominal cramps and diarrhea. But because diarrhea helps rid the patient's body of the toxin, don't expect to give an antidiarrheal during the first 24 hours. Instead, give a mild sedative, such as chloral hydrate, to ease your patient's discomfort.

# Substance Abuse

### Initial care summary

The patient had a history of substance abuse and initially had some of the following signs and symptoms:
- signs of CNS depression (ranging from lethargy to coma)
- signs of CNS stimulation (ranging from euphoria to assaultive behavior)
- hallucinations
- respiratory depression
- seizure activity
- abnormal pupillary size and response
- nausea and vomiting.

# CASE IN POINT:
# FAILURE TO RESTRAIN A PATIENT

Tony Peterson, age 27, arrived in the ED after overdosing on phencyclidine (PCP). The emergency medical technician warned you that Tony was violent en route to the ED, but now, during your assessment, Tony seems calm and in control. After charting his signs and symptoms, you prepare restraints, but Tony convinces you not to use them. Against your better judgment, you leave the restraints tied to the bed frame and move on to your next patient. Within a few minutes, Tony again becomes violent: he starts screaming, knocking over chairs—acting totally irrational. During his fit of rage, Tony sustains a laceration on his face that may leave a permanent scar. When he recovers from the incident, he sues you and the hospital for negligence. Are you liable? Consider this:

*Methodist Hospital v. Knight* (1969) involved a nurse caring for an elderly patient who suddenly became extremely violent; in a struggle with a hospital assistant, the patient's hip was fractured. The court reasoned that the nurse's failure to anticipate a violent reaction from a confused postsurgical patient, and her failure to apply restraints, caused the patient's injuries. The court found the nurse negligent.

To avert legal consequences related to using restraints, follow these guidelines:
• During a patient's acute reaction to—or withdrawal from—a drug overdose, apply restraints judiciously to ensure his safety.
• Although many hospitals' policies require a doctor's order to apply restraints, you may temporarily restrain a patient in an emergency or when you suspect his condition will lead to violent behavior. If you do this, be sure to obtain a doctor's written order afterward.
• Assess and record the patient's condition and behavior that prompted your decision to restrain him. Be sure you also record the time you applied and/or removed the restraints and the type of restraints you used.
• Before you administer sedatives or tranquilizers to a violent patient, make sure he's adequately restrained.
• Once you've applied restraints, you're liable for any injuries the restraints may cause. Use only reasonable force to restrain the patient, and check him often to make sure he doesn't work his way out of the restraints or strangle himself. Reassess him frequently for signs of impaired circulation and skin irritation.

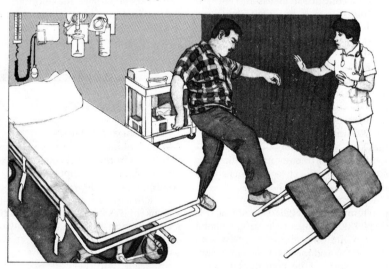

*Methodist Hospital v. Knight,* 1969 CCH Neg. 4571 (Tenn.)

In addition, the patient may have had signs and symptoms specific to the abused substance (see *Nurse's Guide to Commonly Abused Substances,* pages 784 to 789).

If the patient was unconscious, a large-bore I.V. catheter was inserted to replace fluids and to administer $D_{50}W$ and thiamine. Naloxone (Narcan) was also given to reverse the abused substance's narcotic effects. (The I.V. was secured in place with an armboard and gauze to prevent the patient from dislodging it.) If the patient showed signs of respiratory depression, he was given oxygen via a nasal cannula, mask, or intubation and mechanical ventilation. The patient was attached to a cardiac monitor, and a 12-lead EKG was taken. Samples of his urine, blood, and vomitus (if any) were obtained for toxicology screening. Restraints may have been applied to prevent the patient from harming himself.

If the patient ingested the abused substance, his gastric contents were emptied by induced vomiting or by gastric lavage. Activated charcoal and a cathartic were administered to help adsorb the substance and to speed its elimination through the patient's GI tract.

### Priorities

Because abused substances often cause severe respiratory depression and can have cardiotoxic effects, your first priority is to reassess your patient's airway, breathing, and circulation. Keep oxygen, suction equipment, and emergency airway equipment nearby, and be prepared to intervene *immediately* if his status deteriorates. Be prepared to give CPR, too, if necessary. (See the "Life Support" section in Chapter 3.)

Check his vital signs for possible indications of shock, such as decreased blood pressure and faint, rapid pulse. If he shows signs of shock, place him in a modified Trendelenburg position and start administering a fluid challenge, as ordered, to replace his blood volume and to prevent circulatory collapse. If his blood pressure's still low after volume replacement, you may need to apply medical antishock trousers (a MAST suit) or to give a vasopressor, as ordered.

### Continuing assessment and therapeutic care

After you've stabilized your patient's vital functions, perform a thorough assessment and obtain a detailed history of his substance abuse emergency. If he's suffering from a *drug overdose,* what drug(s) did the patient take, how much, and when? (Remember, he may use a street name to identify the drug. See *Nurse's Guide to Commonly Abused Substances,* pages 784 to 789.) If he has *alcohol poisoning,* did he combine drugs with alcohol? Question the patient's family or friends, or rescue personnel, thoroughly to get a reliable history. You may not be able to get accurate information from the patient because of:

• drug-induced amnesia
• depressed level of consciousness
• deliberate attempts to mislead or misinform (especially with a suicidal patient)
• ignorance about the type of drug taken (a suicidal patient may have taken any drugs he could find, without identifying them first).

For help in identifying the drug your patient took, see *Nurse's Guide to Commonly Abused Substances,* pages 784 to 789. This chart offers guidelines for identifying abused substances according to the signs and symptoms they produce.

You'll get definitive information about the patient's substance abuse emergency after the quantitative results of initial toxicology screening are available—but this may not occur until several hours after you first see him. In the meantime, continue assessing him for possible complications.

Reassess your patient's respiratory status and auscultate his breath sounds frequently. Be alert for dyspnea and tachypnea—signs that may give early

## NURSE'S GUIDE TO COMMONLY ABUSED SUBSTANCES

| SUBSTANCE | SIGNS AND SYMPTOMS | ASSESSMENT AND INTERVENTION |
|---|---|---|
| **Amphetamines**<br>• amphetamine sulfate (Benzedrine)—bennies, greenies, cartwheels<br>• methamphetamine (Methadrin)—speed, meth, crystal<br>• dextroamphetamine sulfate (Dexedrine)—dexies, hearts, oranges | • Dilated reactive pupils<br>• Altered mental status (from confusion to paranoia)<br>• Hallucinations<br>• Tremors and seizure activity<br>• Hyperactive tendon reflexes<br>• Exhaustion<br>• Coma<br>• Dry mouth<br>• Shallow respirations<br>• Tachycardia<br>• Hypertension<br>• Hyperthermia<br>• Diaphoresis | • If the drug was taken orally, induce vomiting or perform gastric lavage; give activated charcoal and a sodium or magnesium sulfate cathartic, as ordered.<br>• Acidify the patient's urine by adding ammonium chloride or ascorbic acid to his I.V. solution, as ordered, to lower his urine pH to 5.<br>• Force diuresis by giving the patient mannitol, as ordered.<br>• Expect to give a short-acting barbiturate, such as pentobarbital, to control stimulant-induced seizure activity.<br>• Restrain the patient to keep him from injuring himself and others—especially if he's paranoid or hallucinating.<br>• Give *haloperidol (Haldol)* I.M., as ordered, to treat agitation or assaultive behavior.<br>• Give an alpha-adrenergic blocking agent, such as *phentolamine (Regitine)*, for hypertension, as ordered.<br>• Watch for cardiac dysrhythmias. Notify the doctor if these develop, and expect to give *propanolol* or *lidocaine* to treat tachydysrhythmias or ventricular dysrhythmias, respectively.<br>• Treat hyperthermia with tepid sponge baths or a hypothermia blanket, as ordered.<br>• Provide a quiet environment to avoid overstimulation.<br>• Be alert for signs and symptoms of withdrawal, such as abdominal tenderness, muscle aches, and long periods of sleep.<br>• Observe suicide precautions, especially if the patient shows signs of withdrawal. |
| **Cocaine**<br>• "free-base"<br>• cocaine hydrochloride | • Dilated pupils<br>• Confusion<br>• Alternating euphoria/apprehension<br>• Hyperexcitability<br>• Visual, auditory, and olfactory hallucinations<br>• Spasms and seizure activity<br>• Coma<br>• Tachypnea<br>• Hyperpnea | • Calm the patient down by talking to him in a quiet room.<br>• If cocaine is ingested, induce vomiting or perform gastric lavage; give activated charcoal followed by a saline cathartic, as ordered.<br>• Give the patient a tepid sponge bath and administer an antipyretic, as ordered, to reduce fever.<br>• Monitor his blood pressure and heart rate. Expect to give *propranolol,* for symptomatic tachycardia.<br>*(continued)* |

| SUBSTANCE | SIGNS AND SYMPTOMS | ASSESSMENT AND INTERVENTION |
|---|---|---|
| **Cocaine**<br>• "free-base"<br>• cocaine hydro-chloride<br>*(continued)* | • Pallor or cyanosis<br>• Respiratory arrest<br>• Tachycardia<br>• Hypertension/hypoten-sion<br>• Fever<br>• Nausea and vomiting<br>• Abdominal pain<br>• Perforated nasal septum or oral sores | • Administer an anticonvulsant, such as *diazepam (Valium),* as ordered, to control seizure activity.<br>• Scrape the inside of his nose to remove residual amounts of the drug.<br>• Monitor his cardiac rate and rhythm—ventricular fibrillation and cardiac standstill can occur as a direct cardio-toxic result of cocaine. Defibrillate and initiate CPR, if indicated. |
| **Hallucinogens**<br>• lysergic acid di-ethylamide (LSD)—hawk, acid, sunshine<br>• mescaline (Peyote)—mese, cactus, big chief | • Dilated pupils<br>• Intensified perceptions<br>• Agitation and anxiety<br>• Synesthesia<br>• Impaired judgment<br>• Hyperactive movement<br>• Flashback experiences<br>• Hallucinations<br>• Depersonalization<br>• Moderately increased blood pressure<br>• Increased heart rate<br>• Fever | • Reorient the patient repeatedly to time, place, and person.<br>• Restrain the patient to protect him from injuring himself and others.<br>• Calm the patient down by talking to him in a quiet room.<br>• If the drug was taken orally, induce vomiting or perform gastric lavage; give charcoal and a cathartic, as ordered.<br>• Give *Valium* I.V., as ordered, to control seizure activity. |
| • phencyclidine (PCP)—angel dust, peace pill, hog | • Blank staring<br>• Nystagmus<br>• Amnesia<br>• Decreased awareness of surroundings<br>• Recurrent coma<br>• Violent behavior<br>• Hyperactivity<br>• Seizure activity<br>• Gait ataxia<br>• Muscle rigidity<br>• Drooling<br>• Hyperthermia<br>• Hypertensive crisis<br>• Cardiac arrest | • If the drug was taken orally, induce vomiting or perform gastric lavage; instill and remove activated charcoal repeatedly, as ordered.<br>• Force acidic diuresis by acidifying the patient's urine with ascorbic acid, as ordered, to increase excretion of the drug.<br>• Give *Valium* and *Haldol*, as ordered, to control agitation or psychotic behavior.<br>• Administer diazepam, as ordered, to control seizure activity.<br>• Expect to continue to acidify his urine for 2 weeks, because signs and symptoms may recur when fat cells release their stores of PCP.<br>• Provide a quiet environment and dimmed light.<br>• Give *propranolol (Inderal)*, as ordered, to treat hypertension and tachycardia. If the patient's hypertension is severe, give nitroprusside, as ordered.<br>• Closely monitor his urine output and serial renal function tests—rhabdomy-olysis, myoglobinuria, and renal failure may occur in severe intoxication.<br>• If the patient develops renal failure, prepare him for hemodialysis. |

*(continued)*

## NURSE'S GUIDE TO COMMONLY ABUSED SUBSTANCES *(continued)*

| SUBSTANCE | SIGNS AND SYMPTOMS | ASSESSMENT AND INTERVENTION |
|---|---|---|
| **Tricyclic anti-depressants**<br>• imipramine hydrochloride (Tofranil)<br>• amitriptyline hydrochloride (Elavil) | • Dilated pupils<br>• Blurred vision<br>• Altered mental status (from agitation to hallucinations)<br>• Loss of deep tendon reflexes<br>• Seizure activity<br>• Coma<br>• Anticholinergic effects (dry mucous membranes, diminished secretions)<br>• Tachycardia<br>• Hypotension<br>• Nausea and vomiting<br>• Urinary retention | • Expect to induce vomiting or perform gastric lavage if the patient ingested the drug within the past 24 hours. (Anticholinergic effects of these drugs decrease gastric emptying.) Give activated charcoal and a magnesium sulfate cathartic, as ordered.<br>• Replace fluids I.V. to correct hypotension, as ordered.<br>• Give *sodium bicarbonate* and *sodium physostigmine* I.V., as ordered, to correct hypotension and dysrhythmias; if bifascicular or complete heart block occurs, assist with insertion of a temporary transvenous pacemaker.<br>• Treat seizure activity with *diazepam* or *phenobarbital* I.V., as ordered. |
| **Alcohol (ethanol)**<br>• beer and wine<br>• distilled spirits<br>• other preparations, such as cough syrup, aftershave, or mouthwash | • Ataxia<br>• Seizure activity<br>• Coma<br>• Hypothermia<br>• Alcohol breath odor<br>• Respiratory depression<br>• Bradycardia<br>• Hypotension<br>• Nausea and vomiting | • Expect to induce vomiting or perform gastric lavage if ingestion occurred in the previous 4 hours. Give activated charcoal and a saline cathartic, as ordered.<br>• Start I.V. fluid replacement and administer dextrose, thiamine, B-complex vitamins, and Vitamin C, as ordered, to prevent dehydration and hypoglycemia and to correct nutritional deficiencies.<br>• Pad bed rails and apply cloth restraints to protect the patient from injury.<br>• Give an anticonvulsant such as diazepam, as ordered, to control seizure activity.<br>• Watch the patient for signs and symptoms of withdrawal, such as hallucinations and delirium tremens. If these occur, give *chlordiazepoxide (Librium), chloral hydrate,* or *paraldehyde,* as ordered. (Be sure to administer paraldehyde with a glass syringe or glass cup to avoid a chemical reaction with plastic.)<br>• Auscultate the patient's lungs frequently to detect rales or rhonchi, possibly indicating aspiration pneumonia. If you note these breath sounds, expect to give antibiotics.<br>• Perform neurologic assessments, and monitor the patient's vital signs every 15 minutes until he's stable.<br>• Assist with dialysis if the patient's vital functions are severely depressed. |

| SUBSTANCE | SIGNS AND SYMPTOMS | ASSESSMENT AND INTERVENTION |
|---|---|---|
| **Barbiturate sedatives/ hypnotics** • barbiturates— downers, sleepers, barbs • amobarbital sodium (Amytal sodium)—blue angels, blue devils, blue birds • phenobarbital (Luminal)— phennies, purple hearts, goofballs • secobarbital sodium (Seconal)—reds, red devils, seccy | • Poor pupil reaction to light • Nystagmus • Depressed level of consciousness (from confusion to coma) • Flaccid muscles and absent reflexes • Hyperthermia or hypothermia • Cyanosis • Respiratory depression • Hypotension • Blisters or bullous lesions | • Induce vomiting or perform gastric lavage if the patient ingested the drug within 4 hours; give activated charcoal and a saline cathartic, as ordered. • Maintain his blood pressure with I.V. fluid challenges and vasopressors, as ordered. • If the patient's taken a phenobarbital overdose, give *sodium bicarbonate* I.V., as ordered, to alkalinize his urine and to speed the drug's elimination. • Apply a hyper- or hypothermia blanket, as ordered, to help return the patient's temperature to normal. • Prepare your patient for hemodialysis or hemoperfusion if toxicity is severe. • Perform frequent neurologic assessments and check your patient's pulse rate, temperature, skin color, and reflexes often. • Notify the doctor if you see signs of respiratory distress or pulmonary edema. • Watch for signs of withdrawal, such as hyperreflexia, grand mal seizures, and hallucinations. • Protect the patient from injuring himself and provide symptomatic relief of withdrawal symptoms, as ordered. |
| **Nonbarbiturate sedatives/ hypnotics** • methaqualone (Quaaludes)— ludes, soapers, love drug | • Dilated pupils • Nystagmus • Disorientation • Slurred speech • Hypertonicity • Ataxia • Twitching and seizure activity • Coma • Dry mouth • Anorexia • Nausea, vomiting, or diarrhea | • Expect to induce vomiting or perform gastric lavage if the patient ingested the drug within the past 2 to 4 hours. Give activated charcoal and a cathartic, as ordered. • Maintain his blood pressure with I.V. fluids and vasopressors, as ordered. • If the patient has severe toxicity, prepare him for hemodialysis or hemoperfusion. • Give *diazepam* initially, as ordered, to treat hypertonicity. If hypertonicity doesn't improve, expect the doctor to give curare and to place the patient on a mechanical ventilator. • Give *diazepam, phenytoin,* or *phenobarbital,* as ordered, to control seizure activity. • Auscultate his lungs frequently. Note rales, rhonchi, or decreased breath sounds, possibly indicating aspiration pneumonia. Give supplemental oxygen |

*(continued)*

### NURSE'S GUIDE TO COMMONLY ABUSED SUBSTANCES *(continued)*

| SUBSTANCE | SIGNS AND SYMPTOMS | ASSESSMENT AND INTERVENTION |
|---|---|---|
| **Nonbarbiturate sedatives/ hypnotics** <br> • methaqualone (Quaaludes)— ludes, soapers, love drug *(continued)* | | and antibiotics, as ordered. <br> • Watch for signs of withdrawal, such as hyperreflexia, grand mal seizures, and hallucinations. <br> • Give *pentobarbital* or *phenobarbital*, as ordered, to treat withdrawal signs and symptoms. |
| • glutethimide (Doriden)—cibas, CD, blues | • Small, reactive pupils <br> • Nystagmus <br> • Drowsiness <br> • Irritability <br> • Impaired thought processes (memory, judgment, attention span) <br> • Slurred speech <br> • Twitching, spasm, and seizure activity <br> • Hypothermia <br> • CNS depression (unresponsive to deep coma) <br> • Apnea <br> • Respiratory depression <br> • Hypotension <br> • Paralytic ileus <br> • Poor bladder control | • If the drug was taken orally, induce vomiting or perform gastric lavage; give activated charcoal and a cathartic, as ordered. <br> • Maintain the patient's blood pressure with I.V. fluid challenges and vasopressors, as ordered. <br> • Assist with hemodialysis or hemoperfusion if the patient has hepatic or renal failure or prolonged coma. <br> • Administer an anticonvulsant, such as *diazepam,* for seizures, as ordered. <br> • Perform hourly neurologic assessments: coma may recur because of the drug's slow release from fat deposits. <br> • Be alert for signs of increased intracranial pressure, such as decreasing level of consciousness and widening pulse pressure. Give *mannitol* I.V., as ordered. <br> • Watch for signs of withdrawal, such as hyperreflexia, grand mal seizures, and hallucinations. <br> • Protect the patient from injuring himself, and provide symptomatic relief of withdrawal symptoms. |
| **Anxiolytic sedative hypnotics** <br> • benzodiazepines (Valium, Librium) | • Confusion <br> • Drowsiness <br> • Stupor <br> • Decreased reflexes <br> • Seizure activity <br> • Coma <br> • Shallow respirations <br> • Hypotension | • Induce vomiting or perform gastric lavage; give activated charcoal and a cathartic, as ordered. <br> • Give supplemental oxygen to correct hypoxia-induced seizure activity. <br> • Administer fluids I.V., as ordered, to correct hypotension; monitor the patient's vital signs frequently. <br> • If the patient's severely intoxicated, give *physostigmine salicylate (Antilirium),* as ordered, to reverse respiratory and CNS depression. |

| SUBSTANCE | SIGNS AND SYMPTOMS | ASSESSMENT AND INTERVENTION |
|---|---|---|
| **Narcotics**<br>• heroin—smack, H, junk, snow<br>• morphine—mort, monkey, M, Miss Emma<br>• hydromorphone hydrochloride (Dilaudid)—D, lords | • Constricted pupils<br>• Depressed level of consciousness (but the patient's usually responsive to persistent verbal or tactile stimuli)<br>• Seizure activity<br>• Hypothermia<br>• Slow, deep respirations<br>• Hypotension<br>• Bradycardia<br>• Skin changes (pruritus, urticaria, and flushed skin) | • Repeat *naloxone (Narcan)* administration, as ordered, until the drug's CNS depressant effects are reversed.<br>• Replace fluids I.V., as ordered, to increase circulatory volume.<br>• Correct hypothermia by applying extra blankets; if the patient's body temperature doesn't increase, use a hyperthermia blanket, as ordered.<br>• Reorient the patient frequently.<br>• Auscultate his lungs frequently for rales, possibly indicating pulmonary edema. (Onset may be delayed.)<br>• Administer oxygen via nasal cannula, mask, or mechanical ventilation to correct hypoxemia from hypoventilation.<br>• Monitor cardiac rate and rhythm, being alert for atrial fibrillation. (This should resolve spontaneously when the hypoxemia's corrected.)<br>• Be alert for signs of withdrawal, such as piloerection (goose flesh), diaphoresis, and hyperactive bowel sounds. |
| **Antipsychotics**<br>• phenothiazines<br>• chlorpromazine (Thorazine)<br>• thioridazine (Mellaril) | • Constricted pupils<br>• Photosensitivity<br>• Extrapyramidal side effects (dyskinesia, opisthotonus, muscular rigidity, ocular deviation)<br>• Dry mouth<br>• Decreased level of consciousness<br>• Decreased deep tendon reflexes<br>• Seizure activity<br>• Hypothermia or hyperthermia<br>• Dysphagia<br>• Respiratory depression<br>• Hypotension<br>• Tachycardia | • Expect to perform gastric lavage if the patient ingested the drug within the past 6 hours. (Don't induce vomiting, because phenothiazines have an antiemetic effect.) Give activated charcoal and a cathartic, as ordered.<br>• Give *diphenhydramine (Benadryl)* or *benztropine (Cogentin)*, as ordered, to treat extrapyramidal side effects.<br>• Give *physostigmine salicylate, as ordered, to reverse the drug's anticholinergic effects in severe cases.*<br>• *Replace fluids I.V., as ordered, to correct hypotension; monitor the patient's vital signs frequently.*<br>• *Monitor his respiratory rate and give supplemental oxygen to treat respiratory depression.*<br>• *Give an anticonvulsant, such as diazepam,* or a short-acting barbiturate, such as *pentobarbital sodium (Nembutal)*, as ordered, to control seizures.<br>• Keep the patient's room dark to avoid exacerbating his photosensitivity. |

warning of impending respiratory complications, such as pulmonary edema or aspiration pneumonia. A patient with rales who's pale, diaphoretic, and gasping for air may have pulmonary edema. A patient with rhonchi or decreased breath sounds probably has aspiration pneumonia. If you detect any of these signs, call the doctor *immediately*. If your patient has pulmonary edema, expect to decrease his I.V. infusion rate and to give him furosemide (Lasix), as ordered. For a patient who has aspiration pneumonia, expect to administer antibiotics and mini-nebulizer treatments to diffuse the medication through his lungs.

Carefully monitor your patient's cardiac rhythm and rate. If you see dysrhythmias, such as ventricular fibrillation or cardiac standstill, be prepared to perform advanced cardiac life-support techniques, including defibrillation and CPR, and to administer such drugs as epinephrine and calcium. (See the "Life Support" section in Chapter 3.) If your patient's not intubated already, expect to assist with endotracheal intubation now. The doctor will probably order propranolol if your patient has tachydysrhythmias, lidocaine if he has frequent PVCs, or atropine if he has bradydysrhythmias.

If your patient's receiving a fluid challenge to correct hypotension, insert an indwelling (Foley) catheter and start monitoring his output hourly. His output and his blood pressure should increase with treatment.

You may detect *hypertension* in a patient who's taken an overdose of a CNS stimulant. If so, expect to treat his hypertension by administering diazoxide (Hyperstat) or phentolamine (Regitine) through an I.V. push.

Your patient's neurologic status will change frequently as his body metabolizes the poison, so perform frequent neurologic assessments. If you note seizure activity, this may be due to the poison's toxic effect on the patient's brain tissue or to hypoxia from poison-induced respiratory depression. To control seizure activity, expect to give diazepam (Valium). If the abused substance affects your patient's temperature-regulating center (hypothalamus), you may note hypo- or hyperthermia. To help return your patient's body temperature to normal, expect to use either extra blankets and a hyperthermia mattress or antipyretics and a hypothermia mattress, as ordered.

Take the appropriate steps to stop further absorption of the abused substances. For example, if your patient's taken cocaine, gently scrape his nostrils to remove any remaining traces of the drug. With other types of substance abuse, you may be asked to begin forced diuresis, to alkalinize or acidify the patient's urine, or to assist with hemodialysis or hemoperfusion. (See *Nurse's Guide to Commonly Abused Substances,* pages 784 to 789.)

Remember: Your patient may be afraid, confused, or disoriented. If his overdose was intentional, he's probably suicidal. As you care for him, do what you can to calm and orient him. Explain the procedures you're performing, using a quiet, reassuring manner of speaking, and keep his environment as nonstressful as possible. (Of course, if your patient's suicidal, observe your hospital's suicide precautions.)

# A FINAL WORD

In the United States, the number of people who suffer toxic effects from poisons or substance abuse and overdose *each year* is estimated at between 2 to 10 million. Of these, about 4,000 die, and many who survive are left with permanently damaged organs, mental capacities, or psychosocial functioning. These are frightening statistics.

Of course, you're doing your part, as an alert and concerned nurse, to stem the tide of this virtual epidemic. And the American Association of Poison Control Centers' hot lines are now available to provide prompt and accurate information for managing poisoning and substance abuse emergencies. Other recently developed aids include:

• *drugs*—Narcotic antagonists, such as naloxone (Narcan), counteract narcotic overdose; nonnarcotic antagonists, such as acetylcysteine (Mucomyst), counteract acetaminophen overdose; pralidoxime chloride (Protopam) acts to reverse the effects of organophosphate poisoning.

• *toxicology screening techniques*— Spot-testing procedures for blood and urine, and thin-layer chromatography for analyzing gaseous or dissolved chemical materials, can help you identify—within minutes instead of hours—the toxic substance a patient's ingested.

All these advances help you provide quicker, better care for a patient with a poisoning or substance abuse emergency. But you should be aware that efforts to *prevent* these emergencies are also under way. For example, data analysis services such as the Drug Abuse Warning Network (DAWN) have been established to study trends in substance abuse. These studies have helped many communities target educational programs related to specific substance abuse problems; the studies have also highlighted ways to prevent occupational injuries and accidental poisonings. So community efforts to combat these types of emergencies are on the rise.

As a nurse, you can contribute to these efforts. For example, you can provide your patients with information on how to "child-proof" their homes by keeping toxic substances out of reach. And you can make sure your patients understand drug dosage instructions and the potential for abuse of prescribed narcotics and other medications. That way, you can help ensure that at least some poisoning and substance abuse emergencies never occur.

## Selected References

Arena, Jay M. "The Treatment of Poisoning," *Clinical Symposia* 30(2):3-47, 1978.

Arnold, Robert E. *Poisonous Plants*. Jeffersontown, Ky.: Terra Publishing, 1978.

*Assessment*. Nurse's Reference Library. Springhouse, Pa.: Springhouse Corp., 1983.

Budassi, Susan A., and Barber, Janet M. *Emergency Nursing: Principles and Practice*. St. Louis: C.V. Mosby Co., 1981.

*Critical Care Quarterly* Issue on Poisonings and Overdose. 4(4): April 1982.

Czajka, Peter A., and Duffy, James P. *Poisoning Emergencies: A Guide for Emergency Medical Personnel*. St. Louis: C.V. Mosby Co., 1980.

*Diagnostics*. Nurse's Reference Library. Springhouse, Pa.: Springhouse Corp., 1983.

Dreisbach, Robert H. *Handbook of Poisoning: Prevention, Diagnosis, and Treatment*, 11th ed. Los Altos, Calif.: Lange Medical Pubns., 1983.

*Drugs*, 2nd ed. Nurse's Reference Library. Springhouse, Pa.: Springhouse Corp., 1984.

Goldfrank, Lewis R., and Kirstein, Robert. *Toxicologic Emergencies: A Comprehensive Handbook in Problem Solving*, 2nd ed. East Norwalk, Conn.: Appelton-Century-Crofts, 1981.

Haddad, Lester M., and Winchester, James F. *Clinical Management of Poisonings and Drug Overdose*. Philadelphia: W.B. Saunders Co., 1983.

Hofmann, Frederick G. *A Handbook on Drug Abuse and Alcohol Abuse: The Biomedical Aspects*, 2nd ed. New York: Oxford University Press, 1983.

*Topics in Emergency Medicine*. Issue on Poisonings and Overdose. 1(3): October 1979.

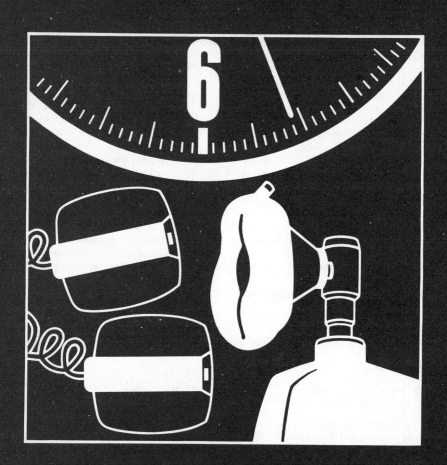

# Appendices
and Index

# Nurse's Guide to Pediatric Emergencies

You know, of course, that a child is not a "small adult"—that, instead, his developing body is uniquely susceptible to numerous disorders. For example, a child's at increased risk for respiratory problems from trauma, infection, and aspiration of foreign materials. In fact, in a child, even an apparently minor respiratory system problem may quickly become life-threatening. Here's why:

• A child's airway is smaller in diameter than an adult's and contains a greater proportion of soft tissue. This makes airway obstruction more likely if excessive mucus formation or edema occurs.

• Because a child's mucous membranes are loosely attached to his airway, they're easily irritated. This may cause edema and coughing.

• An infant's larynx is located two or three cervical vertebrae higher than an adult's, increasing the risk of airway obstruction by aspiration.

• A child's smaller respiratory tract allows

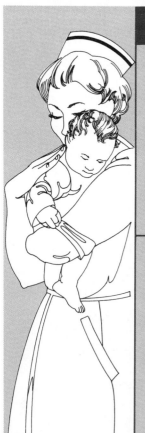

| CONDITION | SIGNS AND SYMPTOMS |
|---|---|
| **Bronchiolitis**<br>A viral infection that inflames the lining of the small bronchioles, bronchiolitis causes airway obstruction and overdistention of the lungs. It's most common in children ages 2 months to 2 years—with a peak incidence at 6 months—and usually follows a mild cold. It occurs most often in the winter and spring and is highly contagious to other young children. | • Rhinitis<br>• Fever<br>• Paroxysmal, hacking cough<br>• Dyspnea and nasal flaring<br>• Tachypnea<br>• Intercostal and subcostal retractions<br>• Rales, wheezing, and decreasing breath sounds<br>• Hyperexpanded lungs with scattered consolidation seen on X-ray<br>• Lethargy or restlessness and irritability from hypoxemia<br>• Possible dehydration<br>• Impaired ability to eat and sleep |
| **Acute laryngotracheobronchitis (viral croup)**<br>Upper airway obstruction results from this viral infection, which causes severe inflammation of the larynx, trachea, and bronchi. It's most common in children ages 3 months to 3 years who've had an upper respiratory infection. It usually occurs in the fall and winter. | • Mild fever or hypothermia<br>• Hoarseness<br>• A barking, brassy cough<br>• Tachycardia<br>• Dyspnea<br>• Laryngitis<br>• Inspiratory stridor and expiratory wheezing<br>• Substernal and suprasternal retractions<br>• Rales, decreased breath sounds, and rhonchi<br>• Pallor or cyanosis<br>• Restlessness or irritability from hypoxemia<br>• Fatigue |

bacteria and other microorganisms to travel easily into his lungs.

• A child's lungs contain fewer alveoli than an adult's. So when his lungs become congested, he suffers greater loss of oxygen and carbon dioxide exchange. Yet, because of his more rapid metabolism, he needs even more oxygen than an adult needs.

• In addition to his increased risk of respiratory problems, a child's more vulnerable to alterations in fluid and electrolyte balance than an adult; more likely to become dehydrated and go into shock from excessive diarrhea or vomiting, polyuria, fever, or fluid loss from burns; and more susceptible to epiphyseal plate fractures that can disrupt bone growth.

• Because a child's immune system isn't well developed, he has fewer defenses against infection.

This chart will help you identify pediatric emergencies and intervene appropriately.

## NURSING INTERVENTIONS

• Follow your hospital's isolation procedures to avoid spreading infection.

• Monitor the patient's respiratory rate and pattern; report nasal flaring, retractions, wheezing, tachypnea, or any change in level of consciousness.

• Keep his nostrils open; using cotton-tipped applicators to clear them of mucus will alleviate respiratory difficulty and reduce mouth breathing.

• Prepare him for chest X-rays to determine the presence of pulmonary hyperinflation, and draw venous and arterial blood, as ordered, for laboratory studies.

• Place him in a mist tent, on his stomach, to aid mucus drainage and to compress his distended lungs during expiration. Or place him in a semi-Fowler position, with his neck slightly extended, to open his airway and to aid lung expansion.

• Administer oxygen via the tent if needed.

• Monitor the patient's arterial blood gases (ABGs); notify the doctor of any decrease in $PaO_2$ or increase in $PaCO_2$, and be prepared to assist with intubation and mechanical ventilation.

• If the patient has increased tachypnea and dyspnea when eating, give him nothing by mouth and expect to administer I.V. fluids.

• Keep an accurate intake and output record, and check the child's urine specific gravity regularly for evidence of dehydration.

• Begin antibiotic therapy as ordered for secondary bacterial infection.

• Monitor the patient's respirations; place him in a sitting position while you listen for his breath sounds.

• Place the patient in a cool mist tent, administer oxygen, and administer racemic epinephrine by inhalation for temporary relief of respiratory distress, as ordered.

• Draw blood for ABG analysis, as ordered.

• Insert an I.V. and begin fluid replacement as ordered, if the patient's unable to take liquids orally.

• Prepare to assist with an emergency intubation or tracheostomy if the patient develops these signs of impending respiratory failure: increased heart rate, decreased respiratory rate, and decreased or absent breath sounds.

• Prepare the patient for X-rays of the chest (to rule out bronchiolitis) and cervical trachea (to rule out epiglottitis).

*(continued)*

## NURSE'S GUIDE TO PEDIATRIC EMERGENCIES *(continued)*

**Epiphyseal plate fractures (Harris-Salter type I-V fractures)**

Separation of the epiphyseal plate from the bone shaft and the epiphysis causes stunting of that bone's growth. Epiphyseal plate fractures occur in children of all ages, usually from trauma but also from bone diseases such as cancer.

Signs and symptoms include:
- pain, edema, deformity, and redness of the extremity around the fracture
- decreased range of motion and refusal to move the affected arm or leg or to put weight on it.

If your patient has an epiphyseal plate fracture, expect to:
- immobilize and protect the injured arm or leg.
- assist the doctor with a closed reduction and cast application, or prepare the patient for surgery.
- elevate the arm or leg to control edema after the cast is applied.
- frequently check the pulses of the affected extremity and the color, warmth, sensation, and movement in the extremity's toes or fingers.
- administer pain medications as ordered.
- teach the patient and his parents to keep the cast clean and dry, to prevent cast softening and malpositioning of bones, and emphasize the importance of medical follow-up.

| CONDITION | SIGNS AND SYMPTOMS |
|---|---|
| **Epiglottitis (bacterial croup)** A bacterial infection of the epiglottis and surrounding area, epiglottitis rapidly causes inflammation, edema, induration, and—if not treated—complete airway obstruction. It's most common in children ages 2 to 7 who've had an upper respiratory infection. It may occur in any season. | • Sudden onset of high fever<br>• Sore throat and dysphagia<br>• Drooling<br>• Unusual body positioning: the child leans forward, head hyperextended, jaw thrust forward, mouth open, and tongue protruding<br>• Severe respiratory distress with inspiratory stridor; nasal flaring; intercostal, suprasternal, supraclavicular, and subcostal retractions; and paradoxical breathing<br>• Rhonchi and diminished breath sounds<br>• Cherry red, irregularly swollen epiglottis<br>• Apprehension, restlessness, and anxiety from hypoxemia<br>• Pallor or cyanosis |
| **Intussusception** This condition involves the telescoping of one section of the intestine into another, causing inflammation, edema, intestinal obstruction, hemorrhage, and—unless treated within 24 hours—death. It usually occurs in children ages 3 months to 2 years, and it may be related to disturbances in intestinal motility, such as cystic fibrosis or acute enteritis. | • Colicky abdominal pain that causes the infant to scream and draw his legs up to his chest<br>• Vomiting<br>• Diarrhea consisting of bloody, mucous stools—the classic "current jelly" stool (or, in some patients, constipation)<br>• A distended, tender abdomen<br>• A palpable, sausagelike mass in the right upper or lower quadrant<br>• Fever and diaphoresis<br>• Tachycardia |
| **Reye's syndrome** An acute, often fatal encephalopathy, Reye's syndrome causes increased intracranial pressure and fatty infiltration of the liver, kidneys, and brain. It affects children from infancy to adolescence and frequently follows an acute viral infection such as an upper respiratory infection, influenza, or chicken pox. | • Recurrent vomiting<br>• Progressive changes in level of consciousness from drowsiness and lethargy to stupor and coma<br>• Fever, diaphoresis, and dehydration<br>• Hyperactive reflexes<br>• Respiratory distress, progressing from hyperventilation to Cheyne-Stokes and apneic respirations<br>• Unilateral or bilateral fixed and dilated pupils, with severe encephalopathy<br>• Seizures<br>• Decorticate or decerebrate posturing<br>• Elevated liver enzyme levels, hyperammonemia, hypoglycemia |

## NURSING INTERVENTIONS

- Don't use a tongue depressor to visualize the epiglottis in a seriously ill child. Doing so may cause a laryngospasm and complete airway obstruction.
- Place the child in a sitting position to ease his respiratory difficulty. Assess his vital signs and respirations frequently, and report any changes. *Never* leave him alone—he may develop total airway obstruction at any time.
- Assemble the equipment for possible intubation or tracheotomy (tracheotomy may be done prophylactically), and prepare to administer humidified oxygen.
- Calm the child during X-rays of his chest and cervical trachea.
- Keep external stimuli to a minimum.
- Start an I.V. for antibiotic therapy and fluid replacement, and draw blood for laboratory studies, as ordered.
- Keep an accurate intake and output record, and monitor the patient's urine specific gravity.

---

- Assess the infant's vital signs (take an axillary temperature to prevent rectal injury).
- Insert an I.V. line, draw blood for laboratory studies, and begin fluid replacement, as ordered.
- Insert a nasogastric (NG) tube, as ordered, to empty the patient's stomach.
- Monitor his input and output; watch for rectal bleeding or signs of dehydration.
- Prepare him for hydrostatic reduction or surgery.

---

- Monitor the patient's vital signs and neurologic status.
- Be alert for any signs of increasing intracranial pressure: widened pulse pressure, decreased pulse rate, and any change in respiratory pattern.
- Keep the head of the patient's bed elevated.
- Insert an NG tube, an indwelling (Foley) catheter, and arterial and central venous pressure (CVP) lines, as ordered. Be prepared to begin intracranial pressure monitoring.
- Draw blood for laboratory studies.
- Keep accurate intake and output records; limit fluids to prevent cerebral edema.
- Start an infusion of hypertonic glucose, and administer mannitol or glycerol for cerebral edema, as ordered.
- Maintain seizure precautions, and be prepared to administer an anticonvulsant.
- Be prepared to assist with intubation if your patient's mental status or respiratory status deteriorates.

*(continued)*

## NURSE'S GUIDE TO PEDIATRIC EMERGENCIES *(continued)*

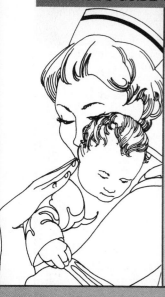

| CONDITION | SIGNS AND SYMPTOMS |
|---|---|
| **Acute dehydration due to diarrhea** Acute dehydration is a loss of 10% or more of total body weight within 24 to 48 hours. | • Prolonged diarrhea (over 24 hours) • Anorexia and vomiting • Oliguria or anuria (less than 1 ml/kg/hr) • Excessive thirst • Dry, cracked mucous membranes; sticky, thick saliva; poor skin turgor; dark discoloration around the eyes; depressed fontanelles • Restlessness and irritability that may progress to coma • Tachycardia and hypotension from progressive hypovolemia • Muscle weakness • Lethargy • Abdominal distention • Fever |

# Recognizing Child Abuse

Whenever an injured child is brought to the ED, be sure to assess him for possible abuse. Remember, too, that the law requires reporting of all incidents of suspected child abuse to designated authorities.

### ASSESSMENT
Your assessment of an injured child should always include an evaluation of:
• his injuries
• his general appearance
• his behavior *and* the behavior of whoever accompanies him.

First, carefully assess the child's injuries. Suspect child abuse if you see:
• multiple bruises, abrasions, or lacerations
• fractures (especially Salter type II or "bucket handle" fractures, or rib fractures)
• burns from immersion in very hot water or from cigarettes; "branding" appearance of burns
• head trauma, facial injuries, or retinal hemorrhage
• internal injuries
• signs of genital or rectal trauma—discharges, bruises, or lacerations.

Note the location of burns, bruises, and lacerations; on an abused child, common areas for these injuries include the cheeks, trunk, genitals, buttocks, thighs, and arms.

Note the child's general appearance. An abused child is likely to come to the hospital dressed inappropriately for the weather, and he may have a dirty, unkempt appearance. He's likely to be shorter and to weigh less than the average for his age. And he may have several cuts and bruises, in various stages of healing, or unusual skin markings or scars. If he's been beaten, these markings may be in the shape of the object used, such as an electrical cord, a hand, a wire hanger, a coiled rope, or a broad strap or belt.

Observe the child's behavior. An abused child is likely to:
• be underactive or hyperactive
• have a blank look
• seem especially fearful of his parents or cling to them in terror
• be extremely passive or drowsy or display other erratic or inappropriate behavior, indicating possible drug intoxication
• move away when you try to touch him.

Finally, note the parents' behavior, if they're the ones who've brought the child for treatment. Abusive parents are frequently uncooperative. They may hesitate or refuse to give you any information, refuse to give consent for diagnostic studies, or try to remove the child from the hospital before you can do a thorough examina-

## NURSING INTERVENTIONS

• If an infectious condition caused the diarrhea, follow your hospital's procedures for handling excreta and for laundry disposal.
• Draw blood as ordered for laboratory tests.
• Begin I.V. fluid replacement as ordered; expect to administer an isotonic electrolyte solution based on the child's weight. The doctor may change the replacement fluid or rate of infusion, depending on the severity of the child's fluid and electrolyte imbalance and his response to initial treatment.
• Check the patient's neurologic status and

vital signs frequently, watching for signs of impending shock. Report changes in level of consciousness, and follow seizure precautions.
• Keep an accurate intake and output record, documenting the amount, color, consistency, and odor of each stool. Save the patient's stools and urine for laboratory analysis, and check his urine specific gravity regularly. Weigh the patient daily.

tion. They may demand instant treatment, complain about their own problems and other problems unrelated to the child's injury, and generally over- or underreact to the seriousness of the situation.

Other abusive parents may react inappropriately by appearing totally uninterested in their child's problem; by giving you a history that doesn't explain the child's injury; by presenting contradictory or inconsistent versions of the injury-causing incident to different hospital personnel; or by blaming a third party, such as a sibling or neighbor, for the child's injury.

Still other abusive parents will admit that they caused their child's injuries, yet defend their actions as justified punishment for the child's behavior.

When you talk to the parents, use a nonjudgmental approach, and focus on their concerns rather than on their child's. Remember, you don't know *for sure* that they've abused their child, no matter how strong your suspicions are. Keep in mind that parents may be indirectly asking for help when they voice insistent complaints or bring their child's injuries to attention.

### DOCUMENTING AND REPORTING
If your assessment findings lead you to suspect that the child's a victim of abuse, inform the doc-

tor on duty of your suspicions. Expect him to order total body X-rays, a blood coagulation profile, and toxicology studies of the child's blood and urine.

If you continue to suspect child abuse after receiving the test results and talking with the parents, follow your hospital's protocol for notifying the appropriate state agency. (Many states impose a criminal penalty for failure to report.) State laws vary, so be sure you're familiar with the laws of your state.

Assist the doctor in explaining to the parents that their child's history and physical findings cause you to suspect abuse and that you must report your suspicions. If they become alarmed, offer support and explain that you're making the report because the law requires it for protection of all children who may be abused. Be careful to maintain a nonjudgmental attitude.

Finally, document all your findings carefully, completely, and objectively. Include the information you've gathered, the information you've given to the parents, and your subsequent actions, such as reporting the incident. Remember that, in a court hearing, deciding factors could include:
• your description of the child's injuries
• the information you obtain from his parents
• your impressions of the parent-child interaction.

# Understanding Colloid and Crystalloid Solutions

You'll use plasma volume expanders—colloids and crystalloids—to treat patients whose emergency conditions result in compromised hemodynamic stability. These agents work by refilling the vascular space, increasing the patient's cardiac output, and perfusing his tissues. Volume expanders can't carry oxygen or replace blood, but they *can* provide volume expansion, protein, and electrolytes in an emergency.

Crystalloid solutions have low-molecular-weight particles that *quickly* expand the plasma. These electrolyte-rich solutions take effect more quickly than colloids, but they last only a short time in the plasma. So you'll administer them more frequently. Crystalloids are also less expensive than colloids.

Colloids are higher-molecular-weight solutions that take effect more slowly than crystalloids but

| TYPE OF SOLUTION | DOSAGE | ADVANTAGES |
|---|---|---|
| **SYNTHETIC COLLOIDS** | | |
| **dextran** (Dextran 40, Dextran 70, Dextran 75) | For shock: <br>• Infuse 500 ml of 10% Dextran 40 solution rapidly. <br>• Infuse remaining dose slowly for a total daily dose of 2 g/kg body weight. <br>• After 24 hours, infuse no more than 1 g/kg daily. <br>• Continue for no more than 5 days. <br><br>For venous thrombosis and pulmonary embolism: <br>• Infuse 500 ml of 6% Dextran 70 or 75 solution at a rate of 20 to 40 ml/minute. <br>• Don't exceed the 1.2 g/kg total dose for the first 24 hours. | • Decreases blood viscosity and improves blood flow through microcirculation <br>• Remains in the vascular bed for 12 to 18 hours (Dextran 40) or 2 to 3 days (Dextran 70 or 75), so less fluid is needed <br>• Coats red blood cells (RBCs) and platelets, causing antisludging effect in capillaries <br>• Is inexpensive and readily available |
| **hetastarch** | For shock: <br>• Infuse 500 to 1,000 ml of 6% hetastarch in saline solution. <br>• Infuse no more than 1,500 ml/day. <br>• Infuse up to 20 ml/kg hourly for a patient with hypovolemic shock. | • Remains in circulation for 24 to 36 hours <br>• Rarely causes hypersensitivity reactions—if it does, they occur early in infusion <br>• Doesn't interfere with blood typing or cross matching <br>• Is inexpensive and has a long shelf life |
| **NATURAL COLLOIDS** | | |
| **serum albumin** (5% and 25%) | For shock: <br>• Infuse 25 g of 5% or 25% | • 5% albumin is equivalent to plasma oncotic pressure |

have a longer life in the plasma; this means that you won't have to repeat the dosage as often. Colloids are particularly helpful in the management of patients with hypovolemic or cardiogenic shock, but keep in mind that they carry a high risk of fluid shift and adult respiratory distress syndrome (ARDS). All colloids are more expensive than crystalloids, with natural colloids more expensive than synthetic ones. Synthetic colloids are more likely to cause hypersensitivity reactions and other adverse effects.

Depending on your patient's condition, you'll infuse colloids, crystalloids, or both to achieve hemodynamic stability even before blood transfusions begin. Review this chart to help you increase your understanding of the common uses of colloid and crystalloid solutions.

| DISADVANTAGES | NURSING CONSIDERATIONS |
|---|---|
| • May cause fluid overload<br>• May cause anaphylaxis or a hypersensitivity reaction<br>• May cause renal failure by blocking the tubules<br>• May impair blood clotting and increase bleeding time by disturbing platelet and fibrinogen function<br>• May cause RBCs to clump, making subsequent cross matching impossible<br>• May cause increased urine viscosity<br>• May increase levels of serum glutamic-oxaloacetic transaminase and serum glutamic-pyruvic transaminase | • Don't administer dextran to a patient who's hemorrhaging or who has a bleeding disorder.<br>• Use cautiously in a patient with congestive heart failure (CHF) or pulmonary edema.<br>• Draw blood samples before infusing Dextran because it coats the RBCs.<br>• Watch for signs and symptoms of fluid overload—dyspnea, rales, increased central venous pressure (CVP), increased pulmonary capillary wedge pressure (PCWP), increased heart rate, and diaphoresis. Stop the infusion immediately and notify the doctor if they occur.<br>• Watch for signs and symptoms of a hypersensitivity reaction—urticaria, pruritus, hives, facial swelling, chills, nausea, vomiting, fever, or dyspnea. Stop the infusion immediately and notify the doctor if they occur.<br>• Monitor the patient's urine flow during infusion. If oliguria develops, stop the infusion and give an osmotic diuretic.<br>• Check his hemoglobin and hematocrit values. Don't allow the hematocrit level to fall below 30%.<br>• Discard partially used containers. |
| • May cause fluid overload<br>• May cause a hypersensitivity reaction<br>• May alter coagulation if infused in large volumes<br>• May also cause headaches and lower leg edema | • Don't administer hetastarch to a patient who's hemorrhaging or who has a bleeding disorder.<br>• Use cautiously in a patient with CHF or renal failure.<br>• Watch for signs and symptoms of fluid overload—dyspnea, rales, increased CVP, increased PCWP, increased heart rate, and diaphoresis. Stop the infusion immediately and notify the doctor if they occur.<br>• Watch for signs and symptoms of a hypersensitivity reaction—urticaria, pruritus, hives, facial swelling, chills, nausea, vomiting, fever, and dyspnea. Stop the infusion immediately and notify the doctor if they occur.<br>• Check the patient's clotting studies and hemoglobin and hematocrit values. Don't allow the hematocrit level to fall below 30%.<br>• Discard partially used bottles. |
| • May cause a hypersensitivity reaction | • Don't administer albumin to a patient with severe anemia or cardiac failure. |

*(continued)*

## UNDERSTANDING COLLOID AND CRYSTALLOID SOLUTIONS *(continued)*

| TYPE OF SOLUTION | DOSAGE | ADVANTAGES |
|---|---|---|
| **serum albumin** (5% and 25%) *(continued)* | serum albumin undiluted or diluted in saline solution or dextrose 5% in water.<br>• Repeat dosage after 15 to 30 minutes if necessary.<br>• Infuse no more than 250 g within 48 hours.<br><br>For hypoproteinemia:<br>• Infuse 5 to 10 ml/minute of 5% solution or 2 to 3 ml/minute of 25% solution.<br>• Infuse no more than 100 g/day.<br><br>For burns:<br>• Vary dosage according to extent of burns.<br>• Maintain plasma albumin level at 2 to 3 g/100 ml. | • Draws 3.5 times its volume into vascular space (25% albumin)<br>• Elevates plasma protein levels<br>• Has no hepatitis viruses<br>• Rarely causes hypersensitivity or hypotensive reactions<br>• Doesn't interfere with blood coagulation<br>• Reduces edema by drawing fluid from the interstitial space to the intravascular space and by enhancing renal excretion |
| **plasma protein fraction (PPF)** (Plasmanate) | For hypovolemic shock:<br>• Infuse 250 to 500 ml of 5% PPF solution no faster than 10 ml/minute.<br><br>For hypoproteinemia:<br>• Infuse 1,000 to 1,500 ml of 5% PPF solution daily no faster than 8 ml/minute. | • Temporarily compensates for protein deficiencies<br>• Has no hepatitis viruses<br>• Can act as a plasma replacement without typing or cross matching (but doesn't contain clotting factors as fresh-frozen plasma does) |
| **CRYSTALLOIDS** | | |
| **0.9% sodium chloride solution** (normal saline solution) | For shock:<br>• Replace estimated volume loss based on the patient's fluid and electrolyte losses and salt depletion. | • Can be infused rapidly while patient's blood is being typed and cross-matched<br>• Doesn't cause hypersensitivity reactions<br>• Is inexpensive and readily available |
| **Ringer's lactate** (Hartmann's solution) | For shock:<br>• Infuse dosage I.V. over 18 to 24 hours.<br>• Dosage is highly individualized and based on fluid volume and electrolyte losses. | • Contains sodium, chloride, potassium, calcium, and lactate and closely approximates normal blood electrolyte contents<br>• Doesn't cause hypersensitivity reactions<br>• Can be infused rapidly while the patient's blood is being typed and cross-matched<br>• Is inexpensive and readily available |

| DISADVANTAGES | NURSING CONSIDERATIONS |
|---|---|
| • May cause fluid overload<br>• May impair salt and water excretion<br>• May cause bleeding<br>• May cause ARDS from albumin transudation into the pulmonary interstitium<br>• May cause blood pressure variations, pulse abnormalities, and respiratory effects with repeated doses<br>• May be expensive | • Use cautiously in patients with low cardiac reserve, an adequate albumin level, or restricted salt intake.<br>• Make sure the patient's well hydrated before infusion.<br>• Don't use any serum albumin solution that's cloudy or contains sediment.<br>• Watch for signs and symptoms of fluid overload—dyspnea, rales, increased CVP, increased PCWP, increased heart rate, and diaphoresis. Stop the infusion immediately and notify the doctor if they occur.<br>• Watch for signs and symptoms of a hypersensitivity reaction—urticaria, pruritus, hives, facial swelling, chills, nausea, vomiting, fever, and dyspnea. Stop the infusion immediately and notify the doctor if they occur.<br>• Watch for signs of bleeding when the vascular space refills after surgery.<br>• Monitor the patient's intake and output. Check his hemoglobin, hematocrit, serum protein, and electrolyte values.<br>• Don't freeze the bottles—they could crack. |
| • May cause fluid overload<br>• May cause a hypersensitivity reaction<br>• May cause a hypotension reaction if administered too quickly<br>• May also cause hypersalivation and headaches<br>• May be required in large volumes | • Don't administer PPF to a patient who's undergoing a cardiopulmonary bypass or who has severe anemia.<br>• Don't use PPF if the solution's been frozen, looks cloudy, has sediment, or has been open for more than 4 hours.<br>• Consider using PPF while cross matching is being done.<br>• Watch for signs and symptoms of fluid overload—dyspnea, rales, increased CVP, increased PCWP, increased heart rate, and diaphoresis. Stop the infusion immediately and notify the doctor if they occur.<br>• Watch for signs and symptoms of a hypersensitivity reaction—urticaria, pruritus, hives, facial swelling, chills, nausea, vomiting, fever, and dyspnea. Stop the infusion immediately and notify the doctor if they occur.<br>• Monitor the patient's blood pressure frequently, and discontinue the infusion if hypotension develops. |
| • May cause fluid overload<br>• May aggravate CHF<br>• May cause edema or pulmonary edema if too much solution's given too rapidly<br>• May cause electrolyte disturbances and loss of potassium | • Use cautiously in a patient with CHF, circulatory insufficiency, or renal dysfunction.<br>• Use cautiously in a patient with hypoproteinemia.<br>• Check serum electrolytes during therapy.<br>• Watch for signs and symptoms of fluid overload—dyspnea, rales, increased CVP, increased PCWP, increased heart rate, and diaphoresis. Stop the infusion immediately and notify the doctor if they occur. |
| • May cause fluid overload<br>• May be required in large volumes | • Don't administer this solution to a patient with renal failure, except as an emergency volume expander.<br>• Use cautiously in a patient with CHF, circulatory insufficiency, renal dysfunction, and pulmonary edema.<br>• Use cautiously in a patient with hypoproteinemia.<br>• Watch for signs and symptoms of fluid overload—dyspnea, rales, increased CVP, increased PCWP, increased heart rate, and diaphoresis. Stop the infusion immediately and notify the doctor if they occur. |

# Coping with Psychiatric Emergencies

Regardless of what's causing your patient's psychiatric emergency—drugs, alcohol, or a functional disorder such as schizophrenia—if he's violent, suicidal, or having an acute psychotic episode, and you have to manage him, you need to know how to respond appropriately.

Your response may be as basic as establishing rapport with the patient or as complicated as applying leather locking restraints to confine his movements so you can start caring for him. Your specific initial interventions will vary with each emergency condition, but expect to follow these general guidelines:

• Assure the safety of your patient, yourself, and others. Have security personnel assist you in removing from the patient, and the area, anything he could use to harm himself or others (razors, glasses, belts, electrical cords).

• Minimize stimuli in the area that may contribute to the patient's behavior. Turn off the television or radio, and dim the lights. Have any people who may upset the patient leave the area.

• Attempt to establish a rapport with your patient, to gain his trust and cooperation. If he's violent or psychotic, speak firmly but calmly in a nonthreatening way. If he's suicidal, try to express your concern.

• Assist the doctor in performing diagnostic tests to determine if an underlying physical condition is causing the patient's psychiatric emergency.

Here are some special nursing considerations to keep in mind when the patient you're caring for is violent, suicidal, or having an acute psychotic episode.

## The Violent Patient

A patient who's violent directs his anger toward others and is used to expressing his feelings physically.

• *Seclude and restrain the patient if he becomes combative.* Don't try to subdue him yourself. If hospital security officers aren't available to take over, get staff members to help you. Watch for indications that he's also suicidal.

• *Give any medications, as ordered.* Expect to give your patient haloperidol (Haldol) to control his violent behavior; in some cases, you may give chlorpromazine hydrochloride (Thorazine).

## The Suicidal Patient

A suicidal patient typically has severe depression and low self-esteem and directs his anger inward.

• *Attempt to determine his suicide potential.* Is this a gesture—a way to manipulate others—or is it a real attempt at suicide? How upset or disturbed is your patient? Did he choose a suicide method that was likely to succeed?

• *Arrange for follow-up counseling.* Contact the local suicide prevention center or a psychiatrist for a referral.

## The Patient Having an Acute Psychotic Episode

• *Try to assess the patient's orientation.* Use simple terms in short, direct sentences. Ask if he knows his name, the date, and where he is. Reorient him if necessary, and don't threaten him by getting too close to him or to his belongings.

• *Give any medications, as ordered.* Expect to give your patient lithium carbonate (Lithane) P.O. or haloperidol (Haldol) I.M., as ordered, to control his psychotic behavior.

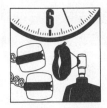

# Acknowledgments

**Chapter 4**    **New Advances in Respiratory Monitoring—Oximetry**
p. 117—Illustration adapted from photograph courtesy of
Bioximetry Technology Inc., Boulder, Colo.

**Chapter 6**    **What Are D.S.A. and M.R.I.?**
pp. 260-261—Photographs courtesy of Robert A. Zimmer-
man, MD, Chief of Neuroradiology, Hospital of the University of Pennsylvania, Philadelphia.

**Special Color**    **EMERGENCY! Atlas of Major Injuries**
**Section**    p. 560—Photograph 1 courtesy of C. Edward Hartford,
MD, Medical Director of the Burn Treatment Center,
Crozer-Chester Medical Center, Chester, Pa.

pp. 560-562—Photographs 2-7, 9-10 courtesy of Geoffrey
G. Hallock, MD, Lehigh Valley Hospital Center, Allentown,
Pa.

p. 562—Photograph 8 courtesy of *Emergency Medicine*
13(21):38, December 15, 1982.

p. 563—Photographs 11-15 courtesy of Sherman A. Minton,
MD, Indiana University School of Medicine, Indianapolis.

p. 564—Photographs 16-18 courtesy of Isadore Mahalakis,
MD, Forensic Pathologist, Lehigh Valley Hospital Center,
Allentown, Pa.

p. 564—Photographs 19-21 courtesy of Thomas A. Farrell,
MD, Director of General Ophthalmology Service Clinics,
Wills Eye Hospital, Philadelphia.

Special thanks to Richard L. Cutshall for coordinating
Lehigh Valley Hospital Center's contributions to the
Special Color Section.

# Index

## A

Aaron's sign, 335
ABCs, 58. See also Airway;
    Breathing; Circulation
Abdomen
    in abruptio placentae, 531
    in acid ingestion, 779
    in burns, 667, 670
    in coma, 240
    in diabetic ketoacidosis, 441
    in gastrointestinal
        emergencies, 308-309
    in kidney trauma, 582
    penetrating wounds, 78-79
    physical assessment, 73-75
    in poisoning, 749
    in pregnancy, 511, 513
Abdominal mass, 573
Abdominal pain
    in appendicitis, 308
    in ectopic pregnancy, 523
    in endocrine emergencies,
        436
    in gastrointestinal
        emergencies, 304-305
    in genitourinary
        emergencies, 571
    in intestinal obstruction, 329
    in poisoning, 748-749
    in pregnancy, 511, 513
Abdominal trauma
    blunt, 314-317, 556
        acute abdomen in, 315-
            316
        peritonitis in, 314
        seat belt syndrome, 315
        warning signs and
            symptoms in, 317
    penetrating, 310-311, 313-
        314, 559
    peritoneal fluid in, 312,
        313
ABO incompatibility, 489
Abortion
    complete, 520
    incomplete, 520, 521
    inevitable, 515, 520, 521
    missed, 520-521
    septic, 521, 522
    spontaneous, 515, 520-523
        RhoGam after, 523
        types, 521
    threatened, 515, 521, 522
Abruptio placentae, 529-531
Abscess, peritonsillar, 424
Accidents. See also Trauma
    comparing causes of death
        due to, 565
    mechanisms of injury in,
        76-78t, 79-80
    motorcycle, 77t

Accidents (cont'd)
    motor vehicle, 315, 549-550
        genitourinary trauma in,
            571
        occupant injuries, 76t
        pedestrian injuries, 77t,
            549, 550
Acetaminophen overdose,
    757-758
Acetazolamide
    adverse effects, 731
    in altitude illness, 731
    in retinal artery occlusion,
        415
Acetohydroxamic acid, 595
Acetylcysteine, 757, 758
Acid(s)
    burns. See also Burns,
        chemical
    lavage for, 694
    ingestion, 777-779
    inhalation, 777
Acid-base disorders
    in hypovolemic shock, 628
    in renal failure, 580
    in salicylate intoxication,
        753
Acidification of urine
    in amphetamine abuse,
        784t
    in PCP intoxication, 785t
Acidosis
    in carbon monoxide
        poisoning, 766
    in heat-related illness, 724
    in hypothermia, 714
    metabolic, 465
        after acid ingestion, 779
        in cardiogenic shock, 634
        in poisoning, 748
    in near-drowning, 728
    respiratory, 150t
        in hypovolemic shock,
            628
Acrolein inhalation, 693t
Acromioclavicular separation,
    355, 356
Acute abdomen. See
    Abdominal pain
Addison's disease, 461. See
    also Adrenal crisis
Adrenal crisis, 461-466
    corticosteroids in, 464, 466
    dysrhythmias in, 464
    electrolyte imbalances in,
        459
    hypovolemia in, 431
Adult respiratory distress
    syndrome, 157-163
    heart failure in, 159
    nursing interventions in,
        162t
    after pulmonary contusion,
        131

ARDS (cont'd)
    in septic shock, 645
    stages of, 162t
Advanced cardiac life support
    (ACLS), 55, 60-61, 93
    flow sheet for, 57
Afterload, 199
Against medical advice, 41
Airway
    in anaphylactic shock, 612
    artificial, 58, 99
    in burn patient, 659-660
    in cardiovascular
        emergencies, 173-174
    in endocrine emergency,
        430-431
    in environmental
        emergencies, 703-704
    in eye, ear, nose, and throat
        emergencies, 394-395
    in genitourinary
        emergencies, 568
    in hematologic
        emergencies, 475
    in musculoskeletal
        emergencies, 344
    nasopharyngeal, 99, 227
    in obstetric-gynecologic
        emergencies, 508-509
    obstruction, 55, 58, 116,
        118, 147-150
        in burns, 659
        cricothyrotomy in, 100-
            101
        in gastrointestinal
            emergency, 299, 302
        in infants and children,
            126, 794
        in inhalation injury, 692
        in neurologic emergency,
            226
        in pediatric patient, 83,
            86
        percutaneous
            transtracheal
            catheter ventilation
            in, 101
        upper tract, 147-148, 150
        wheezing in, 703
    opening of, 55, 58, 98, 116,
        118
        in multiple trauma, 81, 82
        in neurologic
            emergencies, 226-
            227
    oropharyngeal, 99
    in pediatric patient, 794
    in poisoning, 745-746
    primary assessment of, 55,
        58-59
    in shock, 612
    in status epilepticus, 279
Albumin therapy, 483t, 800-
    803t

t refers to a table

t refers to a table

# O

t refers to a table

# WHEN DISASTER STRIKES

In terms of patient care, a disaster is any event that injures more people than your hospital's emergency department can routinely manage. Whether the disaster occurs inside or outside the hospital, all or most of the hospital's staff will respond, following previously established protocols. As part of a community disaster-response network, your hospital—and you—may be involved in:
• an internal disaster in the hospital (for example, a fire or a bomb threat)
• A community disaster (for example, a hotel fire)
• the local response to a countywide disaster (for example, a tornado)
• the local response to a statewide or national disaster (for example, a hurricane or a nuclear accident).

Be sure you're thoroughly familiar with your hospital's disaster-response protocols, which should resemble the general guidelines presented here.

### A COMMUNITY DISASTER OCCURS

Be sure you know your hospital's disaster mobilization codes, such as "Signal D," for general community disaster, or "Dr. Black" for a specific disaster (tornado).

**If you're called to respond:**
• If you're at the hospital, go to the designated command post to receive instructions.
• If you're at home, go to the hospital (but only if road conditions are reasonably safe), as quickly as possible. Take your nursing license and hospital employee identification with you.
• At the command post, pick up an identifying tag, vest, or armband and a disaster action card specifying your assignment to a triage or treatment team.

### A HOSPITAL FIRE OCCURS

**If you discover the fire:**
• Activate the alarm system and notify the hospital switchboard operator.

**If you're at the scene:**
• Use a fire extinguisher to fight a small or contained fire.
• Turn off oxygen tanks and wall units in the area.
• Shut windows and doors to contain the fire.
• Seal doors with wet cloths to prevent smoke from escaping.

### A HOSPITAL BOMB THREAT OCCURS

**If you receive the call:**
• Keep the caller on the line as long as possible. While you're talking, have someone notify the switchboard operator and hospital administration. They'll alert local authorities so a trace can be started immediately and bomb technicians can be called in.
• Does the caller's voice give clues to his identity? (Young or old, male or female, with or without an accent?) Note any background noises—music, other voices, traffic, motors—that may help determine where he's calling from.
• Ask where the bomb is, what explosives it contains, what it looks like, and when it's going to explode. Write down any information you can get and pass it along to the authorities immediately. *Keep the caller talking,* if possible, until the trace is completed.